Magic and Medicine of Plants

Reader's Digest

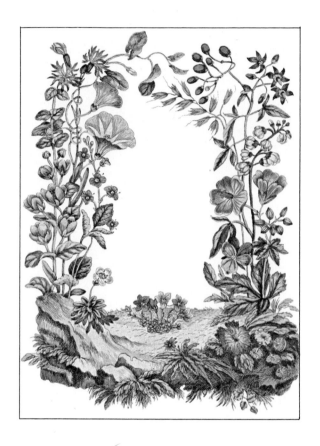

Magic and Medicine of Plants

The Reader's Digest Association, Inc.

Pleasantville, New York   Montreal

Magic and Medicine of Plants

STAFF
Project Editor: Inge N. Dobelis
Project Art Director: Gerald Ferguson

Senior Editors: James Dwyer
David Rattray
Associate Editor: Gayla Visalli
Research Editor: Hildegard Anderson
Editorial Assistant: Dolores Damm

READER'S DIGEST GENERAL BOOKS
Editorial Director: John A. Pope, Jr.
Managing Editor: Jane Polley
Art Director: Richard J. Berenson
Group Editors: Norman B. Mack, John Speicher,
David Trooper (Art), Susan J. Wernert

CONSULTANTS
Norman R. Farnsworth, Ph.D., Director, Program for Collaborative Research in the Pharmaceutical Sciences, University of Illinois at Chicago
Dr. Susan Levitzky, Attending Physician, Beth Israel Medical Center, New York, New York
Djaja D. Soejarto, Ph.D., Associate Professor of Pharmacognosy, College of Pharmacy, University of Illinois at Chicago; Research Associate, Department of Botany, Field Museum of Natural History, Chicago, Illinois
Dr. William C. Steere, President Emeritus and Senior Scientist, The New York Botanical Garden, Bronx, New York

Contributing Editors: Lea Guyer Gordon
Edmund Harvey

Rebecca Chaitin
Donald Earnest
Wendy Murphy

Contributing Writers: Thomas A. Christopher
Alexandra Hoffman

Oliver Allen
William Bake
Donna Dannen
Kent Dannen
Josh Eppinger
Carolyn Fisher
Walter Fox
Guy Henle
Peter Limburg
Lilla Pennant
Carl Proujan

Contributing Artists: Mary Kellner
Sej

Contributing Researchers: Amelia Daly Forbert
Mary Hart
Mary Lyn Maiscott
Jozefa Stuart

Indexer: Sydney Wolfe Cohen

Reader's Digest Fund for the Blind is publisher of the Large-Type Edition of Reader's Digest. For subscription information about this magazine, please contact Reader's Digest Fund for the Blind, Inc., Dept. 250, Pleasantville, N.Y. 10570.

The credits and acknowledgments that appear on page 464 are hereby made a part of this copyright page.

Library of Congress Cataloging in Publication Data: page 464

WARNING

The information in this book is primarily for reference and education. It is not intended to be a substitute for the advice of a physician. The editors do not advocate self-diagnosis or self-medication; they urge anyone with continuing symptoms, however minor, to seek medical advice. The reader should be aware that any plant substance, whether used as food or medicine, externally or internally, may cause an allergic reaction in some people.

About This Book

In these days of fast foods, plasterboard houses, and synthetic clothing, which of us does not long to return to a more natural way of life? No longer a back-to-nature fad but a growing philosophy, this wish to put nature back in our lives applies above all to those two most important of human concerns: getting healthy and staying healthy.

From time immemorial man has relied on plants to treat sicknesses and soothe aches and pains. The same herbs, trees, and shrubs employed by ancient peoples have continued to be valued through the ages—by the Egyptians, Greeks, and Romans, by apothecaries and physicians in the Middle Ages and later, by the settlers who came to North America, by the Indians who met them here, and even by our own grandparents. Many of these plants are still used today; nearly half of all medicines currently prescribed are derived from members of the plant kingdom.

Over the ages, many magical and mystical powers were ascribed to such plants. Occasionally these beliefs were mere superstitions; more commonly they were based on keen observation. For although people knew that certain plants had indisputable healing powers, they could not explain how the plants' medicinal powers worked, and so attributed them to supernatural forces. Today we understand many of the underlying physical and chemical principles that account for the medicinal properties of plants. Yet plants still do possess a magical quality—their beauty and the astonishing variety of their forms. This book is your guide to the wonderful world of magical, medicinal plants.

You can enjoy this wonder and beauty without stepping outside your home. Start by turning to the book's central "Gallery of Medicinal Plants." Here you will find specially commissioned paintings of more than 280 North American species. Here you can pore over breathtaking representations of the flowers, trees, herbs, and shrubs that have bewitched and beguiled mankind over the millennia.

Or use the gallery as a field guide. The paintings, as accurate as they are beautiful, provide all the details you need to identify the plants in the wild—or in a garden. Each is accompanied by a full-color photograph that shows what the plant looks like in its natural habitat and by a description of its growth habits, its geographic range, and the specific environment in which it grows.

You will also learn each plant's story—how it was used by ancient peoples, what magic and myths they associated with it, and, not least, what today's scientists are learning about its medicinal properties.

Other self-contained sections offer the knowledge accumulated by the scientists, historians, anthropologists, and others who have explored the worlds of botany and medicine. In "Exotic Plants" you can read the fascinating stories of many plants of incomparable value that are native to parts of the world outside the United States and Canada. In "Plants in Myth and Magic" you'll learn how, in the struggle to gain mastery over nature, mankind has used plants as a magical force. Healers, not knowing how, or why—or even if—their medicines would work, employed magic spells, incantations, elaborate rituals, and charms to aid their cures. Not just among primitive peoples, but in advanced civilizations such as those of the Greeks and Romans, and even in recent times, plants have been thought to have supernatural attributes that make them effective medicines.

"ABC's of Plants" tells you how to find plants in the wild, how to identify them, how to collect and preserve them. It's a quick and easy course in botany covering the parts of a plant from root to flowering shoot, and it also describes the way plants manufacture medicinal substances.

"Plants, People, and Medicine" tells the fascinating story of mankind's relationship to plants from prehistoric times to the present. Archeologists and anthropologists have contributed their knowledge of civilizations far removed from us in time or space; historians of the more recent past; and doctors and herbalists of today's developments. Finally, in the section called "Growing and Using Herbs" you'll learn how to grow your own healthful herbs, and discover the many useful and delightful ways that you can employ them in cooking, crafts, and cosmetics.

MAGIC AND MEDICINE OF PLANTS offers you a world of pleasure and knowledge. It is a portal to the endless variation of the plant kingdom, a repository of the myths and legends surrounding even the most inconspicuous plants, and an introduction to the fascinating world of herbal medicine.

The Editors

✿ Contents ✿

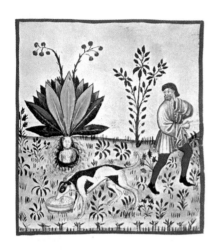

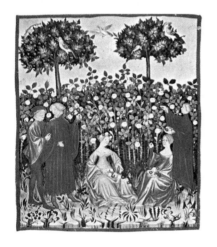

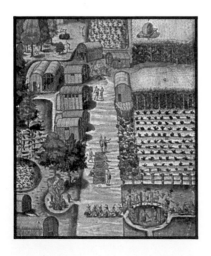

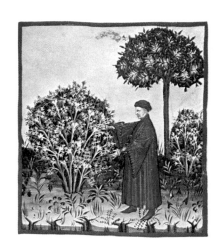

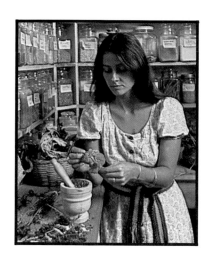

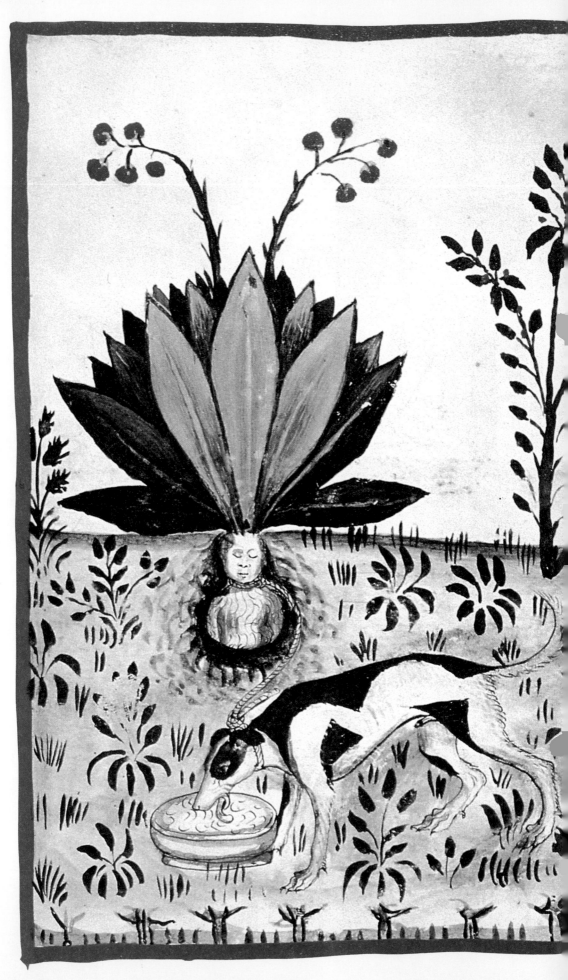

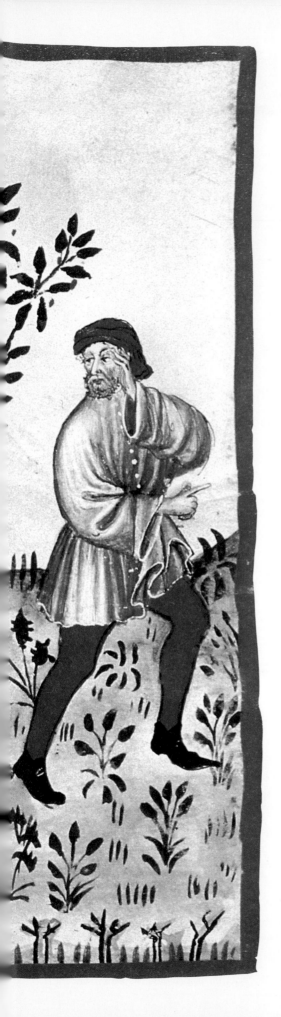

Plants in Myth and Magic

In the long struggle to achieve mastery over the powerful forces of nature, man has always turned to plants for help—for food, shelter, clothing, weapons, and healing, and even for relief from the hardships of life. Plants provide all these and something more: an astonishing display of vital energy in their growth and seasonal rebirth. No wonder then that, from the most primitive societies to the most advanced, plants have been invested with magical power. No wonder that so many myths attribute to plants an intimate personal relationship with our daily lives and with our destinies.

9

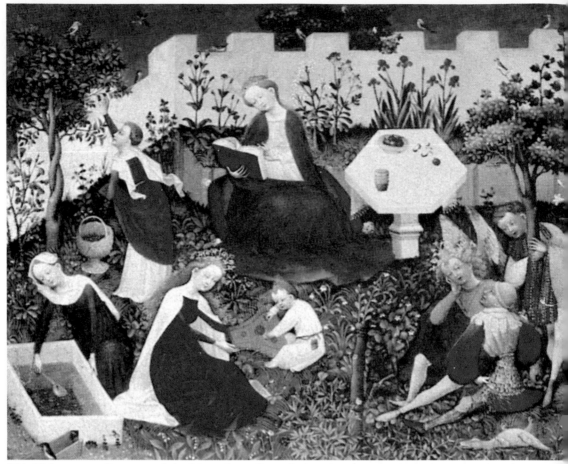

This 15th-century German artist's vision of paradise is lush with plants both medicinal and mythical.

How could early man doubt that plants were magical? Lacking the vantage of science, how else could he explain the mysteries of the plant kingdom? Every autumn in temperate climes, prehistoric human beings watched the forests die: the trees shed their leaves; grasses and flowers withered; only a few evergreens retained a semblance of summer's vitality. Yet come spring, all were reborn: buds burst into leaf, and fresh shoots sprouted from the earth. Surely any beings that resurrect themselves each year must be filled with magic.

In the tropics, there was no killing winter chill. A huge variety of plants grew, reproduced, and spread, with a vigor and speed that must have seemed no less miraculous than the seasonal cycle of growth and dormancy.

Our distant ancestors did not need to be trained botanists to observe and appreciate the remarkable energy and diversity of the plant world. Necessity made them diligent students of the local flora. Plants furnished foods, medicines, clothing, and shelter. Some plants' behavior must also have filled our ancestors with wonder. Why did the sunflower's blossom turn to track the sun moving across the sky? Why did the morning glory's trumpets open only at daybreak? Unable to find any apparent cause for such behavior, our early ancestors used their imagination. They populated the countryside with nymphs and dryads. They animated trees and flowers with guardian spirits both benign and evil. In Peru, for example, sun worshipers venerated the sunflower as the earthly embodiment of the sun. And in Japan, morning glories became "jewels of heaven" because their beauty lured the sun-goddess back into the sky at dawn.

Already dependent upon plants for material needs, human beings turned naturally to the plant kingdom for aid in the daunting struggle to achieve mastery over their environment and fate. Plants appeared to have magical power: if this could be harnessed and directed, then surely it would afford relief from misfortune and disease, control of the future, and peace with the gods.

Countless plants were tested by sorcerers in the hope of achieving such power. Many plant names still bear testimony to these experiments, long after the plant has lost its supernatural reputation. *Verbena*, for instance, is the generic name of many shrubs and herbs. It recalls the use of one verbena species, *V. officinalis*, or vervain, in sacred festivals of ancient Rome.

Garlic is a plant that has long enjoyed a reputation for white magic—the power to turn back the evil forces of black magic. If magic lies in an ability to prevent malnutrition, then garlic is certainly magical. Over the centuries not only has this homely herb added vitamins and minerals to meals, it was also said to have defended people against vampires and the plague. Even today, Chinese, Greek, and Jewish grandmothers will sometimes present a clove of garlic to their infant grandchildren as protection against the evil eye.

In contrast to garlic's reputation for extraordinary goodness, other plants were marked as evil because of their poisonous or narcotic qualities. These plants all too often served as instruments of human wickedness. Thus belladonna, whose juice is both toxic and sedative, frequently figured in murderers' potions and devilish brews, and came to be known as deadly nightshade, witch's-berry, and sorcerer's-cherry, among other names.

The Goose Barnacle Tree and Other Tales

The tall tales spun by returning travelers and explorers also spawned many a fanciful plant with magical properties. Because of the expense and danger of travel, premodern men rarely ventured far from their homelands, and the few brave souls who did see the world could inflate their experiences with little fear of being found out. To impress the stay-at-homes, these voyagers populated the world with monsters and marvels, including exotic plants that had fantastic attributes.

One of the most durable of these stories was that of the goose barnacle tree. This extravagantly imaginary bit of flora was a seaside tree that bore shells, or barnacles, containing live geese as its fruit. It may have grown out of sailors' quite factual descriptions of the long-necked barnacles that are found attached to ships' hulls. In any case, the goose barnacle tree gained wide celebrity among landlubbers. Enthusiastic chroniclers placed it in such remote spots as the Irish coast or the Scottish Hebrides, and asserted that the trees were the source of a marsh goose, which one writer renamed the barnacle goose. Accepted as fact for centuries, the goose barnacle tree provoked a theological debate. Technically its geese were fruit, not fowl. Therefore some Christians decided that these geese could be eaten on fast days when flesh was forbidden.

Other plant marvels were based on accounts of real plants that had become distorted in the telling and retelling. An example is the legend of the vegetable lamb tree of Scythia (a region that stretched from southern Europe to the Crimea), also known as the Tartarian lamb tree and as the *Borametz*. The legend seems to have begun with a straightforward description of a cotton plant, *Gossypium herbaceum*, by Herodotus, the Greek historian. In the fifth century B.C., he wrote an account of the struggles

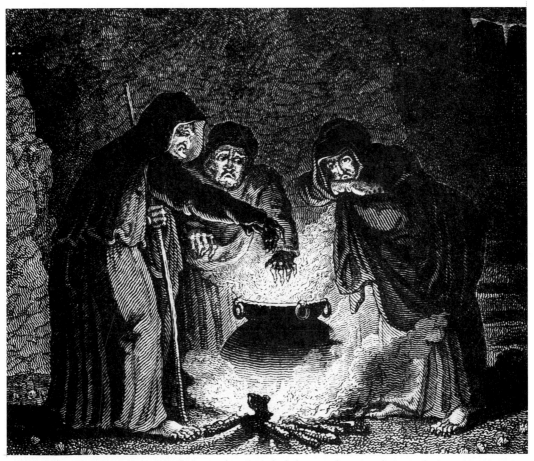

In Macbeth, *Shakespeare dramatized the age-old belief that witches use plants to brew magic potions.*

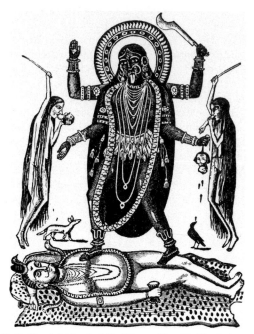

In India nightshade felled the goddess Kali's victims.

between the Greeks and the Asian peoples to the east. His account, titled simply the *Histories,* starts with the Trojan War. The book contains very extensive descriptions of lands outside the boundaries of the civilized world of the Greeks, Egyptians, and Persians. Herodotus reported that "certain trees . . . bear for their fruit fleeces surpassing those of sheep in beauty and excellence, and the natives clothe themselves in cloths made therefrom."

Retold and embellished for centuries, Herodotus' story grew ever more fantastic. Eventually, his "wool-bearing" tree had become a "vegetable lamb plant," a little flesh-and-blood sheep. The tree grew from a melonlike seed. Rooted to the earth by a stem from its navel, this floral cannibal grazed voraciously on the surrounding greenery. When it had devoured all within reach, it withered and died. A 14th-century traveler, whose pen name was Sir John Mandeville, claimed to have tasted the creature's flesh. Despite the protests of generations of scientists, this fable was not laid to rest until 1887.

Sometimes such tall tales required careful sifting to separate fact from fiction. From the Indian subcontinent, Europeans brought back stories of a plant now known to science as *Datura metel,* which is related to the nightshades. They described the metel's flower as so powerful that its fragrance alone would fell passersby. This story has a basis in truth. Though the metel's unsavory perfume is not intrinsically fatal, the aroma can stupefy those who breathe it. Like other members of the nightshade family, including the American jimsonweed, metel contains scopolamine. This alkaloid acts as a powerful sedative and soporific. It was allegedly used by the Thugs,

an Indian secret society, to drug chance wayfarers, whom they robbed and then strangled, in sacrifice, people said, to the goddess Kali.

Mystique of the Mandrake

Even a familiar plant could develop a supernatural reputation if its habits were sufficiently bizarre. An example of this kind of elaborate embroidery involves the mandrake, or mandragora, a small perennial herb common throughout the Mediterranean region.

Like other nightshades, the mandrake derives its reputation for magical power partly from its toxicity. This potent herb can kill the unwary, although it has also served as an important source of therapeutic medicines. Adding to the mandrake's mystique is the appearance of its root. Thick and tuberous, it can be imagined to look like a little human being, a coincidence that deeply impressed some contemporaries of the ancient Greek botanist Theophrastus. They were the *rhizotomoi,* or "root cutters." The herbalists of their day, these root cutters supplied herbs to physicians. There was even more to the mandrake's magical appeal. It is a plant that phosphoresces. Sometimes at night, chemical substances in its berries react with the dew to give a pale light. A phenomenon that today is explained by science our ancestors attributed to spirits and magical forces.

Flavius Josephus, a Jewish general, statesman, and historian of the first century A.D., described the perils of harvesting the mandrake. While its glow made it easy to locate, the herb shrank back whenever approached; and merely touching it could prove fatal. One way to collect the herb was to dig carefully all around it until only a small portion of the root remained covered. The collector would then lash a dog to the root and walk away. The dog would pull the root free in a suicidal effort to rejoin its master. But in exchange for the dog's death, according to Josephus, the master obtained an infallible charm against demons. Other people said the mandrake protected against battle wounds, cured all diseases, brought luck in love, promoted fertility, guaranteed perfect marksmanship, and unearthed hidden treasures.

A remarkable thing about plant magic is how it runs through many periods of human experience. As long as ignorance kept people enslaved to superstition, the idea of magical plants remained powerful. Infiltrating every activity from romance to agriculture, herbal magic was acknowledged as instrumental to health, happiness, and success. Though nations sneered at the credulity of their neighbors—and new generations laughed at the ignorance and gullibility of the old—each in turn wove its own new fantastic tissue of herbal taboos, tales, and lore. The tradition of the mandrake root, for instance, kept a firm hold

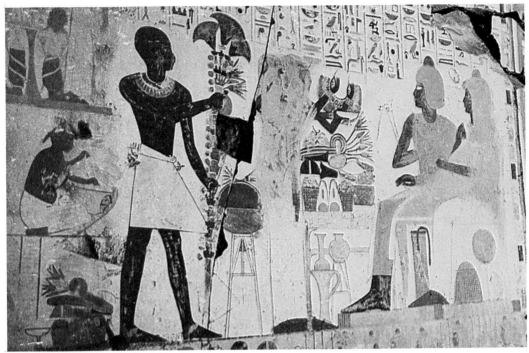

In a tomb painting at Thebes, a subject makes a funerary offering of papyrus.

on people's imagination, if not belief, for many centuries. "Go, and catch a falling star,/Get with child a mandrake root," were among a long list of impossible tasks set forth by the 17th-century poet John Donne.

Sacred Botany of the Pharaohs

An ancient Egyptian might spend his entire life preparing for the next world, his daily routine dominated by priests and ritual. According to Herodotus, who had sailed up and down the Nile exploring their grandiose temples and observing their burial customs, the Egyptians were unique. "They are of all men the most excessively attentive to the worship of the gods," he wrote. Such a land was an ideal breeding ground for plant magic.

Everywhere the Egyptians looked they found evidence of divine presence. In the blue and white lotuses that sprouted from the Nile's muddy shallows they saw a symbol of nature's irrepressible fertility. It was a lotus blossom, they believed, that had emerged from the ocean at creation. Papyrus, the prolific reed of the Nile, not only furnished the Egyptians with paper but became their symbol of freshness, youth, and vigor. A papyrus-shaped amulet ensured long life to its wearer. Papyrus bouquets adorned religious rites. Papyrus columns—stone pillars formed to look like bundles of the plant—endowed the ancient temples with the reed's spiritual virtues.

Another plant revered by the Egyptians was the onion. Though it was a favorite dish in ancient Egypt, it served as much more than a vegetable. In the onion's fragrant bulb the Egyptians found a symbol of the universe. Just as each layer of the onion was wrapped in another, so, they believed, was the nether world enveloped by the earth and, in turn, by heaven. As some people today might swear on a Bible, the Egyptians took their oath on an onion. They also presented onions to their gods as sacrificial offerings.

In this arid country trees were sacred, and groves were customarily planted around temples for the enjoyment of the gods. Egyptians filled even crypts with flowers. Their mummies have been found with the remains of wreaths of such familiar plants as sweet marjoram, chrysanthemums, narcissus, and roses.

Plant collecting was an important activity on Egyptian military and commercial expeditions. In 1475 B.C., for instance, when the pharaoh Thutmose III won his first campaign in Syria, exotic plants constituted an important part of the booty sent back to Egypt. Later, in the third campaign, Thutmose III dispatched his chief treasurer Ray to the new territories to collect "all the plants that grow, all flowers that are in God's-Land [Syria]." Upon Ray's return, the proud pharaoh offered the exotic specimens to the god Amon and decorated a room in Amon's great temple at Karnak with wall carvings of the foreign plants.

Myrrh Trees From the Land of Punt

Even more remarkable was the venture of Thutmose III's aunt, Queen Hatshepsut. Amon informed her in an oracle that he wanted myrrh trees planted around his temple. Myrrh played a vital role in the Egyptians' religious ceremonies. When burned, it releases a fragrant odor that the Egyptians believed pleased the gods. Since myrrh trees were not to be found in Egypt, Hatshepsut sent five ships south to the Land of Punt, a region in equatorial Africa known for its myrrh production. When her sailors finally reached Punt, they encountered there a strange tribe living in domed huts set atop pilings. In a deal reminiscent of the Dutch colonists' purchase of Manhattan Island, the Egyptians bartered an ax, a knife, and some bangles, necklaces, and rings for ebony, ivory, gold, cinnamon, cattle, apes, dogs, panthers, slaves, sacks of myrrh, and 31 fresh myrrh saplings.

Delighted with the mission, Queen Hatshepsut had it depicted in a series of reliefs on the walls of a temple she was building to enclose her own tomb. After formally offering the saplings to Amon, she used them to create "a Punt in his house . . . according as he commanded." She ordered terraces built around the temple, reproducing in miniature the hilly landscape of Punt. As legend has it, Amon was so satisfied as he walked abroad in his new garden that he promised Hatshepsut "life, stability and satisfaction . . . forever."

Plants in Greek Mythology

Even if, as Herodotus felt, no nation exceeded the Egyptians in religious fervor, his countrymen, the Greeks, certainly excelled in the inventiveness of their plant superstitions. Their myths, like all mythology, are stories created either to account for natural phenomena (such as the change of seasons) or to define the role of the supernatural in everyday life.

Twelve great gods ruled the heavens, earth, sea, and underworld, according to the Greeks, and they made their home on the summit of Mount Olympus in northern Greece. Members all of one family, each of these Olympians had distinctive attributes and a special personality, and each had favorite plants. Zeus, the

chief of the gods, had adopted the oak as a symbol of his enduring might. His son Ares, god of war, preferred the ash, the tree that supplied shafts for spears. Athena, goddess of wisdom, chose the olive, an invaluable tree of her own creation, which furnished not only timber but also fruit and oil.

In Greek literature and art, these plants served as their respective gods' symbols. The plants also were seen as living links to the gods. An oak grove at Dodona, in northwestern Greece, became the oracle of Zeus. There, by listening to the rustling of oak leaves, priests interpreted Zeus' divine will. Another even more famous oracle was Apollo's shrine at Delphi, where a priestess foretold the future in a trance, a state she reputedly attained by breathing the hallucinogenic smoke of smoldering secret herbs.

Demeter was the Greeks' goddess of agriculture. She could deny harvest to the farmer. To win her favor, the Greeks courted her with seeds of the corn poppy, which, they thought, must be Demeter's favorite flower, since she was said to wear a garland of poppies interlaced with barley and wheat.

Poems and stories told how some familiar plants had provided havens for the persecuted. When the nymph Daphne, whose father was a river, sought to escape the amorous pursuit of the powerful sun-god Apollo, she entreated her father for help. He transformed her into a bay, or laurel tree, which became sacred to Apollo.

Flowers could also serve as lures. When Demeter's daughter, Persephone, went gathering flowers in Sicily, she saw a blossom more beautiful than all the rest. The Greek name for this flower comes from *narke*, meaning "numbness," and translates as "narcissus."

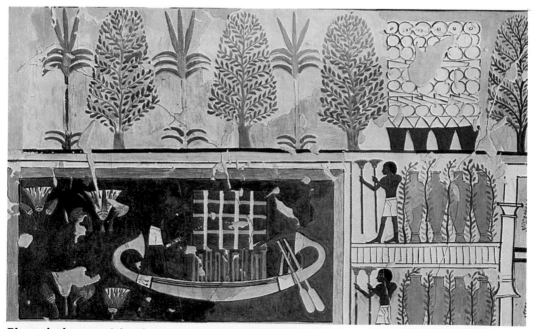

Plants, both terrestrial and aquatic, dominate this 15th-century B.C. Egyptian tomb painting.

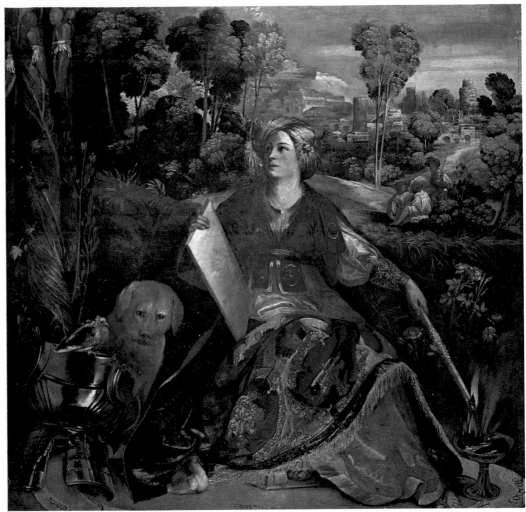

Homer's Odyssey *relates the plant magic of Circe, here portrayed by 16th-century Italian Dosso Dossi.*

Thus it may indicate a species of the genus much later scientifically named *Narcissus*, which includes daffodils. In any case, when Persephone reached for the flower, a chasm opened, and Hades, god of the underworld, grabbed the girl and carried her down to become his bride. Persephone should have known better, for the narcissus had infernal connotations. Greek physicians knew of its ability to deaden the senses, and the flower often adorned tombs as an offering for the deceased.

The story does not end with Persephone's abduction. Demeter, in rage and then despair at the fate of her daughter, let the world become cold and barren. Nothing would grow. The human race was about to die out from famine. It would have happened had not Zeus realized that, without human beings, the Olympians would lose the gifts and sacrifices provided by mortals. The farsighted Zeus ordered Persephone's release. But there was a problem. While living in the underworld, Persephone had eaten a pomegranate seed, which committed her to be forever married to Hades. At this point, Zeus worked out a compromise between Persephone's mother

and husband. Persephone would spend one-third of the year with Hades. Each year, when Persephone descends to the underworld, Demeter plunges the world into winter.

Sorceresses are active in some of the Greek myths. Compared with the typical witches of later legends, the Greek sorceresses were beautiful, passionate women. Yet they made perilous companions. One victim of their charms was Odysseus, the wily creator of the Trojan horse. Sailing back from Troy, he and his men stopped at the island home of Circe, mistress of the occult. By feeding them the "juice of magical herbs," Circe changed into swine all the men Odysseus had sent out to reconnoiter. The "juice" would probably have been made from henbane or mandrake. Odysseus escaped only by keeping with him the herb moly (usually identified as garlic), an antidote supplied by a friendly god.

Apparently, herbal sorcery was a family business, for Circe's niece, Medea, was also an expert practitioner. Medea's occult skills won the golden fleece for her lover Jason. The fleece was her father's most treasured possession, and he refused to surrender it unless Jason could overcome two bulls and a crop of

15

superhuman warriors that had sprung from a dragon's teeth. To help her lover gain victory, Medea selected a plant grown from the blood of the god Prometheus. This plant yielded an ointment that, when rubbed on his body, would make Jason invulnerable for one full day. Applying the salve, the young man won both the contest and the golden fleece.

Rome: Pliny's Cornucopia

Of all the collections of plant lore that have survived from ancient times, the most outstanding comes from the Roman era. It is called the *Natural History*, by Gaius Plinius Secundus, known to modern readers as Pliny. The collection was based in part on a now lost work by one Quintus Sextius Niger. By profession a lawyer and administrator, Pliny was a wealthy man and a friend of the Roman emperors Vespasian and Titus. He had a lifelong interest in every aspect of the natural world. Indeed, so great was his commitment to this study that it may have killed him. Pliny died witnessing an eruption of Mount Vesuvius, the same eruption that overwhelmed Herculaneum and Pompeii. Fumes from the erupting volcano felled Pliny. Just two years before, he had completed his monumental 37-volume compilation of natural history.

To supplement his own observations in this great work, Pliny claimed in his preface to have drawn upon 100 previous authors, and to have extracted from their works "20,000 noteworthy facts." (Actually that claim is modest, for Pliny uses many more sources and items of information.) Many of these, however, are not facts at all. They are legends, embroideries, and superstitions, and therein lies much of the fascination of Pliny's work for students of antiquity as well as for the general reader.

Typical is Pliny's discussion of amber, the fossil resin prized by the ancients as a gem. He devotes two chapters to the lore of amber, covering himself at the outset by mentioning "falsehoods" the Greeks told about it. From this account we learn that some of the ancients believed amber to be tears shed by exotic birds or by the daughters of the sun or to be the solidified urine of a species of lynx.

Though Pliny did identify amber correctly as an exudation from trees, he gave it many properties it does not have. Worn at the neck, he wrote, a piece of amber wards off tonsilitis and goiter. It also makes fever go away. Furthermore, amber amulets were meant to benefit babies in some general way and protect people of all ages from "attacks of wild distraction" and strangury (slow, painful urination). Pliny's own account of the source of amber is, however, almost entirely accurate and in line with modern standards of objectivity. Thus misinformation is continually mixed with kernels of scientific fact here and there. For example, Pliny's mention of Indian "amber" is

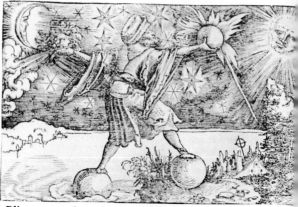

Pliny covers the universe: the herbalist-astrologer as depicted in the 15th century.

now seen as a garbled reference to shellac, a product relatively unknown in Pliny's world, since it was derived then from the resinous secretion of an Indian insect.

Amazing "facts" are sprinkled throughout Pliny's *Natural History*. Spiked loosestrife when woven into a garland and hung around oxen's necks, the reader learns, will make the beasts pull together as a team. Thunder causes truffles to grow. *Silphium,* a member of the composite family that Pliny describes as a purge, first sprang up after the ground had been soaked with a "rain the color of pitch." Cucumbers creep toward water but away from oil. Grapevines abhor radishes and must never be planted near them. Turnips provoke lust.

Pliny's work contains a great deal about the medicinal uses of trees, herbs, and flowers. Drawn from the foremost medical authorities of the age, this information covers much that is genuinely scientific. But it also includes many curious practices whose origins are in superstition and whose benefits are at best questionable. To aid conception, for instance, Pliny transmits the recommendation that a woman bind to her body a cucumber seed that had never touched the ground. If that same seed was preserved and later wrapped in ram's wool and tied to the woman's loins before delivery, it would ease her labor pains. Leaves of maidenhair fern, if steeped in the urine of a young boy, pounded with saltpeter, and applied to a woman's abdomen, would protect her from wrinkles. Even the humble barley possessed special powers in the folklore of Pliny's day. If a man afflicted with a boil would take nine grains of barley, trace a circle around the boil three times with each grain, and then throw the barley into a fire with his left hand, he would be cured at once.

Toxicology, too, was covered in Pliny's *Natural History.* Eating mushrooms, the book warned, could be risky because many were poisonous. Even the nonpoisonous ones, if breathed upon by a venomous snake, would turn toxic, readers of Pliny learned. In Pliny could be found both instructions for rubbing radishes on the skin to stop venomous creatures from biting and recommendations of plants for healing if one was bitten anyway by a scorpion, spider, snake, or mad dog.

For some of Pliny's plant sorceries, applications are difficult to imagine. Did anyone actually drink bull's blood, and so stand in need of a cabbage seed antidote? Many of the charms, of course, did address real needs, but whether or not they met those needs is another question. Did Pliny's recipe for an asparagus-based talisman against bee stings, for example, actually work? And if basil really did reinforce the procreative urge of donkeys and horses, as the naturalist claimed, then the Roman stockman would want to know about this herb; but the same question arises. Love potions are always in demand, and if, as Pliny reported, the carrot does in fact have aphrodisiac properties, what a blessing for the lovelorn! In an age that believed in witchcraft (as even educated Romans did), who could ignore the learned author's advice to ward off evil spells with a bunch of squill in the doorway?

From Moses to Mistletoe

The Bible reveals that plant magic often played a part in the lives of the men and women whose stories the scripture relates. During Moses' conversion, a bush became the oracle through which God spoke: an angel of the Lord appeared in the flame of the miraculous bush that burned but was not consumed. Later, with God's help, Moses bested the Egyptian magicians. With a rod that his brother Aaron had once changed into a serpent, Moses divided the Red Sea and struck water from a desert rock. The burning bush is not the only plant oracle in the Bible. It was a balsam tree, for instance, that told David to begin the attack on the Philistines.

In the Song of Solomon, there is an allusion to the aphrodisiacal properties of the mandrake, when the maiden invites her lover into the fields where "mandrakes give forth fragrance"; and the Book of Genesis tells that Leah and Rachael, the daughters of Laban, both wished to bear sons for Jacob, the man for whose affections they persistently competed. Rachel was successful only after taking a dose of mandrake roots.

Further on in Genesis, Laban agrees to give all his striped and spotted livestock to Jacob. That did not amount to many animals, but Jacob had a magic trick up his sleeve. He "took fresh rods of poplar and almond and plane, and peeled white streaks in them, exposing the white of the rods." Jacob then placed the peeled rods in front of the watering troughs, and "the flocks bred in front of the rods and so . . . brought forth striped, speckled, and spotted [offspring]." This story reflects a belief that piebald offspring could be produced by

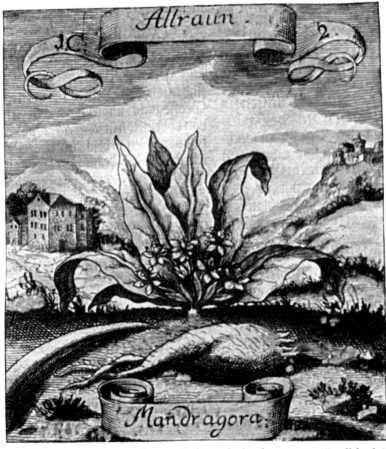

An 18th-century German book called mandrake the strongest "troll herb."

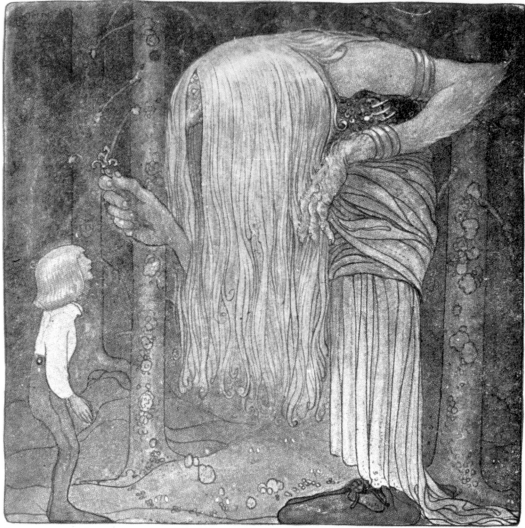

In a scene evoking Norse folklore, a witch in a dark wood offers a magic herb to an innocent boy.

setting striped sticks in front of female animals' eyes while the females were breeding.

Apart from Judeo-Christian traditions, other peoples developed their own independent and fascinating mythologies involving plants. Of these perhaps none has a more striking symbol than Yggdrasil, the great ash tree of Norse (Teutonic) mythology. Evergreen and immortal, this tree was inconceivably huge, with branches reaching right up into heaven and foliage that shaded the entire world. In this "tree of destiny" lay the fate of the universe. It tapped the fountains of youth and wisdom while sheltering and feeding all manner of beasts. Yet one of its roots penetrated right into hell and was gnawed ceaselessly by an evil serpent. When, at last, Yggdrasil came crashing down, all life would cease.

Another rich tradition of plant lore originated with the druids, the priests of the ancient Celts. Though the druids used herbs in their rites, trees were the object of their special veneration. When the forces of darkness had threatened man, trees had come to his defense. In the ensuing battle, the forest giants had won three gifts for man: the dog, the deer, and the

lapwing. In gratitude, the druids took the Celtic word for tree as their name, and made trees the basis of their alphabet. For their A, they drew a stylized elm (or *ailm* to them); for B, a birch, and so on.

One example of druidic lore found its way into Pliny's volumes. It concerns the mistletoe. This was almost certain to interest educated Romans, because the mistletoe is the famous "golden bough" of Virgil's *Aeneid*, written less than a century before Pliny's work.

A strange little parasite, the mistletoe has singular habits that elicited the druids' worship. It seemed to defy nature by living its entire life aloft in the branches of trees, never descending to the earth, a plant's natural habitat. Equally strange, mistletoe appeared to spring from nowhere (whereas, in fact, new mistletoe colonies are established as birds traveling from tree to tree expel the seeds in their droppings). To the casual observer, the plant's reproduction and spread seemed spontaneous. The druids declared it—and the oak tree on which it grew—sacred. The druids viewed oaks as their greatest allies.

Six days after the new moon, white-robed

druid priests entered the oak groves to gather mistletoe. One of the priests climbed up into the tree to harvest the mistletoe with a golden sickle, a symbol of the sun. Other priests, waiting below, caught the falling sprigs in a white cloak. If the cuttings touched the ground, so it was believed, they would lose their heaven-sent virtues. Finally, with prayers, spells, and the sacrifice of two white bulls, the magical crop was brewed into a mysterious potion with special health-giving properties.

After the Romans conquered what is now France and Britain, the religion of the druids faded. For centuries afterward, however, mistletoe retained its therapeutic reputation; and despite the lack of any proved medicinal value, it continued to be an ingredient in many treatments. In Sweden, for example, mistletoe was supposed to lend a special potency to a tonic called *aqua hirundinum* ("swallows' water"). It was an appalling concoction, made of a mixture of peony, lily of the valley, elderberry, linden, coriander, nutmeg, cubeb, and of course mistletoe, all distilled together with 24 live baby swallows. Recommended as a remedy for sore throats, swallows' water remained in favor until 1757, when it was mercifully struck from the pharmacopeia by an official act of the Swedish government.

In the past, a bunch of mistletoe was hung in homes as insurance against all sorts of ills: witchcraft, disease, bad luck, and fire. Today it hangs as a holiday decoration in many American homes, where it effects another kind of magic, the encouragement of holiday kisses.

Martyrs and Missionaries

Among the laws that God gave to Moses at Mount Sinai was the one stating, "You shall not permit a sorceress to live." It was a law that many medieval clerics would enforce ruthlessly, condemning most suspects to torture and then death. The earlier Christian church, however, did not enforce the law nearly so strictly.

Many plants, especially flowers, were exorcised of their pagan connotations by a new association with Christian saints and martyrs. To many pre-Christian peoples, the rose's beauty had suggested divinity. The Greeks had associated the rose with Aphrodite, the goddess of love; and the Egyptians had offered the rose to the souls of their dead pharaohs. Rather than ban this lovely blossom, the church fathers reconsecrated it to the Virgin Mary. Thus, as the Christian missionaries spread across Europe, they converted flowers as well as people.

Vervain, a plant of the *Verbena* genus, had played a part in the religious rites of early Germans and Celts. The missionaries rechristened it herb-of-the-cross, claiming it had stanched Christ's wounds on Calvary. The holly underwent a similar transformation. This evergreen, the druids taught, provided a winter refuge for the wood spirits and so protected against bad fortune; and the Celts decorated their huts with holly branches. Under Christian influence, the holly became for some a symbol of Christ's sacrifice: the spiny leaves recalled His crown of thorns, and the scarlet berries the blood of His passion.

Christian priests effectively used plants and flowers as teaching tools. For the most part, their flocks consisted of illiterate peasants, and the parish priests could not reach them with written tracts. But as farmers, the peasants were very familiar with the weeds that infested their fields and with the wildflowers that filled their meadows. Seizing the opportunity, the priests found a Christian lesson in many weeds and wildflowers.

Shamrocks, as St. Patrick pointed out, illustrate the concept of the Trinity: three distinct leaves, yet joined to make a whole. Every Irishman knows that story, but not so well remembered is the significance of the alchemilla, *Alchemilla vulgaris*. Its flowers set seed without fertilization, since the male parts wither before the female parts mature. Today, scientists know this to be a perfectly natural process called parthenogenesis; but early Christians saw in it a miraculous virgin birth, a commemoration of Jesus' virgin birth. Renaming the plant lady's-mantle, they created a perpetual reminder of the Virgin Mary's immaculate purity.

One unforeseen consequence of the christening of *A. vulgaris* was the reputation for magical powers that it brought this unprepossessing herb. Alchemists distilled the essence of lady's-mantle in the hope that it could turn dross into gold. (Its alchemical popularity was later to give the plant its scientific generic name, *Alchemilla*.) Moreover, during the Renaissance, the herb was believed to contain the secret of eternal youth and to be the source of a miracle cure that would restore virginal beauty to an old woman's body.

Christian missionaries associated certain plants, according to their period of bloom, with the holy feasts. Monks called the wood sorrel, or shamrock, alleluia. They did so because it flowered between Easter and Whitsuntide, a season when the Psalms read in their services all ended with that exclamation. Similarly, Michaelmas daisies flower about the feast of St. Michael, September 29, and so on. By watching for these and other blossoms, the faithful could punctually observe the holidays, even if they could not read a calendar.

As happened with so many other plants, the Christian role of St. John's wort, *Hypericum perforatum*, was connected to pagan origins. Its golden hue and its habit of being in bloom at the time of the summer solstice had made the herb a totem of sun worshipers throughout the ancient world. The Romans burned it in bonfires that were part of the celebrations on

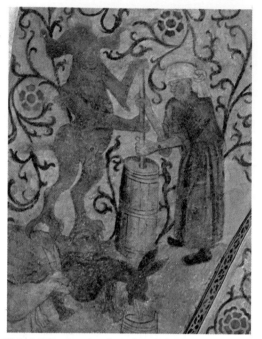

This 1450's drawing in a Swedish church warned against potions mixed by the Devil (left).

Midsummer Day. Under Christianity, since the plant's association with the summer solstice (about June 21) linked it to the day celebrated as the birth of John the Baptist, June 24, Christian priests rededicated the plant to that martyr. After its conversion, St. John's wort continued to be hung in doorways to repel evil demons and witches, a custom rooted in pagan beliefs. This did not seem to bother the Christian priests, who collected the holy herb to use in casting out devils.

A Witch's Garden of Herbs

While medieval churchmen used flowers to spread the gospel, there were others who employed them to less holy ends. Throughout the Middle Ages, and indeed until the present day in many parts of the world, a few questions in the right places to the right people could lead one to a witch. This was a man or woman who would, for a fee, cast a spell, concoct a magic potion, or manufacture a charm. Witches have been known to be good as well as evil; and the reputation of a "good witch" often stemmed from the ability to come up with herbal brews that satisfied people's wants or needs.

A typical parish priest did not look kindly on this competition. He damned such sorcery as black magic and accused the witches of a compact with the Devil. Yet even the most systematic repression could not put the witches down. They provided services that the priest could not. If a woman found herself pregnant with an unwanted child, the witch, for a price, provided her with a concoction sure to cause a miscarriage. If a young man found his beloved cold and unresponsive, the witch

could sell him a potion guaranteed to soften the lady's heart. Had the family cow dried up? Was the baby ailing for no known reason? No doubt they were bewitched, and if a priest's prayers could not help, then perhaps the witch's incantations could.

Because discovery could mean death, witches conducted their business in strictest secrecy. Much of what little witches' lore survives is found in the transcripts of their trials. These transcripts contain testimony extracted under torture, together with descriptions from the witch hunters' manuals, fanciful accounts that seem to owe more to the prosecutors' lurid imaginations than to fact. From such sources, we gather that witches were heirs to ancient lessons about the medicinal properties of many substances found in nature. The witches preserved and continued to use plant lore that the Christian church had suppressed as "heathen" mysteries. In patches hidden deep in the woods, witches grew forbidden plants.

Many of the witches' herbs were poisonous, plants now recognized as containing potent drugs and toxins. Most also had ancient reputations. The familiar henbane and mandrake were witches' standbys. By special treatment, however, witches tried to endow these old plant servants with new powers.

Thus, the witches preferred to harvest mandrakes from beneath a gallows tree. The hanged man had to have been a "pure youth." That meant a congenital criminal who had been wicked from conception and devoted his whole life to crimes. The newly harvested root had to have special treatment. It had to be bathed in wine, clothed with silk and velvet, and fed every week, preferably with a sacramental wafer stolen during communion.

Another favorite plant of the witches was Jupiter's bean, or henbane. Harvested at night when the moon was in the proper phase, this deadly member of the nightshade family served the witch as an ingredient of her flying ointment. After blending the herb with such nauseating ingredients as bat's blood, vipers, toads, and the fat of dead children, the witch would rub the mixture into her skin. Soon the witch would start to hallucinate, imagining that she was soaring through the air or dancing with demons. Later her recollections gave rise to tales of magical flights and black Sabbats.

The witch did not always reserve the nightshades' powers for her own use. Many of the brews she served her customers or victims had active ingredients derived from henbane and other nightshades. Sometimes the result was innocent enough. The juice of one nightshade became for a time a favorite beauty aid of ladies, who dropped it in their eyes to dilate their pupils—a look they considered attractive. The scientific name of this nightshade species is *Atropa belladonna*; *belladonna* means "fair lady" in Italian.

A relative of the deadly nightshade, the thorn apple (*Datura stramonium*), later called jimsonweed, appealed to lovers of a more aggressive disposition. This "love will" was supposed to make the object of one's desires lose all powers of resistance and become, against his or her will, passionately aroused.

Some witches are supposed to have hired out regularly as assassins, a trade that earned all witches, good and bad, a frightening reputation. For a fee, the village witch would eliminate a rival or hasten an inheritance— whatever a client desired. If her curses did not suffice, then the witch dispatched the victim with a "magic" potion, a deadly brew made of toxic plants such as the nightshades.

Plants furnished the witch with the materials for her magic; they also were seen as the best defense against evil witchcraft. Angelica, for example, came to be known as root of the Holy Ghost. That person of the Christian Trinity was said to have revealed to a monk the special power of angelica: protection against any kind of witchcraft.

A yew tree planted at the southwest corner of a house also protected the dwelling from evil though it did seem to involve some risk of attracting witches as well. Shakespeare relates that Macbeth's three witches threw into their bubbling brew, among other items, "slips of yew sliver'd in the moon's eclipse."

Many of the herbs from the witch's garden have reappeared later in different roles. During World War II, the Germans developed— but never used—a particularly effective nerve gas. It was colorless, odorless, and almost instantly fatal. The only known antidote was a preparation made from belladonna. Another of the witches' poisons was the common foxglove, or witch's bells. It later served as the source of a valuable cardiac medicine, digitalis. Indeed, this medicine's scientific discovery is linked to an 18th-century English concocter of herbal folk remedies (such a practitioner was often referred to as a witch, in the benign sense). Her herbal tonic had gained a reputation for treating the excessive fluid retention (edema) associated with certain heart problems. The witch's tonic attracted the attention of a local doctor, William Withering, who correctly concluded that it was foxglove that made the tonic effective against edema.

A Magical Melting Pot

In America, many traditions of plant myth and magic came together. On the North American continent, descendants of various black peoples passed on to the whites elements of black beliefs (including voodoo and its related cult religion, obeah). In exchange, whites passed back not only their own religious traditions, principally Christian, but the rich plant folk-

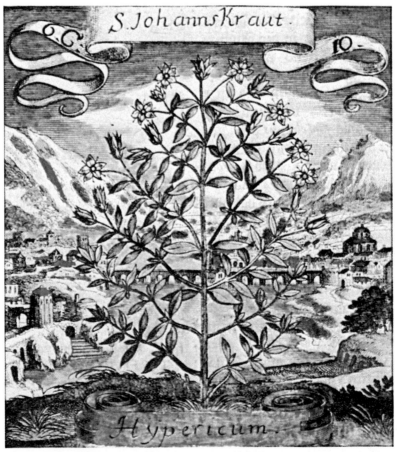

By the 18th century, St. John's wort was a Christian not a pagan herb.

21

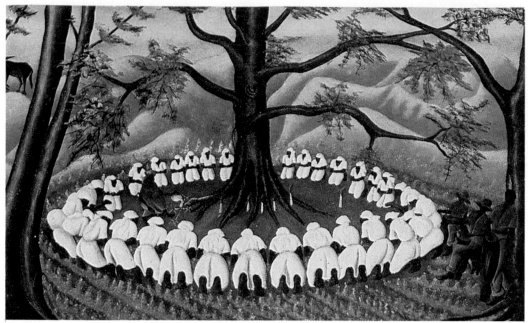

A silk-cotton jumby ("ghost") tree is the centerpiece of this 20th-century voodoo ceremony in Haiti.

lore inherited from their European ancestors. In turn, Indians traded medicinal lore with both blacks and whites. From this intermarriage of traditions sprang many new beliefs.

When Hernando Cortez and the Conquistadores burst into Mexico in 1519, they found a culture rich in herbal knowledge and lore. Aztec emperors encouraged learning about every aspect of their region's flora. Into every corner of their domains, Aztec lords sent their gardeners to collect rare and valuable plants. Artisans painted pictures of those plants on palace walls. In the emperors' gardens, doctors experimented with new remedies and gardeners tested new varieties.

Surprisingly, some of this knowledge survived the destruction of Aztec civilization. Struck by the beauty and utility of the Aztec gardens, the Spaniards spared them. In 1570, Philip II of Spain sent his personal physician, Francisco Hernández, to catalog and describe the Aztec plant collections. The book this Spanish scholar wrote was to serve as the basis of modern botanical texts on the flora of Mexico. Aztec plant magic met a harsher fate: ruthless suppression.

Although much of the written tradition of Aztec plant magic perished on the Spanish pyres, relics were preserved in the encyclopedic compilations of a handful of 16th-century missionaries. This work was aided by Indians, whom the missionaries had educated in the ways of European book learning. The resulting works are the primary source of information about Aztec civilization.

In one such tract, *The Treatise on Superstitions*, Father Hernando Ruiz de Alarcón listed the prayers the Indians made to tobacco. These prayers invoked tobacco's aid in everything from woodcutting to planting new crops.

"It can be very well seen and proven," Ruiz de Alarcón wrote, "how they worship [tobacco], for they confide in it, ask for its aid, and entrust it with the task. May God free us through His mercy from him [the Devil] who for our perdition disguises and whitewashes his lies and presumptions under the cover and mask of the tobacco. Amen." By contrast with this prayer, the U.S. surgeon general's warning on cigarette packages seems tame.

Psychoactive plants—peyote, certain kinds of mushroom, and morning glory seeds—fascinated the Aztecs as windows into another existence. The Aztec name for hallucinogenic mushrooms means "flesh of the gods."

Here is how a Franciscan friar, Bernardino de Sahagún, described a mushroom feast. "They ate the mushrooms with honey and when they began to feel excited . . . the Indians started dancing, while some were singing and others weeping. . . . Others, however, saw in a vision that they died and thus cried; others saw themselves being eaten by a wild beast; others imagined that they were capturing prisoners of war; others that they were rich or that they possessed many slaves; others that they committed adultery and had their heads crushed for this offense; others that they had stolen some articles for which they had to be killed. . . . When this mushroom intoxication had passed, the Indians talked over amongst themselves the visions they had seen."

Because of its psychoactive properties, peyote has earned a reputation as "strong medicine" among the Indians. It was these properties that often gave plants a sacred or magical reputation among Indians.

Yet many tribes revered plants for much more general reasons. For example, the Cherokees of the Appalachian Mountains saw plants as their allies. Long ago, according to a Cherokee myth, the Indians had gone through a period of very rapid population growth. To feed their increasing numbers, hunters killed so much game that the animals began to fear for their own survival. The bears, birds, deer, fishes, insects, and reptiles decided to strike back. They loosed upon their human tormentors a host of painful and fatal diseases; but the beasts had not counted upon the intervention of the plant kingdom:

"When the plants, who were friendly to man, heard what had been done by the animals, they determined to defeat the latter's evil designs. Each tree, shrub, and herb, down even to the grasses and mosses, agreed to furnish a cure for some one of the diseases named, and each said: 'I shall appear to help man. . . .' Thus came medicine; and the plants, every one of which has its use if we only knew it, furnish the remedy to counteract the evil wrought by revengeful animals. Even weeds were made for some good purpose. . . . When the doctor does not know what medicine to use for a sick man the spirit of the plant tells him."

Voodoo and "Rootwork"

In the ships that brought them across the Atlantic, Africans kidnapped into slavery were forced to lie so close together that they could hardly breathe. They owned nothing, not even themselves, nor did their new masters allow them any room for baggage. Yet these Africans contrived to bring treasures with them: music, dance, crafts, and folklore.

They brought their magic, too. Out of their midst came the various cults that would inspire voodoo and obeah in the New World. The Afro-American magicians, or "doctors" as they came to be called, were experts at "rootwork"—performing magic with roots and other plant parts. Culling herbs from the southern countryside, they hoodooed their enemies; rescued family, friends, and clients from rival witches; and conjured away all manner of ills.

As recently as the middle of the 20th century one researcher, Harry M. Hyatt, found this tradition still flourishing in the rural South, and it extended to the northern black ghettos as well. The occult doctors believed implicitly in their "shields," as they called their favorite roots and cuttings. In their pockets these doctors carried bottles full of those herbs, each with different powers. A tea made from Sampson's snakeroot would "kill" any poison. Mixed with the milk of a black cow, green gourd seed freed one witch doctor's client, an old woman, from the clutches of another doctor who had been "riding" her. And an old man, conjured almost to death by his landlord, was healed by washing his feet in a bath of running brier and pokeweed root.

Mountain Magic

Rich lore also lay in the Ozark and Appalachian mountains. A natural refuge for rebels and individualists, this rugged terrain was home to groups with diverse backgrounds and ethnic origins. Each of these groups brought a different tradition, which mixed with the others to produce the region's complex plant lore. Buckeyes—the large nutlike seeds of horse chestnuts—were prized by both Indians and whites. A buckeye in his pocket, the white hillman believed, warded off rheumatism and hemorrhoids, while to lose this talisman brought bad luck. Respect for the horse chestnut and its buckeyes was apparently passed on to the white settlers from the Osage Indians, who made a fish poison from the tree's root. Devil's-shoestring, a conjure root of black doctors, was used by the Cherokees to make a shampoo. They believed it would make their hair as thick and tough as the plant itself.

Another plant the Cherokees held in high esteem was the cedar. Its wood was sacred, said to be stained with the blood of a wicked magician. Too special for an ordinary campfire, the wood of this "medicine tree" was burned only on ceremonial occasions when, the Cherokees believed, its smoke would drive off ghosts and evil spirits.

One tradition that white settlers brought from Europe was the belief that the moon's phases told the best times to plant different crops. This belief was still strong in the Ozarks as recently as the 1930's. So strong, it caused one farmer to remove his son from the village high school. Upon hearing that the local farm agent advised planting potatoes on March 17, regardless of the moon's phase, the outraged father stormed: "If education doesn't learn a man better than that, I don't want it in my family!" That may sound like ignorant stubbornness, but planting by the moon's phases, rather than by an arbitrary calendar date, had served farmers fairly well for many millennia.

Such practices, however, have not held up well against the pressure—and often outright ridicule—of increasing numbers of farm agents, agricultural experts, and others armed with statistics and technical data. Education and increasing contact with the outside world are rapidly eroding most of the old ways and beliefs, even in the most remote mountain hollows. Yet as faith in the traditional lore wanes, recognition of its importance grows. Aged mountaineers, who not so long ago were derided for their "superstitious ignorance," are now being sought out, as anthropologists, psychologists, and historians begin to recognize that one key to our past and to human imagination lies in traditional customs and beliefs. Plant magic may not produce miracles, but it can help point modern man in the direction of something equally valuable and saving: self-knowledge.

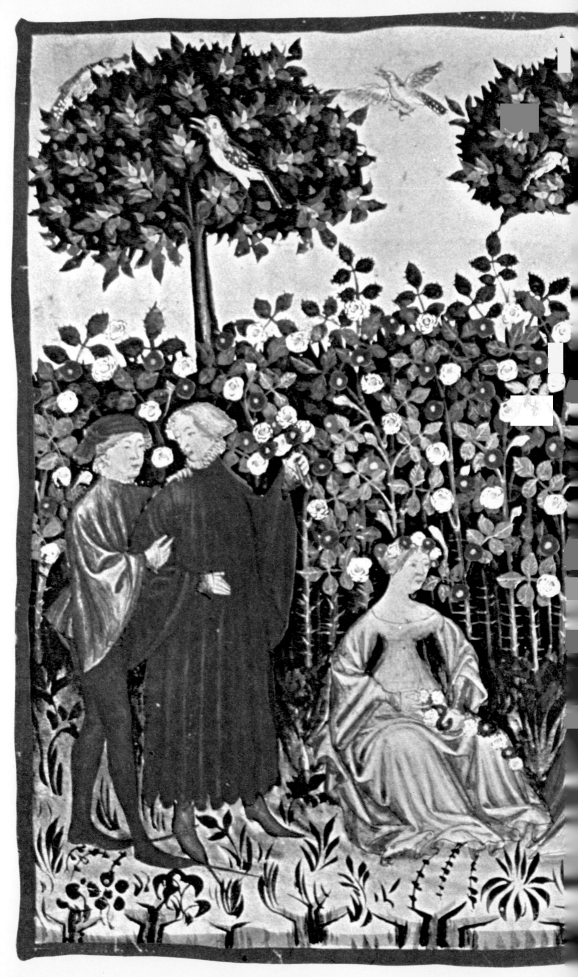

24

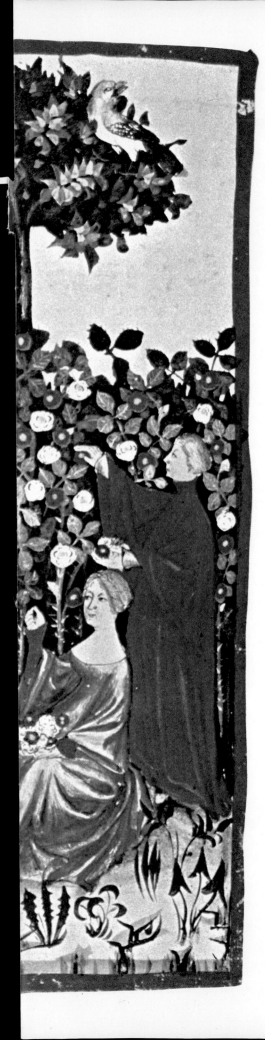

ABC's of Plants

For those intrigued by healing herbs—and the magic and myth associated with them—another rich experience beckons. To know herbs is to gain an intimate knowledge of the flora in one's area, and to become a student of the fascinating science of botany. In this chapter you will find the pointers needed to become not just an armchair expert on herbs but a scientific herbalist in the field.

Finding Plants in the Wild

Plants are both prisoners and shapers of their environment. The key to finding a particular species is to know the environmental conditions—the habitat—most favorable to the plant. For readers of this book, the search is made easier by the brief habitat descriptions accompanying each of the hundreds of featured plants. Here are just a few general considerations to keep in mind.

Each kind of plant can prosper only in the places where its particular growing needs are met. Soil can be soggy or well drained, for example, composed of hard-packed clay or coarse sand. It can be acid or alkaline, or it can be rich or poor in the mineral nutrients most needed for a certain species' well-being. The area, moreover, can be sunny or shady, amply watered or dry, always temperate or subject to harsh climatic extremes. The particular combination of such factors in any given place determines the kinds of plants that are able to survive there.

For all that, plants are supremely adaptable. Few places on earth are completely devoid of vegetation. Over the course of time, different species have evolved and developed means of colonizing even the most unlikely habitats. Some desert plants have many-branched root systems that reach far down for water through packed, parched layers of soil and subsoil. Others, such as cacti, store water in their stems and draw on this reserve to survive dry spells.

Above the timberline on high mountains, many species grow in dense, ground-hugging cushions that protect individual plants from high winds and sub-zero temperatures. Other alpine plants survive almost year-round snow cover and the brief summer growing season by maturing quickly and producing seeds within just a few weeks. Some of these seeds begin to sprout while still covered with snow.

Narrowing the Search

Though plants can be found almost anywhere, finding any particular one takes a little knowledge and some common sense. It would almost surely be a waste of time, for instance, to look for marsh marigolds on a dry hillside. As their name suggests, these plants are most likely to inhabit swamp edges and soggy streambanks. True water lovers, they often grow with their stems partly submerged.

Blue flag and cankerroot are other examples of plants that thrive in marshes and similar damp places. In contrast, the growing needs of yarrow, mullein, and Queen Anne's lace are best met in open, sunny places—fields, pastures, roadsides—and it is there that one should look for them.

It would be unrealistic, too, to expect to find marsh marigolds fringing every marshland; or to expect to find mullein on every sunny roadside. Be sure to check a species' natural range, consulting the brief notes for each plant described in this book. If a plant's range is limited to the southeastern United States, there is not much point in looking for it in the Rocky Mountains. And don't forget that the

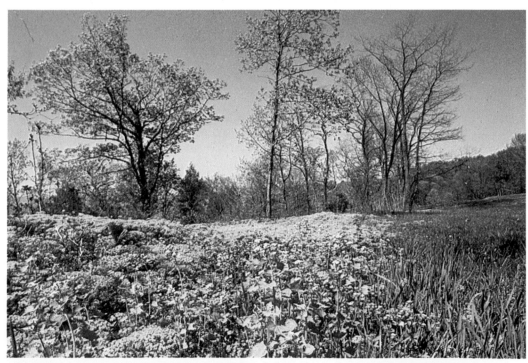

If the place is a well-drained northeastern meadow and the season is spring, look for rocket and mustard.

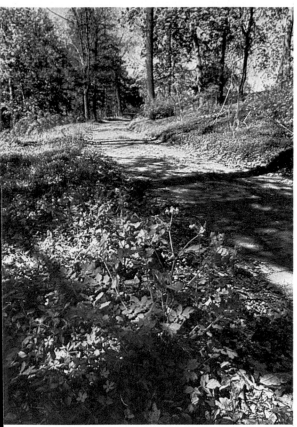

Celandine and periwinkle have established themselves on roadsides but not in deeper woods.

appearance of a plant can change dramatically from season to season: many beginning naturalists have failed to identify a plant with which they are really well acquainted because they know the characteristics identifying it at only one time of the year.

Whatever and wherever the species, it is a good rule of thumb to collect medicinal plants where they are reasonably abundant and growing vigorously. Note, however, that growth lush to the point of overcrowding can alter the properties and strength of medicinal compounds. Furthermore, the same species' medicinal strength can vary from region to region and sometimes from one site to another within the same region. Other factors that can affect medicinal strength are the season and a plant's stage in its growth cycle. That is one reason why pharmacologists and other authorities on herbal medicine warn against gathering and using herbs for self-medication.

Baffling Identities

Sometimes even a botanist may be baffled by a plant that seems to be a member of a certain species, but has some characteristics that are not typical. Or a collector may identify a certain plant in a region where authoritative sources say it has never grown before.

It happens for a number of reasons. First, no two individual plants look exactly alike. They can vary in height, leaf shape and size, flower color, or any of a number of other characteristics. This phenomenon, called biological variation, is the result of differences in the genetic makeup of individuals. In some cases the differences are caused by hybridization between closely related species. As for plants in the "wrong" place, similar environments may be hundreds or even thousands of miles apart, but if a plant from one somehow manages to reach the other—naturally or through human intervention—it has a good chance of taking hold in the new area. As one botanist remarked, some plants "have never read the book" defining what their habitat and range should be. Finally, if a new habitat has certain conditions that are different from those in the plant's former habitat, then these new conditions may cause differences in the size, color, shape, rate of growth, and other characteristics used to identify the species.

Natives, Escapes, Aliens

Plants that originated in a given place and have long grown there are called **native,** or **indigenous,** to that area. A plant that starts out under cultivation but subsequently grows wild on its own without human attention is called an **escape.** If a plant is introduced from a distant geographical area (say, from another continent) and takes hold, it is called an **alien** where it is introduced. If aliens take hold in great numbers and become part of the native flora, they are said to have become **naturalized.**

Probably the greatest invasion of alien plants in historical times occurred with the European settlement of North America. Europeans brought hundreds of species from their homelands and introduced them to the New World. On a somewhat smaller scale, the settlers who populated the American West introduced species from both Europe and eastern North America. Some species were carried intentionally because they were favorites of settlers; others went along by accident, as seeds stuck in the fur of animals, for example, or clinging to packing materials. Many of these plants found new environments that were favorable, and they became naturalized and are now considered wild plants of the particular region.

Even today, this process of escape and assimilation continues. Cultivated flower species escape from gardens, colonize a local area, and grow just like wildflowers, without human help. It may take a very experienced botanist to tell the difference between a garden plant and an escape, a native and an alien. However, as a general rule, most of the plants growing in established woods, pastures, and meadows are natives. They occupy their own self-contained niches, where aliens find it difficult to enter and compete successfully. Naturalized aliens are more commonly found in recently disturbed soil, such as that along highways and close to human habitation.

Making Your Own Herbarium

To become knowledgeable about plants, there is no surer, more satisfying course than to create one's own herbarium. The term today means what the 18th-century Swedish naturalist Carolus Linnaeus called an *herbarium vivum:* a collection of plants or plant parts that are picked in the wild or garden, pressed and dried, and then mounted for permanent display and reference.

An Education in Itself

The activities involved in creating an herbarium—searching for, identifying, collecting, pressing, and drying plants—are really a hands-on education in the diversity of forms and structures of plants and how species differ. Beginning with just a few species, a student of plants can expand the herbarium to an ever larger collection. Each new positively identified species becomes a permanent reference against which to compare specimens gathered on future field expeditions. An herbarium thus is more than an attractive display. It can be a working research tool, showing the differences between species as well as the often confusing differences that may occur among individual members of the same species.

Two parts of this book are especially helpful in getting started on an herbarium. The simple diagrams on pages 32–41 help train the eye to find distinguishing features of plants in general, while the book's central gallery (pages 74–

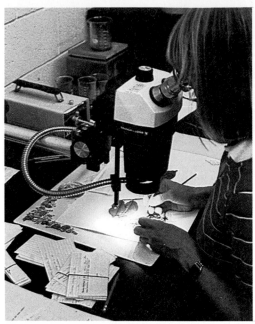

Dried specimens yield secrets to a botanist at the New York Botanical Garden.

354) describes close to 300 individual medicinal plants and where to look for them. Be sure to read very carefully all information on poisonous plants, heeding warnings about the handling and use of species that may be toxic in one way or another.

Heed, too, the pleas of conservationists to treat gently both individual living plants and the environments they inhabit. Removing or causing the destruction of any plant (in some cases even any part of any plant) is prohibited in most parks and nature reserves, whether public or private. On public property, check with the responsible authority for rules if they are not posted; on private property, don't collect anything without getting the owner's permission. Threatened or endangered species should never be molested: a list and description of an area's protected species can usually be obtained from state or local conservation officials, garden clubs, nature groups, and the like. Finally, even if a species appears in weedlike abundance on unrestricted property, collect sparingly to avoid long-term damage to the habitat.

Collecting

No fancy, expensive equipment is needed to collect plants for an herbarium. To cut off shoots or branches, use a pocket knife with a strong, sharp blade—or a pair of sturdy handheld pruning clippers. Take a garden trowel for digging up roots or underground stems. Carry along some plastic bags (for toting specimens home) and a notebook and pencil. That

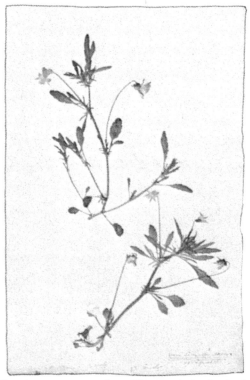

Pansies grace a page from Linnaeus' own herbarium at Sweden's Museum of Natural History.

is all you need for essential gear. The cautious collector will also wear gloves to guard against skin scratches or contact with toxic plants such as poison ivy.

How much of a plant to cut or dig for later mounting in an herbarium? It depends mainly on the size of the plant press and of the mounting sheets the collector plans to use. Here again, a local garden club, botanical society, or nature group can give valuable tips. Smaller plant presses—typically 6 or 8 inches square—are often sold ready-made through gardening and craft shops and mail-order houses. Some collectors carry along small presses like these on field trips, to begin pressing immediately after specimens are cleaned and wiped dry. Such presses are fine for most individual leaves and flowers.

University and museum botanists prefer somewhat larger herbarium sheets—11½ by 16½ or 12 by 18 inches—which allow more room for the display of plants and their parts. Ideally, an herbarium sheet would exhibit, intact, every significant part of a collected specimen: root, stems, leaves (tops and undersides) on stalks, buds, flowers, fruits. To preserve such specimens, botanists use various pressing and drying methods, including some large and elegant plant presses. But at little or no cost (see page 30), anyone can assemble a serviceable plant press to do the same work.

A little extra effort on field trips will save time in the long run and also increase the herbarium's value as a research tool. For example, since some species are identified by the arrangement of their leaves, be sure to cut enough of a stem or branch to show how leaves grow on it. Because plants change from season to season, it makes sense to collect specimens in the same spot three or four times a year. Herbarium pressings of a plant's spring flowers, for example, nicely complement its fall fruits. For trees and woody shrubs, make a winter expedition to cut a few twigs that show the structure and arrangement of dormant, overwintering buds.

Accurate records are at the heart of scientific collections. Don't put off taking notes with the excuse that "later," when you have more time, will be better. Right at the gathering site, make notebook entries of the date, the place, the kind of habitat (woodland, grassland, etc.), specific growing conditions (shade or sun, moist or dry, neighboring species), and other observations such as the plant's abundance in the area and the apparent effect (if any) of human activity on its environment. Other information about the plant itself that may be lost when the specimen is dried and mounted (height, smell, color) should be noted to help in positive identification. Both the bark and the overall shape of trees are important identification clues; these can be described in words or by rough sketches in the notebook.

Keep the notes with the specimen right up until mounting. The notes are the raw data for the label that will describe the mounted herbarium specimen. Botanists give consecutive numbers to all the plants they collect; a plant's number corresponds to the number heading of field notes kept in a book.

Once gathered, specimens should be carefully handled to prevent breaking, cracking, drying, and wrinkling. Keeping specimens fresh in their plastic bags is preferable to exposing them to the drying effect of air; but this buys only a little time. The faster a collector can begin pressing, the better the finished herbarium specimens are likely to look. Some botanists advise refrigerating or freezing specimens to kill any insect pests; but get expert advice before doing this because exposure to cold can ruin a specimen.

Making and Using a Plant Press

No matter how large or elaborate, all plant presses have two simple features in common. One is a material for absorbing moisture. The other is a source of pressure. For instance, you can use newspapers for absorbing moisture and heavy books for pressure.

Making a basic plant press is hardly more

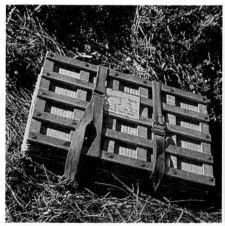
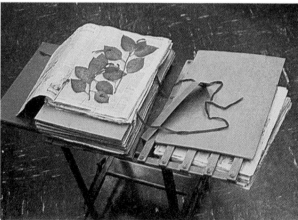

Portable plant presses come in many shapes and sizes. This one, which handles the larger specimens preferred by botanists, is shown in the field (left) and opened on return from a collecting trip.

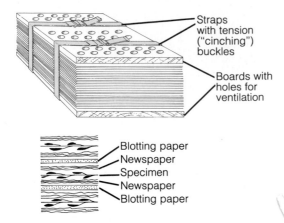

Blotting paper
Newspaper
Specimen
Newspaper
Blotting paper

Straps exert pressure and papers absorb moisture in this version of a basic plant press.

complicated. Put aside a stack of old newspapers. (Although not absolutely necessary, sheets of ordinary blotting paper may be used together with the newspapers.) Then obtain two pieces of plywood about 11 by 14 inches—roughly the size of the standard tabloid newspaper page or of the larger newspaper page folded in half horizontally. Some collectors prefer the plywood to have holes, so that it gives the press more ventilation. For applying pressure, two straps with tension buckles will serve nicely, as will two old belts, or even two pieces of strong twine.

Lay one plywood board over the straps, and put four or five newspaper sheets (folded to approximately 11 by 14 inches) on top of the board. Now arrange one or more plant specimens—how many depends on their size and shape—on the topmost sheet.

The position and arrangement of specimens at this point should be considered permanent, since as a specimen dries, it becomes brittler and harder to rearrange without breaking. Most collectors opt for as natural a look as possible—that is, one most like the living, undisturbed plant. Longer stems can be bent in zigzags, curled, or cut into sections. Some leaves should be laid topside up, others underside up, since both sides may be needed for positive identification. Thick parts, such as stems, should be sliced into sections to speed drying and avoid unmanageable lumps in the press. And be sure to tuck the field notes right in with the drying specimen: don't *ever* risk misplacing those valuable observations. For protection against excess moisture and stains, the notes can be placed in a moisture-resistant transparent envelope or in a clear plastic bag of the kind used to wrap food leftovers. (Many botanists also place an *empty* transparent envelope with the specimen. This provides a handy place to put any pieces of the specimen that may fall off as a result of drying and handling.)

On top of the first specimen, add four or five more layers of newspaper, then the next specimen or specimens. Continue adding layers of newspaper and specimens until the stack is perhaps 6 inches high—a little more or less will not matter. It is a good idea to put extra layers of paper around the thicker specimens, both to make them dry faster and to keep them from poking through and damaging more delicate specimens in the press. Some collectors feel they get best results by inserting blotting paper between every two or three newspaper sheets. Sheets of corrugated cardboard at intervals will allow air to circulate through the stack and speed drying. Finally, put the second plywood board on top of the stack and secure the straps snugly around the whole press.

Store the press in a dry, warm, well-ventilated place. If a specimen was extra thick or juicy, check the newspapers around it every day or so and replace them, if they are quite damp, with dry ones. After a week or two in the press, almost all specimens should be dry enough for mounting, and even the juiciest plant parts should be ready in no more than a month.

Provided a specimen is not damaged by too much heat or removed before drying is complete, the quicker the drying, the better. Specimens can get moldy and deteriorate if the drying process is prolonged by poor ventilation, for example, that does not waft enough moisture out of the press. Fleshy specimens are particularly vulnerable. Leaving plants that are being pressed in the sun—or in an artificially heated place—can speed up drying. A fan also helps keep the air circulating.

Mounting

Before preparing final herbarium sheets, the collector may wish to call a local botanical garden, university, botany department, or botanical society, and talk with an expert about dos and don'ts. Although a beginner would surely benefit from such contact with professional standards, no special body of knowledge is required to create an attractive and useful herbarium. Other than dried plant specimens, the necessary materials are available at most stationery or school-supply stores.

Neatly glue or tape each specimen to a sheet of heavy white paper or cardboard. Use a clear-drying paste or glue or transparent tape.

When arranging specimens on the herbarium sheet, remember to leave room for the label, which most collectors stick at the lower right-hand corner. It should give scientific name (genus and species in Latin), common name or names, date and place of collection, and any other significant information from the field notes. The specific circumstances of when, where, how the plant was collected are very important. A specialist will be able to identify the specimen many years later, but only the collector can relate its "personal history"—a good reason for the collector to sign the label proudly with his or her name.

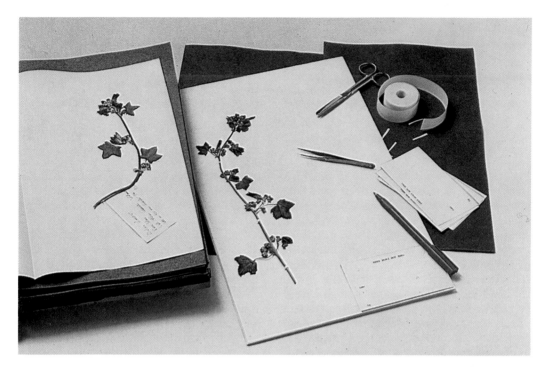

Mallow (right) enters an herbarium with the help of scissors, tape, tweezers, labels (above).

Clear plastic wrap can be used to protect mounted specimens. Store them in any convenient manner—for example, laid flat in drawers—so long as they are protected against crushing and bending. And some system of arranging is a must, whether by scientific classification, by environment or habitat, or by another logical scheme, such as alphabetical order. It will make the collection easily accessible—and all the more enjoyable.

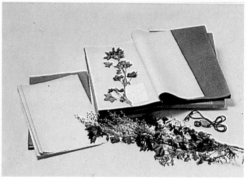

How About Photography?

Photographs can effectively complement—but not replace—the herbarium as a research and reference tool. They are especially useful for documenting the living plant—its colors, its environment, its seasonal transformations. Any good 35-mm single-lens reflex (SLR) camera will yield sharply detailed studies. An SLR lets you see the exact image you will get—a special concern when you are photographing a small subject at close range.

You may want to move in even closer than the camera normally permits. An inexpensive way to take closer views is with supplementary close-up lenses, which screw into an SLR's lens like filters. Photo stores sell sets of different magnifications in sizes to fit most lenses. And if you have a zoom lens, it may have a useful "macro" (close-up) mode.

When a subject is magnified in a close-up, any movement it or the camera makes is also magnified. A faint breeze that flutters a plant or an unsteady grip on the camera can result in a blurred image. Professionals mount their cameras on tripods and often stake a plant or rig a cardboard windbreak. An easier alternative is to use high-speed film, like one of the popular ISO 1000 films. The film's extra sensitivity lets you freeze motion with a fast shutter speed of $\frac{1}{500}$ second or $\frac{1}{1000}$ second. The gain in convenience that high-speed film brings more than offsets the very slight loss in image quality.

Nevertheless, to insure that your subject is sharp and well framed, work on calm days and hold your camera steady. The softer light of overcast days is ideal for photographing plants; bright sunlight is all right but will give harsher, more contrasty images.

Photography can never replace an *herbarium vivum*. Only specimens can convey a plant's texture and feel and, for many species, provide positive identification. This is especially true of closely related species, where examination under a microscope (sometimes even an electron microscope) may be necessary to determine a plant's identity. Yet the two techniques—photography and *herbarium vivum*—work together wonderfully. Seeing a page of skillfully mounted specimens, followed by a page of color pictures of the plant, would make Linnaeus himself turn green with envy.

31

The Anatomy of Plants

In the bewildering profusion of the plant world, certain patterns repeat themselves. These patterns—as set out in these 10 pages of diagrams—are a guide when you search woods and fields for plants—whether to use them or to admire them for their beauty.

Roots

Roots anchor a plant to the soil, from which they absorb water and dissolved mineral nutrients. The root then transports these substances from the point of absorption (root tip) to the stem. In many species, roots are food-storage organs. Some have medicinal or nutritional value; others are poisonous. Primary root systems develop from the seedling's embryonic root into either a dominant taproot or a cluster of fibrous roots. An adventitious root system develops from a plant part other than a root, such as a stem (see next section), that sends down roots to produce new plants. Adventitious systems usually have fibrous roots. Both primary and adventitious roots can have fleshy parts that are sources of food and medicine.

Primary Root Systems

1. A taproot is a dominant root with many smaller secondary roots and rootlets branching from it. The dividing line between the root and the stem (or shoot) is called the collar. At the root's other, or distal (underground), end is a root cap, shielding the new growth of the root tip from contact with the soil through which the root pushes. Behind the tip are ranks of

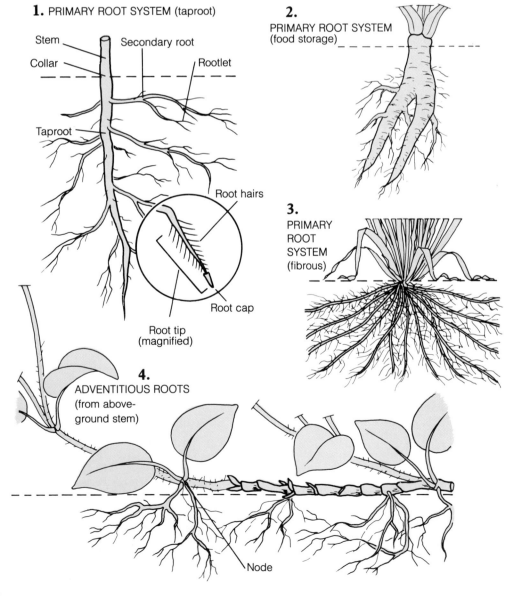

1. PRIMARY ROOT SYSTEM (taproot)

Stem
Secondary root
Collar
Rootlet
Taproot
Root hairs
Root cap
Root tip (magnified)

2. PRIMARY ROOT SYSTEM (food storage)

3. PRIMARY ROOT SYSTEM (fibrous)

4. ADVENTITIOUS ROOTS (from above-ground stem)

Node

threadlike root hairs. They "pump" in water for eventual use by the whole plant.

2. Some taproots that store food have long been important in the human diet. Examples are carrots, radishes, and parsnips.

3. Primary roots may also develop into a cluster of fibrous roots, all about the size of the seedling's primary root. Cereal grains and grasses are examples of plants with fibrous roots. The erosion-resistant sod beneath a healthy lawn or prairie is a tangle of fibrous roots, usually interlaced with the underground stems called rhizomes.

Adventitious Root Systems

4. Many herbs have ground-hugging stems that send down fibrous adventitious root clusters at intervals marked by nodes; new shoots grow from these clusters. Adventitious roots also grow on underground stems.

Stems

The stem supports the leaves that catch the sunlight needed for photosynthesis. Stem tissues conduct water, minerals, and organic nutrients throughout the plant. Aerial stems grow above ground, underground stems spread below ground; but the distinction between them is not always obvious. The same plant, and even the same stem, may have both aerial and subterranean stem parts. Moreover, in form and function, underground stems are easy to confuse with roots. Some rootlike food-storage organs, for example, are really stems. Herbal writers do not always make such distinctions, since these authorities are mostly concerned with indicating which part—in this case, the underground one—of a plant to use.

Aerial Stems

5. Branches and branchlets, spreading from an aerial stem, form a plant's distinctive aboveground shape, or crown, characteristic of the species. (A plant's entire aboveground portion is often called its shoot or shoot system.) Herbaceous plants, such as grasses and most annuals, have fleshy and short-lived aerial stems, in contrast to the trunks of trees, which are woody and perennial aerial stems.

6. Strawberries, wild thyme, and certain other plants produce aerial stems called stolons, or runners. They creep over the ground, then root (adventitiously) to produce a plant like the parent plant. This plant sends out a runner that roots and makes another clone, and so on.

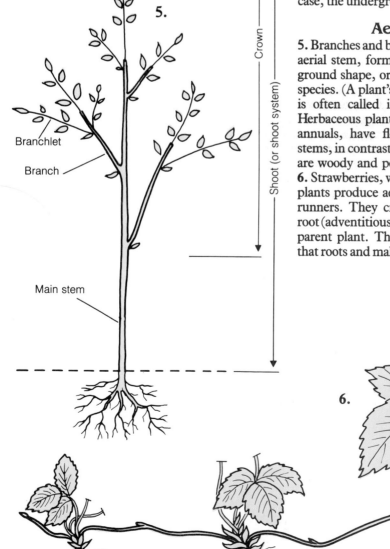

Underground Stems

7. Rhizomes, which are also known as rootstocks, are stems that burrow beneath the soil, producing at intervals both adventitious roots and aerial stems and leaves.

8. Thick and fleshy rhizomes—such as those of the iris—can be rich sources of potentially useful chemical compounds.

9. Common white potatoes are tubers—thickened ends of rhizomes.

10. The lily bulb, like all true bulbs, is an underground bud that stores food in fleshy bulb scales (modified leaves). They encase the base of the stem and may be individually prominent as in the lily, or form a smoother wrap as in the tulip. The gladiolus and crocus rely on an underground stem called a corm, which does not have the true bulb's nourishing scales but sends down an adventitious root as its growth season begins.

11. Onions are bulbs whose food-storage leaves (scales) form overlapping rings.

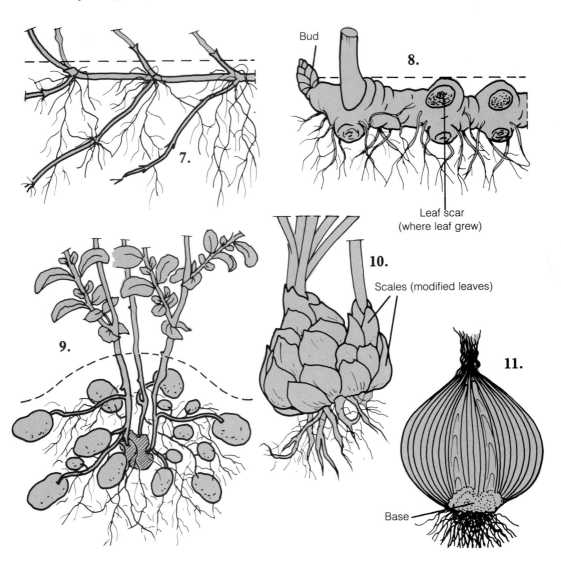

Bud

8.

Leaf scar
(where leaf grew)

10.

Scales (modified leaves)

9.

11.

Base

Leaves

Appendages of the stem, leaves are the main organs of photosynthesis, the process by which a leaf's green chlorophyll pigments absorb solar energy and use it to make organic molecules from carbon dioxide in the air and water in the soil. The simplest of these organic substances are carbohydrates and sugars such as glucose; but with mineral elements from the soil added, more complex organic compounds, such as amino acids and fatty acids, are manufactured. These organic compounds are the building blocks of all living matter. As by-products of this manufacturing process arise the medicinal compounds found in plants. Photosynthesis can be carried out by plant parts that are neither green nor leaves. Some nongreen pigments of algae have photosynthetic ability, as do the green stems of some plants. Nature's best adaptation for capturing the energy of sunlight, however, remains the green leaf in its myriad shapes and sizes, from pine needles to giant jungle fronds.

Leaf Structure and Attachment

12. Most leaves consist of a blade and a stalk, or petiole. A blade's waxy upper surface helps retard the evaporation of water. The petiole connects blade and stem; on its base may be found outgrowths called stipules, which protect the budding leaf. Axillary buds form in the angle (axil) between petiole and stem; terminal buds, at the growing end of a stem. A node is where a leaf is (or was) attached, and the interval between one node and another is called the internode. At the node, the leaf may form a sheath partly or wholly enclosing the connecting portion of the stem.

13. Sessile leaves have no petiole; the blade attaches directly to the stem.

14. The sessile leaves of the plants in the grass family form a sheath around the stem as they grow from the node.

Veins

15. Extensions of the leafstalk, veins serve as the leaf's supporting skeleton and its network for the inflow and outflow of water, minerals, dissolved gases, and organic compounds. The parallel veins of grass and lily leaves are one pattern of venation.

16. Another venation pattern—a single vein running the leaf's entire length—is found in pine needles. (Vein indicated by dotted line.)

17. A very common venation is pinnate, characterized by a dominant central vein (midrib) with smaller branching veins.

18. Maple leaves have palmate venation; that is, several veins of about the same size radiate from the petiole, or leafstalk.

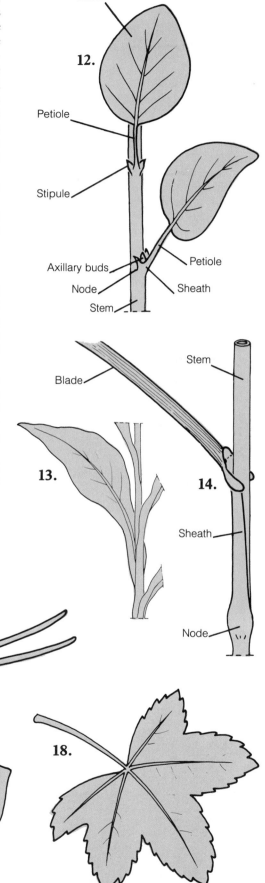

35

Simple and Compound Leaves

19. Simple leaves have a single blade. A simple entire leaf is one with a smooth edge (margin), like that of the lilac.

20. A simple toothed leaf, such as the chestnut leaf, has more or less regularly spaced little teeth on its margin.

21. Simple toothed leaves may also have teeth that form an irregular, wavy margin. Examples: great burdock, aspens, cottonwoods.

22. Simple lobed leaves have gaping indentations along their edges, as in oaks.

23. Compound leaves have a number of leaflets supported by one petiole. Leaflets of pinnately compound leaves grow on each side along an axis (rachis) extending from the petiole, as in walnuts and ashes. Each leaflet may have its own stalk, or petiolule.

24. On palmately compound leaves, such as those of horse chestnuts, leaflets emerge from a single point at the top of the petiole.

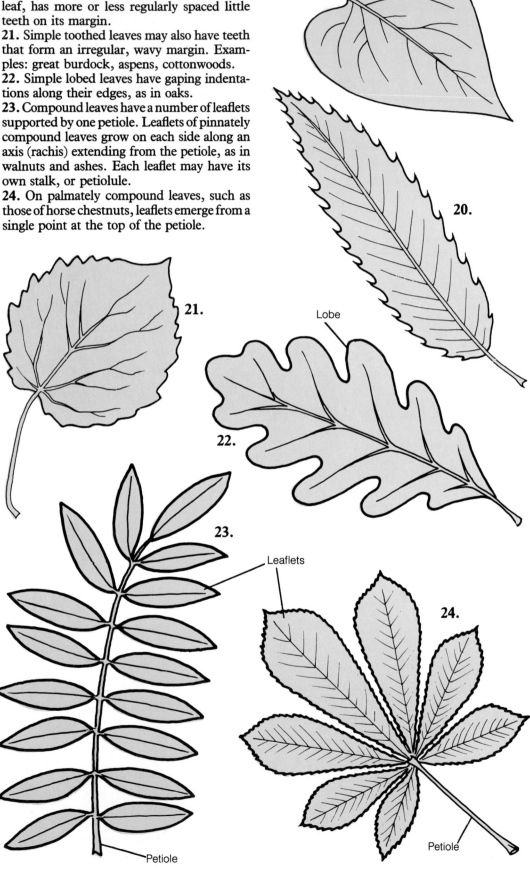

19.

20.

21.

Lobe

22.

23.

Leaflets

24.

Petiole

Petiole

Leaf Arrangements

25. Opposite leaves grow in pairs at the stem node; the two leaves are opposite one another on different sides of the stem.

26. Alternate leaves grow singly at intervals along the stem, usually from defined points located in a spiral along the stem.

27. Whorled leaves grow in groups of three or more from the same node.

28. On some plants, such as the foxglove, leaves form a rosette (radiating cluster) at the base of the stem.

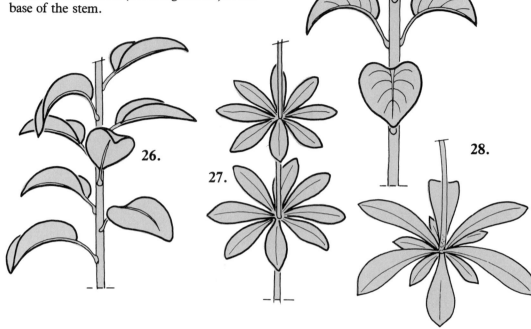

Flowers

The flower is an organ for sexual reproduction. What botanists call a perfect flower contains its own bisexual reproductive system: it has both male (stamens) and female (pistils) sex organs. Imperfect (unisexual) flowers, such as those of willows and corn, have one or the other kind of sex organs, not both.

Flower Parts and Structure

29. A flower is called complete when it has sepals, which are usually green and collectively form the calyx; petals, which usually give the species its characteristic flower color and collectively form the corolla; a set of stamens, or pollen-producing male organs; and one or more pistils (also called carpels, a term some authorities prefer), the pollen-receiving, seed-producing female organs. Almost invariably the arrangement of these floral parts follows the same order, from the outside to the inside: sepals, petals, stamens, pistil. The technical term for flowers that lack any of these parts is "incomplete."

A stamen consists of a filament (stalk) and an anther, where pollen grains are produced. The pistil (with either one carpel or several

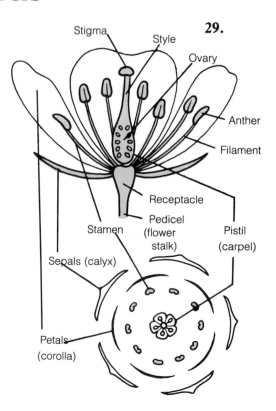

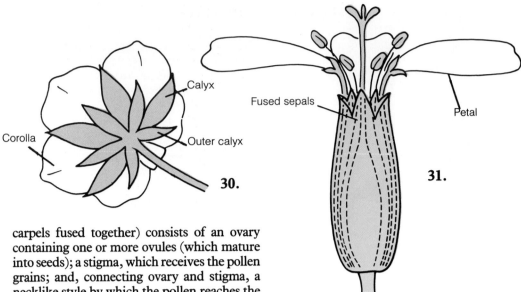

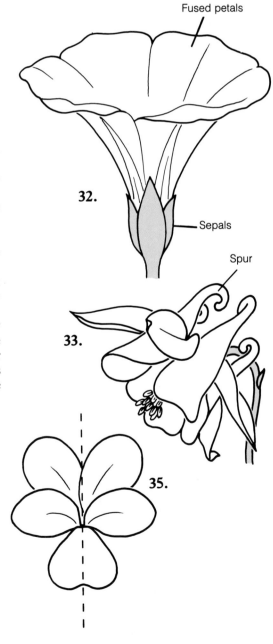

carpels fused together) consists of an ovary containing one or more ovules (which mature into seeds); a stigma, which receives the pollen grains; and, connecting ovary and stigma, a necklike style by which the pollen reaches the ovary. Calyx (sepals) and corolla (petals) together are called the perianth. The flower's stalk is the pedicel, whose tip forms the receptacle, a platform to which the floral parts are attached. A flower lacking a pedicel is called sessile.

Some Common Variations

30. Seen from where the pedicel meets the floral parts, the perianth's calyx and corolla are most clearly visible. Some species have an outer calyx (epicalyx), as shown.

31. The sepals of bouncing Bet fuse into a tube around the inner parts of the flower.

32. In morning glories, it is the petals that fuse to form a funnel-shaped structure.

33. Columbine petals form projecting spurs. Insects probe for nectar in the spurs, pollinating the plant.

34. Regular flowers have radial symmetry: their parts are arranged evenly around a center, giving many planes of symmetry.

35. Irregular flowers such as violets display bilateral symmetry: they have only one plane of symmetry. Their two halves form mirror images of each other only if the flower is divided along one specific axis (the dotted line in the diagram).

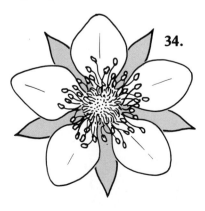

Flower Clusters

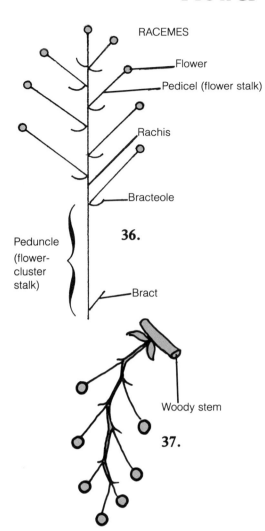

RACEMES

Flower

Pedicel (flower stalk)

Rachis

Bracteole

Peduncle (flower-cluster stalk)

36.

Bract

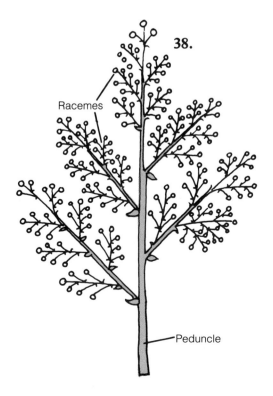

Woody stem

37.

38.

Racemes

Peduncle

Many species, such as poppies and tulips, bear their flowers singly, one flower on a stalk. On other plants, flowers occur in a cluster, or inflorescence, borne at the end of a peduncle (stalk of a flower cluster). The names of such clusters differ, depending on the arrangement of their individual flowers. In a flower cluster, each flower is supported by a small leaflike structure called a bracteole; the structure that supports the whole cluster is called a bract.

Racemes

36. The kind of inflorescence called a raceme has a main stalk (rachis) on a peduncle; the rachis supports many flower-bearing pedicels, all of about equal length.

37. The raceme of the currant or of the wild gooseberry droops in a flowery cluster from the plant's woody stem.

38. A compound, many-branched raceme—racemes on racemes—is called a panicle. The lilac's blossoms form a pyramidal panicle.

Spikes

39. A spike is an elongated inflorescence whose flowers are sessile (lacking individual pedicels and supported only by bracteoles), being attached directly to the main stalk as in gladiolus. A simple spike has only one flower at each point of attachment.

40. A compound spike has more than one flower at each point of attachment.

41. A catkin is a long spike, usually drooping and densely covered with flowers of one sex.

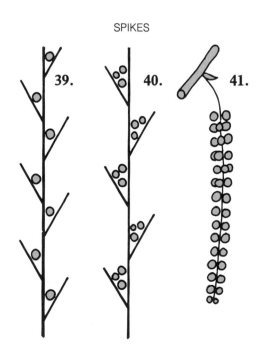

SPIKES

39. **40.** **41.**

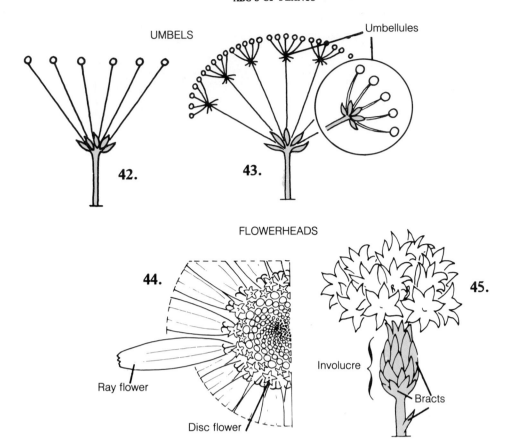

UMBELS

Umbellules

42.

43.

FLOWERHEADS

44.

45.

Ray flower

Disc flower

Involucre

Bracts

Umbels

42. In an umbel, many individual flower stalks (pedicels) arise from the same point at the tip of a stem or peduncle.

43. A compound umbel is a flower cluster of many smaller umbels (umbellules), as in Queen Anne's lace, or wild carrot. The scientific name of the carrot family is Umbelliferae, meaning "umbel-bearing."

Flowerheads

44. Dense, compact clusters of flowers at the tip of a peduncle are called flowerheads. Characteristic of the composite, or sunflower, fam-

ily, they resemble a single flower but really are many individual flowers. The white "petals" of daisies, for example, are flattened ray, or marginal, flowers ringing the margin of the head. The central "button" is a dense mass of individual yellow disc flowers. A flowerhead is enclosed by many flower-leaves, or bracts. The collective term for these encircling bracts is involucre.

45. Cornflowers, or bachelor's-buttons, are flowerheads that lack ray flowers. But the base of the flowerhead—like that of all members of the composite family—is surrounded by an involucre, or ring of overlapping bracts.

Fruits

A fruit is the mature product of a fertilized ovary or ovaries. The ovules within the ovary have matured into seeds, which are ready to germinate and give rise to other plants of the same species.

Fleshy Fruits

46. In the type of fleshy fruit known as a drupe, or stone fruit, one single seed is protected within a hard-walled stone, itself embedded in a juicy pulp surrounded by a somewhat tougher outer skin. Olives are typical.

47. Cherries too are drupes. Their mature ovary wall develops into a structure called a pericarp, which has three distinct layers: the epicarp (also called exocarp), or outer skin; the

mesocarp, or juicy flesh; and the stony endocarp enclosing the seed.

48. Peaches are drupes with an exceptionally thick, hard endocarp.

49. Apples are examples of the fleshy fruits called pomes. Their mature ovary wall is less distinct than that of drupes and forms only the inner core, a papery layer around the seeds (matured ovules). The apple's edible flesh develops from the floral cup that surrounded the ovary.

50. Berries—which include grapes and tomatoes but not strawberries (see page 41)— are fleshy fruits with many seeds embedded right in the juicy pulp, which is a pericarp that lacks the distinct layers found in drupes.

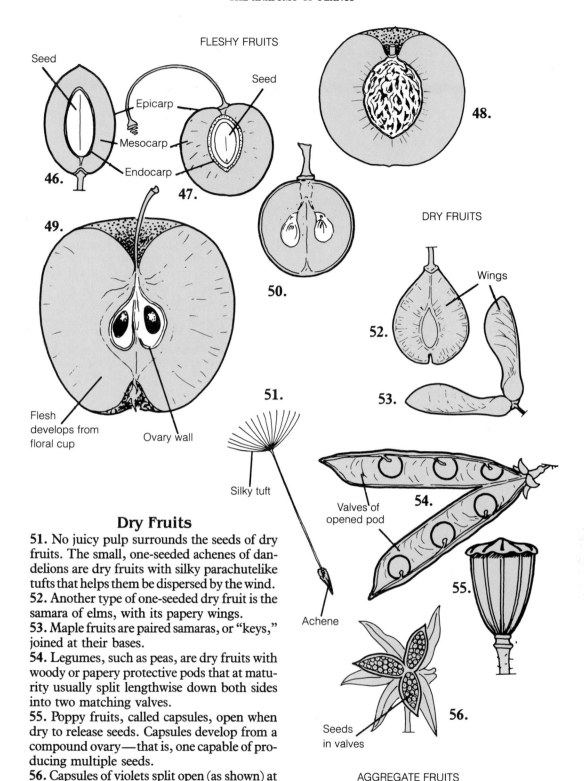

FLESHY FRUITS

Seed

Seed

Epicarp

Mesocarp

Endocarp

46.

47.

48.

49.

50.

51.

DRY FRUITS

Wings

52.

53.

Silky tuft

Flesh develops from floral cup

Ovary wall

Valves of opened pod

54.

55.

Achene

Seeds in valves

56.

Dry Fruits

51. No juicy pulp surrounds the seeds of dry fruits. The small, one-seeded achenes of dandelions are dry fruits with silky parachutelike tufts that helps them be dispersed by the wind.
52. Another type of one-seeded dry fruit is the samara of elms, with its papery wings.
53. Maple fruits are paired samaras, or "keys," joined at their bases.
54. Legumes, such as peas, are dry fruits with woody or papery protective pods that at maturity usually split lengthwise down both sides into two matching valves.
55. Poppy fruits, called capsules, open when dry to release seeds. Capsules develop from a compound ovary—that is, one capable of producing multiple seeds.
56. Capsules of violets split open (as shown) at maturity to release seeds.

Aggregate Fruits

57. Aggregate fruits form from a single flower that has many separate pistils. Each tiny spherical segment of a raspberry, for example, is a drupelet (tiny drupe) that has developed from its own ovary.
58. The fleshy part of a strawberry develops from the receptacle, the tip of the stalk where the flower was attached. Each "seed" is an achene from a separate ovary.

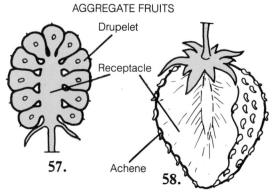

AGGREGATE FRUITS

Drupelet

Receptacle

57.

Achene

58.

Nature's Chemical Industry

The manufacture by plants of medicinal substances is just one part of the grand scheme of life's intricate chemistry. Within plant cells a great many interconnected chemical reactions proceed silently and persistently. The most important reaction is photosynthesis, carried on mainly by the green leaves of plants. This process is fundamental to life on earth, for it provides both our world's food and the oxygen we need to breathe.

The Magic of Photosynthesis

In a typical photosynthetic reaction, carbon dioxide from the air combines with water from the soil to make simple carbohydrates (compounds of carbon and hydrogen), precursors of sugars such as glucose, fructose, and sucrose. A by-product of the reaction is oxygen. Described another way, photosynthesis begins the transformation that turns inorganic (non-living) molecules into organic molecules, the molecules associated with life. In the bargain, life-supporting oxygen is produced.

Photosynthesis slows or shuts down in the dark. It needs power to drive it, and the power comes from the almost inexhaustible radiant energy of the sun. As any indoor gardener knows, artificial light also powers photosynthesis, but such light always derives from the sun. An electric light bulb, for example, recycles solar energy from one of its many earthbound forms, such as fossil fuels.

Plants can accomplish photosynthesis because they have certain substances—catalysts—that initiate and guide the process. By far the most significant of these is the green pigment chlorophyll, which gives plants their green color. But photosynthesis works with certain nongreen catalysts, too, such as the pigment phycobilin in red algae. (The green chlorophyll in the leaves of some species —copper beeches, for example—is masked by nongreen pigments such as carotene and xanthophyll, which help capture the light and forward it to chlorophyll pigments.)

The primary organic products of photosynthesis—simple carbohydrates or sugars— are soon worked upon by a battery of plant enzymes. These enzymes are special proteins, which activate processes that make the simple carbohydrate molecules grow in size and complexity. At the same time, new chemical elements (such as nitrogen) arrive through the root from the soil and are introduced into the carbohydrate structures.

Inexorably, as enzymes operate in the miniature chemical laboratories of living plant cells, an almost infinite variety of different organic compounds are produced. Some of these compounds are transported down the stem into areas such as fleshy roots or tubers, there to be stored as a complex carbohydrate such as starch. Some simple carbohydrates are transformed into cellulose and lignin, which form the tough walls of plant cells and give the whole plant its supporting skeleton.

Carbohydrates combine with nitrates (compounds of nitrogen, hydrogen, and oxygen) and other chemical elements (phosphorus, potassium, sodium, calcium, iron, for example) to form more complex organic compounds. Profoundly important are the amino acids, the building blocks of all life's proteins. Still other carbohydrate molecules are rebuilt and recombined to form fatty acids, the building blocks of the fats and oils found in plants.

Medicinal Compounds

With their stocks of amino and fatty acids, living plant cells are abundantly equipped with the raw materials for building thousands of compounds that have medicinal properties. One broad class of such compounds is the **glycosides.** Some of these, such as the compounds of prussic (hydrocyanic) acid found in the leaves of wild cherry trees, have a bitter-almond flavor and have been used in cough remedies and patent medicine tonics. (But these same prussic acid compounds can also poison and kill livestock that eat quantities of wilted black cherry leaves.) Another glycoside is digitoxin, a powerful heart medicine produced by foxgloves. A third example of a medicinal glycoside is salicin, found in the bark of certain willows. It was salicin that gave chemists the idea of synthesizing aspirin.

Alkaloids are another important group of medicinally active compounds produced by plants. In general, the alkaloids may be therapeutic in small doses and in special formulations but can poison—or kill—otherwise. Among the better-known medicinal alkaloids are quinine, codeine, morphine, nicotine, caffeine, and strychnine.

Plants also manufacture myriads of **essential oils.** These impart characteristic odors to a plant's leaves, fruits, and flowers. Slight variations in the chemical makeup of essential oils create a whole olfactory universe: from the pungent aroma of pine needles, to the sweet scents of clover and roses, to the bracing fragrances of the mints and citrus fruits. Not surprisingly, in addition to a great many medicinal applications, essential oils are used in making perfumes.

Tannins, yet another natural product of plants, give brown, red, or yellow hues to wood and are used in dyes and for tanning, the process of preparing leather from animal hides. Medicinally, tannins are valued for their

(continued on page 44)

The Plant as a Factory

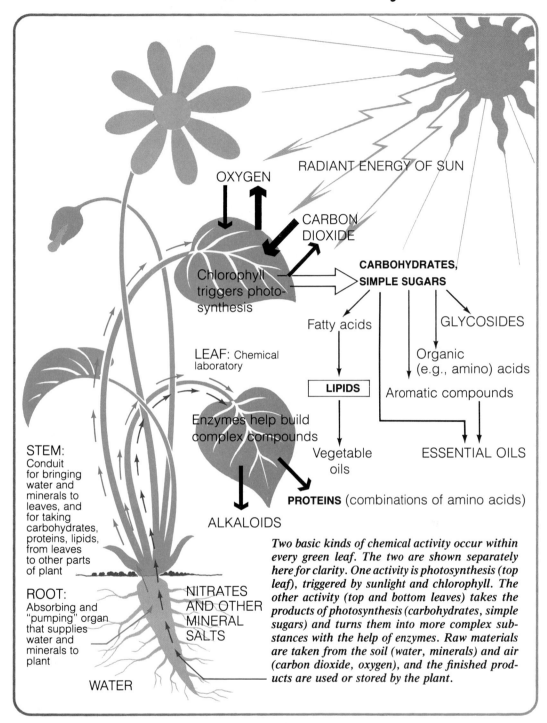

RADIANT ENERGY OF SUN

OXYGEN

CARBON DIOXIDE

Chlorophyll triggers photo-synthesis

CARBOHYDRATES, SIMPLE SUGARS

LEAF: Chemical laboratory

Fatty acids

GLYCOSIDES

Organic (e.g., amino) acids

LIPIDS

Aromatic compounds

Enzymes help build complex compounds

Vegetable oils

ESSENTIAL OILS

STEM: Conduit for bringing water and minerals to leaves, and for taking carbohydrates, proteins, lipids, from leaves to other parts of plant

ALKALOIDS

PROTEINS (combinations of amino acids)

ROOT: Absorbing and "pumping" organ that supplies water and minerals to plant

NITRATES AND OTHER MINERAL SALTS

WATER

Two basic kinds of chemical activity occur within every green leaf. The two are shown separately here for clarity. One activity is photosynthesis (top leaf), triggered by sunlight and chlorophyll. The other activity (top and bottom leaves) takes the products of photosynthesis (carbohydrates, simple sugars) and turns them into more complex substances with the help of enzymes. Raw materials are taken from the soil (water, minerals) and air (carbon dioxide, oxygen), and the finished products are used or stored by the plant.

The medicinal substances found in plants are the products of natural processes. These manufacturing processes are common to all plants, but each species has its own particular variation. One species may need more or less light, more or less water, more or less of a mineral than another species needs. Given these variations, each plant species produces chemical compounds slightly different from those of another. Some plants produce medicinally useful compounds, such as glycosides and alkaloids, while others do not.

As indicated by the diagram above, green leaves are the site of a great deal of the chemical activity that goes on in plants, including the most fundamental process of all: photosynthesis. But leaves are far from independent laboratories. They need the support and the raw materials supplied by the root and stem to carry on their work. Among the general classes of plant chemicals that have long been used for medicinal purposes are the alkaloids, the glycosides, and the essential oils.

astringent properties—that is, their ability to make the skin and blood vessels constrict. They have also been used as antidotes for certain poisons. **Flavonoids,** yellow pigments whose chemical structure resembles that of tannins, also have medicinal uses.

Plants are nature's source of most of the **vitamins** needed to sustain human health and life. Almost all of the essential vitamins can be naturally synthesized only by plants. Thus human beings must eat plants, or animals that have eaten plants, in order to get essential vitamins. (Artificially synthesized vitamins—whether in pills or some other man-made form—can supplement but not, over the long term, satisfactorily replace vitamins occurring naturally in a well-balanced diet.) Equally essential to human nutrition are **mineral elements**—zinc, iron, cobalt, manganese, and others—supplied by plants in a form that can be digested by the human body.

Among other useful medicinal compounds arising from plant metabolism are **antibiotics** produced by certain species. Examples are sulfur compounds from garlic; some of the glycosides produced by mustards; and alkaloids found in some water lily species.

Key Medicinal Parts

Sometimes the whole plant, including its root system, is used for medicinal purposes. More commonly, medicinally active substances tend to be concentrated in one part of the plant or another. Frequently it is the **leaves.** The site of much of a plant's chemical activity, including photosynthesis, leaves are often rich in the various glycosides, alkaloids, and essential oils that have been found to have therapeutic effects on human beings.

Stems serve mainly for support and as conduits for sap (mineral and organic nutrients and metabolic by-products in watery solution) moving through the plant. But the stems of some woody species do contain medicinal compounds, particularly in their bark and sapwood (the layer between the inner heartwood and outer bark). For instance, an antispasmodic is prepared from extracts of the bark of the black haw, or stagbush, a shrub or small tree common in eastern North America. And the bark of the white oak, *Quercus alba*, has been used to make astringents.

Buds of perennial species may also reward the seeker for medicinal compounds. Those of the black poplar, *Populus nigra*, have long been valued for their antiseptic properties. And the buds of the Chinese pagoda tree, familiar as an ornamental tree in the United States, are used in the Far East to treat hemorrhages, fevers, and seizures.

In some **flowers** the medicinally active constituents are found with pigments that give the blossoms their distinctive color. The yellow petals of broom, for example, contain flavon-oids, and red rose petals are full of tannins. Many other flowers, such as marshmallow and German chamomile, are rich in essential oils. The pollen of some species has a relatively large amount of vitamins and minerals.

The rind and the seeds of **fruits** may be rich in substances with potential medical uses. The seedlike dry fruits of many members of the carrot family—for example, dill, fennel, anise, caraway—supply flavorful essential oils. Fleshy fruits usually contain large reserves of vitamins, organic acids, and sugars and so play an important part in human nutrition—and in treating the many diseases and disorders caused by nutritional deficiencies.

Medicinal parts of plants can also be found underground. The **roots** of both North American and Asiatic ginseng have been credited by herbalists with having a wide variety of therapeutic effects. Dug up in the autumn and dried, the roots of six- to eight-year-old ginseng plants are coveted for their reputed ability to improve all-round health and mental powers. (Because the roots can bring high prices ginseng has become so rare in North America that many states protect the species, and location of wild patches is usually a jealously guarded secret.) Many kinds of roots are also important as foods because they accumulate large stores of starches and sugars and are the source of vitamins and other nutrients.

Rootlike underground structures—**rhizomes, bulbs, tubers,** for example—also contain stores of food that ensure the plant's survival over the winter after the aboveground parts have died. A familiar specific example is the tuber of the white potato, which is filled with starch. Onion and garlic bulbs contain medicinally active sulfur compounds. Garlic cloves in particular have a reputation among some peoples as an almost magical cure-all. Among the powers attributed to them are those of warding off all manner of germs and diseases, improving one's general health, stimulating stomach and gall bladder secretions, and killing intestinal parasitic worms. They are said to function both as an antispasmodic and as a vasodilator, or substance that widens the blood vessels and so helps the flow of blood through them. Scientific studies have substantiated a number of claims made for garlic—for example, its antiseptic properties—and research indicates that it may help reduce blood pressure and blood cholesterol levels. The cloves are rich in vitamins A, B_1, B_2, and C.

Finally there are various kinds of plant secretions, especially **gums** and **resins,** with therapeutic applications. The resins of pine, spruce, and balsam fir have been much used medicinally. Gums such as gum arabic (from certain African acacias) are employed as stabilizers intended to improve or maintain the texture and consistency of mixed foods such as ice cream, jellies, and cough drops.

About Plant Names

Angelica, church steeples, eyebright, Queen Anne's lace—the common names of many plants have a charm and poetry of their own. Some describe outstanding features of a plant. Bindweed, for example, is a vine that entangles any plant it grows upon. Butterfly weed does seem to be irresistible to butterflies, which are drawn to the nectar in its orange blooms.

Other plants get their names from the use people have made of them. Down through the centuries the wood of boxwood was fashioned into decorative boxes, woundworts were used to treat wounds, snakeroots to treat snakebite.

Confusion!

Yet common names can be a source of confusion. Frequently the same plant has more than one name: butterfly weed, for example. Because it was once used to treat pleurisy (an inflammation of the membranes covering the lungs and lining the chest cavity), butterfly weed is called pleurisy root in some areas. Bouncing Bet, a common roadside wildflower brought to America by European settlers, is also known as soapwort: its leaves and rhizomes boiled in water make a lather for laundry and bathing. Other names for bouncing Bet are fuller's-herb and lady's-washbowl.

Just as confusing as having a plant with more than one common name is having the same name applied to two or more different species. Across North America there are a number of completely unrelated plants called snakeroots. And the name squawroot refers to different species in different areas.

The Scientific Solution

To avoid such confusion, scientists use a standardized two-part naming system called binomial nomenclature for both plants and animals. This nomenclature was pioneered by the 18th-century Swedish naturalist Carolus Linnaeus. His system grew into the rules now set down in the *International Code of Botanical Nomenclature*, a book on international botanical naming conventions. The first part of a plant's name gives its genus, the group to which it belongs and with which it shares many features. Violets, for example, belong to the genus *Viola*, roses to the genus *Rosa*.

The second part of a plant's name tells its species—the particular kind of plant in a genus. Thus *Rosa multiflora* is the scientific name for the multiflora (many-flowered) rose, and *Rosa canina* is the internationally recognized botanical name of the dog (canine) rose.

A botanical name is often followed by an abbreviation of the name of the person who classified the plant scientifically. (See "Botanists and Their Abbreviations," next page.) Thousands of plant names, for example, are followed by the initial "L." for Linnaeus.

Speaking Botanical Latin in Five Minutes

Botanical names are easier to pronounce than they may appear to be. With few exceptions, you simply say the word as you would any English word. No matter how many syllables the word has, just say each syllable, one after the other, the way you would if you were asked to pronounce any ordinary word slowly and distinctly. As for the question of which syllables to stress, even botanists may differ—but they always manage to understand one another, nevertheless. In the following examples, the syllables usually stressed are printed in capital letters. If you spend five minutes pronouncing your way through the words that follow, you will begin to get the knack of speaking Botanical Latin. The quasi-phonetic respellings after each item give only a rough-and-ready *suggested* style of pronunciation, helping solve typical kinds of problems you may encounter in speaking botanical names or hearing them spoken. Note, for example, the preferred pronunciations of *ch*, *cn*, and *cy*.

Abies balsamea
  AY-beez ball-SAY-mee-ah
Achillea millefolium
  ah-KILL-ee-ah MILL-i-FOH-lee-um
Cheiranthus cheiri
  KYE-ran-thus KYE-rye
Cnicus benedictus
  NYE-kus ben-i-DIK-tus
Cynoglossum officinale
  SY-noh-GLOSS-um off-fiss-i-NAY-lee
Cypripedium calceolus
  SIP-ri-PEE-dee-um kal-SEE-oh-luss
Euonymus europaeus
  you-OH-nim-us you-roh-PEE-us
Glycyrrhiza lepidota
  GLIS-sir-RYE-zah lep-ID-oh-tah

Iris pseudacorus
  EYE-ris soo-DAY-koh-rus
Ligustrum vulgare
  li-GOO-strum vul-GAY-ree
Lycopodium clavatum
  lye-koh-POH-dee-um klah-VAY-tum
Lysimachia nummularia
  lye-si-MAY-kee-ah NEW-mew-LAY-ree-ah
Medicago sativa
  MED-i-KAY-goh sah-TIE-vah
Ruta graveolens
  ROO-tah gray-VEE-oh-lens
Stachys palustris
  STACK-is pah-LUSS-tris
Tussilago farfara
  tuss-i-LAY-goh FAR-far-ah

Genera that share significant characteristics are grouped into botanical families, usually ending in the suffix "-aceae." Plants of the genus *Lilium* (common lilies), for instance, are placed with the genus *Hemerocallis* (daylilies) in the lily family, or Liliaceae.

Latin and Greek Demystified

Plants' scientific names are based on Latin and Greek, but this does not, in any way, make these names forbiddingly complicated. Many Latin and Greek genus names, in fact, have become the familiar, everyday names of plants: iris, geranium, and nasturtium are examples.

Some genus names, such as *Achillea*, *Artemisia*, and *Asclepias*, come from the names of mythological figures. Others Linnaeus simply borrowed from the Latin or Greek common name, making *Alnus* the generic (genus) name for alders, *Populus* for poplars, and so on.

Still other genus names were coined to honor somebody. The genus *Kalmia*, which includes the North American mountain laurel (*Kalmia latifolia*), was named for Peter Kalm, a student of Linnaeus's who traveled in North America to collect plants for him.

The second (species) part of a botanical name, more often then not, describes something specific about the plant. Sometimes it tells the color of a plant's flowers: *alba* for white, *rubrus* for red, *purpureum* for purple. Or it may describe foliage: *grandifolia* for large leaves, *rotundifolia* for round leaves, *millefolium* for thousand- or many-leaved. Or it may describe some other salient characteristic: *erectus* for upright, *hirsutum* for hairy, *odorata* for fragrant, *myrtilloides* for myrtlelike. Some specific (species) names describe where a plant is typically found: *montana*, on the mountain; *maritima*, by the sea; *aquatilis*, in the water. And others tell how people have used the plants: *edulis*, edible; *cathartica*, cathartic.

"Officinalis" Species

One specific name, *officinalis* (sometimes *officinale*), deserves special comment because it is part of the scientific name of many medicinal plants. It means "of the workshop." The allusion is to apothecaries' shops, and the name signifies that any *officinalis* plant was once prized by the apothecary, forerunner of today's licensed pharmacist or druggist. Thus balm is *Melissa officinalis*; the dandelion is *Taraxacum officinale*; eyebright is *Euphrasia officinalis*, to give just three examples. Here again, the scientific name, far from being mystifying, gives a useful bit of information about the plant, inviting us to learn more.

Botanists and Their Abbreviations

The names of plant classifiers appear, usually abbreviated, after the plant's botanical name. If a name is later changed for certain reasons, the original classifier is noted in parentheses. Below are the abbreviations, the names they represent, and data on the botanist-classifiers.

ACH. Ascharius, Erik, 1757–1819, Swedish. Physician.

A.CHEV. Chevalier, Auguste Jean Baptiste, 1873–1956. French.

A.GRAY Gray, Asa, 1810–1888. American. Professor, Harvard University, Cambridge, Mass.

AIT. f. Aiton, William Townsend, 1766–1849. English. Mgr., Royal Botanic Gardens, Kew, England.

A.RICHARD Richard, Achille, 1794–1852. French.

BAILL. Baillon, Henri Ernest, 1827–1895. French. Dir., Botanical Garden, Paris.

BAKER Baker, John Gilbert, 1834–1920. English. Curator, Royal Botanic Gardens herbarium, Kew, England.

BALF. Balfour, John Hutton, 1808–1884. Scottish. Dir., The Botanical Garden, Edinburgh.

BART. Barton, Benjamin Smith, 1766–1815. American. Physician, naturalist.

BARTR. Bartram, William, 1739–1823. American.

BEAUVOIS Beauvois, Ambroise Marie François Joseph Palisot de, 1752–1820. French. Explorer.

BENTH. Bentham, George, 1800–1884. English.

BERNH. Bernhardi, Johann Jacob, 1774–1850. German.

BERTONI Bertoni, Moisés Santiago, 1857–1929. Paraguayan.

BLUME Blume, Carl Ludwig, 1796–1862. Dutch. Dir., the Government Herbarium, Leiden, Holland.

B.MEY. Meyer, Bernhard, 1767–1836. German. Physician, pharmacist, ornithologist.

BRITT. Britton, Nathaniel Lord, 1859–1934. American. Founder, The New York Botanical Garden, New York City.

BROT. Brotero, Felix de Avellar, 1744–1828. Portuguese. Dir., Botanical Garden, Ajuda, Portugal.

BURM.f. Burman, Nicolaas Laurens, 1733–1793. Dutch.

CHAIX Chaix, Dominique, 1730–1799. French. Abbot.

CHAM. Chamisso, Adelbert von, 1781–1838. German. Dir., Berlin Botanical Garden, Berlin.

COV. Coville, Frederick Vernon, 1867–1937. American. U.S. Dept. of Agriculture.

CRAIB Craib, William Grant, 1882–1933. Scot.

CYRILLO Cirillo, Domenico Maria Leone, 1739–1799. Italian. Statesman.

DC. Candolle, Augustin Pyramus de, 1778–1841. Swiss.

DRYAND. Dryander, Jonas Carlsson, 1748–1810. Swedish.

EHRH. Ehrhart, Jacob Friedrich, 1742–1795. German. Pharmacist.

ELL. Elliott, Stephen, 1771–1830. American. Planter, banker, statesman, editor.

ENDL. Endlicher, Stephan Ladislaus, 1804–1849. Austrian. Dir., The Botanical Garden and Institute, University of Vienna.

FARW. Farwell, Oliver Atkins, 1867–1944. American.

FERN. Fernald, Merritt Lyndon, 1873–1950. American. Curator and Dir., Gray Herbarium, Harvard University, Cambridge, Mass.

FORSK. Forsskål, Pehr, 1732–1762. Swedish.

FORST.f. Forster, Johann Georg Adam, 1754–1794. German. Naturalist, professor.

FRIES Fries, Elias Magnus, 1794–1878. Swedish.

GAERTN. Gärtner, Joseph, 1732–1791. German. Physician.

GAILL. Gaillon, François Benjamin, 1782–1839. French.

G.DON Don, George, 1798–1856. English.

GREENE Greene, Edward Lee, 1843–1915. American. Theologian.

GILIB. Gilibert, Jean Emmanuel, 1741–1814. French. Professor.

HARMS Harms, Hermann August Theodor, 1870–1942. German.

HOLMES Holmes, Edward Morell, 1843–1930. English.

HOOK.f. Hooker, Sir Joseph Dalton, 1817–1911. English. Dir., Royal Botanic Gardens, Kew, England.

HUDS. Hudson, William, 1730–1793. English. Pharmacist.

HULL Hull, John, 1761–1843. English. Physician.

JACQ. Jacquin, Nicolaus Joseph von, 1727–1817. Austrian. Physician, Dir., Gardens of Schönbrunn Palace, Vienna, Austria.

J.S.PRESL Presl, Jan Swatopluk, 1791–1849. Czech.

KER Ker (Ker-Gawler), John Bellenden, 1764–1842. English.

KURZ Kurz, Wilhelm Sulpiz, 1834–1878. German. Curator, Royal Herbarium, Calcutta, India.

L. Linnaeus, Carolus, 1707–1778. Swedish. Biologist, famous for devising a system for classifying all known plants and animals.

LABILL. La Billardière, Jacques Julien Houtton de, 1755–1834. French.

LAMK. Lamarck, Jean Baptiste Pierre Antoine de Monet de, 1744–1829. French. Zoologist.

LINK Link, Heinrich Friedrich, 1767–1851. German. Dir., Botanical Garden, Berlin, Cofounder, German Horticultural Society.

MARSH. Marshall, Humphrey, 1722–1801. American.

MAXIM. Maximowicz, Karl Johannes, 1827–1891. Russian. Curator and Chief Botanist, Botanical Garden, St. Petersburg.

MEDIC. Medikus, Friedrich Kasimir, 1736–1808. German.

MERR. Merrill, Elmer Drew, 1876–1956. American. Dir., Arnold Arboretum of Harvard University, Cambridge, Mass.

MICHX. Michaux, André, 1746–1802. French.

MILL. Miller, Philip, 1691–1771. English. Dir., Chelsea Garden, England.

MOENCH Moench, Konrad, 1744–1805. German. Chemist.

MUHL. Mühlenberg, Gotthilf Henry Ernest, 1753–1815. American. Clergyman.

MURR. Murray, Johan Andreas, 1740–1791. Swedish. Physician, professor.

NEES Nees von Esenbeck, Christian Gottfried Daniel, 1776–1858. German.

NEWM. Newman, Edward, 1801–1876. English. Publisher.

NUTT. Nuttall, Thomas, 1786–1859. English-American. Professor.

OEDER Oeder, Georg Christian, 1728–1791. German. Provincial Governor, Oldenburg, Germany.

PLANCH. Planchon, Jules Émile, 1823–1888. French.

PURSH Pursh, Friedrich Trautgott, 1774–1820. German-Canadian.

RAEUSCH. Räuschel, Ernst Adolph, worked 1772–1797. German.

R.BR. Brown, Robert, 1773–1858. English. Keeper, Botanical Collections, British Museum, London.

ROSCOE Roscoe, William, 1753–1831. English. Founder, Botanical Garden, Liverpool, England.

ROXB. Roxburgh, William, 1751–1815. Scot. Physician, Founder, The Calcutta Botanic Garden, Calcutta, India.

RUSBY Rusby, Henry Hurd, 1855–1940. American.

ST.-HIL. Saint-Hilaire, Augustin François César Prouvençal de, 1779–1853. French. Explorer.

SAVI Savi, Gaetano, 1769–1844. Italian.

SCHERB. Scherbius, Johannes, 1769–1813. German.

SCHOTT Schott, Heinrich Wilhelm, 1794–1865. Austrian. Dir., Gardens of Schönbrunn Palace, Vienna, Austria.

SCOP. Scopoli, Giovanni Antonio, 1723–1788. Austrian. Naturalist.

SIBTH. Sibthorp, John, 1758–1796. English. Physician.

SMITH Smith, Sir James Edward, 1759–1828. English. First Pres., Linnean Society, London.

SPRENG. Sprengel, Kurt Polycarp Joachim, 1766–1833. German. Physician, Dir., Botanical Garden, Halle, Germany.

STAPF Stapf, Otto, 1857–1933. Austrian-English. Dir., Royal Botanic Gardens herbarium, Kew, England.

SWARTZ Swartz, Olof Peter, 1760–1818. Swedish. Professor.

TORR. Torrey, John, 1796–1873. American.

VAHL Vahl, Martin, 1749–1804. Danish.

WALLICH Wallich, Nathaniel, 1786–1854. Danish-English. Physician, Dir., The Calcutta Botanic Garden, Calcutta, India.

WALT. Walter, Thomas, 1740–1789. American.

WATS. Watson, Sereno, 1826–1892. American.

W.D.J. KOCH, Koch, Wilhelm Daniel Joseph, 1771–1849. German. Physician, Dir., Botanical Garden, Erlangen, Germany.

WEBER Weber, Georg Heinrich, 1752–1828. German. Professor.

WILLD. Willdenow, Karl Ludwig, 1765–1812. German. Dir., Botanical Garden, Berlin.

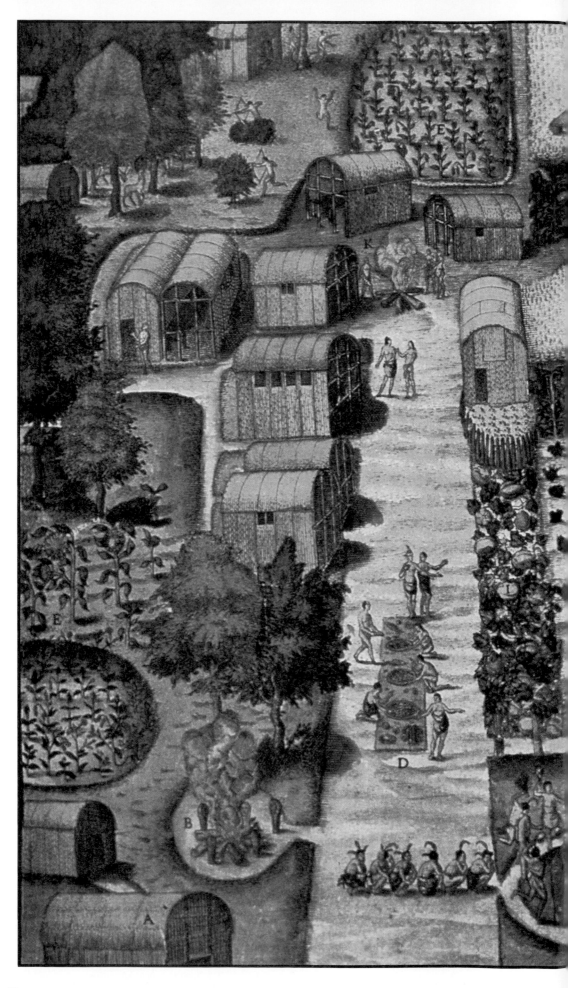

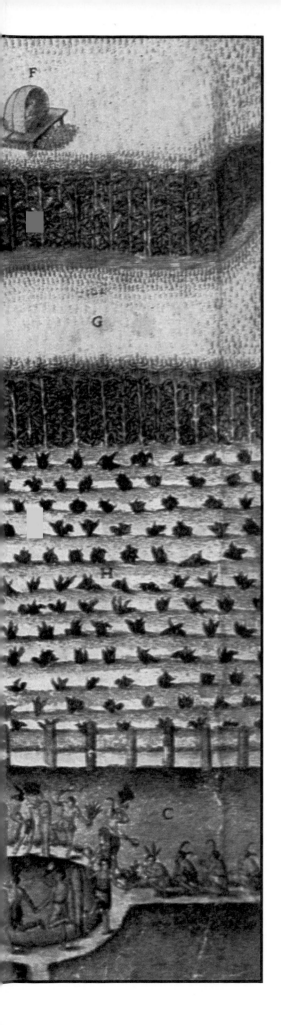

Plants, People, and Medicine

When pain or injury or disease struck, early man had little choice but to turn to plants. Developed empirically, by trial and error, many herbal treatments were nevertheless remarkably effective. Then medicine became more theoretical. The belief arose that the harsher the treatment, the better. Herbal medicine fell out of favor, branded as ignorant superstition. Change came only when formal medicine opened its doors and let the light of modern science shine in. Now, the new medical science is reaffirming much of the old herbal lore and extending the horizons of botanical medicine.

In this scientific age, it is easy to mistake pseudoscience for the real thing. Misconceptions or myths arise, which then pass as scientific truths. One such myth concerns medicines. It says, "Synthetic is best." If a medicine does not contain purified chemicals, expensively made in gleaming laboratories by highly trained scientists in starched and sanitized white coats—so the myth goes—it cannot possibly be a medicine that works.

Like all myths, this one grows out of a certain body of human experience and is true up to a point. Gone are the days when nobody could ever be sure exactly what substances a medical potion contained, or precisely which of the substances, in what strength or combination, might actually help anybody feel any better. Modern science provides precise techniques of analysis, separation, and measurement. Scientists now test the effects and side effects of a medicine before it is released for wide public use. These modern procedures have made the medicines we buy safer. But unfortunately there is still room for tragic errors, such as the one in the late 1950's involving thalidomide, a sedative that caused serious birth defects in the babies of pregnant mothers for whom it was prescribed.

Medicines That Work

The myth also ignores the simple truth that many botanical remedies *worked*, consistently and effectively—in some cases as well as or better than the products of today's laboratories. Finally, there is the fact that many of the drugs and medicines we buy at the pharmacy —often in fancy packages, at fancy prices— contain the same active ingredients as healing plants used by prescientific cultures. In other words, people in "primitive" societies were using basically the same medicines for the same maladies that bring us to our physicians and pharmacists today. Examples abound. To mention just two:

• Tea brewed from the stems of a low shrub the Chinese call mahuang will relieve asthma, colds, and coughs. The stems are a natural source of ephedrine, the active ingredient of many medicines, including decongestants that "unclog" breathing passages.

• The leaves of a plant that grows along roads and in fields contain a substance that is highly effective in treating congestive heart failure. The plant is common foxglove (*Digitalis purpurea*), the source of a chemical substance that aids the functioning of heart muscle.

Through the centuries, sick people have been helped over and over again by remedies that did not arise out of the formal doctrines and procedures of the medical profession. The use of plants to treat sickness is probably as old as mankind; formal medicine and medical degrees are, of course, much more recent. Yet if medicine is broadly defined as the attempt to

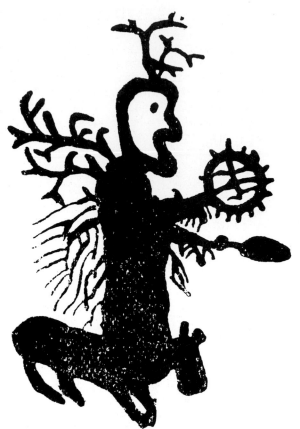

Prehistoric drawing of a medicine man.

treat and cure human illness, then the human beings who first grew and collected plants they thought useful—herbalists—and the first people to try to heal by the use of herbs—also called herbalists, or herb doctors—must surely rank as pioneers of modern medicine.

This is not to say that "good, old-fashioned herbal remedies" are better or safer than the laboratory-made chemical prescriptions that are in favor today, nor that herbalists are somehow superior to today's physicians. Nor is it meant to suggest that readers start dosing themselves with "natural" medicines—to do so would invite not only the risk of accidental poisoning but the dangers arising from self-diagnosis.

The fact remains that plants do produce a variety of chemical substances that act upon animal tissues. One remarkable example is a pretty pink flower that blooms on the island of Madagascar off the coast of Africa. Extracts from this flower can stop the progress of Hodgkin's disease and childhood leukemia. The flower, a periwinkle, contains two substances—known as vincristine and vinblastine—that physicians prescribe to fight certain types of cancer. But there is no need to travel to Madagascar to find medically useful botanical specimens. More than a few familiar plants— including a number of the herbs that are basic items in spice racks—are commonly used in pharmacy today.

Learning From Medicine's Past

Through most of human existence, plants (together with animal substances and mystical rites) were virtually all that was available to healers and those who hoped to be healed. This is still largely true outside the developed world. Not until the present century did advances in pharmacology, chemistry, and technology make possible the synthesis of many of the compounds currently used in medicine. Even so, roughly 25 percent of modern pharmaceuticals are derived from some parts of higher plants. (The figure approaches 50 percent when pharmaceuticals made from microbial organisms are included.) In most cases, today's use of the modern pharmaceutical product is similar to the traditional use of the plant from which it is derived.

Furthermore, scientists are finding that the purified active ingredients of some "new" pharmaceuticals may cause undesirable side effects that the "old," unpurified, botanical medicines did not cause. Could it be, ask these scientists, that some plants may have built-in safety factors, long ignored, that could minimize some of the side effects of their active ingredients? In the hope of answering such questions, many researchers are looking back at the ways of herbal doctors and medicine men and women of bygone eras, as well as scrutinizing the practices of contemporary folk healers. Such investigations keep pointing to the hypothesis that herbalists have been using the same plant remedies for countless generations for the simple reason that those remedies happen to work.

Earliest Treatments

In most past societies (and some present ones), sickness was viewed as a punishment from the gods. Early medicine men treated the sick with prayers and rituals that included what may have been considered "magic potions." Most of these medicinal preparations were concocted from local herbs. Though it may be true that the herbs were selected first because of their color, odor, shape, or rarity, what followed could hardly have been a process guided by whim alone. Rather, the application of any one herb or mixture of herbs to a specific disorder must have been the result of much trial-and-error experimentation over many generations. How else to explain the fact that, oceans apart from one another, different civilizations learned to use closely related medicinal plants in almost identical ways?

Archeological discoveries at a 60,000-year-old Neanderthal burial ground in Iraq point to the use of several plants that still figure in folk medicine—among them marshmallow, yarrow, and groundsel. Mexican Indians of thousands of years ago used peyote cactus. Possibly then, as now, peyote was valued for its hallucinogenic properties, and equally possibly for its active medicinal substances, which are still used to heal bruises and wounds, and are now known to have antibiotic properties.

The Sumerians inhabited an area around the Tigris and Euphrates rivers (in what is now Iraq) about 4000 B.C. From their cuneiform writings on clay tablets we know that their medicines included opium, licorice, thyme, mustard, and the chemical element sulfur. The Babylonians who followed apparently expanded the Sumerians' stock of medicinal substances, adding senna leaves, saffron, coriander, cinnamon, and garlic, among other herbs, to their formulary. From such herbs and from plant resins such as galbanum and storax they made medicinal decoctions (extracts), wines, poultices, salves, and liniments.

Ancient Egyptian Medicine

Out of the next great civilization, the Egyptian, came Imhotep, a skilled physician who later became the Egyptian god of healing. Ancient Egypt also gave the world one of its first medical texts, the Ebers Papyrus, named for the German Egyptologist Georg Ebers. He bought it, in 1873, from an Arab who claimed to have found it in the necropolis outside Thebes. The papyrus is believed to have been written in the 16th century B.C. It contains some 800 recipes and refers to over 700 drugs, including aloe, wormwood, peppermint, henbane, myrrh, hemp dogbane, castor oil, and mandragora. With such ingredients, the Egyptians prepared decoctions, wines and infu-

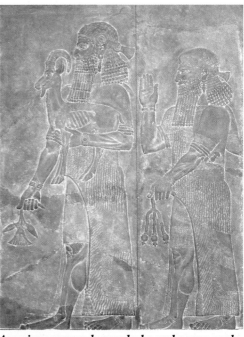

Assyrians gave gods mandrake and poppy seeds.

sions, as well as pills, salves, and poultices.

The Ebers Papyrus mentions a recipe that suggests the Egyptians had a treatment for diabetes. It also advises putting mud or moldy bread over sores to keep them from becoming infected. Not until millennia later was it discovered that mud and molds often contain certain microorganisms—filamentous bacteria and filamentous fungi—that produce one class of antibiotic wonder drugs.

Chinese, Hebrew, Sanskrit Writings

Ancient Egypt was not alone in recording the healing powers of plants. At least 2,000 years ago (according to the rather hazy system that is traditionally used to date events of ancient China), the earliest known Chinese pharmacopeia, the *Pen Tsao*, appeared. Attributed to the legendary emperor Shen Nung, this work described the use of chaulmoogra oil from trees of the *Hydnocarpus* genus to treat leprosy. The *Pen Tsao*, like pharmacopeias that followed it, attempts to give an authoritative, up-to-date survey of the age's medicinal preparations. Among its many other plant listings are hemp dogbane and opium poppy, as well as rhubarb and aconite. These ancient Chinese first recorded the use of the desert shrub called Chinese ephedra, or mahuang, to improve circulation, reduce fevers, help urinary function, suppress coughing, and relieve lung or bronchial disorders. Its active ingredient was nearly lost to modern medical science until its rediscovery earlier in this century. We now know it as ephedrine, the key ingredient in modern pharmaceuticals used to relieve breathing difficulties and other symptoms of asthma, hay fever, and the common cold.

The Jews of the Old Testament period are remembered for their high standards of public health and hygiene. Yet among these people of the rugged terrain at the eastern end of the Mediterranean, the use of plants for medicinal purposes was an accepted custom. The Book of Ecclesiasticus (or Sirach) in a sense authorizes and encourages this practice: "The Lord created medicines from the earth, and a sensible man will not despise them." Dozens of plants from juniper to mandrake, from cotton to mustard, yield substances that were used medicinally in Old Testament times.

In India, many generations of medical tradition were formalized in the *Ayurveda*, a collection of Hindu medical lore that was probably first put into writing about the time of Christ. The doctrine itself goes back to the much earlier *Rig Veda* and its hymns dedicated to the medicine-god-narcotic Soma, since identified as the narcotic and hallucinogenic mushroom *Amanita muscaria*. The *Veda*s, written down originally in Sanskrit, made many references to healing plants, including the snakeroot *Rauvolfia serpentina*, used in India to treat snake-

bite, epilepsy, mental disorders, and other illnesses. *R. serpentina* is the source of reserpine, a tranquilizer and hypotensive agent used widely in modern pharmacy. The *Charaka Samhita*, a comprehensive Indian herbal, cites more than 500 plant remedies.

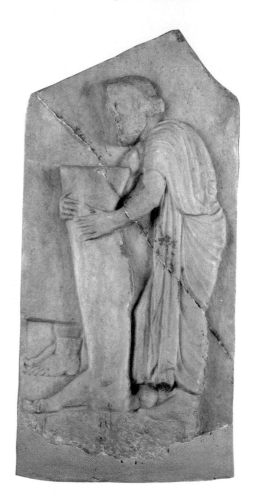

Thanks for cure: a Greek donates image of leg.

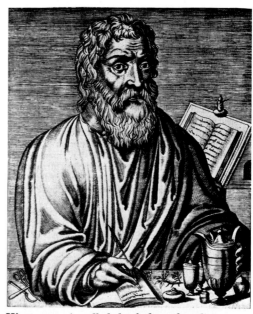

Hippocrates is called the father of medicine.

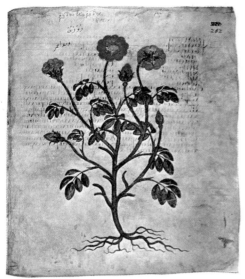

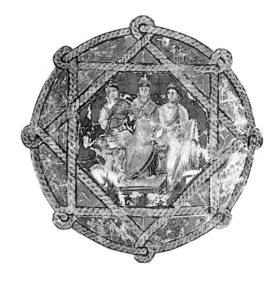

Dioscorides' De Materia Medica: *pages from an* A.D. *512 manuscript. Dioscorides may be the man depicted in the center of the illustration at right.*

The Greek Contribution

Ancient Greece produced a god and several mortals whose names figure prominently in the early history of medicine. The god was Aesculapius, the god of healing. His sign was a snake curled around a staff—the caduceus, still a symbol of medicine today.

In ancient Greece, medicine was practiced by priests, called Aesculapiads. The sick sought these priests' help in temples built in Aesculapius' honor. Treatment was a religious ritual full of incantation and mystery, carried out over several days of fasting and bathing. It culminated in the "temple sleep." (Fasting may help botanical and other medicines work. In modern times, patients are frequently told to take a medication on an empty stomach or so many hours before or after meals.) After sufficient bathing and fasting, the patient entered the holiest room in the temple and lay down on the bloody hide of a sacrificial animal. During the night, the priest, representing Aesculapius and having with him the sacred snake, awakened the patient. Assisted by priestesses, the Aesculapiad interpreted the patient's dreams and advised on medical treatment and day-to-day regimen. If they recovered, patients frequently "paid their bill" by sending the temple an image of the part of the body that was cured.

About 400 B.C., a Greek named Hippocrates moved the healing profession away from the realm of mysticism and religion. He asserted that medicine was a science and an art. For this he is called the father of modern medicine.

The teachings of Hippocrates, contained in the Hippocratic Collection, place great emphasis on diet, life-style, exercise, sunshine, and water. His underlying principle was that the "important thing is to do no harm." His famous oath, which scholars now think was a group effort rather than Hippocrates' own,

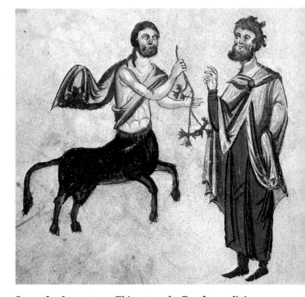

In myth, the centaur Chiron taught Greeks medicine.

suggests strong humanitarian concerns among a number of the Greek physicians of the era.

Hippocrates believed that the four elements—fire, water, earth, and air—were represented in the human body by yellow bile, phlegm, black bile, and blood. One's health depended on the balance of these four humors, or "cardinal juices"—that is, on their respective strengths in the body. When the balance became upset, sickness was the result. Health could be restored only by ridding the body of excess "juices" through bleeding, enemas and laxatives, diuretics, sweating, or vomiting. As laxatives, physicians of the time used aniseed, asses' milk, and castor beans. Plants employed to increase urine flow were parsley, thyme, fennel, and celery. In all, Hippocrates' writings name some 300 to 400 healing plants.

After Hippocrates came Aristotle, whose far-ranging scientific work included an effort

53

to catalog the properties of the various medicinal herbs. Less well known is Aristotle's pupil Theophrastus, a botanist whose treatise *Inquiry Into Plants* was to influence both botany and medicine for centuries to come.

In the first century A.D., Greece produced the forerunner of all modern pharmacopeias and the authoritative text on botanical medicine for over a thousand years, *De Materia Medica*. This work featured hundreds of medicinal plants. Its author was Dioscorides, one of the last of the ancient Greeks who cast giant shadows forward to modern medicine.

Roman Advances

Before Dioscorides, to the west, Rome had begun its rise to power in Europe and the lands around the Mediterranean Sea. With Roman hegemony came two of history's most impor-

Theophrastus (c. 371–c. 287 B.C.)

History's first scientific botanist was the Greek philosopher Theophrastus. Extending to plants a classification scheme developed by his teacher Aristotle, Theophrastus wrote *Inquiry Into Plants* and *Growth of Plants*. These works—covering some 550 plants from Europe to India—were the first to classify plants by form and structure, and prefigure the Linnaean system used today (see page 66). Theophrastus was a first-rate observer as well: his description of germinating seeds, for example, was long unsurpassed. Yet he also transmitted fantasies that were to haunt natural science down to modern times, such as the idea that plants were put on earth solely for man's use, a notion implicit in the doctrine of signatures. As to his reason for mixing figment with fact, Theophrastus wrote: "Fabulous tales are not made up without reason."

tant public health measures: fresh drinking water, distributed through the aqueducts, and a sewage system.

As for private health, medical practice in the first century A.D. seems to have included three approaches: diet, pharmacy, and surgery. Most infectious diseases were treated with diet and rest. In the tradition of Hippocrates, body "balances" were restored by surgery, which often involved some method of drawing blood from the body. Along with such procedures, botanical treatments were also prescribed to correct body imbalances. Besides honeys and wines, many other herbal medicines such as dill and coriander were used. These included plants that acted to purge the digestive tract.

This, too, was the age of the theriac (from the Greek *theriakon*, a remedy for animal bites). A theriac was a combination of many different herbs, primarily opiates and antispasmodics. It was given as a general cure-all. Most likely, what a theriac actually did was to relieve symptoms while nature took its course.

"Mithridates' Antidote" was the name of

Mithridates (died 63 B.C.)

A special place in the story of medicinal plants belongs to Mithridates VI, king of Pontus. Because he is said to have made himself invulnerable to poisoning by taking progressively larger doses of poison, his name lives on in the term *mithridatism*, "acquired tolerance of a poison." Facing capture by Roman enemies, he reputedly tried in vain to poison himself and had to get a slave to stab him to death. Accounts written after his death portray Mithridates as a diligent biological investigator who knew 22 languages and studied medicine as well. An antidote called the mithridate bore his name in medieval pharmacology. Mithridates' physician Crateuas was famous in antiquity for his lifelike botanical paintings, now thought to have been the basis for illustrations in Dioscorides' *De Materia Medica*.

one famous theriac. It was devised, probably in the first century B.C., by Mithridates Eupator, king of Pontus, a kingdom on the shores of the Black Sea that was conquered by the Roman general Pompey in 66 B.C. Mithridates lived in fear of being poisoned by his enemies. (His fear was apparently not just paranoia, since he seems to have devoted a morbid amount of time and energy to murdering friends and relatives, including his immediate family.) Legend has it that Mithridates concocted an antidote out of many poisonous ingredients, including blood from ducks that had been raised on toxic plants. He then reputedly took small, but increasingly larger, doses of the mixture in an effort to make himself immune to poisons.

Other than for his curious antidote and bizarre behavior, Mithridates Eupator is remembered today because an entire plant genus, *Eupatorium*, with between 40 and 1,000 species (depending on the authority consulted), bears his name.

Dioscorides (first century A.D.)

The most influential pharmaceutical writer of antiquity was the Greek physician Dioscorides, born near Tarsus (in modern Turkey) probably shortly after the time of Christ. Little is known about Dioscorides' personal life, other than that he may have served as a doctor with the Roman army. His pharmaceutical guide, *De Materia Medica*, deals with more than 600 plants, 35 animal products, and 90 minerals used in medicine. Illustrated manuscripts of this work circulated over the next 1,600 years throughout the West and the Middle East. One of its earliest print editions was published by the great Renaissance botanist-naturalist Pietro Mattioli in Venice in 1544. The Mattioli edition is regarded as a cornerstone of modern botany. A great many of the scientific and everyday plant names we use today can be traced back to Dioscorides.

Nor did Mithridates' Antidote die with him. Its composition was reblended and "improved" by Andromachus, Nero's personal physician, until it became Andromachus' theriac. This was a mixture of approximately 70 vegetable, mineral, and animal substances (on the theory that if one ingredient did not help the patient, another would). Included were opium; a lizard, prized as an aphrodisiac; and snake flesh, representing Aesculapius. This apothecaries' brew figured in medicine for over 1,500 years.

Pliny's *Natural History,* published in the first century A.D., was a compilation of thousands of Greek and Roman treatises. Much of what Pliny wrote down eventually passed into the folklore of Europe and the New World. The *Natural History* stated a proposition, held by many cultures, before and since, that nature is the servant of man. That is, plants exist to meet man's needs, and all plants not clearly useful for man's food, clothing, and shelter may possess medicinal properties.

Out of this same period came yet another great figure of medicine, Galen, a Greek physician who practiced in Rome during the second century A.D. Galen's primary fame is associated with the fauna, not the flora, of his time and place. He revolutionized medicine by performing animal experiments, out of which he developed the first medical theories based on scientific investigations. Although many of Galen's theories proved wrong because they assumed animal studies would apply directly to human beings, his place as the founder of experimental medicine is unchallenged. His followers were called eclectic because they treated disease with whatever they found to work. Most frequently what worked for Galen were herbal remedies, but his followers also used mineral potions. Later, the divergent medical theories of allopathic (cure a disease by its "opposite") and homeopathic ("like cures like") medicine would both grow out of Galen's doctrines.

Medicine Under the Church

From about A.D. 400 to 1500, a period that included the Crusades and the Inquisition, the church controlled almost all medical knowledge and aspired to absolute power in its domain. Medicine, as the treatment of human illness, became an extension of church teachings. Since sickness and disease were often seen as punishments for sin, they could be cured mainly by prayer and repentance. But much Greek and Latin medical knowledge was nevertheless preserved, as scholars in monasteries transcribed ancient documents.

Although the church made a point of discrediting much of what non-Christian scholars had advanced, its official strictures did not reach into the herb gardens of the monasteries and country people. There, herbalism contin-

Pliny (A.D. 23/24–79)

"To live is to be awake" was the credo of the Roman administrator and natural historian Pliny. His *Natural History* in 37 books was a major source for herbalists and botanists from medieval times through the 17th century. Books 12 through 19 of the *Natural History* deal with botany, and Books 20 through 27 with plant pharmacology. Pliny and the Greek doctor Dioscorides, his contemporary, have been cited by writers on medicinal plants down to the present century. Generations of authors passed along Pliny's words without attributing them to him—so that a number of his statements of fact and fancy have entered the folklore of plants. Pliny died in a way befitting a true naturalist: he went to investigate an eruption of Vesuvius, and on a beach near Pompeii succumbed to the sulfurous fumes. A vivid account of this final scene exists in a letter written by Pliny's nephew, who is called Pliny the Younger to distinguish him from his uncle, who is sometimes known as Pliny the Elder.

Galen (C. A.D. 130–200)

The most famous physician of his day and a prolific medical writer, Galen found his intellectual inspiration in Greek thought: the medicine of Hippocrates, the science of Aristotle, the philosophy of Plato. Born in Pergamum (now Bergama, Turkey), Galen determined when he was 16 years old to bring precision to the study of medicine. He studied and traveled for the next 12 years, spending probably several years at Alexandria, the chief medical center of the age. After returning to Pergamum and serving as a physician to the gladiators there, Galen went to Rome, about 161. He soon numbered influential Romans among his admiring patients and thus began his long association with Rome's rich and powerful. Although he taught the now antiquated concept of medicine as adjusting the body's basic humors, Galen also believed in testing medicines empirically, a very modern stance. Not until the 16th and 17th centuries did challenges arise to his medical authority. The terms "galenicals" and "galenic products" today refer to medicinal substances extracted from plants by methods associated with Galen.

ued largely undisturbed, albeit with an increasingly Christian orientation. It was during this period, for example, that many plants acquired names linked to Jesus, the Virgin Mary, saints, and martyrs.

Moreover, in the latter part of the medieval period, the church actively encouraged two major advances in medicine. One was the hospital, a system of caring for the sick without charge, established in Byzantium by charitable Christians largely in reaction to the high fees charged by Greco-Roman physicians. The Christian hospitals followed the example of the "storehouse of piety" founded during the fourth century A.D. by Basil the Great, bishop

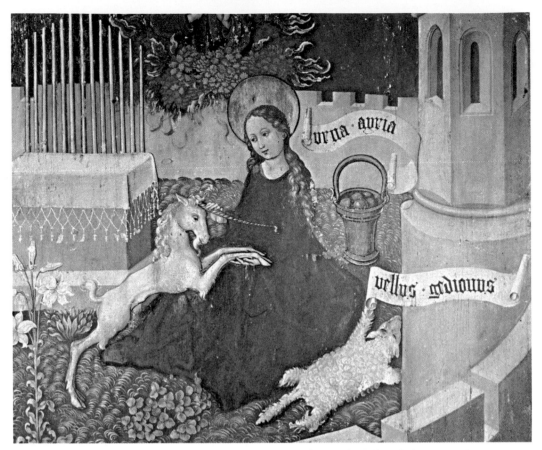

In the Middle Ages, Christian and pagan beliefs mixed, allowing herbal medicine to survive.

of Caesarea (now Kayseri, Turkey), to provide care and shelter for the sick—primarily lepers—and for travelers.

Christianity's second great contribution to medicine was the establishment of the first university medical schools. According to some reports, students were admitted to these schools without regard to creed or nationality. The famous medical school at Salerno was founded by four men, known to tradition as Adale the Arab, Salernus the Latin, Pontus the Greek, and Elinus the Jew.

Students at the Salerno school were apparently active experimenters with the medicinal properties of plants. One of their concoctions was an anesthetic—used in amputations—that contained opium, mandragora, and henbane in equal parts, pounded and mixed with water. Pressed under the nostrils on a wet cloth, it reportedly put a patient into a deep sleep, impervious to pain.

Arab Medicine and Alchemy

Outside the Christian world, the culture of Islam was rediscovering the medical works of the Greeks. Translating these original works into their own language, the Arabs made refinements based on their own experience. They added plants such as camphor, saffron, and spinach to the classical pharmacopeia.

Rhazes, a physician born in Persia in the late ninth century, wrote a famous treatise correctly describing smallpox and measles for the first time. And a hundred years later, Islam gave to history the "prince of physicians," Avicenna. His *Canon of Medicine* contains many references to the teachings of Galen and Aristotle. The *Canon* was used as a textbook in medical

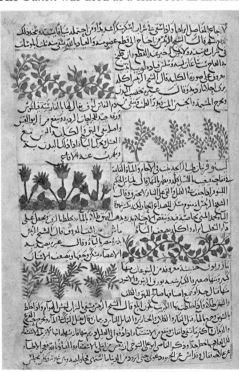

Old Arabian herbal: beauty and precision.

56

schools throughout Europe well into the 17th century and is still studied in the East. In it, Avicenna described meningitis, tetanus, and many other disorders.

Islam created secular hospitals, formalized medical education, and began to require examination and licensing of physicians. A Jewish physician and philosopher practicing in Cairo in the 12th century, Maimonides (or Moses ben Maimon), was part of this tradition. His principles of medical ethics and his aphorisms are still quoted today.

Through the Arabs, also, came the peculiar mixture of philosophy and chemistry known as alchemy, whose origins, in such widely separated parts of the world as ancient Alexandria and China, are still not fully known. Despite

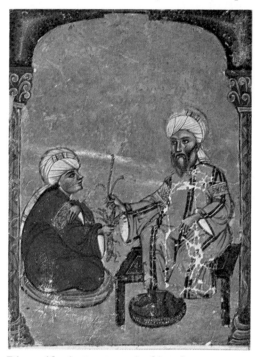

Dioscorides instructs an Arabian doctor.

Avicenna (980–1037)

When he was barely out of his teens, the Persian philosopher-statesman Avicenna earned a reputation as a healer by curing a ruler of a critical illness. Thereafter he was in demand as a physician and adviser to princes. For the rest of his life, he worked by day as a minister of state and wrote by night on an encyclopedic range of subjects: medicine, natural history, physics, chemistry, astronomy, mathematics, music, economics, political science, and theology. His poetry is quoted in the Arab world to this day. The most important of his 131 authenticated works is the voluminous *Canon of Medicine,* based on the Greek writings of Hippocrates, Aristotle, Dioscorides, Galen, and others. To their work Avicenna added his own theoretical and empirical observations. Book 2 of the *Canon* contains Avicenna's pharmacology of herbs. He also discussed various remedies such as chicory, oxymel, and balsam. Latin translations of the *Canon* existed within a century after Avicenna's death, and it was the basic medical text at all medieval universities both Christian and Moslem. The scientific revolution of the West was cruel to Avicenna. Leonardo da Vinci (1452–1519) rejected his anatomy; the Swiss physician Paracelsus (1493–1541) burned a copy of the *Canon* while teaching medicine in Switzerland; and William Harvey (1578–1657), the English physician who discovered the circulation of the blood, demolished Avicenna's theories on this important subject.

its shroud of secrecy, alchemy had become well established in Europe by the 13th century. Alchemy's goal was to use the laboratory to penetrate the secrets of nature and the universe. Alchemists worked with many materials, including metals. This led to the popular conception of alchemists as trying to turn base metals into gold.

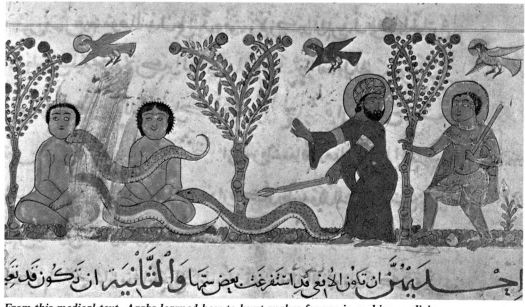

From this medical text, Arabs learned how to hunt snakes for use in making medicine.

Pietro Mattioli (1501–77)

A typical Renaissance man, the Italian physician-naturalist Pietro Mattioli published a number of works in poetry and prose on a wide range of subjects, including botany and pharmacology. After studying as a youth in Padua and Rome, he began a lifetime career as a practicing physician, first to the cardinal of Trent and then, later in his life, to the court of the Holy Roman emperor in Prague. All during these years, he devoted a great deal of time to the study of plants and "materia medica," or medicinal substances. The publication that made Mattioli famous was his Italian edition of Dioscorides' *De Materia Medica.* Its purpose was to give Italian physicians and pharmacists systematically organized information that would enable them to identify the medicinal plants discussed in the ancient Greek doctor's herbal, then a still highly trusted source. The book was a best-seller from its first printing, in 1544. A decade later, Mattioli issued an expanded edition in Latin. It included the plant names and their synonyms in various languages, a much expanded commentary, and many illustrations. Conceived as a practical reference tool, the book was so successful that it went into an uninterrupted series of reprints over the next 200 years. Mattioli continued to publish books on related subjects, including a lengthy work on identifying and collecting medicinal plants.

Many Arab physicians, including Rhazes and Avicenna, were alchemists. They experimented with medicinal uses of minerals, trying to turn them into forms that would work more effectively. Chief among these minerals was mercury, which they used extensively in treating skin diseases. Thus began mercury's long, widespread, and often disastrous use in the treatment of many illnesses, including most notoriously syphilis.

The golden age of Arab medicine came to an end with the invasion of the Mongols in the 13th century. The medical school at Salerno had begun to decline, but one at Montpellier, France, and another at Paris were in full flourish. Meanwhile, perhaps the most famous medical school of all had been founded at the University of Bologna. The first dawn of the Renaissance was starting to light the European sky, and medicine began to free itself from the strictures of the church.

The Renaissance

In the theater at the University of Bologna, at the end of the 13th century, dissections of human cadavers were being done. This was the beginning of truly scientific studies of the human body by physicians. But it was an artist, not a physician, who a century later would revolutionize the science of anatomy.

The great Leonardo da Vinci, driven by a desire to learn more about the structure of the human body, performed many dissections. The result was one of the world's greatest artistic and scientific treasures—more than 750 drawings by Leonardo that accurately illustrated human anatomy. Leonardo's works were followed by those of Andreas Vesalius, a physician who was a professor of medicine at the University of Padua. Vesalius' dissections resulted in the first scientific anatomy text, *On the Fabric of the Human Body,* published in 1543. It became the basis of modern anatomical studies, correcting and superseding much of Galen's work. The works of Leonardo and Vesalius transformed surgery. In the vanguard of this transformation was Ambroise Paré, a 16th-century French army surgeon, who is known as the father of modern surgery.

Herbal medicine also experienced a kind of rebirth in the new editions of Dioscorides, most notably those published by Pietro Mattioli (sometimes Latinized as Mattheolus).

Paracelsus' Influential Ideas

Yet another figure from the Renaissance would influence the underlying philosophy of medicine for centuries to come: Theophrastus Bombastus von Hohenheim, a Swiss physician better known as Paracelsus. He is generally regarded as a popularizer of the famous doctrine of signatures—or at any rate, as its prominent exponent in Europe during the Renaissance. In this very man-centered view of nature, not only are plants created for man's use, but also each plant displays a clear sign— a signature—of the purpose for which it is intended. Thus, Chinese lantern, with its calyx shaped like a bladder, is meant to cure urinary disorders; a plant with heart-shaped leaves is meant for treating heart disease, and so on. Whatever the merit of the doctrine of signatures, Paracelsus is regarded by many as the father of chemical pharmacology. He was the first to champion the importance of chemistry in preparing drugs.

A student of alchemy, Paracelsus advocated the internal use of metals, such as mercury and antimony, until then used almost exclusively as external medications. Unfortunately, many of those who later prescribed metals (and other dangerous substances) for internal use failed to remember the care and caution with which Paracelsus measured and administered the doses of medicine he gave patients. "It depends only upon the dose," Paracelsus wrote, "whether a poison is poison or not." Paracelsus' philosophy of prescribing dosages has been described as "a lot kills, a little cures."

Paracelsus is also regarded as a founder of homeopathy, the system of medicine based on the proposition that like cures like. Some 300 years later, a German physician named Samuel Hahnemann introduced homeopathic practice on a large scale. Homeopaths believe that symptoms are the body's way of ridding itself

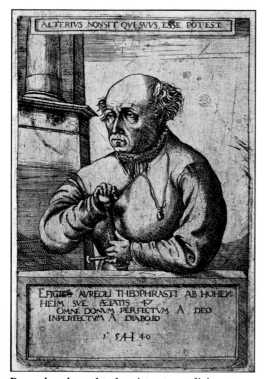

Paracelsus brought chemistry to medicine.

Paracelsus (1493–1541)

The prime mover of a new direction in medicine was named at birth Theophrastus Bombastus von Hohenheim, but later took the name Philippus Aureolus Paracelsus. The Swiss-born physician, who was also an able chemist, realized that the virtues of medicinal plants came from their chemical makeup. He pioneered in the extraction of plant essences and the use of tinctures, a revolutionary advance over the pharmacology of his day, which settled for less meticulous ways of producing drugs. Paracelsus was educated in botany, mineralogy, natural philosophy, and the occult, and he traveled widely, ministering to the poor wherever he went. He was fired from his position at the University of Basel for disrespect for the establishment. His published pharmacological research and his unfinished herbal, *On the Virtues of Plants, Roots, and Seeds*, reveal his extensive work with botanical medicine both in the laboratory and in his practice. The doctrine of signatures in plants—that in the appearance of plants can be found a divine sign of their curative powers—appears often in his works and in the writings of his influential followers. The doctrine left an enduring imprint on herbal medicine.

of disease. Thus, minuscule doses of drugs that produce the same symptoms as a disease will stimulate a healthy person's defense mechanisms for fighting that disease.

Toward Modern Medicine

The scientific curiosity awakened during the Renaissance was gradually adding to man's knowledge of himself. In the early 1600's, William Harvey produced the first true explanation of how blood circulates. The development of the microscope in the late 1600's by the Dutch scientist Anton van Leeuwenhoek made possible the study of microorganisms. In 1796, Edward Jenner used cowpox to immunize a young boy against smallpox, and the science of immunology was born.

The pace of medical discovery quickened dramatically in the 19th century. The germ theory of disease was established by Louis Pasteur and Robert Koch. Antiseptic surgery was introduced, thanks to Ignaz Semmelweis, who first stressed the need for cleanliness in childbirth, and Joseph Lister, who actually made the connection between cleanliness and the absence of germs. In the 1840's, William T. Morton, a dentist, demonstrated the value of ether as a relatively safe anesthetic, thus making difficult operations easier and less risky. In 1895, Wilhelm Roentgen reported the discovery of what was to become one of medicine's most valuable diagnostic tools—X-rays. Three years later, in 1898, Marie and Pierre Curie discovered the radioactive element radium, used in the treatment of cancer and other diseases.

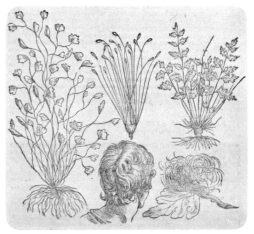

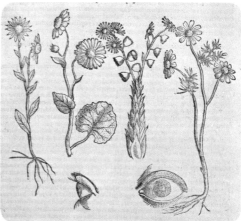

"Doctrine of signatures": hairlike plants made hair grow; eyed flowers gave sharp vision.

59

The Persistence of Herbal Medicine

Alongside this burst of scientific and technological discovery, the story of plants as medicine had continued to unfold, however quietly and independently. Rich herbal traditions reach far back in Europe. During the eighth century, for example, the emperor Charlemagne named a group of herbs to be grown within his domain. Among them was houseleek, to be planted on the rooftops as a protection against lightning (still done in some regions), as well as roses and lilies.

Europe's Great Herbals

In Britain, following its fifth-century invasion by Germanic tribes, the medical texts were Anglo-Saxon translations of Latin manuscripts, called leech books. These were essentially herbals, books about herbs and their medicinal uses. The name came from *laece*, an Old English word meaning "physician." One of the best known of these Anglo-Saxon herbals is *Bald's Leechbook*. (Bald was the name of the manuscript's first owner.) Written in the 10th century, Bald's book combines the herbal lore of ancient Britain with prescriptions from the East. These had been sent by the patriarch of Jerusalem to Alfred the Great, king of the West Saxons at the end of the ninth century.

British herbalists at this time knew upwards of 500 medicinal plants. Their use, as recorded by Bald, was closely involved with the myths and superstition of pagan rites.

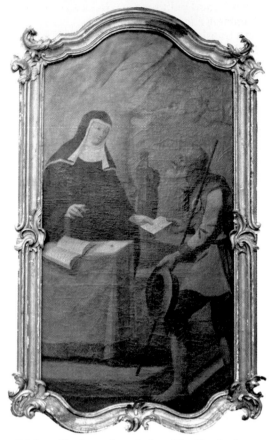

Hildegard had vast knowledge of healing herbs.

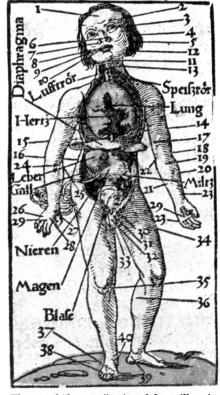

Theory of "humors" reigned for millennia.

However, it was not pagan institutions but Christian monasteries that were the repositories of medical knowledge during the Middle Ages, and this knowledge encompassed medicinal plants and their applications. In the 12th century, Hildegard of Bingen, a German abbess, compiled a *Book of Healing Herbs*. Her book described a wide range of plants and their applications in healing, as well as the origin and treatment of various diseases.

As the Age of Exploration began to widen Europeans' geographical horizons, it was inevitable that their scientific horizons should also expand. Travelers to far-off lands discovered diverse civilizations, each with its own customs and practices, which included medicine based on local plants. Along with other treasures, explorers brought back samples of native botanical specimens. Later, as colonists settled in the new lands, the exchange of botanical samples between continents became, for a time, a flourishing business.

The influx of never-before-seen plants sparked a tremendous fascination with botany among Europeans. One result was a "golden age of herbals." The most famous herbals in the English language were published in Britain during the 15th, 16th, and 17th centuries. The *Grete Herball* was published anonymously in 1526, followed, in the mid-16th century, by an herbal written by William Turner, considered to be the father of English botany. In 1597, John Gerard published the *Herball or Generall Historie of Plantes*. This was in large part based on a translation of a book written by Rembert Dodoens, a botanist who lived in what is now Belgium. To Dodoens's work Gerard added his own observations of familiar plants, and the

Hildegard of Bingen (1098–1179)

A medieval pioneer in natural science was the mystic Hildegard of Bingen, abbess of the Rupertsberg convent in the Rhineland. A Benedictine nun from age 15, Hildegard was taught the ancient doctrine of the humors, according to which the "cardinal juice" called phlegm caused most illness. She added her own broad knowledge of folk medicine, her interest in nature, and her highly developed powers of intuition. (Visions commanded her: "Write what you see and hear.") Her writings on the natural world include much on healing herbs. She is often called St. Hildegard although she was never formally canonized.

Herball included 1,800 woodcut illustrations. A surgeon and an apothecary (mixer and dispenser of drugs, the forerunner of today's pharmacist), Gerard had his own garden of medicinal herbs in London.

Kindly, Controversial Culpeper

Possibly the most famous herbal of all was *The English Physician*, written by Nicholas Culpeper and published in 1653. In 1649 Culpeper's English translation of the Latin *Pharmacopoeia* of the College of Physicians had been published. These books were extremely controversial and played a major role in the ultimate schism that developed between formal medicine and the practice of herbalism. Part of the blame for this lies in the fact that Culpeper was a believer in astrology, which led him to write that the planets governed both diseases and the plants used to treat them. But the controversy Culpeper provoked can also be attributed partly to the self-interest and narrow-minded dogmatism of the era's medical establishment.

Nicholas Culpeper was studying medicine at Cambridge when his fiancee was killed in a thunderstorm. Evidently overwhelmed by this tragedy, he gave up his studies and apprenticed himself to an apothecary. Eventually Culpeper set up his own healing practice near London. He was struck and saddened by the hardship of the working people he saw around him. To help these people, he began to sell them medicines cheap.

In Culpeper's London, restrictions governing who could, or could not, treat illness were not nearly so strict as they are today. Physicians who had received formal training at university medical schools practiced side by side with apothecaries, alchemists, and other dispensers of medicines, including all manner of quacks.

As for herbal remedies, they still made up the major portion of the medicines and drugs listed in the pharmacopeias of the day. However, medical fashion was swinging toward the use of various nonbotanical medications, some of which had been experimented with, off and on, since antiquity. Mercury (usually in the form of mercurous chloride, or calomel), arsenic, copper sulfate, iron, and sulfur began to come more into vogue among 17th-century physicians. Thus some treatments—such as botanicals and metals—were dispensed with equal license by formally schooled physicians and by apothecaries like Nicholas Culpeper. The physicians probably resented the competition and proceeded to try to discredit the popular Culpeper.

To some, Culpeper's theory of astrology was reason enough to discredit him. Even today, though, there are passionate defenders of Culpeper who argue that his astrology was no more ridiculous—and a lot less harmful—than the physicians' idea of curing a disease by letting huge amounts of blood out of a patient's veins, or the practice of administering powerful laxatives and emetics to purge one and restore one's humors to balance, or feeding a patient massive doses of mercury, now known to cause severe, permanent damage when it does not kill.

Furthermore, astrology was enjoying wide favor in Culpeper's England as well as in other parts of northern Europe. The German mystic Jakob Böhme (1575–1624) had connected the movements and positions of heavenly bodies with herbal healing in his book *The Signature of All Things*. Böhme was not the first to associate astrology and the practice of medicine. Such

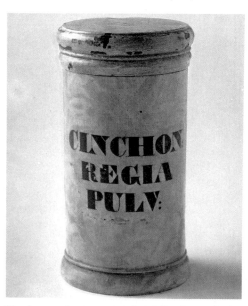

Cinchona: plant source of quinine for malaria.

Nicholas Culpeper (1616–54)

"He is arrived at the battlement of an absolute atheist, and by two years' drunken labor hath gallimaufred the apothecaries' book into nonsense, mixing every receipt [recipe] therein with . . . rebellion or atheism, besides the danger of poisoning men's bodies." Thus did the English medical establishment, in the royalist periodical *Mercurius Pragmaticus*, greet the publication of *A Physical Directory, or a Translation of the London Dispensatory,* by Nicholas Culpeper. His mistake was to have translated the Latin pharmacopeia into everyday language, thus threatening the near monopoly on medical knowledge that the College of Physicians enjoyed. A clergyman's son, Culpeper attended Cambridge University and was well versed in Greek, Latin, and both classical and contemporary medical authors. About 1640 he set up as an apothecary-astrologer-healer in Spitalfields, near London. He fought against the royalists in the English Civil War, suffering a chest wound that may have hastened his early death from consumption. Besides *A Physical Directory,* Culpeper published *The English Physician,* which included "369 medicines made of English herbs." He wrote many other works, all of which sold well and angered the medical establishment.

views reach perhaps as far back as 2000 B.C. to the ancient Babylonians.

So it seems that Culpeper may have incurred the wrath of the College of Physicians far less for his theories of medicine than because first, he came from outside their ranks, and second, his *A Physical Directory* made the secrets of their Latin *Pharmacopoeia* more accessible to the English folk. Furthermore, because he felt that the traditional herbals relied too much on foreign plants, he told his patients where to find local species that worked just as well. And he charged lower fees than the physicians did.

Two other famous herbals entered the medical literature in the 17th century: *Theatrum Botanicum,* published in 1640 by John Parkinson, a renowned British herbalist and apothecary; and *The Art of Simpling,* by William Coles, who enthusiastically espoused the doctrine of signatures put forward by Paracelsus. ("Simpling" in Coles' title derives from an old sense of the word *simple,* "medicinal herb.") Nevertheless, it is Culpeper's *The English Physician* that is best known today. Periodically reissued under different titles and sometimes updated with modern commentary, it continues to inform and delight students of herbalism and plant lore.

Culpeper himself was greatly loved by the people of England, very likely in return for his genuine concern for them. The colonists took his herbal with them to the New World both as a medical reference and, because of its astrological commentary, as a guide to when to plant and when to harvest.

The Great Plant Trade

Early settlers in North America quickly discovered that many plants that had always been familiar to them and were recommended in their herbals could not be found in their new home. As a result, a business developed in the importation of seeds and plants from Europe. Many of these eventually escaped cultivation to become naturalized in the New World.

This plant migration was not one-sided, for botanists were eager to expand their knowledge. As new plants were discovered in the colonies, samples were dispatched to the Old World. In 1577 a London merchant named John Frampton published *Joyful Newes out of the Newe Founde Worlde,* an English version of a book by the Spanish physician Nicolás Monardes. The "joyful news" was of the vast array of medicinal plants that explorers and colonists had found in America.

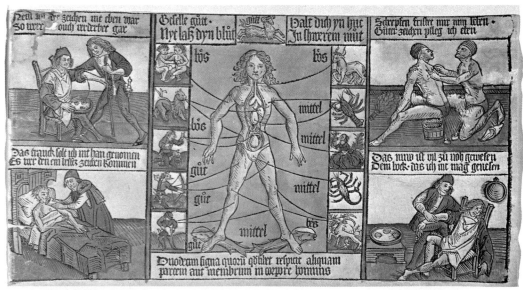

Not only did 16th-century doctors bleed their patients, they also relied on astrological signs.

Schism: Academics Versus Healers

The period from the dawn of the Renaissance to modern times was one of heated disputes in medicine. The establishment of university medical schools and of a system of formal medical education, coupled with the increasingly accurate understanding of human physiology, was changing the practice of medicine from an art into a science and a profession. But long before this metamorphosis was complete, an ugly schism opened between the new, academically trained physicians and the traditional healers. With hindsight, today's scholars see right and wrong on both sides of this conflict, which lasted into the 20th century.

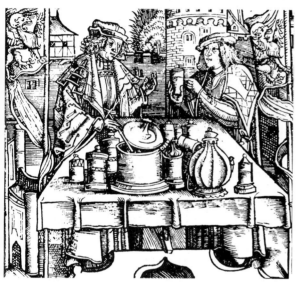

Medicine-maker stirs up potent brew, 1500's.

The Boerhaave Model

To complicate matters further, not all the academic, or "regular," physicians agreed with one another regarding the proper approach to diagnosis and treatment. About the beginning of the 18th century, a Dutch academic physician named Hermann Boerhaave set forth a theoretical approach to medicine. He maintained that health was the proper interaction of body solids and fluids, and developed a system of medicine based on that concept. Boerhaave's medical views reflected many recent scientific discoveries. He has been called the father of clinical medicine for his insistence that all theory must be confirmed by clinical observation, a dictum that many academic physicians unfortunately disregarded.

Boerhaave's theories of medicine influenced medical practice for the next several generations. Thus a typical 18th-century European physician was very likely a theorist trained according to Boerhaave's principles. Such a Boerhaave disciple believed that to heal his patient the physician must prescribe not for the symptoms, but for the underlying condition: blood too viscid or too thin, humors too acidic or too oily, body fluids circulating too freely or stagnating. The Boerhaave disciple typically disassociated himself from the nonacademic traditional healer, who prescribed herbs known to be effective against the symptoms at hand.

Moderates Versus Extremists

Meanwhile, a heated battle was raging within the profession of academic medicine. On one side were the Galenics, who adhered to the practice of botanic medicine as set forth by Galen in ancient times. On the other side were Paracelsans, who appear to have come to a somewhat selective understanding of Paracelsus' dicta. These latter-day Paracelsans felt that medicinal plants were generally inferior to the stronger medicine of nonbotanic chemicals, often administered in doses that would have horrified Paracelsus. To give them their due, these Paracelsans were quite willing to administer a plant drug, provided its action was powerful enough. They were fondest of narcotics and purgatives such as opium, belladonna, aconite, scammony, jalap, henbane, hemlock, and other poisonous plants because of their high level of "activity," as it was called.

Terrible Diseases, Terrible Cures

The plagues that swept Europe from the Middle Ages to early modern times were beyond the power of contemporary human medical specialists to cure. Yet strangely these terrible epidemics helped to further the belief that the stronger and more agonizing the cure, the more effective. Since mercury did seem effective against syphilis, Paracelsans were soon prescribing it indiscriminately, for everything, evidently under the impression that if a little is good, a lot is better.

It is probably an exaggeration—but not a great one—to say that between the 15th and the 20th century, more people were bled, purged, or poisoned to death by physicians than ever died of the diseases that physicians were supposed to cure. Despite the fact that many people of the time, including a lot of physicians, seem to have recognized this fact, regular medicine continued to consist for generations of mercury (or antimony or some equally dangerous brew) and a sharpened lancet for making surgical incisions and drawing blood. Many physicians must have known that metals sometimes killed patients. Yet if the disease would kill anyway, a metal potion might at least give the afflicted a chance.

It was not, incidentally, some breed of ignorant country folk who so trustingly presented themselves for this kind of medical treatment. Everybody, high and low, was sus-

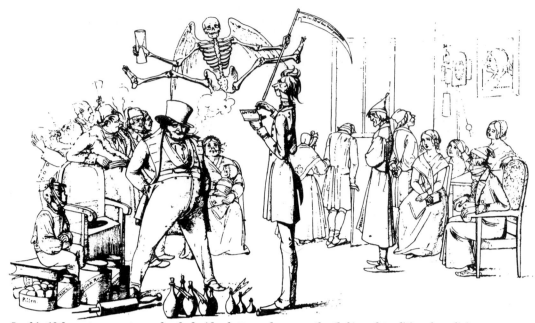

In this 19th-century cartoon, death decides between homeopathy (left) and traditional medicine.

ceptible to it because it seemed to be the best medicine available. Even such giants of science as Robert Hooke (1635–1703), the English experimental scientist who discovered plant cells, and Isaac Newton (1642–1727) dosed themselves regularly with concoctions that contained turpentine, metals, and a number of other noxious ingredients.

Alternative Systems

So traumatic were these approved cures, so agonizing for the patient, that eventually an array of alternative systems of medicine began to spring up both within the medical profession and without. One of the most influential of these was homeopathy. Rooted in Paracelsus' theory that like cures like, the homeopathic system of medicine was developed in Europe by a German physician named Samuel Hahnemann in the early 19th century and spread later to the United States. Homeopathy grew out of Hahnemann's observation that cinchona (Peruvian bark, the source of quinine) made people sweat profusely, just as patients did when they had malaria. He experimented by dosing himself with cinchona and eventually built up his own collection of drugs, each of which he and his pupils "proved," or tested on themselves in precisely the same manner that he had tested cinchona. A few of the drugs were from animals and minerals, but the majority were from plants.

In using any drug, Hahnemann was ever mindful of Paracelsus' caveat against overdosing his patients. Hahnemann frequently diluted his doses to the point that there was little of the active drug left. The science of immunology has long since confirmed the basis of Hahnemann's philosophy—that triggering the body's defense mechanisms is a key to curing illness. Such modern medical practices as vaccination and desensitization therapy for allergies reflect the validity of some homeopathic principles. As for the principle of the effectiveness of the minimal dose, consider radiation therapy for cancer, a treatment where minimal dosage is absolutely necessary to protect the life of the patient.

Another alternative system of medicine was eclecticism, established in New York by Dr. Wooster Beach. It eventually spread throughout the United States. In practicing eclecticism, Dr. Beach attempted to combine what was good in the old medicine with what was good in the new. His treatments relied heavily on plant drugs.

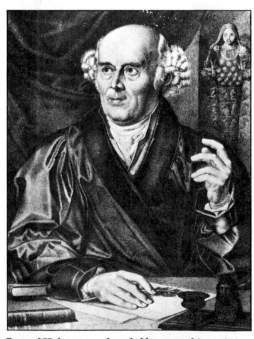

Samuel Hahnemann founded homeopathic medicine.

Samuel Hahnemann (1755–1843)

A towering figure in herbal tradition is that of the German chemist-physician Samuel Hahnemann, founder of the system of alternative medicine known as homeopathy. As a young man he retired from conventional medical practice in disgust at the excessive procedures—bleedings, debilitating purges, and dangerous drugs—that were then routinely prescribed. During the 1790's, Hahnemann made the discovery that Peruvian bark (also called cinchona, the source of quinine) was effective in treating malaria, and from this discovery deduced the basic principle of homeopathy: "Like cures like." What this meant, in practice, was that a minuscule dose of a drug capable of producing in a healthy person a response similar to a disease's primary symptom may produce a reaction that will overcome the disease in a sick person's body. This and related tenets set forth in Hahnemann's *Organon of Medicine* (1810) form the conceptual basis of homeopathy. An empirical basis was then provided by Hahnemann's monumental *Materia Medica Pura*, comprising detailed summaries of "provings" (proofs of effectiveness) for many, mainly plant, substances. Hahnemann's denunciations of the medical establishment and pharmaceutical industry, his use of plant tinctures, and his counsels of moderation in diet and the ingestion of coffee, tea, alcohol, and tobacco presage views heard in the late 20th century.

Thomson's Herbal Sweats

Not all of those who championed alternative medical systems were trained physicians. Samuel Thomson was a New England healer who attracted thousands of followers in the United States in the 1820's and 1830's. He had cured his daughter of a serious illness after the family doctor had given her up. Noticing that the child was struggling for breath, Thomson held her over a bath filled with steaming water for 20 minutes until she breathed easily. (It was a technique he may have learned from the Indians, whose sweat lodges were part of their medical tradition.)

Thereafter, Thomson traveled the New England states advocating the use of steam and roots and herbs to cure. His favorite plant drug was a lobelia, Indian tobacco, which he used as an emetic. The Indians also used it for this purpose and as an aid to respiration in treating asthma and similar breathing disorders.

Thomson used approximately 65 plants in his herbal practice, but his place in history is as the advocate of steam and lobelia to cure nearly everything. Unfortunately, although his original motivation was largely altruistic, he eventually became as dogmatic about his system of medicine as the medical establishment was about the use of mercury and mercury compounds such as calomel.

Proponents of various other alternative systems proselytized on both sides of the Atlantic. Some of them were physicians, others folk healers like Thomson. Almost all these alternative healers displayed refreshing elements of open-mindedness, common sense, and human kindness; yet many, like Thomson, eventually closed their minds to theories other than their own —rather like the medical establishment and its mercury.

Just as there were many quacks poisoning people with metals and toxic plants, there were an appalling number of regular physicians doing precisely the same thing. The conflict was not really over what would cure, but rather over who had a legal license to kill. So while the botanic doctors may have had less understanding of pathology than did the regular physicians, their medicines were rarely fatal and occasionally made their patients feel better.

Enter Linnaeus

Meanwhile, there had been scholarly efforts to catalog and classify ailments, work begun by

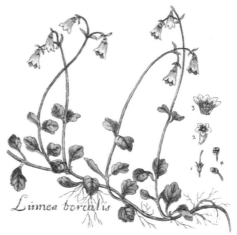

A genus named for Linnaeus: botany and herbal medicine were never the same after his work.

the English physician Thomas Sydenham in the 17th century. Contributors to this science of nosology, as it is called, included the Swedish physician and naturalist Carolus Linnaeus, who had already developed a system of classifying plants according to their mode of reproduction. In his *Systema Naturae* he divided plants into 24 classes, mostly according to the number of stamens (male reproductive parts) each possessed. Each class was then divided into orders, according to the number of pistils (female parts); then into genera, based on the way the stamens and pistils functioned; and finally into species. Thus, a plant with the designation *Anchusa officinalis* L. would be the species *officinalis* of the genus *Anchusa*, as classified by Linnaeus (L.). The *Systema Naturae* extended this classification system to animals too, and though it was not always accurate, it established the basis of modern

Carolus Linnaeus (1707–78)

No less an ambition than to name and to categorize everything in the "three kingdoms" of nature—plants, animals, and minerals—inspired young Carolus Linnaeus (or Carl von Linné). Aiming so high, this great Swedish scientist fell short, but he put his stamp on all future botanical study. Linnaeus' preeminence in the intellectually rigorous field of botanical taxonomy—plant classification—has tended to obscure his joyful enthusiasm for roaming the Scandinavian countryside on collecting expeditions. Nor is it generally remembered that Linnaeus received his doctorate in medicine in Holland and lectured at the University of Uppsala (Sweden) on such subjects as how to cope with the pressures of modern life. Although his criteria for classifying plants have undergone revision, binomial nomenclature—his system of two-part names, genus and species—has continued to serve science well. His preoccupation with taxonomy, some say, set back other aspects of botanical study, such as plant physiology. Linnaeus' fame was assured as much by his devoted students, who traveled the world collecting plants in his behalf, as by his written works such as *Systema Naturae* and *Philosophia Botanica*.

taxonomy, the science of classification.

Linnaeus moved botany a giant step in the direction of modern science, just as others were moving medicine in the same direction. Yet in some ways the schism between medicine and botany was never deeper than it was in the 18th and 19th centuries.

Withering's Herbal Science

The story of William Withering, a young physician in 18th-century England, illustrates both the depth and the folly of the distrust between the regular physicians, Withering's peer group, and the herbal healers. Had he not begun to collect plants for the woman patient whom he later married, Withering might never have become familiar with some of the herbs used by folk healers in the English countryside where he and his wife settled down to live. And so he might never have paid attention to the secret cure for dropsy administered by an old woman in Shropshire.

On further investigating the old woman's secret cure, Withering recognized the action of foxglove, and he began to study its use in treating the fluid retention, called edema or dropsy, that can be a sign of congestive heart failure. After years of careful experimentation,

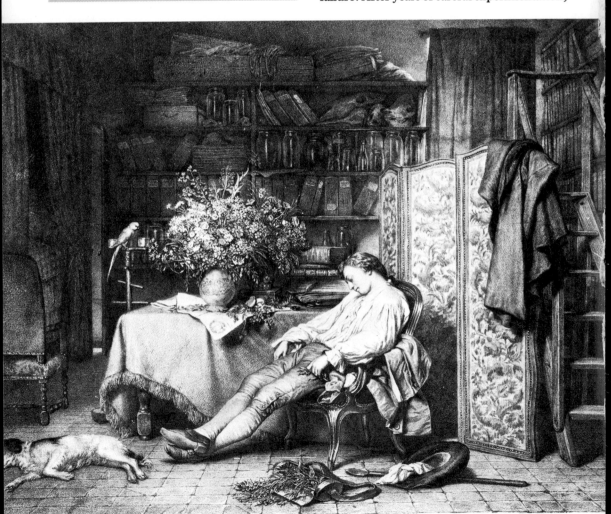

Linnaeus' capacity for work awed friends. In this painting, he catnaps after collecting.

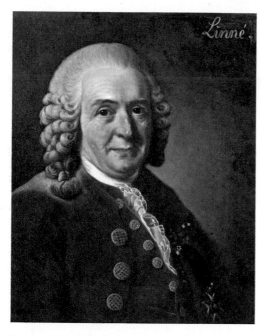

Linnaeus was the father of modern taxonomy.

he standardized procedures for gathering, preparing, and administering the drug in proper doses and gave to the world its active ingredient, digitalin (also commonly called digitalis), which would later become, for a time, the principal medicine used to treat this type of heart disease. Despite Withering's long and careful clinical trials, which proved both the efficacy of foxglove and its danger when improperly prescribed, organized medicine generally ignored his findings and continued to use it as a powerful purgative and emetic, or as a sedative. When their patients died from overdoses, physicians condemned the drug.

New World, Same Medicine

This same kind of behavior permeated the medical establishment of the New World as well. The fact that scurvy wrought havoc among the white settlers but rarely affected the Indians led few regular physicians to wonder whether the Indian diet of fresh fruit and vegetables or the Indians' habit of drinking spruce tea had anything to do with the Native Americans' freedom from the devastating effects of vitamin C deficiency.

Like their European counterparts, North American physicians relied on bleeding, mercury, antimony, and powerful plant purges to treat any and all illnesses. One account tells how physicians treated the final illness of George Washington. Suffering from sore throat, chills, and fever, the man citizens of the United States call "the father of our country" sent for his physicians. They extracted over four pints of blood from his 67-year-old body (enough to send him into acute shock), dosed him with mercury and antimony, gave him a cathartic enema, and blistered his throat and feet. Washington was dead within 24 hours.

What the Indians Taught

On the farms and vast frontiers of the new land, there were few doctors. The settlers, forced to attend to their own illnesses, learned much by listening to and watching the Indians.

The Native Americans had extensive knowledge of medicinal plants and their uses. They could also teach white settlers about surgical techniques, setting fractures and replacing dislocations, healing wounds, and making birth safer. They were less accomplished in treating infectious diseases, because few Indian medicines were effective against the ravages of chicken pox, diphtheria, malaria, measles, scarlet fever, smallpox, typhoid, tuberculosis, and other sicknesses introduced by the white man.

The Indians' knowledge of medicine was empiric. It was empiric despite the insistence of their shamans (medicine men and women) that the secrets of healing came from dreams, and despite the Indians' belief in their own doctrine of signatures, which held that every plant, bush, and tree had a special use, frequently proclaimed (so they believed) by the plant's appearance.

For Indians, the ultimate test of a medicine's value was its effect on the human body.

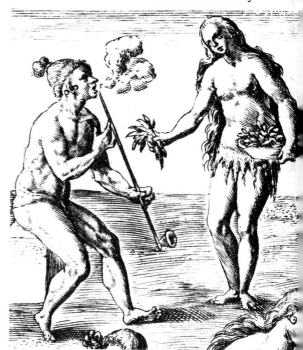

Florida's Indians smoked tobacco as medicine.

This was determined through trial and error and careful observation: in other words, through empiric and clinical procedures. Occasionally, a potential cure turned out to be poison. But when a remedy worked, it remained in the Indians' pharmacopeia, which was typically small but effective.

Indian medical training has parallels in modern organized medicine. Among the Chippewas, for example, the aspiring young shaman received a broad education in the various types of plant medicines and their uses. Then the student began to specialize, learning all about one disease or group of related diseases and about the plants that were effective in treatment. This knowledge represented the accumulated medical experience of the tribe.

The Indians added many drugs to our modern pharmacopeia, including cascara sagrada, Indian tobacco, American ginseng, joe-pye weed, mayapple, goldenseal, sassafras, and witch hazel, to name but a few. In South America, Indians taught Spanish colonists the medicinal uses of ipecac, Peruvian bark (the source of quinine), and coca.

Heyday for Patent Medicines

American frontiers also represented golden territory for enterprising purveyors of quack remedies and bottled cure-alls, for many communities had no physicians at all, or else were served by "doctors" who had served as apprentices to physicians or perhaps had no training all. Patent medicines were already becoming popular in England, and many were imported to America. Among these were Dover's Powder (containing opium and ipecac), Duffy's Elixir (senna, a plant laxative), and James Fever Powder (antimony).

Probably the most common ingredient of these medicines—few of which were actually

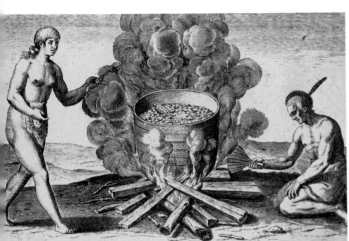
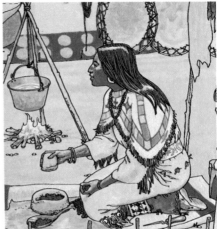

In Virginia (left), then in the West (right), Europeans benefited from Indian medicine.

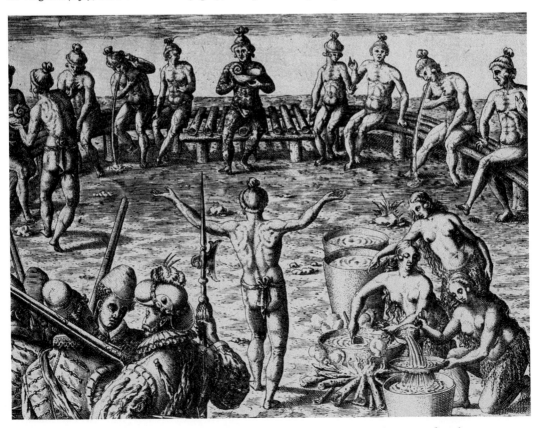

At Timucua councils, downing strong herb tea, which caused copious sweating, proved one's competence.

patented, incidentally—was alcohol: their alcohol content was commonly 25 percent, or 50 proof. These frontier cocktails were trustingly quaffed by teetotaling pioneers and administered to children and infants. One of the most popular claims for patent medicines was that they "purified the blood"—a term that was carried over from the days when medicine was given to purge toxic materials and evil spirits from the body. Such medicines were touted as cures for everything from dropsy to cancer.

Observing the close bonds between the frontier people and their horses, patent-medicine peddlers were quick to concoct potions that could be used by both: liniments for sore muscles, both horse and human; and medicines to be swallowed according to the prescription "one for a man, two for a horse."

Eventually American apothecaries began to make up their own herbal preparations, many of whose ingredients would made a modern physician or pharmacist pale.

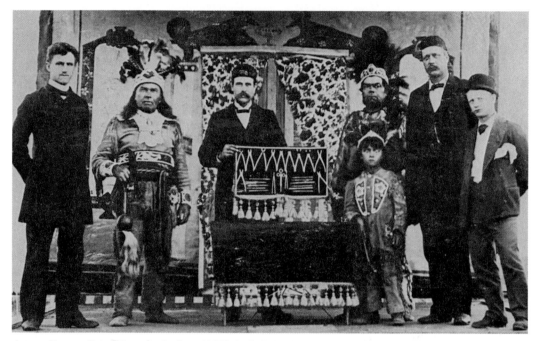

A traveling medicine show in the late 1800's included Indians who could demonstrate herbal treatments.

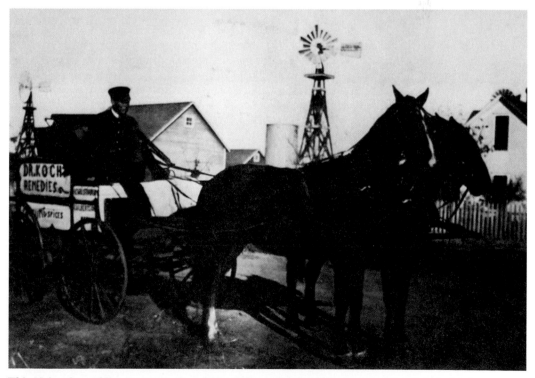

This Nebraska peddler was part of an $80-million-a-year business in patent medicine's heyday.

Medicine Becomes a Science

While vast backwaters of ignorance, dogmatic self-interest, and quackery continued to exist, the main current of medicine had entered its modern period by the early 20th century. The invention of the microscope, the germ theory of disease, the use of diagnostic X-rays, and many other technological advances brought a truer understanding of how the human body functions, what disease is, and how it is caused. Chemists had learned first, how to isolate the active substances in plants, and second, how to synthesize these chemicals in the laboratory. A true science of pharmacy developed, devoted to understanding how drugs work and why the body responds to them as it does.

New Medical Standards

At this time, too, moves were begun to standardize medical practice. In 1910, under the auspices of the Carnegie Foundation for the Advancement of Teaching, the American educator Abraham Flexner surveyed 155 medical schools in the United States and Canada. Flexner's conclusion: only Johns Hopkins Medical School in Baltimore provided an acceptable medical education. This led to important reforms.

Birth of Pharmaceutical Chemistry

The days of mercury and antimony and bleeding were past. The same fate—or so it seemed in the first heady years of pharmaceutical chemistry—was just around the corner for botanical medicines.

About 1805, Friedrich Sertürner had isolated the opium poppy's painkilling substance, morphine, a plant alkaloid. Soon his technique was being used to isolate the active substances in other plants. From such beginnings grew a pharmaceutical industry that not only could isolate the basic constituents of natural drugs, but could synthesize new substances in laboratories and supply them to physicians in stable, standardized doses.

These synthetics became almost an obsession with the fledgling medical science. "Made in the laboratory" came to connote more effective, more reliable, safer medicines than those that came from field or garden. Nor was this bias altogether misguided, having much common sense and solid evidence to support it.

William Withering, in his work with foxglove, had understood that the strength of an herb would vary at different periods of its growth. In order to insure the stability of his

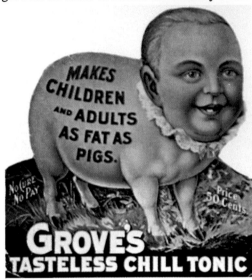

If plump meant healthy, this was one's tonic.

digitalis, he had always gathered his herb during its flowering period—when, he reasoned, its chemical activity would be at its peak. Others were not so intuitive. Gathering an herb too early or too late in its growth cycle, using dried instead of fresh, using different populations of the same plant or closely related species—all these factors might affect the stability of a drug. Chemicals made in laboratories were certainly likely to be more uniform.

Herbal Medicine Today

In the last few decades, a curious thing has happened to botanical medicine. Instead of being killed off by medical science and pharmaceutical chemistry, it has made a comeback. Botanical medicine has benefited from the objective analysis of medical science: while fanciful and emotional claims for herbal cures have been thrown out, herbal treatments and plant medicines that *work* have been acknowledged. And herbal medicine has been found to have some impressive credentials. No laboratory has yet produced a substitute for digitalis. The penicillin that replaced mercury in the treatment of syphilis and put an end to so many of the deadly epidemics comes from plant molds; it was discovered accidentally as it destroyed a bacterial culture that Alexander Fleming was trying to grow in his laboratory. Belladonna still provides the chemicals used in ophthalmological preparations and in antispasmodics used to treat gastrointestinal disorders. In fact, plant substances remain the basis for a very large proportion of the medications used today for treating heart disease, hypertension, depression, pain, cancer, asthma, neurological disorders, and other ailments.

Has medical science yet more to learn from the folk doctors? It seems likely. Consider *Rauvolfia serpentina*, the Indian snakeroot. Its active ingredient, reserpine, was the basic constituent of a variety of tranquilizers first used in the 1950's to treat certain types of emotional and mental problems. Though reserpine is seldom used today for this purpose, its discovery was a breakthrough in the treatment of mental illness. It is also the principal ingredient in a number of modern pharmaceutical preparations for treating hypertension. But reserpine can have a serious side effect— severe depression. On the other hand, a tea made of *R. serpentina* has been used in India as a sedative for thousands of years.

Or consider again the Chinese ephedra mentioned at the beginning of this chapter. For at least 2,000 years, traditional Chinese herbal doctors have been prescribing ephedra, or mahuang, tea to treat coughs, colds, asthma, bronchitis, and other respiratory problems. Its active ingredient, ephedrine, is used in modern pharmaceutical preparations for asthma and other respiratory problems because it clears the air passages and permits the patient to breathe more easily. But many patients cannot tolerate these preparations because ephedrine also makes the heart beat more rapidly and raises blood pressure. A physician practicing in Tucson, Arizona, however, gives his patients a tea made from an American species of ephedra that contains no ephedrine. This brew, the Tucson doctor says, gives his patients relief from asthma without the side effects associated with ephedrine.

The Synergy Question

Could the very purity of laboratory-isolated substances be a drawback? Do some natural plant medicines have ingredients that prevent dangerous side effects in human use? Perhaps. It is a research avenue that many scientists are now exploring. The idea certainly has popular appeal. A great many people, fearing the harmful effects of chemical substances, are leaning toward anything "natural," including medicinal plants and their products.

At Harvard University and at the University of Illinois at Chicago (among other institutions), scientists have reopened the field of botanical medicine and folk remedies. They are asking questions for which modern science, as yet, has no answers.

Why have certain plants been used to heal since prehistoric times? Do they really do what folk legend claims they will? If they do, precisely what makes them work?

And among the most fascinating questions of all: Is there sometimes a synergistic effect when the whole plant, as opposed to just the purified chemicals derived from it, is used? Could less pure extractions from the whole herb be more effective because the plant's constituents work synergistically: that is, make the total beneficial effect of the botanical medicine greater than what could be predicted by simply adding up the effects of its individual chemical constituents? In other words, is the action of a whole plant sometimes more than the sum of its chemical parts? Do some plants contain substances that neutralize the negative effects of the active chemical?

For scientific answers to the riddles of how plant medicines really work, researchers are seeking out shamans and folk healers practicing in remote corners of the world, particularly where trained physicians and hospitals are in short supply. There, most likely, is where folk doctors keep alive the age-old traditions of herbal medicine.

America's Practicing Herbalists

In the rural areas of Missouri's Ozark Mountains, many people are folk healers of sorts. Ozark gardens and woods and fields are filled with herbs that have been used in medicine as long as anyone can remember. The people brew their own remedies for use at home, and make up herbal teas to sell in shops. Local physicians sometimes prescribe plant medicine, with the caution that proper diagnosis must come first, or the would-be healer is likely to use the wrong herb to treat the wrong disease. In fact, this can be a deadly mistake in other ways, too, for many plants are poison, and even the safest of plants may be useless if not used properly.

In ancient times, garlic was looked upon as almost a cure-all, prescribed for a multitude of ills, including cardiovascular disorders. Today, Ozark herbalists continue to prescribe it to lower blood pressure.

The juice of the aloe vera plant, an ingredient in many suntan and skin lotions, is squeezed on burns to soothe and promote healing, and on poison ivy to stop itching. Mullein is smoked as a decongestant. The milky juice of wild lettuce is recommended to make a wart fall off. The inside bark of the slippery elm, dried and pounded to powder, is used to make a drink to soothe the throat and stomach. Violet leaves are used to make a "blood purifier," and dandelions are prescribed for kidney trouble.

In New Mexico, *curanderos* and *curanderas* use the manzanilla, a local chamomile, to treat colic and other infant ailments. They make a tea of yerba buena, a mint, to treat stomachache. A salve of comfrey is applied to pimples. A dandruff shampoo is made from yucca root. The osha root is chewed for toothache, headache, and indigestion; made into a poultice for sores; brewed into a tea for colds; and drunk prophylactically to prevent hangover. The *curanderos*' pharmacopeia includes sage and purple sagebrush, Mormon tea, and many less generally familiar plants such as *canutillo*,

71

mariola (an aster), and *yerba de la negrita* (a mallow), used to treat everything from rheumatism, urinary and kidney disorders, and congestion to skin ailments and fevers. They also mix wild cinnamon with a plant called *calabazilla* to make a pesticide, claiming it drives insects and mice out of the house.

The Papago Indians of Arizona generally use a team approach to medical practice. Actual procedures vary depending on the village and the medicine men in charge. Typically, a Papago diagnostician might speak to the patient about his illness, then sing and meditate until a diagnosis is revealed to him. The second member of the medical team is a singer, who in addition to singing, administers the remedy recommended by the diagnostician. Third is an herbalist, who prescribes plant medicines if the first two members of the team have not cured the patient. One such medicine might be yucca roots, mashed and boiled, which the Papagos use to treat diabetes.

Physicians at the Indian Hospital of the U.S. Public Health Service on the Papago Reservation work side by side with folk healers. The hospital staff cooperates fully when a patient's family decides to call in a medicine man for diagnosis or treatment, and the hospital is always open to traditional healers.

There is probably nowhere in the United States where folk medicine is more widely practiced than in the Appalachian Mountains. It is also one of the country's principal sources of medicinal herbs. Goldenseal, for sores, and American ginseng, the universal tonic, are among the most popular herbs of the region. Goldenrod and boneset are prescribed for colds, fever, and flu. Alfalfa tea is drunk for arthritis, blackberry juice is given for diarrhea. Yellowroot, white and black oak, wild cherry, horehound, and other plants are gathered, each in its right season, and dried, pounded, chopped, boiled, brewed, or prepared according to time-honored recipes.

At the very southern tip of the Appalachians, in Alabama's Cherokee County, a septuagenarian named Tommie Bass was dispensing a wide variety of herbal remedies in the 1980's. His visitors included professors who were impressed as much by Bass's encyclopedic knowledge of the local flora as by his herbal concoctions such as catnip tea for headaches and calamus root for indigestion.

Chinese Botanical Medicine

In China, the ancient tradition of using herbs to heal exists side by side with Western medicine. Since the Communists took power on the mainland in 1949, the government has had to deal with an acute shortage of trained physicians. It has encouraged the practice of "traditional" medicine. The paramedics, or "barefoot doctors," who serve the rural areas are trained in traditional practice, which combines the use of medicinal plants with acupuncture to bring the *yin* and the *yang* back into balance.

The use of ginseng as a tonic and panacea probably originated in China thousands of years ago. Chemical analysis has shown that ginseng contains a number of vitamins, minerals, and medically active substances called saponins. These would account for ginseng's apparent ability to increase resistance to stress and to increase mental and physical capacity.

Like their counterparts in North America, Chinese herbalists use many cooking herbs in their medicines. Among these are mints, cinnamon, orange peel, and licorice and gingerroots (all used to treat headaches). Camphor and angelica are applied to bruises; alpinia berries are used to make a stomach powder; the tassel flower is used to treat fevers.

Latin America's Herbal Riches

Some of the most powerful modern drugs have come from the plants of Central America and South America. Several centuries ago, Spanish priests discovered the power of Peruvian bark—the bark of the cinchona trees of Peru—to control malaria. For over 300 years the bark's active constituent, quinine, was the most widely prescribed drug against this disease. By converting quinine into quinidine, scientists have created a drug to control atrial fibrillation, a type of cardiac arrhythmia.

Peru also gave us cocaine, which has been important in medicine despite being a drug of abuse. From Brazil came emetine, which is extracted from the ipecac root and used to treat amebic dysentery. From South America comes a substance originally used by jungle tribes to poison their arrow tips—curare, used in anesthesia as a muscle relaxant.

But medical science may have barely begun to tap the botanical riches of the South American jungles or the knowledge of the native medicine men and women. In the Amazon Basin, in Peru, grows a plant called *chanca piedra*, from the Inca and Spanish meaning "to break stone." It is prescribed by native doctors to dissolve kidney stones and gallstones. Campa Indians use the yellow sap of the fustic tree to help extract decayed teeth. Natives along the Ucayali River mix the bark of the *hiporuru* shrub with local rum to cure osteoarthritis. To heal the most severe burns in a few days and without scarring, Witoto Indians bind the burned areas with strips of fresh bast (phloem) from the sweet cassava tuber. Another plant of the same family, a vine called *Amwebe*, is said to heal old, infected burns without scarring.

Searchers for a safe, long-lasting contraceptive cannot ignore the practices of Indian tribes in the Amazon Basin. Canelos Indian women drink medicinal preparations made from sedges of the genus *Cyperus*, locally called *piripiri*, in order to prevent conception, as do

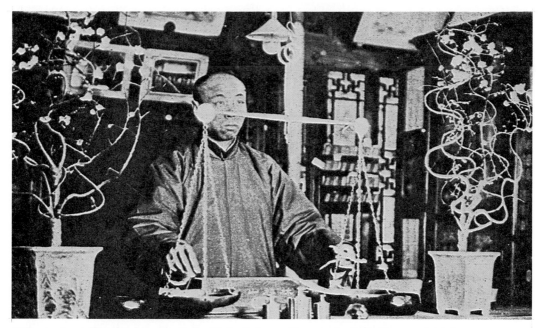

Chinese shops like this one, stocked with herbal remedies, survived the Communist takeover.

women of several other tribes. The precise recipes for these concoctions differ from tribe to tribe, but the effect is reportedly the same— sterility, for a year or longer, depending upon how many doses are taken, the potency of the particular plant, and the woman's age. And apparently menses do not cease during the time of sterility.

Among the Witoto, females traditionally marry as children. At puberty, girls are given one or another of several local contraceptive herbs to render them infertile for about six years. Another herb known locally as *amor seco* not only prevents conception among women of the Campa tribe for three years, but also seems to prevent the discomforts of menopause.

Given the questions surrounding presently available oral contraceptives and drugs for relieving menopausal distress, the practices of these Indians of the Amazon Basin of South America clearly invite scrutiny.

The Future

As these few examples suggest, there would appear to be much more to be learned from folk customs dealing not only with medicinal plants but also with many aspects of maintaining health and treating illness and disease. In rural Scotland, the old women used to say that if you had a yellow baby, you should put it in a bed by the window so the sun would shine on it. Today it is common hospital practice to place such babies in the artificial sun of special lamps over their isolettes. These babies have a potentially dangerous condition called biliru- binemia, which involves an excess of a chemi- cal, bilirubin, that gives their skin an orange- yellow cast. The hospital lamps break down the excess bilirubin—just as the sun had done for the Scottish infants.

And hundreds of years ago, people in Asia and Europe picked a scab from a smallpox victim and rubbed it into a scratch in a healthy person's skin. Folklore said this would bring resistance to the disease: crude, perhaps risky, but a form of vaccination all the same.

Vaccination began the medical revolution that found treatment after treatment, cure after cure, and brought tens of millions of human beings longer, healthier, happier lives. After vaccines came antibiotics and a host of other wonder drugs. Yet now that botanists and physicians (and pharmacists, too) are fi- nally working together, following the guide- lines of modern science, it is very possible that greater medical discoveries lie ahead.

Plants may offer a medical revolution of another kind to 4 billion inhabitants of the world who rely primarily on traditional medi- cine for their health care needs. These people are a special concern of the World Health Organization's Collaborating Center for Tradi- tional Medicine at the University of Illinois at Chicago. There, scientists have identified 90 species of plants that provide drugs in 62 therapeutic categories including laxatives, cough medicines, analgesics (painkillers), an- esthetics, sedatives, antidepressants, and med- icines for heart disease, high blood pressure, gout, and contraception. What these scientists propose gives a vast new dimension to the term "alternative medicine" for developing nations, where Western-made pharmaceutical prod- ucts are prohibitively expensive and where advanced medical technology has not yet de- veloped. Such nations, the scientists indicate, could in effect "raise their own medicines" from the plants that already exist in their countries and perhaps from cultivating species imported from other lands.

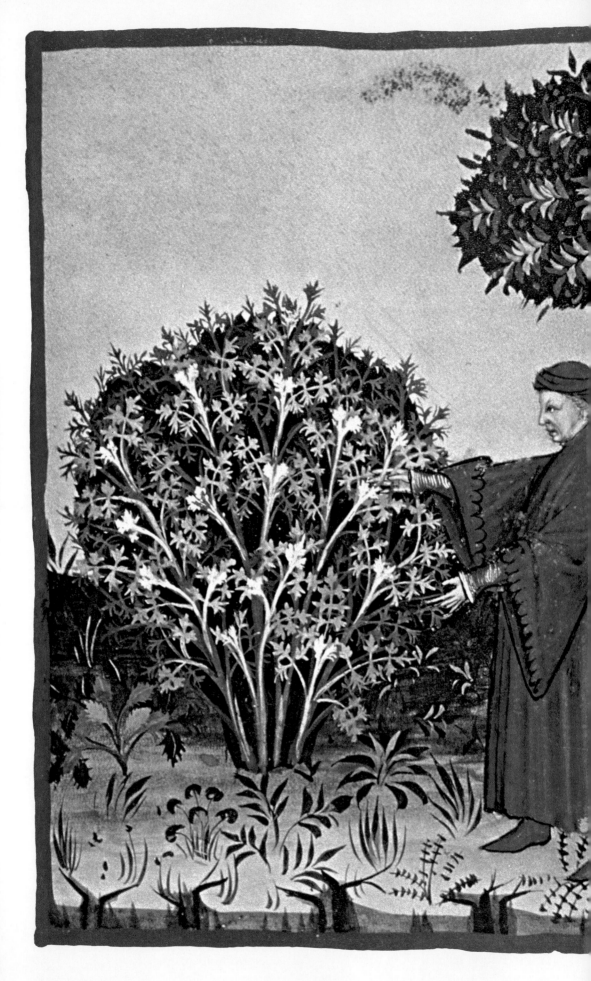

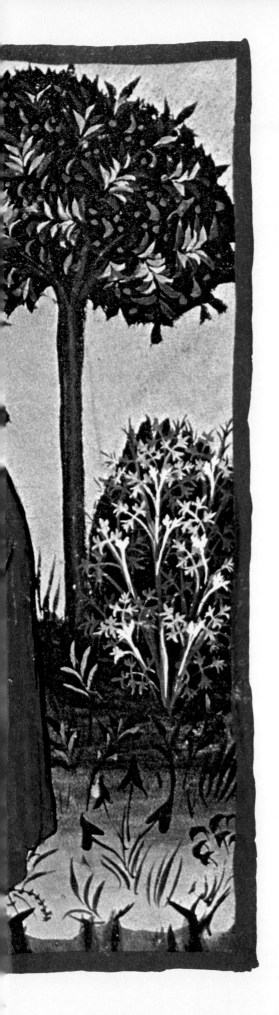

Gallery of Medicinal Plants

Since prehistoric times man has turned to plants for healing and the relief of physical discomfort. The plants in this gallery number nearly 300 and include the most popular medicinal plants that have been used in folk medicine in North America.

Introduction

Plants were the earliest source of medicine, and until comparatively recent times, they remained mankind's chief method of healing. Even now, in an age dominated by scientific and technological marvels, by miracle drugs and miracle cures, botanicals—or their synthetically derived equivalents—account for the majority of prescription and nonprescription medicines.

Archeological evidence indicates that the use of plants for healing dates far back into prehistory. Digs at the Shanidar cave in northern Iraq have revealed the 60,000-year-old grave of what appears to have been a Neanderthal medicine man. Arrayed around the body were the remains of eight species of flowers. Seven of them are used to this day for medicinal purposes by inhabitants of the region.

The 282 plants illustrated and discussed in this "Gallery of Medicinal Plants" include the major herbs that have served North Americans as medicines and folk remedies. Many species were brought to this continent by European settlers who wanted to be assured of having their trusted sources of medicine in the new land. Other herbs, native to the New World, had a place in the medical lore of the American Indian. The colonists soon adopted the Indians' use of these plants and also applied them to their own diseases, many of which had been unknown to the Indians.

Neither the settlers nor the Indians considered their botanical medicines to be mere home remedies. Indeed, a large number of those botanicals were listed in English and other European pharmacopeias—official publications that set standards for medicinal products. Pharmacopeias described (as they still do) each drug in such a way that the pharmacist (or laboratory) dispensing it would know exactly what its constituents were and how to attain the proper quality and strength. Many species, both introduced and native to North America, became part of the *U.S. Pharmacopeia*, which was founded in 1820.

Not only did many of the species introduced by European settlers enter the *U.S. Pharmacopeia*, they also became part of the North American countryside. These Old World plants, finding the new habitat hospitable to their growth, established themselves as wild plants when they "escaped cultivation," as botanists say. Seeds blown beyond the confines of a garden would germinate in uncultivated soil, and the process of naturalization, or becoming part of the local flora, would begin.

Herbs in Folklore and Science

The text that accompanies each plant in the gallery explains how Indians and settlers, ancients and moderns, used the herbs for medicinal and other purposes. Most of the herbs have medicinal applications going back hundreds, even thousands, of years. Again and again (with exceptions, of course) these uses have been found valid. Foxglove, belladonna, garden heliotrope, cascara sagrada, wild senna, dill, eucalyptus—all growing wild in North America—are just a few of the species whose traditional medicinal uses have been validated by scientific experiments and fieldwork.

As you read the articles and the "Uses" section of the plant profiles, you will see statements correlating folklore with scientific evidence. This information represents the most accurate observations that modern pharmacology and medical science can now make about the species' efficacy. Many of the statements are based on studies and knowledge of the effects that chemical compounds found in the plants have on human beings. At other times the information is based on the results of experiments on animals. The presumption is that the effect on the animal would parallel the effect on humans. Such presumptions do not always hold true, but they hold true often enough for scientists to make informed judgments based on the laboratory work.

Healthful Herbs Explained

When you have read a number of the gallery articles, you will notice certain patterns. Plants that contain tannin, for example, are astringent, causing the small blood vessels of the skin and mucous membranes to contract. Tannin-rich plants have therefore been used to help stop minor bleeding and to control diarrhea. Seeds of a number of species in the carrot family, such as caraway and dill, have been used for relieving flatulence and gas pains. So have the leaves of many mint species. This effect comes from the essential oils in the seeds or leaves. Other plants are often cited for relieving coughs, either by helping to loosen phlegm or by soothing the tickling feeling in the respiratory tract. These plants owe their effectiveness to the presence of mucilage. Still other species help ease the pains of rheumatism or arthritis when they are applied as a liniment; usually they work because they contain an aspirinlike substance called salicin.

In Search of the Healthful Herb

The gallery is both a field guide to medicinal plants growing in the United States and Canada (see page 78, "How to Use the Gallery") and a summary of current knowledge about the species—history, legend, myth, and scientific facts. Do not view any of the information in the gallery as a recommendation, explicit or implied, that you experiment with medicinal plants, whether to maintain or improve health, to cure an illness, or to remedy an injury. There are good reasons for heeding this advice:

1. Before one can be cured, one must be properly diagnosed.

2. Many of the species described here are no longer found in the *U.S. Pharmacopeia*. One reason for loss of official sanction might be that the plant has toxic properties or undesirable side effects that made its use unnecessarily risky once a safe substitute was found. Some plants have been replaced by more effective drugs (although this does not mean that a deleted species was ineffective).

3. Gathering herbs for medicinal use requires expert knowledge. Identification must be accurate. And a plant yields its active principle only at certain stages of its growth, at a certain season, or when growing in certain types of soil.

4. Even the right plant, properly harvested and applied to a correctly diagnosed illness, can cause harm or be ineffective if it is improperly administered. How much of the leaves or roots should you use? How long after harvesting should you wait before using the plant? For how long should you boil or steep the plant? In other words, how can you be certain that you have a safe, effective dosage?

The Role of Pharmacology

The ancients recognized the need for accuracy and precision in making medicines. There are herbals—books describing plants and their medicinal uses—that date back several thousand years. Pharmacopeias were a further step in promoting the safe and effective prescription of medicinal and other drugs. The *Nuremberg Pharmacopoeia*, published in Germany in 1542, is generally acknowledged as the first such publication in the West. The earliest national pharmacopeia was issued in England in the 19th century.

More than anything else, however, it was the development in the early 19th century of pharmacology—the study of the effects of chemicals on living things—that changed the prescribing of medicine from an art into a science. With the knowledge of chemistry, scientists could analyze the composition of plants and other products and determine the effect of their components. Physicians prescribing drugs could be confident that the patient would receive from the pharmacist the right substance, in the required state of purity, and in the correct dosage. Drugs could also be made synthetically, with many benefits. Synthesis in the laboratory produced purer drugs. In many cases, pharmacologists no longer had to rely on natural supplies of drugs such as ephedrine, whose availability depended on uncertain overseas sources. Manufacturers no longer had to rely on the vagaries of crops. And in some instances (vitamins are an example), synthetic drugs are cheaper to produce.

Plants in Modern Medicine

In a matter of years synthetic drugs nearly supplanted many of the medicinal herbs that had reigned supreme throughout man's existence. Today about 25 percent of all prescription drugs are derived from higher (flowering) plants, and some 12 percent more come from lower plant forms (the molds that produce penicillin and other antibiotics are the best-known examples). In medical research, while some scientists look to chemistry for cures, others explore the plant kingdom for medical breakthroughs. The Madagascar periwinkle is being used in the treatment of Hodgkin's disease, a form of cancer; *Lippia dulcis,* an herb growing in central Mexico, holds the promise of being a safe sugar substitute; several plants that South American women use to suppress or regulate the menstrual cycle are being studied as contraceptives that may be both safer and easier to use than current products. Much of the work with medicinal plants is done by men and women trained in pharmacognosy— the study of drugs and other economic products obtained from natural sources.

Medicinal Herbs and You

Books on herbal medicine occupy several feet of shelf space in bookstores around the country. You probably do not have to drive far to find a store selling natural products ranging from vitamins to cosmetics to laxatives. If the community you live in is large enough, you may even find a place where you can buy most of the herbs described in this gallery; you can also purchase them by mail order. Supermarkets offer large selections of herbal teas. Still, it pays to be cautious. Heed the warnings in the section "In Search of the Healthful Herb." And remember that even some of the culinary herbs can be harmful if taken in large doses. (For example, certain popular herbs, such as comfrey and borage, have recently been discovered to cause cancer in laboratory animals and thus should not be taken internally in large quantities or over a period of time.) Drink herbal teas sparingly; in many cases no one knows what their long-range effects may be if they are drunk to excess.

WARNING

The information in this book is primarily for reference and education. It is not intended to be a substitute for the advice of a physician. The editors do not advocate self-diagnosis or self-medication; they urge anyone with continuing symptoms, however minor, to seek medical advice. The reader should be aware that any plant substance, whether used as food or medicine, externally or internally, may cause an allergic reaction in some people.

HOW TO USE THE GALLERY

In the "Gallery of Medicinal Plants" are 282 North American species arranged in alphabetical order by the most commonly used popular name. An entire page is generally devoted to illustrating and describing each plant. In addition to the chief popular name of each species, you will find its scientific name (genus and species), a list of its alternative common names, and the English and Latin names of the botanical family to which the plant belongs. The common names of plants are often local in character, varying from one part of the country to another. If you do not find a plant under the name you know it by, check the index beginning on page 450, where you will find listed the various common names of all the plants discussed in this gallery.

The Stories Behind the Plants

In two or three short, fact-filled paragraphs you can read the fascinating story of each plant. Hardly a species does not have some ancient lore associated with it. The lore may be myth, legend, pure superstition—or amazingly accurate knowledge borne out by modern scientific studies. Superstition, for example, accounts for giving the forget-me-not the name scorpion grass. Since the plant's curled flower stalk resembles a scorpion's tail, it was therefore held to be a cure for not only scorpion bites but bites of other venomous creatures too. There is no scientific evidence, however, that the plant has any medicinal value. The opposite is true of belladonna, or deadly nightshade, which because of its lethal properties has been associated in legend with both the Devil and the three Fates of Greek mythology. In Italy centuries ago, women dropped the juice of the plant in their eyes for cosmetic reasons, to enlarge the pupils and make their eyes look dark—a mark of beauty. Modern eye doctors use belladonna derivatives in order to peer through the pupil into the interior of the eye.

Some plants have truly ancient histories—recorded on Egyptian stones, for instance, or pieced together by archeologists from prehistoric remains. Many of the species that colonists and subsequent settlers brought to North America from Europe had medicinal applications going back at least to the early Greeks and Romans and described by their physicians and naturalists in meticulous detail. Still other species, native to North America, were part of Indian pharmacopeias.

Beauty and Botany

As you turn the pages of this gallery you can have the same pleasures that you might enjoy as you walk along roadsides or through fields and woods—a lacy white blanket of Queen Anne's lace, a sea of purple loosestrife, clumps of chicory that defy pollution and brighten the shoulders of highways. The illustrations of each of the plants in the gallery afford the esthetic pleasure that we get from nature and from fine works of art depicting nature. But they do more than that. Each drawing offers a detailed study of the plant or, if the plant is too large, the distinctive part that will help you identify the species in the wild or in a garden. Some illustrations are accompanied by drawings of a detail of the plant—the single flower of a flower spike; the mature fruit, which would not appear on the plant in bloom; the tuber of a plant that is valued for that part. The photographs at the top of each page show the plant in its natural environment. The species is not always easy to discern, for nature sometimes reveals its splendors only to those who look for them diligently.

The Plant Profiles

At the bottom of each page, set off in a box, is a profile of the plant. The profile has two purposes: to aid in identification of the species, for even with the illustration and photo, you may need further information to help you identify it; and to provide the most up-to-date scientific evidence regarding the use of the plant, as follows:

✗ A toxic plant: The part or parts that cause poisoning; the symptoms and effects of the poison; cautions about confusing the species with a similar-looking but poisonous plant.

✗ Ingestion of the plant may cause immediate dire effects.

Habitat: The type of environment that is hospitable to the species and where it may be found in the wild: for example, dry fields and meadows, roadsides; woodlands, meadows, clearings; marshes, bogs, ponds.

Range: The geographical areas in North America where the plant grows wild.

Identification: A botanical description of the plant: annual, bienniel, or perennial; height; description of the stem, leaves, flowers (including the months of blooming), and fruit; other distinctive characteristics such as what kind of smell it has.

Uses: Employment of the plant in herbal folk medicine in present-day North America, as well as its employment in current established medical practice; statements regarding the scientific evidence about the validity of the uses in folk medicine.

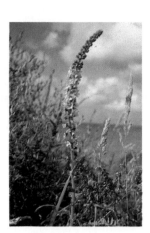

Agrimony

Agrimonia eupatoria L.

Church Steeples, Cocklebur,
Philanthropos, Stickwort
ROSE FAMILY
Rosaceae

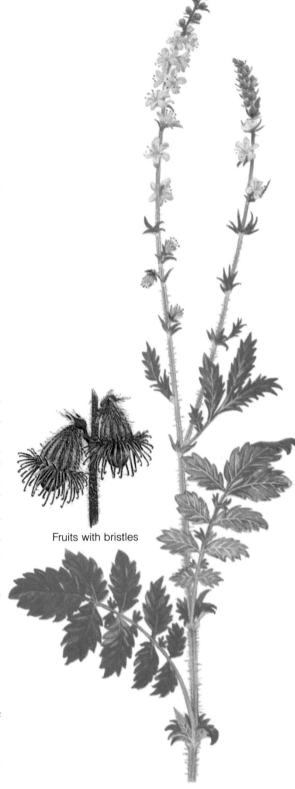

Fruits with bristles

A pretty plant, bearing spikes of tiny yellow flowers (church steeples) and fruit with hooked bristles at the top (cockleburs), agrimony grows wild by roadsides, fields, and woods. Although the plant has no narcotic properties, tradition holds that when placed under a person's head, agrimony will induce a deep sleep that will last until it is removed.

Folklore aside, agrimony has a long history of medicinal use. The English poet Michael Drayton once hailed it as an "all-heal," and through the ages it did seem to be a panacea. The ancient Greeks used agrimony to treat eye ailments, and it was made into brews to cure diarrhea and disorders of the gallbladder, liver, and kidneys. Anglo-Saxons made a solution from the leaves and seeds for healing wounds; this use continued through the Middle Ages and afterward, in a preparation called *eau d'arquebusade,* or "musket-shot water." Later, agrimony was prescribed for athlete's foot.

In the United States and Canada, late into the 19th century, the plant was prescribed for many of these ills and more: for skin diseases, asthma, coughs, and gynecological complaints, and as a gargle for sore throat.

Habitat: Roadsides, waste ground, fields, woods.
Range: Native to Europe, agrimony is cultivated in much of the United States and southern Canada.
Identification: A perennial, growing 2–3 feet high, with an upright mature brown stem covered with soft, silky hairs. The hairy leaves are alternate and pinnately divided, with coarsely toothed leaflets. At the top of the stem grow numerous small yellow flowers (July–August) in long spikes, the blooms opening one above another. Hooked bristles at the upper end of the burlike fruit stick to clothing and animal fur.
Uses: Agrimony's medicinal properties as an anti-inflammatory, antibiotic, and astringent are all due to the presence of large quantities of tannin in the plant. Herbalists today use the flowering stem tips and dried leaves as a tonic and diuretic and for digestive disorders, including diarrhea. The plant is also applied to slow-healing wounds. Agrimony is an ingredient of herb teas.

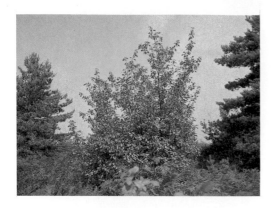

Alder Buckthorn

Rhamnus frangula L.

Arrowwood, Black Dogwood, Glossy Buckthorn
BUCKTHORN FAMILY

Rhamnaceae

Despite its name, alder buckthorn is neither an alder nor is it thorny. The name buckthorn is a translation of the shrub's fanciful but inaccurate Italian name, *spino cervino*, or "stag's thorn." Alder buckthorn was imported from Europe to North America long ago and grows wild in much of the continent's northeast. Nurseries today cultivate a variety named Tallhedge for hedges and windbreaks.

Galen, a Greek physician of the second century A.D., knew of alder buckthorn, although he did not distinguish clearly in his writings between it and other related species. All of these were credited at various times with the power to protect against witchcraft, demons, poisons, and headaches. The ancients ignored the more mundane but true value of the bark as a laxative, and it was not until the 1300's that alder buckthorn was used for that purpose. Buckthorn bark's laxative action is relatively gentle, and it may not have been considered powerful enough to be worthy of attention in a day when violent purgatives were in fashion.

Alder buckthorn wood was formerly used for shoe lasts, nails, and veneer. Its charcoal was prized by makers of gunpowder. The bark yields a yellow dye, and the unripe berries furnish a green dye.

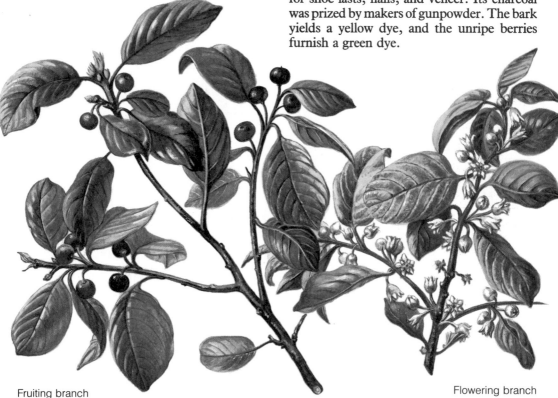

Fruiting branch

Flowering branch

X The berries are slightly poisonous and can cause vomiting.

Habitat: Hedgerows, old fields, woodland edges; prefers well-drained soils.

Range: Native to Eurasia and North Africa, alder buckthorn is naturalized in North America from Nova Scotia to Quebec south to New Jersey and west to Illinois.

Identification: A deciduous shrub or small tree, growing up to 20 feet tall. It has glossy oval green leaves, 1–3 inches long, that are alternate and toothless. The bark is green when young, becoming gray and marked with whitish transverse ridges when older. Small greenish-white flowers (May– July) grow in small clusters at the leaf joints or at the tips of branches. Pea-size berries turn from green to red to black when mature (September).

Uses: Herbalists recommend a tea made from the bark as a laxative. In Europe, the bark is a common ingredient in pharmaceutically prepared laxatives.

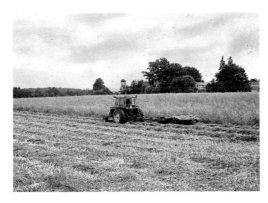

Alfalfa

Medicago sativa L.

Buffalo Herb, Lucerne, Purple Medic
PEA FAMILY
Leguminosae

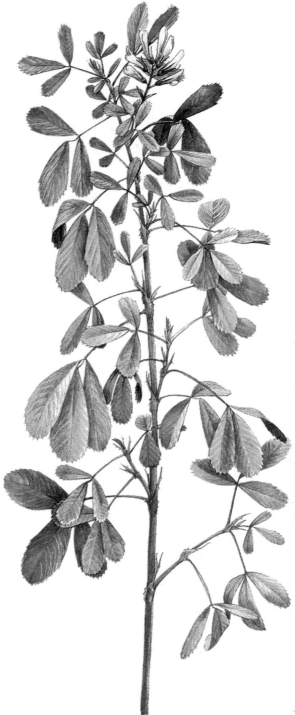

An important forage and hay crop, sweet-smelling alfalfa originated as a wild legume, presumably in the dry uplands of western Asia. The Medes of ancient Persia are thought to have been the first to domesticate the plant, hence its Latin name, *Medicago sativa*, which means "sowed by the Medians." The plant reached Mediterranean Europe by way of the Greeks, who planted it as early as 490 B.C. It pleased the Arabs so well that they dubbed it *al-fasfasah*, "the best fodder." Not only did they feed the leaves, sprouts, and seeds to their horses to give the animals superior speed and strength, but they considered it excellent food for themselves, too. In Spain the Arabic word *al-fasfasah* became *alfalfa*.

Ultimately, alfalfa reached the New World with the Spanish Conquistadores, who planted it in Mexico and Chile. California settlers, calling the novelty Chilean clover, began growing it as fodder in the mid-1800's, and it has been a significant American crop ever since.

Although there is no scientific evidence that alfalfa alters the course of any disorder, herbalists prescribe alfalfa tea and alfalfa tablets, for example, for a variety of complaints, from diabetes to alcoholism to tooth decay. But alfalfa does have a future in human nutrition, particularly as an inexpensive source of vitamins C, D, E, and K.

Habitat: Can be cultivated almost everywhere, even in dry regions. Naturalized varieties spring up along roadsides, in abandoned fields and lots, and in low valleys.
Range: Introduced from Europe, alfalfa has been naturalized in most of North America, especially in the West.
Identification: A bushy perennial 1–3 feet tall. The leaves are alternate and pinnately divided, with three dark green leaflets that are toothed toward the tips. Purple to yellowish flowers (May–October) arranged in heads produce twisted pods containing seeds in the fall.
Uses: Alfalfa's rich nutritional content makes it a valuable food for man as well as animals. In recent years health food advocates have made many extravagant claims for its use—even as a cure for cancer. None of these claims have been substantiated in any way.

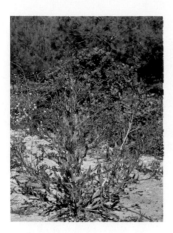

Alkanet

Anchusa officinalis L.

Bugloss, Common Alkanet
BORAGE FAMILY
Boraginaceae

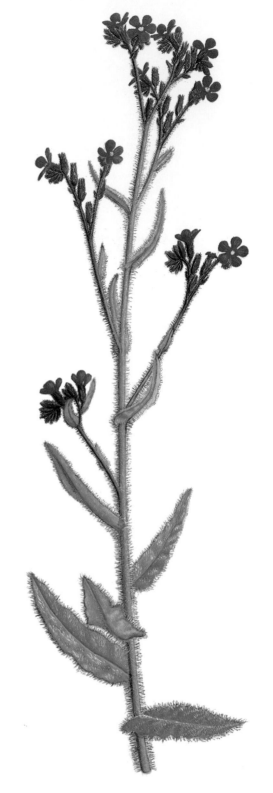

According to Dr. Robert Thornton's *New Family Herbal,* published in England in 1810, "A decoction of the leaves and root of the alkanet is advantageous in inveterate coughs, and all disorders of the chest . . . the expressed juice is given with great success in pleurisy." Dr. Thornton also noted alkanet's "efficacy in the cure of melancholia and other hypochondriacal diseases," and added, "but then it must be steeped in strong ale and wine."

In modern folk medicine an alkanet tea is still specified for the treament of melancholy, to ease coughing, to promote sweating and break a fever, to soften and soothe the skin, and as a diuretic, astringent, and "blood purifier" (an agent that reputedly purges toxic substances from the body).

The name alkanet comes from the Arabic *al-hinna,* or "henna," reflecting an ancient use of this and related plants whose roots contain a red dye. The dye found in this species (which is often known by the common name bugloss) is not as strong as the commercial red dye found in its close relative *Alkanna tinctoria.* For gardeners, alkanet is a rewarding plant because it supplies pretty violet-blue flowers for cutting, and it also attracts bees.

X There is evidence that alkanet may cause cancer if taken internally over a long period of time.
Habitat: Waste places, roadsides.
Range: Introduced from Europe, alkanet may be found growing wild locally from Maine south to New Jersey and west to Ohio and Michigan.
Identification: A biennial herb with coarsely hairy stems and leaves rising from a cluster of basal leaves and growing 1–3 feet tall. The lower leaves are stalked and up to 8 inches long; the upper ones are narrow, oblong to lance-shaped, up to 6 inches long by 1 inch wide, and stalkless. Dainty purplish-blue flowers (late May–October) are tubular, ¼ inch across, and followed by minute nutlike fruits.
Uses: Alkanet is principally employed in herbal medicine today as an expectorant (for bringing up phlegm) and as an emollient (for soothing and softening the skin). Pharmacologists find no evidence that it acts as an expectorant; they have not evaluated its use as an emollient.

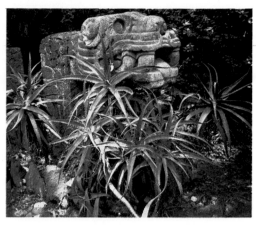

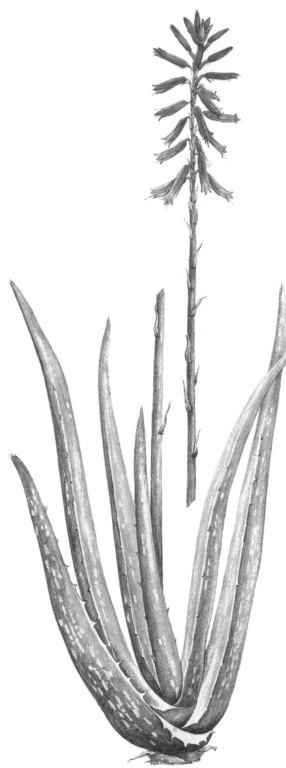

Aloe

Aloe vera (L.) Burm.f.

Aloes, Barbados Aloe, Curaçao Aloe
LILY FAMILY
Liliaceae

Some plants are deservedly popular, and aloe is one of the most deserving of them all. Nearly every cosmetic counter carries shampoos and skin creams containing aloe vera, as it is also called. Aloe's value lies in its ability to regenerate damaged tissues, which it does with dramatic swiftness. The plant originated in the Cape Verde Islands (in the Atlantic west of Senegal) or thereabouts, and by early historical times it had appeared in Egypt, Arabia, and India. The aloe that was used to embalm the body of Christ, according to John 19:39, was possibly *A. vera* or a closely related species. The Roman naturalist Pliny, writing in the first century A.D., cited many uses for aloe: the fresh juice for external application to heal wounds, bruises, and irritations; and a leaf extract to be taken internally as a tonic, purgative, and jaundice remedy. Modern medicine has found new uses for aloe—for example, the fresh juice is employed as a salve for the treatment of radiation burns.

Many people keep a pot of the plant growing on the kitchen windowsill. The fresh juice squeezed from a broken aloe leaf provides instant relief for minor burns and wounds.

Habitat: Dry, sunny places; sandy soils.
Range: Native to Africa and the Mediterranean area, aloe was early introduced to North America and continues to be cultivated in California, Texas, Florida, and Arizona, and as a houseplant.
Identification: A succulent perennial with a rosette of narrow, prickly-edged, fleshy leaves filled with bitter juice, aloe produces a single leafless stalk growing 2–3 feet tall, which terminates in an elongated cluster of downward-pointing yellow to orange-red flowers (June–September).
Uses: The sticky fresh juice of aloe leaves serves as an emollient (skin-softening) ingredient in many skin lotions and creams, salves, and shampoos. It is also used for minor wounds and burns, both in home use of the fresh juice and in various pharmaceutical products. A resinous extract from the dried leaves has been administered internally as a strong laxative. Research indicates that these uses are valid.

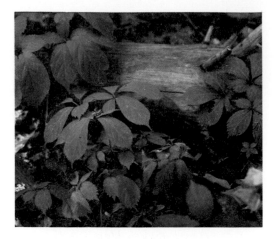

an easy plant to cultivate. It requires much hand labor and takes six years to mature. When the United States resumed trade with China in the 1970's, ginseng was the first commodity to be exported.

Unfortunately, as a result of ginseng's widespread popularity and its value for export, it has been nearly wiped out over much of its former range. Some is still collected in the wild, but the plant has become so rare that it is officially listed as a threatened species in 31 states. Any ginseng found growing wild should be left alone. Admire it for its beauty, marvel at its long and colorful history—and let it be.

American Ginseng

Panax quinquefolius L.

Five-fingers, Tartar Root
GINSENG FAMILY
Araliaceae

Valued by many Indian tribes, American ginseng first attracted the attention of colonists in the early 1700's when a Jesuit missionary in Canada realized that it was almost identical with a medicinal plant much in demand in China. Almost overnight a brisk export trade developed (and continues to this day), as collectors combed the woods in search of ginseng for export to the Orient.

The prize they sought—the plant's contorted, sometimes branching root—vaguely resembles a human body and so was presumed to have general curative powers. The Chinese name for ginseng, *jen-shen*, in fact, means "manlike," as does the Indian name *garantoquen*. Its scientific name, on the other hand, means "five-leaved cure-all," which perfectly reflects ginseng's extravagant reputation. Chinese and Indians alike regarded it as an aphrodisiac, and it has been recommended as a treatment for everything from asthma and anemia to lower back pain.

Today ginseng is grown commercially, mainly in the state of Wisconsin, but it is not

Berries in late summer

Habitat: Rich, cool woodlands.
Range: Formerly found from Quebec to Manitoba and south to Oklahoma, Louisiana, and Florida. Today it is rare in most places.
Identification: A perennial herb, growing 8–24 inches tall. It has three large compound leaves, each composed of five toothed leaflets, atop a straight stem. Flowers (June–July) are tiny (⅛ inch across) and greenish white. They are borne in a single spherical cluster rising above the leaves.

Fruits, produced in late summer, are bright red berries. The root is fleshy and sometimes forked.
Uses: No longer considered a magical cure-all, ginseng today is valued by herbalists primarily as a stimulant and as a tonic taken daily to prevent stress and such minor ailments as colds. Dried ginseng root can be chewed; or it can be powdered and brewed as a tea.

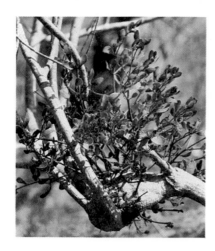

American Mistletoe

Phoradendron flavescens (Pursh) Nutt.

Golden Bough, Mistletoe
MISTLETOE FAMILY
Loranthaceae

In a flash of lightning, mistletoe descends from the sky to alight on the sacred oak, favored host of the succulent parasitic shrub. Fantastic beliefs such as this surrounded the mistletoe with an aura of awe throughout the ancient world from the Mediterranean to the Baltic. In the imagination of Romans, Celts, and Germanic peoples, it was a key to the supernatural. A sprig of mistletoe was the "golden bough" that opened the world of the dead to Aeneas, hero of Virgil's epic poem. To the primitive mind, death's opposites are sex and fertility, and mistletoe stood for these too. Our present-day custom of exchanging kisses under a sprig of mistletoe is a civilized vestige of that primeval connection.

In those times long ago, mistletoe was regarded as a life-giver and a panacea. Later, more specific medicinal virtues were associated with the plant: it was said to cure tuberculosis, stroke, palsy, epilepsy, and the effects of poisoning. Its reputed sedative properties may account for its use in treating epilepsy and palsy. Although American mistletoe belongs to a different species from the European plant, it is heir to some of the same ancient beliefs and medicinal uses. Its display at Christmastime and the New Year dates back to Norse tradition.

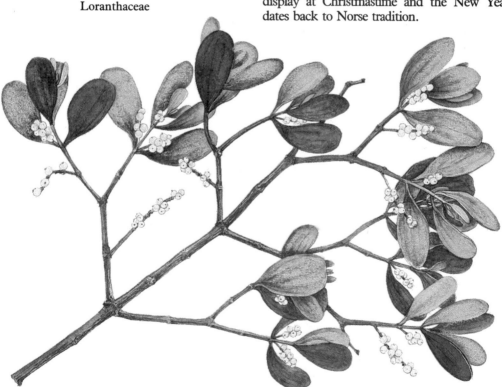

✗ The U.S. Food and Drug Administration lists this plant as "unsafe."
Habitat: Branches of deciduous trees.
Range: New Jersey to Florida, west to the Pacific Coast; coastal British Columbia.
Identification: A parasitic evergreen shrub. Its branching woody stems bear yellowish-green, leathery leaves in opposite pairs. Small whitish flowers (May–July) in spikes mature into fleshy white berries (December) containing single seeds.

Uses: American mistletoe has been used in folk medicine as an antihypertensive and a sedative; research suggests that the plant may have sedative effects. Evidence regarding its effectiveness in treating high blood pressure is inconclusive. There is some evidence that the plant may induce menstruation. It has also showed effectiveness in treating tumors in experimental animals. Because the question of mistletoe's toxicity remains controversial, the plant should not be taken internally.

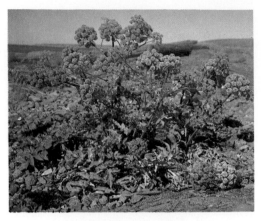

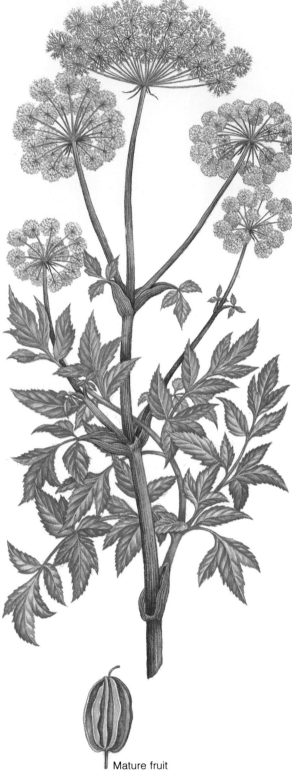

Angelica

Angelica archangelica L.

Garden Angelica, Root of the Holy Ghost
CARROT FAMILY
Umbelliferae

A native of northern Europe, the stately angelica is often grown as a garden herb. Its wild American relative—great angelica, or alexanders (*Angelica atropurpurea*)—is similar in appearance except for its purplish stems and has similar properties and uses.

The name angelica derives from the Medieval Latin *herba angelica*, "angelic herb," so called from its supposed special powers against poison and plague. It was believed to protect against contagious diseases (including the plague), ward off evil spirits and enchantments, bestow long life, and even neutralize the bites of mad dogs. As recently as the end of World War I, people chewed on the root in the belief that it would protect them from the then rampant worldwide influenza epidemic.

Today angelica is valued mainly for its stimulating effects on the digestive system. Ever since colonial times, the aromatic, naturally sweetish stems have been candied for tasty treats and use as pastry decorations. The celerylike leafstalks can also be cooked or eaten raw, and essential oils distilled from the seeds and roots are used in perfumes and as flavorings for gin, vermouth, and various liqueurs such as Chartreuse.

Mature fruit

X Positive identification is essential when collecting the wild species because it resembles some poisonous members of the carrot family.
Habitat: Angelica requires rich, moist garden soil in partial shade. Great angelica prefers wet bottomlands and swamps.
Range: Great angelica grows wild from Labrador to Minnesota, south to Maryland, Indiana, and Iowa.
Identification: A robust perennial herb with thick, hollow stems up to 6 feet tall. The leaves are pinnately compound, with toothed leaflets and enlarged sheaths at the base of the leafstalks. Large globular flowerheads (June–October) consist of many clusters of tiny greenish-white flowers.
Uses: Preparations from stems, seeds, and roots are helpful for calming digestive disturbances and stimulating the appetite and for alleviating coughs. The stems are candied for confections, and the seeds and oils are used in flavorings.

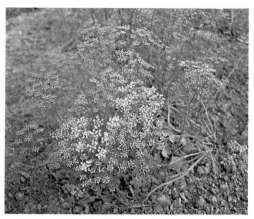

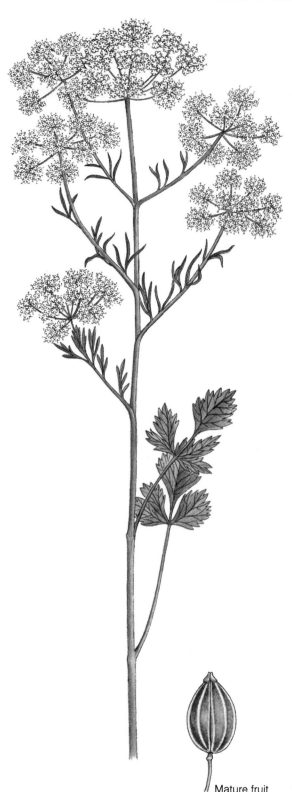

Mature fruit

Anise

Pimpinella anisum L.

Aniseed, Sweet Cumin
CARROT FAMILY
Umbelliferae

The ancient Romans were so fond of the seed of anise, with its spicy aroma and licorice taste, that they made it an ingredient of a special cake, with which they concluded their notoriously enormous feasts. But man's appreciation of anise goes back to much earlier times, for it is one of the oldest known herbs, mentioned in records long before the birth of Christ. The Greeks, including Hippocrates (who suggested it for coughs), the people of Asia Minor, and the Romans found many medicinal applications for it. It was used as a breath sweetener and an aphrodisiac, to relieve flatulence and colic, to stimulate mother's milk, and to combat giddiness and nausea. By the 16th century, Europeans had discovered that anise was an irresistible bait for mice. The oil of the seed has been used to poison pigeons.

Today anise's famous licorice taste is found in both culinary and medicinal products. Its seeds flavor cough medicines, cough drops, baked goods, candies, and liqueurs. Its leaves are added to salads and used as garnishes.

With its dainty white flowers that grow in umbrellalike clusters, anise looks much like Queen Anne's lace, but it is shorter and the flower clusters have no bracts.

Habitat: Warm, sunny gardens with well-drained, moderately rich, sandy soil.
Range: Cultivated throughout North America as a garden plant, anise occasionally escapes from cultivation to be found in the wild.
Identification: An annual growing 1–2 feet high with an erect, smooth stem. Leaves at the base are thick and pinnately divided; the leaflets are oval with toothed edges. The bright green upper leaves are smaller and feathery. Tiny white to yellow blossoms (July–August) grow in umbrellalike clusters. The downy brown seedlike fruits (August–September) produce the essential oil for which this licorice-smelling herb is noted.
Uses: Anise has wide commercial popularity as a fragrance and a flavoring. Its ancient use as a carminative—that is, to relieve gas pains—continues today and is substantiated by modern research in pharmacology.

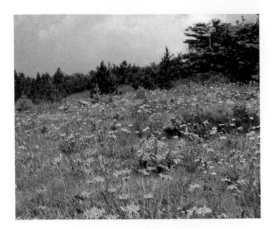

Arnica

Arnica montana L.

Leopard's-bane, Mountain Tobacco

COMPOSITE FAMILY

Compositae

Whether arnica is indeed the bane of leopards and other beasts who eat it remains in dispute, but there is no doubt that it can kill humans. Nevertheless, the plant has been used medicinally in Europe since the 16th century. European physicians prescribed it as a stimulant, particularly for the heart and circulation. In 1565 a Swiss naturalist named Konrad von Gesner tested arnica by taking a dose himself. Then he wrote to a friend declaring that there had been no ill effect. Less than an hour later, Gesner was dead, presumably of arnica poisoning. Not only can overdoses of an extract from the plant cause painful irritation of the stomach and intestines, but arnica is also toxic to the heart and causes increase in blood pressure.

Arnica, in infinitesimally tiny doses, is to this day the standard homeopathic remedy for shock occasioned by a sudden painful injury. But the only safe use for arnica extract is as an ingredient in salves and liniments for bruises and sprains, and even these preparations must be administered by experienced persons and with extreme caution. North American Indians used a related species with similar medicinal properties, *A. fulgens*, externally on wounds and sore muscles.

X Do not use internally or externally. Internal use may cause great pain or even death; external use may irritate the skin.

Habitat: Moist soil in mountains and valleys at elevations from 3,500 to 10,000 feet.

Range: Introduced from Europe to western North America, arnica now grows wild there.

Identification: Arnica resembles many other members of the composite family with yellow-orange sunflowerlike flowerheads (April–September) about 1–2 inches in diameter. Leaves form a basal rosette, with one to four pairs of stem leaves (slightly hairy on top) growing opposite each other; the stems are 4–24 inches tall.

Uses: The plant's chief medicinal virtue lies in its ability to reduce pain and swelling when made into salves or liniments. *Arnica montana* was listed in the *U.S. Pharmacopeia* for such use from the early 1800's to 1960. Today arnica is cultivated as a garden flower.

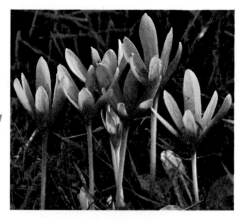

Autumn Crocus

Colchicum autumnale L.

Colchicum, Meadow Saffron, Naked Ladies
LILY FAMILY
Liliaceae

Contrary to two of its popular names, *Colchicum autumnale* is not a crocus nor is it related to the kitchen herb saffron. In fact, to use autumn crocus in cooking would be a fatal error, so deadly is the plant. By some accounts, the Greek naturalist Theophrastus (c. 371–287 B.C.) recognized its toxicity, noting that anyone who took it would not live out the day.

During the fifth century, however, doctors in the Byzantine Empire had a high regard for the plant's effectiveness as a remedy for "conditions of the joints" (probably rheumatism and arthritis), and Arab physicians prescribed it for gout. In England during the 17th and 18th centuries, autumn crocus gained recognition in the *London Pharmacopoeia*, was then dropped, and later reinstated.

The ancient herbalists were correct in their assessment of this plant's value, for modern science has established that colchicine, an alkaloid occurring in autumn crocus, relieves the pain and inflammation of gout. Colchicine is still derived from the plant itself because chemists have not been able to synthesize it inexpensively.

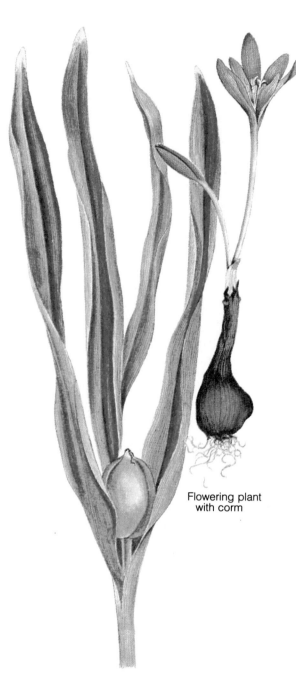

Flowering plant
with corm

Seedpod

X Ingestion of any part of the plant may cause death. The bulb may be mistaken for an onion. Symptoms are a burning sensation in the throat and vomiting, followed by kidney and respiratory failure.
Habitat: Damp meadows, fields, woodlands, and mountainous areas.
Range: Introduced from Europe, autumn crocus is widely cultivated and has escaped in some parts of southern Canada and the United States.
Identification: A perennial herb that rises to a height of 1 foot from a corm (a solid bulb). Large lance-shaped leaves develop in spring, and envelop the previous year's seedpod. In the fall, a leafless flowering stalk produces a solitary white to pale purple crocuslike flower (August–October).
Uses: Autumn crocus has been employed since ancient times to treat gout. It is the source of the modern drug colchicine prescribed by doctors to treat this condition.

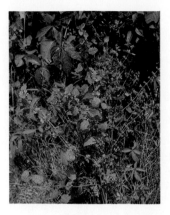

Balm

Melissa officinalis L.

Lemon Balm, Melissa, Sweet Balm
MINT FAMILY
Labiatae

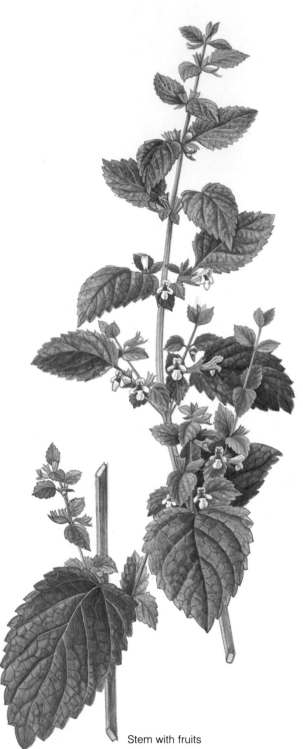

Stem with fruits

The hardy lemon-scented balm has long been used for its soothing medicinal qualities and its aromatic properties as an herb. It was also a favorite of ancient beekeepers, who rubbed its fresh leaves on beehives to encourage bees to return to the hives and bring others with them. In fact, the generic name *Melissa* comes from the Greek word for bee.

The common name also derives from the Greek: *balsamon* means "balsam," an oily, sweet-smelling resin. It was probably the Arabs who introduced balm to medicine, as a remedy for depression and anxiety. The 11th-century Arab physician Avicenna believed it "causeth the mind and heart to become merry" and praised it as an antidote for melancholy. Herbalists still recommend balm as a tonic and as a sedative.

Today the popular balm is used in a variety of ways. A tea made from the fresh or dried leaves is said to soothe menstrual cramps, relieve insomnia, act as a sedative, quiet vomiting, and reduce fever. The leaves contain a volatile oil that is used in the manufacture of perfumes and cosmetics.

Easy to grow under proper conditions, balm has been cultivated for centuries and is often found in herb gardens.

Habitat: Sunny fields and along roadsides with a rich, sandy, loamy soil.
Range: Native to Europe, balm is naturalized in the United States from New England west to Ohio and Kansas, and south to Arkansas and Florida.
Identification: A perennial with upright, hairy, branching stems that can reach 3 feet in height. Light green toothed ovate leaves grow in opposite pairs at each joint. White or yellowish two-lipped flowers (June–September) form in small loose bunches at the axils of the leaves. The leaves give off a strong lemon scent.
Uses: Preparations from leaves are used to treat feverish colds and headaches, to relieve menstrual cramps, and to calm nervous stomachs. The crushed leaves help heal wounds and insect bites. As a culinary herb, balm is used for making teas and cool drinks and as a flavoring in salads, soups, and egg dishes. Commercially, balm is a key element in certain perfumes and cosmetics.

Balsam Fir

Abies balsamea (L.) Mill.

Balm of Gilead Fir, Fir Balsam, Fir Pine,
Sapin, Silver Fir, Silver Pine

PINE FAMILY

Pinaceae

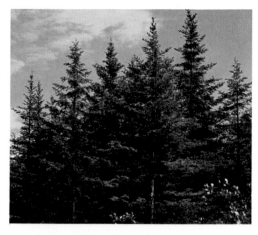

An excellent Christmas tree by virtue of its spicy, delicious fragrance and its ability to hold its needles long after it has been cut, balsam fir goes back further in history than the mid-19th-century introduction of the Christmas tree to North America. It was a veritable dispensary for the American Indians, for whom almost every part of this tree supplied a different medicine. The aromatic resin served them as a salve for cuts, sores, and burns, and they also took it internally for colds, coughs, and asthma. The resin was effective enough to attract the attention of frontier doctors; eventually it found its way into the *U.S. Pharmacopeia*. The inner bark, brewed into a tea, served as a remedy for chest pains, while the twigs, when steeped in water, acted as a laxative. Indians also held bits of the root in the mouth for mouth sores. They managed to use even the needles. Sweat baths, the Indians' saunas, were scented by handfuls of balsam needles on live coals; the bathers inhaled the vapors to clear up the congestion of colds and coughs.

Although balsam fir no longer has a place in established or folk medicine, its esthetic value is undiminished—about 13 percent of all Christmas trees sold each year are balsam firs.

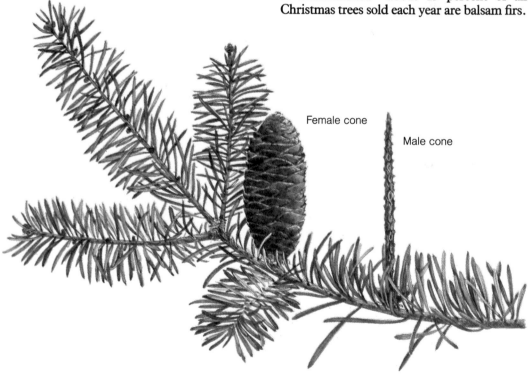

Female cone

Male cone

Habitat: Swamps and bogs to well-drained soils. Mountaintops in the southern part of its range.
Range: Northeastern Canada west to Alberta; in the United States as far west as Minnesota and south through the central Appalachians.
Identification: An evergreen tree growing 40–80 feet tall, balsam fir has dark, shiny green, flattened needles, ¾–1½ inches long, which look as if they were arranged in two rows but actually grow all around the branch. Flowers (May–June) are borne in separate yellow to brown male and green to purple female cones. The young bark is smooth and grayish and is covered with resin blisters that crack into scaly plates when it matures.
Uses: Too soft and perishable to make good lumber, balsam fir wood is used for crates, boxes, and paper pulp. The resin has been used as a source of turpentine and as an adhesive for microscope slides and optical lenses.

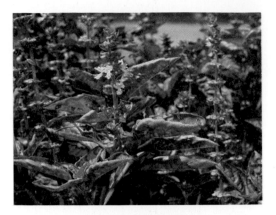

Basil

Ocimum basilicum L.

Common Basil, Sweet Basil
MINT FAMILY
Labiatae

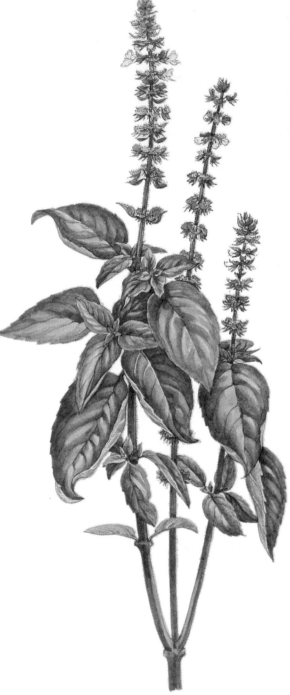

Many cooks would find it hard to do without the leaves of basil—spicy when fresh, sweeter when dried. Yet this popular culinary herb has been alternately praised and excoriated during the course of herbal medical history. Some ancient herbalists asserted that basil damaged the internal organs and the eyes and caused insanity, coma, and the spontaneous generation of worms, lice, and scorpions. Subsequent writers argued that basil did none of these things, but was good both as a condiment and for a variety of medicinal purposes. These opposing viewpoints were argued in herbal medicine through the centuries. The first-century A.D. Roman naturalist Pliny, siding with the defenders, reported that basil relieves flatulence, and this claim is upheld by modern pharmacology.

In folklore as in medicine, basil had a reputation for both evil and good. In some lands it was associated with the legendary reptile known as the basilisk, whose breath and glance could kill. The ancient Greeks believed that basil would grow only if gardeners vilified it while sowing it. Peoples in other countries, however, cherished it as a protection against witchcraft and as a symbol of love.

Habitat: Any well-drained, fairly rich soil.
Range: Native to tropical Asia, basil is now cultivated in most of temperate North America.
Identification: A bushy annual, 2–3 feet tall, with a square stem and numerous branches, basil has opposite, shiny green to purple, toothed leaves, that are elliptical to oval and about 1 inch long. They emit a spicy scent when bruised. Small white or purplish flowers (June–September) grow in whorls of six at the ends of the branches.

Uses: Down to the present day, herbalists have recommended tea made from the leaves of the basil plant for nausea, gas pains, and dysentery. Basil's effectiveness as a carminative (a substance that relieves gas) has been established, and research shows that extracts of the plant inhibit organisms that can cause dysentery. Tea made with basil and peppercorns is a folk remedy reputed to reduce fever. A popular culinary herb, basil is easy to grow and to dry for storing.

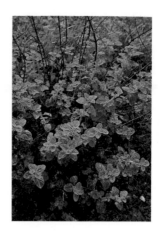

Basil Thyme

Calamintha nepeta (L.) Savi

Calamint, Mountain Mint

MINT FAMILY

Labiatae

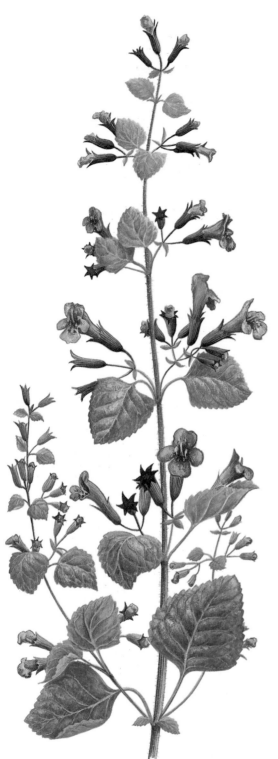

"A common wild plant of great virtue, but too much neglected," Sir John Hill wrote of basil thyme in his *Family Herbal* of 1812. Sir John advised using it as a medicinal tea for weaknesses of the stomach and habitual colic.

The ancients did not neglect this plant. They not only used it, but gave it a place in their legends. A poem attributed to Orpheus states that basil thyme was once a tall fruit tree, until it offended Mother Earth and was shrunk to its present form as a punishment. In a more practical vein the Greek doctor Galen, writing in the second century A.D., said that an application of fresh basil thyme leaves removed the black-and-blue marks of bruises. In his *Herball* (1597), John Gerard wrote that a basil thyme extract would stimulate urine flow; he also stated that it helped to cure jaundice and served as a snakebite remedy. Herbalists of the 20th century have recommended a decoction (extract) of basil thyme for inducing perspiration in order to break a fever, and as an expectorant. Present-day pharmacology has not verified any of these claims.

The common name calamint comes from the plant's ancient Greek name *kalaminthe*, which means "beautiful mint."

Habitat: Well-drained soil in warm locations; herb gardens, rock gardens; waste places, roadsides.
Range: Native to Europe, basil thyme is naturalized and grows wild in North America from Maryland and Kentucky to Georgia and Arkansas.
Identification: A hairy perennial herb growing 1–2½ feet tall, with creeping rhizomes. Bluntly oval leaves are toothed and aromatic, somewhat similar to thyme leaves. The flowers (July–October) range in color from white to pinkish lilac and are about ½ inch long. They are borne in loose clusters at the ends of the stems and branches.
Uses: Basil thyme was prominent in Greco-Roman and early modern herbal tradition. The plant is still recommended by herbalists to break a fever by promoting sweating. They also specify it as an expectorant, but the plant is not widely used in present-day folk medicine.

93

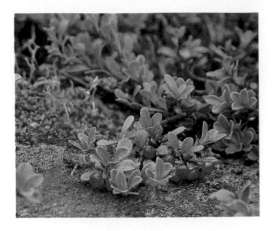

A low, trailing evergreen shrub that resembles a vine, bearberry forms a dense protective carpet on the sandy barrens where it is most often found. The brilliant red berries remain on the plant all winter, affording survival food for bears, birds, and other wild animals when little else is available.

In traditional herbal medicine, however, it is not the berries but the leaves that have held the place of honor. (The berries, while nourishing, are mealy and bland.) Picked in the fall, the leaves were heat-dried for medicinal teas, which folk healers have used for centuries as a tonic and diuretic in many parts of the world. The Cheyenne Indians drank the tea for back sprains, and others used it to treat venereal diseases. Indians and colonists also mixed the dried leaves with tobacco. (The Algonquian name *kinnikinnick* means "mixture.")

Bearberry leaves contain arbutin, a powerful astringent that is thought to have an antiseptic effect on the urinary tract and that may account for bearberry's reputed effectiveness in treating kidney and bladder infections. The leaves are also rich in tannins, which are used for tanning leather.

Bearberry grows abundantly on barren, sandy, or gravelly soils. Its evergreen foliage makes an attractive winter ground cover. The plant is rare or protected in some states.

Bearberry

Arctostaphylos uva-ursi (L.) Spreng.

Bear's-grape, Crowberry, Foxberry, Hog Cranberry, Kinnikinnick, Mealberry

HEATH FAMILY

Ericaceae

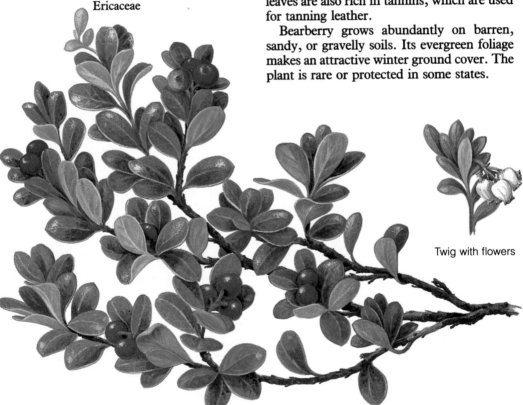

Twig with flowers

Habitat: Dry sandy, gravelly, or rocky soils.
Range: Native to Eurasia, bearberry is naturalized throughout North America as far south as Virginia, west to California.
Identification: A low-growing, trailing evergreen shrub. Dark green leathery alternate leaves, ½– 1½ inches long, are oval and taper toward the base; they have short petioles, or leafstalks. Dense, drooping clusters of pinkish-whitish, waxy, urn-shaped flowers (April–June) are followed by bright red berries that ripen in autumn and last through the winter.
Uses: Because of their reputed diuretic and antiseptic action, the leaves have been used chiefly to treat kidney and bladder infections. Pharmacological studies suggest that the plant may have urinary antiseptic properties, but its reported diuretic effects are questionable.

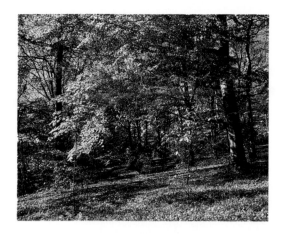

Beech

Fagus grandifolia Ehrh.

American Beech
BEECH FAMILY
Fagaceae

Once a common item on grocery shelves, beechnuts, dried and roasted, were a popular substitute for coffee beans, and a beechnut oil was used in cooking. In parts of the South the emerging leaves served as a potherb. The raw nut itself is sweet and delicious to eat, as not only humans but grouse, squirrels, and other birds and animals know. Because the beech— a tall, handsome tree—grows in loamy soils rich in humus, pioneers who spotted it knew they had found good farmland.

A native tree, the beech has enjoyed a long reputation in America as a source of medicines. The Rappahannock Indians steeped beech bark in saltwater to produce a poison ivy lotion. In Kentucky, beech sap was one ingredient of a syrup compounded to treat tuberculosis. Decoctions of either the leaves or the bark served in folk medicine as an ointment for burns, sores, and ulcers, and when administered internally, as a treatment for bladder, kidney, and liver ailments. A decoction of the root or leaves was believed to cure intermittent fevers, dysentery, and diabetes, while the oil from the nut was given for intestinal worms.

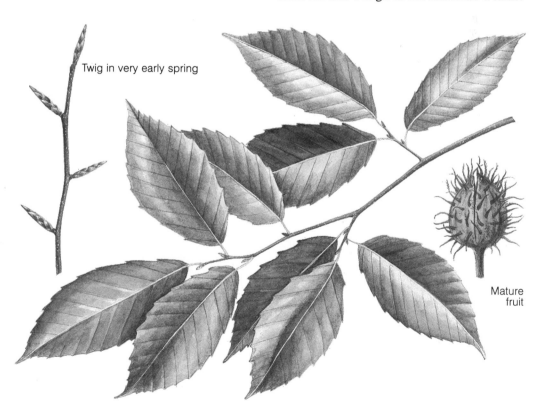

Twig in very early spring

Mature fruit

X Large doses of nuts may be poisonous to humans and animals.

Habitat: Moist, loamy soils.

Range: A native American tree, the beech is found from Nova Scotia to Ontario, south to Florida and eastern Texas, west to Wisconsin and Missouri.

Identification: A medium to large deciduous tree growing to 100 feet or taller. The bark is smooth and light gray to blue-gray. The leaves are alternate, 2½–5½ inches long, with sharp-toothed margins and pointed tips. When mature, the yellowish flowers (April–May) produce spiny fruitlike structures that open late in summer to expose two triangular nuts.

Uses: Beech bark and leaves have astringent and antiseptic properties that account for whatever medicinal effectiveness the plant has. Today beech is valued chiefly for its wood—used in flooring, furniture, crates, and tool handles.

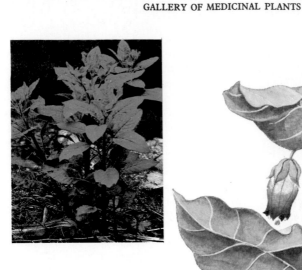

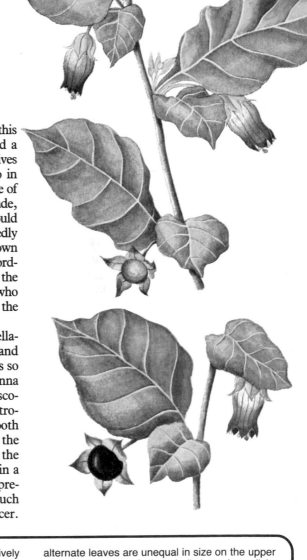

Belladonna

Atropa belladonna L.

Deadly Nightshade, Dwale, Fair Lady
NIGHTSHADE FAMILY

Solanaceae

The Devil himself, it has been said, tends this plant, which is at once a deadly poison and a valuable medicine. Its botanical name derives from one of the three Fates, Atropos, who in Greek mythology cuts the thread of life. One of the plant's popular names is deadly nightshade, and certainly to use it as a home remedy would be deadly folly. Yet despite such a deservedly grim reputation, this plant is universally known as belladonna, or "fair lady" in Italian. According to one story, the name comes from the plant's use long ago by Italian women, who dropped the juice in their eyes to enlarge the pupils and make their eyes more beautiful.

The chemical substance atropine in belladonna does affect the eyes in this manner, and eye doctors today use it to dilate the pupils so that they can examine the retina. Belladonna contains two other valuable substances, scopolamine and hyoscyamine, which, like atropine, are sedatives and act to relax smooth muscle. Individually or in combination, the constituents of belladonna (obtained from the leaves and root) are the basic ingredients in a variety of antispasmodics commonly prescribed today to treat intestinal disorders such as diarrhea, irritable colon, and peptic ulcer.

X Belladonna is extremely toxic; even relatively small doses of it can cause coma and death. Because the ripe berries are not only sweet-tasting but poisonous, children should be expressly warned not to touch them.
Habitat: Woods and wastelands.
Range: Native to Eurasia, belladonna is naturalized in the eastern United States.
Identification: A perennial with a leafy, smooth, branched stem growing about 3 feet tall. Dull green alternate leaves are unequal in size on the upper parts of the stem. Solitary bell-shaped purplish-brown flowers (June–July) arising from the leaf axils are followed by glossy black berries with inky purple juice (September).
Uses: Eye doctors use a belladonna derivative to dilate pupils for eye examinations. The plant is a basic ingredient in medications for colic and peptic ulcers. Externally, belladonna ointment is occasionally applied to treat gout and rheumatism.

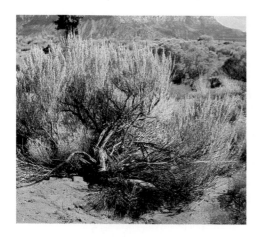

Big Sagebrush

Artemisia tridentata Nutt.

Basin Sagebrush, Common Sagebrush,
Wormwood

COMPOSITE FAMILY

Compositae

The American explorer John C. Frémont noted the appearance of big sagebrush during his westward journey through what is now Wyoming in 1842, calling it by the name of its European relative absinthe. The settlers who followed soon came to regard its presence as a good omen, since where it grew in abundance the soil was fertile enough to support farming.

From prehistoric times, the Indians of the West made use of the treelike shrub, which belongs to the same medicinally important genus of plants as European tarragon, absinthe, and mugwort. They chewed the leaves of sagebrush to ease stomach gas and used a tea made from the leaves to treat other stomach disorders as well as colds and sore eyes. When settlers arrived they took up some of the native uses of the plant and added their own. Sagebrush preparations were used to treat headache, diarrhea, sore throat, vomiting, and even bullet wounds. Some Indians in the Southwest ground the seeds for flour, and many more set great store by a kind of hair tonic made fragrant with sagebrush. Pioneers often used the fast-growing shrub as firewood.

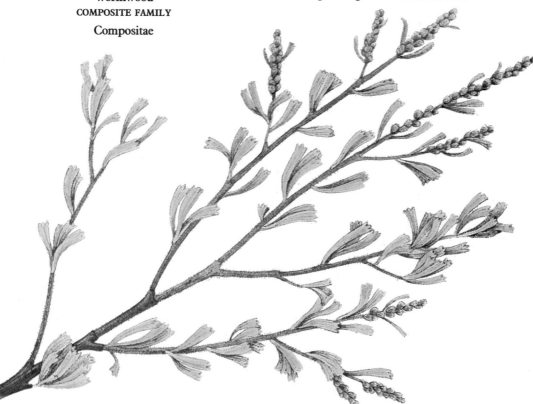

Habitat: Dry gravelly or rocky soils of the plains, high deserts, and lower mountain slopes.

Range: One of the most widely distributed native plants in the American West, big sagebrush is found from British Columbia south to Mexico and east to the Dakotas.

Identification: A woody evergreen shrub, typically 2–10 feet tall. It has a stubby, branched trunk and a grayish-green bark, which shreds with age, and is topped by a rounded crown. Wedge-shaped leaves, about 1 inch long, have three teeth at the tip and are covered with silvery gray hairs that conserve moisture. The leaves emit a pleasantly pungent aroma. Tiny yellow to whitish flowerheads (September–October) grow in dense clusters at the ends of branchlets.

Uses: Big sagebrush is rarely used medicinally today, even in folk medicine. It contains a volatile oil that can be added as an aromatic to liqueurs and hair rinses or used as a bug repellent.

Bindweed

Convolvulus sepium L.

Hedge Bindweed

MORNING GLORY FAMILY

Convolvulaceae

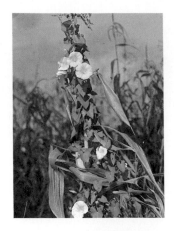

Its scientific name comes from the Latin words *convolvere,* "to entwine," and *sepes,* "a hedge," and that is indeed how bindweed, or hedge bindweed, grows. In hedges or thickets or gardens, wherever it can twine itself, the bindweed spirals, usually counterclockwise, around a neighboring plant or a fence for its support.

As a medicinal plant, bindweed has been valued for the powerful laxative effect of its roots, stem, and leaves. It was also used in folk medicine as a remedy for jaundice.

A relative of the common morning glory (*Ipomoea purpurea*), bindweed is one of the commonest weeds in North America and one of the prettiest. But gardeners do not welcome it, because it strangles neighboring plants, and its huge root system depletes the soil.

Hedge bindweed is just one member of a large family that also includes field bindweed, sea bindweed, jalap bindweed (found in Mexico and South America), and Syrian bindweed (also known as scammony). To a greater or lesser degree these plants have the same cathartic properties, and they also have other characteristics in common: their lovely trumpet-shaped flowers—ranging in color from the white of hedge bindweed to the crimson of jalap, the red-striped rose of sea bindweed, and the sulfur yellow of scammony—and the fact that the flowers of some species close on gray days when the sun does not shine.

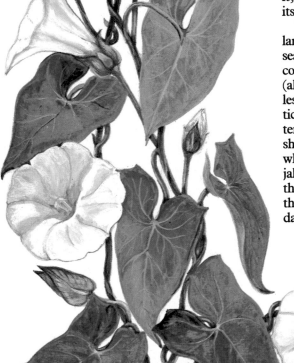

Habitat: Hedges, thickets, waste places, and marshes.
Range: Native to both Europe and North America, hedge bindweed is found in Canada from Newfoundland to British Columbia; and in the eastern half of the United States, extending into Colorado and New Mexico, as well as in parts of the U.S. Pacific Northwest.
Identification: A perennial weed, this trailing member of the morning glory family can grow as high as 15 feet, usually climbing on another plant for support. Large arrow-shaped leaves grow on long stalks. White to pink trumpet-shaped flowers (April–September), 1½–2 inches wide, open in the sun but remain closed on gray days.
Uses: The dried rhizomes (underground stems), roots, and leaves are used in the preparation of laxatives and remedies for gallbladder problems.

The Greek word *lotos* has been given to a number of plants, including the legendary shrub whose fruits were said to inspire happy indolence in those who ate them—the lotus-eaters of mythology. The species name *corniculatus,* meaning "horned," derives from the slender curved tips of the flower bud, which resemble tiny horns. "Bird's-foot" refers to the slender seedpods that look like a bird's foot, and "trefoil" alludes to the plant's similarity to red clover, also known as trefoil.

The medicinal properties assigned to bird's-foot trefoil were discovered in the 19th century by the French herbalist Henri Leclerc. He had recommended an eyewash of sweet clover to treat an attack of conjunctivitis in a countrywoman who also suffered from a nervous condition that caused sleeplessness and heart palpitations. By mistake the distraught patient made a tea of bird's-foot trefoil and drank it. Her nervous troubles reportedly vanished in a week's time!

The plant may have been brought to North America for forage and fodder, a use it still has today. The leaves and flowering tops were once a source of blue and yellow dyes for wool and cotton fabrics, and the flowers are said to furnish an excellent honey.

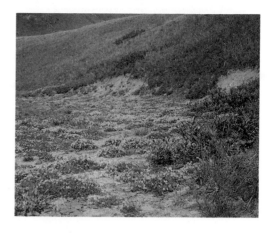

Bird's-foot Trefoil

Lotus corniculatus L.
PEA FAMILY
Leguminosae

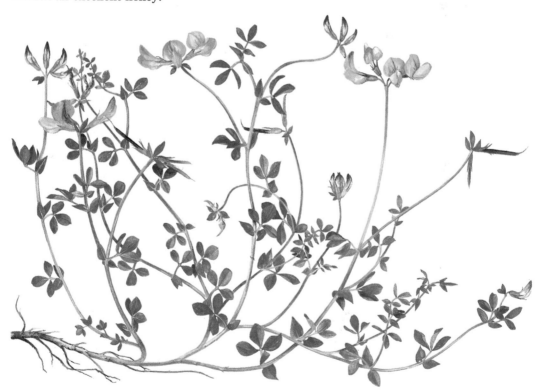

X Leaves and flowers contain cyanide, which may cause paralysis, convulsions, coma, and death.
Habitat: Fields, roadsides, waste places, lawns.
Range: Introduced from Europe, bird's-foot trefoil is now found locally from Newfoundland south to Virginia, west to Ohio and Minnesota, and in northeastern Texas and on the Pacific Coast.
Identification: A low, many-stemmed perennial herb, 6–24 inches high. The leaves are divided into five leaflets, the upper three cloverlike, the lower two in a pair at the base of each leafstalk. Numerous small yellow to orange flowerheads (June–September) are clustered at the ends of long stalks and produce slender seedpods that end in a hornlike tip.
Uses: Herbals classify bird's-foot trefoil as an antispasmodic and sedative and recommend it for the treatment of heart palpitations, nervousness, depression, and insomnia. There is no scientific evidence to validate these uses.

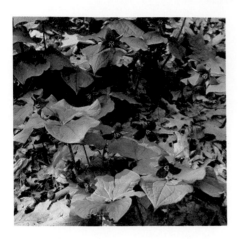

Birthroot

Trillium erectum L.

Bethroot, Indian Balm, Purple Trillium,
Stinking Benjamin, Trillium, Wake-robin
LILY FAMILY
Liliaceae

Walking in woods in early spring, nature lovers will be tempted to pick the pretty, low-growing birthroot. Indeed, its allure is echoed in another of its names, wake-robin, a reminder that the plant is one of nature's early spring offerings. Flower collectors should be warned, however: the plant is rare and threatened in some states. There is another reason for leaving it alone, easily discernible in the nickname stinking Benjamin. Some herbalists found that the plant's odor so much resembled the stench of decaying flesh that they made an ointment from the rhizomes and roots for the treatment of gangrene—on the basis of the once-respected doctrine of signatures, according to which a plant's characteristics indicated its corresponding effectiveness on the human body.

The name birthroot describes the plant's chief medicinal use—to stop hemmorhaging. Specifically, a tea made from the rhizomes and roots was given to new mothers to stop bleeding after childbirth. By association, the tea was also given for uterine disorders. The Indians applied poultices and lotions from the bruised leaves to insect bites and skin irritations.

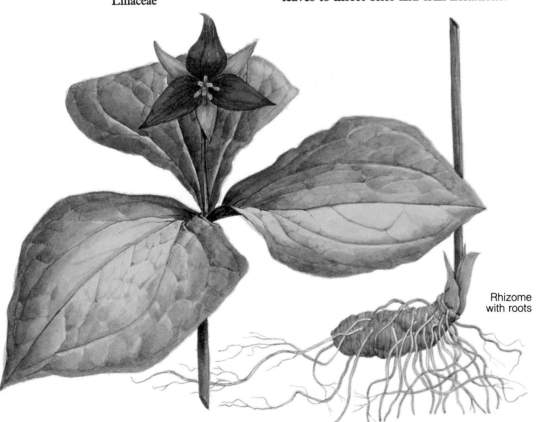

Rhizome
with roots

Habitat: Shady, moist woodlands with rich soil.
Range: Nova Scotia, Quebec, and Ontario south through the eastern and central United States.
Identification: An erect perennial with a smooth, stout stem 8–16 inches high. Its three dark green, diamond-shaped, net-veined leaves, each about 7 inches long, and its solitary, foul-smelling flower (April–June) with three green sepals and three maroon to reddish-brown petals account for the name trillium, from the Latin word for three. The

flower produces an oval, reddish berry. Both the roots and leaves give off a distinctive acrid odor.
Uses: Birthroot remains a popular folk cure for bleeding, snakebite, and skin irritations. Studies indicate that birthroot probably acts as an external astringent and therefore may help external bleeding. No basis has been found to support its use in herbal medicine as an expectorant or an emmenagogue (to promote menstruation). The leaves sometimes serve as a potherb or salad green in Appalachia.

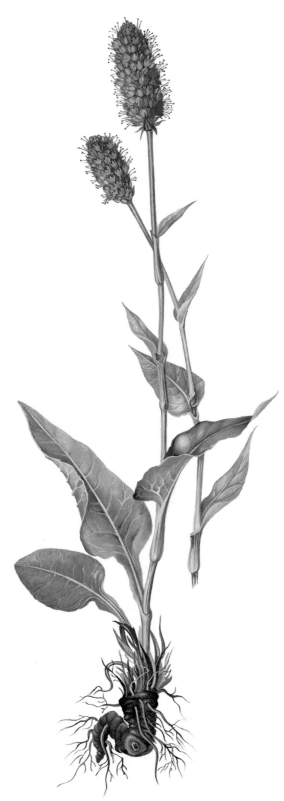

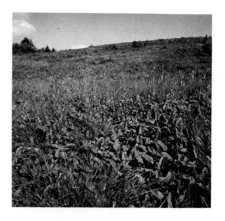

Bistort

Polygonum bistorta L.

Adderwort, Patience Dock, Snakeweed
BUCKWHEAT FAMILY
Polygonaceae

Dense clusters of tiny pink blossoms atop slender stalks in a forest clearing or in a meadow—that is bistort, a common summer sight in the wild throughout the temperate Northern Hemisphere. Two species native to the Old and New Worlds, *P. bistorta* and *P. bistortoides* respectively, are closely akin. The name bistort comes from Latin word elements meaning "twice-twisted." This refers to the gnarled appearance of bistort's dark brown rhizome, or underground stem.

Traditional uses of bistort in herbal medicine are varied. In Shakespeare's day the juice of the plant served as a remedy for nasal polyps. The rhizome, boiled in wine, was used for diarrhea and dysentery. The same decoction reportedly checked heavy menstrual bleeding, stopped vomiting, and healed mouth and throat inflammations. It also had a reputation as a mouthwash that would fasten loose teeth. A common thread unites most of these uses—namely, the plant's high tannin content, which makes it astringent and therefore effective in checking bleeding and diarrhea. Because the rhizomes are starchy, they served as famine food, roasted, boiled in soup, or ground to make flour. Young bistort leaves may be cooked and eaten like spinach.

Habitat: Damp soil, fields, cultivated grounds.
Range: Native to Europe, bistort has been naturalized locally in North America in Nova Scotia and eastern Massachusetts.
Identification: A hardy perennial with slender stems, growing up to 30 inches tall. Each stem is topped by a dense cylindrical cluster of tiny white or pinkish flowers (May–August). Lower down the stem grow long bluish-green leaves that are lance-shaped; higher up, the leaves become smaller.

The rhizome (underground stem) is dark brown to black, thick, knobby, and twisted into an S or double-S shape.
Uses: Bistort is a powerful astringent because of its high tannin content. Herbalists recommend external applications of the powdered rhizome to control bleeding. An extract of the rhizome is suggested for internal use in cases of diarrhea, and herbalists also mention using the extract externally as a wash, or lotion, for sores.

101

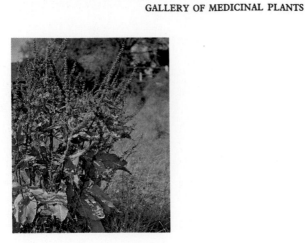

Bitter Dock

Rumex obtusifolius L.

Blunt-leaved Dock, Broad-leaved Dock,
Common Dock, Red-veined Dock,
Round-leaved Dock

BUCKWHEAT FAMILY

Polygonaceae

To most North Americans today, dock is known as a garden weed, and a particularly tenacious one. There are more than 20 species of dock in the New World, some of them introduced from Europe. Leading members of the group are bitter dock, yellow dock, and patience dock. These vary in size, flower, fruit, and leaf, but their medicinal and culinary uses overlap. In folk usage they are not clearly distinguished. As early as classical antiquity, herbalists knew of the docks' effectiveness as laxatives. Centuries later, in Anglo-Saxon England, physicians used a mixture of the leaves, other herbs, ale, and holy water to cure people believed to have been made ill with "elf sickness" by witchcraft. Another old English folk belief holds that the crushed leaves cure nettle rash when accompanied by an incantation such as the following:

Nettle out, dock in,
Dock remove the nettle sting.

By the 17th century, a tea made from dock roots was held to alleviate toothache when taken orally and to cure the itch when used as a wash. The herbalist Nicholas Culpeper stated that dock extract cleared up skin blemishes.

Plant with fruits

Cut stem with root

Mature fruit

Habitat: Meadows, roadsides, waste places.
Range: Native to Europe, the plant now grows wild throughout the United States.
Identification: A perennial herbaceous plant 2–5 feet tall, bitter dock has an erect, greenish stem, often with red streaks. Its large basal leaves are up to 14 inches long and have blunt or heart-shaped bases; the upper leaves are shorter and more slender. Tiny greenish flowers (June–September) occur in dense clusters on tall stalks at the top of the plant. The small one-seeded fruit is enclosed in three winglike and deeply toothed valves.
Uses: Scientific studies have validated the traditional prescription of bitter dock tea as a laxative. The young leaves of bitter dock may be eaten fresh as a salad or cooked like spinach. The root yields a yellow dye.

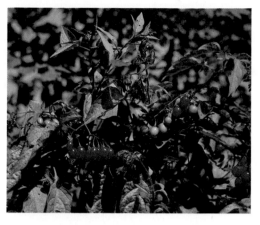

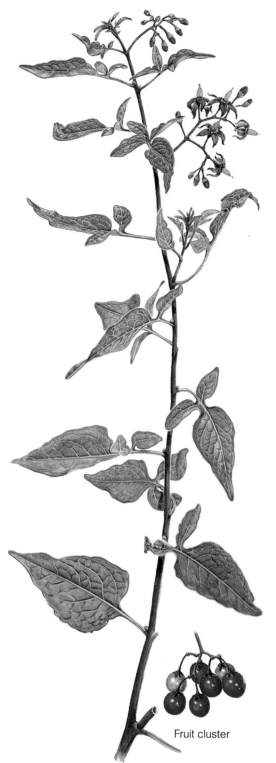

Fruit cluster

Bittersweet Nightshade

Solanum dulcamara L.

Bitter Nightshade, Bittersweet,
Felonwort, Violet-bloom, Woody Nightshade
NIGHTSHADE FAMILY

Solanaceae

An aggressive and persistent weed, bittersweet nightshade, or bittersweet, is one of the poisonous black sheep of a botanical family that also includes such paragons of respectability as the potato and the tomato. Despite its toxicity, bittersweet was once employed as an external remedy for skin diseases and as a treatment for sores and swellings, especially felons—inflammations around the fingernails and toenails. Doctors abandoned the plant's use long ago, but recent research indicates that bittersweet contains a tumor-inhibiting agent, beta-solamarine, which may have some promise in treating cancer. Herbalists have prescribed extracts made from the stems to be taken internally as a sedative, pain reliever, and diuretic and in the treatment of asthma.

The plant's species name, *dulcamara*, refers to the flavor of the berries, which is first bitter, then unpleasantly sweet. An import from Europe, bittersweet has a native American relative, the horse nettle (*S. carolinense*), whose yellow berries have been used to treat convulsive disorders and menstrual problems.

X The whole plant is poisonous and should not be used without medical supervision.
Habitat: Damp places, streambanks, thickets.
Range: Native to Eurasia, bittersweet is naturalized in the United States and temperate Canada.
Identification: A vinelike perennial with trailing or climbing stems up to 10 feet long, bittersweet has alternate heart-shaped to oval leaves, which usually have two earlike segments at their bases. Its star-shaped flowers (April–September) are pinkish purple with bright yellow stamens; they are followed by green berries, which turn bright red.
Uses: Pharmacologists have studied bittersweet's use in herbal medicine as an internal antirheumatic, diuretic, narcotic, and sedative, and as an external astringent. They find little evidence to validate any of these uses, but they find that extracts of the plant do show antibiotic activity, which explains their effectiveness in external use for sores and inflammations.

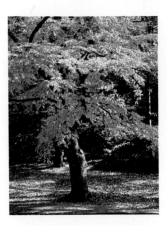

Black Birch

Betula lenta L.

Cherry Birch, Mountain Mahogany, Sweet Birch
BIRCH FAMILY
Betulaceae

With its delightfully clean wintergreen scent and its delicate papery leaves, black birch flourishes especially in the Appalachian Mountains, and it was there that the species came close to annihilation in the 19th century, when the local people learned that an oil made from the bark and twigs could be sold for cash. The oil, it was discovered, was identical in taste, odor, and chemical composition to oil of wintergreen, used to give a pleasant taste to medicines and as a liniment and a flavoring for candies. But the tiny wintergreen plant yielded only minute quantities of oil; far greater amounts could be obtained from birch bark and twigs. Whole families, it is said, went into the business of chopping down the trees, boiling the bark to extract the oil, and selling it by the quart to storekeepers, who acted as the drug manufacturers' middlemen. Subsequently oil of wintergreen (still used as a flavoring) was made synthetically, and the black birch was thus spared further exploitation.

In folk medicine a tea made from the twigs and bark was taken as a remedy for rheumatism and other sorts of aches. Externally the oil from the bark was applied as a pain reliever for wounds and sprains.

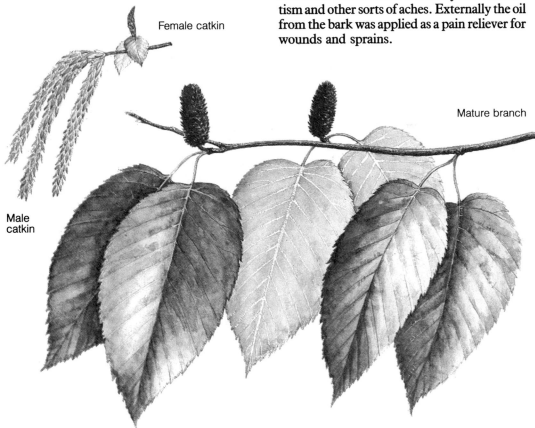

Female catkin

Mature branch

Male catkin

Habitat: Favors moist, rich, rocky hill and valley soils but can occur on drier slopes.
Range: Native to North America, the black birch grows from southern Canada south through the Appalachian Mountains and as far west as Ohio.
Identification: Averaging 50–60 feet tall, with a trunk 2–3 feet in diameter, black birch is known for its wintergreen scent and mahogany-red to gray bark. Slender branches bear thin, pointed leaves 2–5 inches long and hairy underneath. Reddish-brown male flowers (April–May) grow in dangling clusters (catkins) on the same tree with pale green female ones. One-inch cones contain numerous tiny winged seeds (the true fruits).
Uses: Black birch bark has astringent properties, which account for its effectiveness in treating wounds, and it contains methyl salicylate, which explains its usefulness as a pain reliever. When applied externally, the oil is an excellent counterirritant to alleviate the pain of sore muscles.

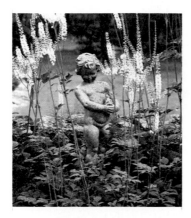

Black Cohosh

Cimicifuga racemosa (L.) Nutt.

Black Snakeroot, Bugbane, Squawroot
BUTTERCUP FAMILY
Ranunculaceae

The strong odor of black cohosh flowers acts as an insect repellent, hence the alternative name bugbane. The botanical name *Cimicifuga* is Latin for "bug repellent."

But the more significant part of this native American plant is its hard, knotty rootstock, or rhizome, which has been used for a wide variety of medicinal purposes. The name cohosh comes from an Algonquian word meaning "rough," a reference to the feel of the rhizome when handled. A brew made from it was a favored Indian remedy for menstrual cramps and the pains of childbirth, uses commemorated in the vernacular name squawroot. The Indians also used a poultice made from the rhizome as a snakebite remedy.

In the 19th century a tincture from the rhizome was deemed helpful for treating rheumatism. Laboratory experiments suggest that extracts of the rhizome have an anti-inflammatory effect and that its use in the treatment of neuralgia and rheumatism may therefore be well founded.

Large doses of black cohosh cause symptoms of poisoning, particularly nausea and dizziness, and can also provoke miscarriage.

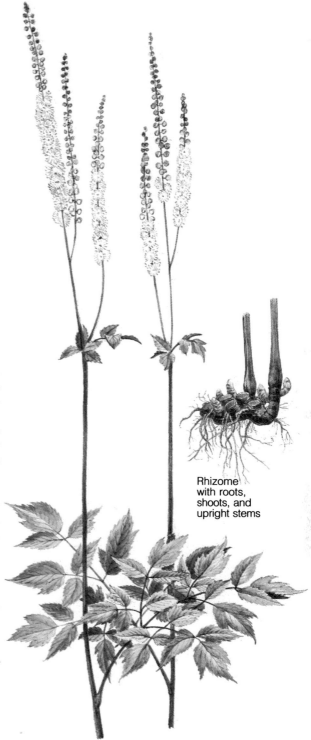

Rhizome
with roots,
shoots, and
upright stems

X Poisonous in large doses.
Habitat: Open woods, edges of dense woods, and recently cleared hillsides.
Range: From Ontario south to Georgia and Tennessee; Massachusetts west to Missouri.
Identification: A stately perennial, 3–8 feet tall, topped by a long plume of white flowers (June–September). The leaves are large and pinnately compound; the leaflets are irregularly shaped with toothed edges. That a plant with prominent white

flowers should be named "black" is often a point of confusion—the "black" refers to the dark color of the rhizome.
Uses: The primary traditional use of black cohosh has been as a relaxant, sedative, and antispasmodic. Its effectiveness as a remedy for dysmenorrhea has not been successfully proven, but research suggests a pharmacological basis for its use in treating rheumatism and neuralgia.

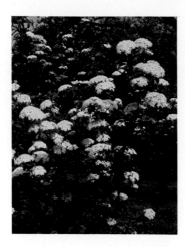

Black Haw

Viburnum prunifolium L.

American Sloe, Cramp Bark, Stagbush
HONEYSUCKLE FAMILY

Caprifoliaceae

In early fall hikers often pause to enjoy the sweet fruits of the black haw tree. The Indiana poet James Whitcomb Riley (1849–1916) extolled their virtues, writing: "What is sweeter, after all, than black haws, in early fall?"

Indian uses of this native tree are not well documented, but one source mentions that they employed a decoction, or extract, from the boiled bark to treat venereal disease. Black haw's service as an early American home medicine, by contrast, is well recorded. Although the plant was used in the early 1800's, the first published mention of it appeared in 1857, in the *American Family Physician,* by Dr. John King, who described it as a "uterine tonic." Doctors largely prescribed a decoction of the bark to prevent miscarriage or threatened abortion. Black haw was also recommended for the relief of painful menstruation and the afterpains of childbirth. As a result of growing demand and repeated articles in medical and pharmaceutical journals, black haw bark gained a place in the *U.S. Pharmacopeia* in 1882 and was listed there until 1926.

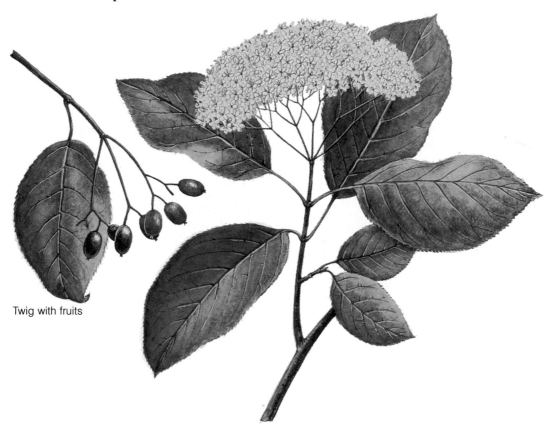

Twig with fruits

Habitat: Rocky hillsides, thickets, woods, shores, borders of streams.

Range: Connecticut to Michigan, south to Florida and Texas.

Identification: A shrub or tree growing up to 30 feet tall. The gray- to reddish-brown bark is rough and cracked into small plates on older trees. Heavily veined, finely toothed leaves are elliptical and grow in opposite pairs. Tiny white flowers (April–May) in round-topped clusters are followed by fruits that turn bluish black when they are ripe.

Uses: An extract of boiled black haw bark has traditionally been employed as a uterine tonic (a substance that aids in childbirth by stimulating the muscles of the womb) and as a medicine to prevent abortion or miscarriage. Research indicates that a bark decoction probably acts as a uterine sedative (an agent that relaxes uterine muscles and hence alleviates menstrual cramps), but they doubt it can prevent abortion or miscarriage.

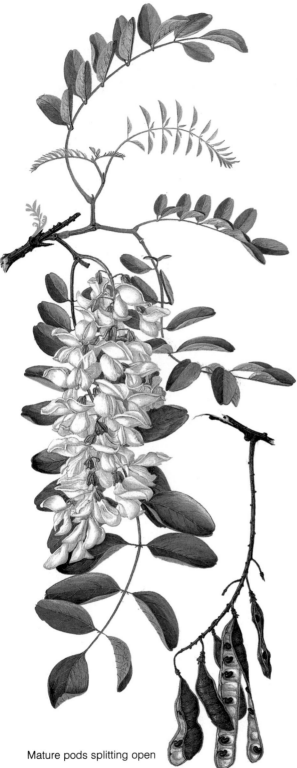

Mature pods splitting open

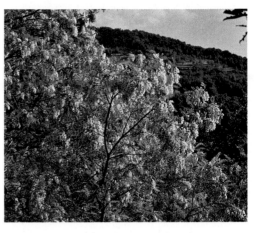

Black Locust

Robinia pseudoacacia L.

False Acacia, Yellow Locust

PEA FAMILY

Leguminosae

The fragrant white pealike flowers and the seedpods of the black locust identify it as a member of the pea family. A North American native, the black locust is believed to have originated in the Appalachian Mountains. At one time, it is said, some American Indians prepared emetics and strong laxatives from the bark; but because the tree contains mildly toxic substances, it never enjoyed wide medicinal use. Its sterling qualities as building timber, however—locust posts set in the ground will remain sturdy for 50 years—led settlers to spread its range, so that it is now widely established in North America. The stately tree was also planted in Paris from seeds sent to Jean Robin, botanist and landscaper to the king of France at the beginning of the 17th century—hence its scientific name, *Robinia*. Since then, the black locust has been planted from England to eastern Europe, becoming the most important timber tree in Hungary and Romania.

Europeans also experimented with black locust for medicinal purposes. A tea made from the flowers was tried for headaches, stomach pains, and nausea, and locust blossoms steeped in wine were used to treat anemia.

X The seeds may cause vomiting, nausea, and dizziness and may dangerously slow the heartbeat.
Habitat: Prefers deep, rich, moist soils but will grow almost anywhere.
Range: Nova Scotia to Ontario, and throughout the United States from Maine to California.
Identification: A deciduous tree 60–80 feet tall, with a thick, deeply furrowed, dark brown bark and crooked, forking branches. Compound, feathery leaves 8–10 inches long consist of oval leaflets 1–2½ inches long. A pair of approximately ½-inch-long thorns forms at the base of each leaf. White, sweet-scented flower clusters (May–June) resemble pea blossoms. Smooth, dark brown pods 3–4 inches long contain poisonous seeds.
Uses: The black locust is no longer used medicinally. The hard, very durable wood is made into fence posts, railroad ties, and mine timbers. Because the trees grow fast, conservationists favor them for erosion control.

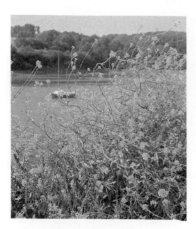

Black Mustard

Brassica nigra (L.) Koch
MUSTARD FAMILY
Cruciferae

In spring endless acres of yellow-blossomed black mustard plants brighten waste areas across the land. In time the graceful flowers produce brown to black seeds that are among the most powerful caustic agents known. The seeds contain two chemical compounds, myrosin and sinigrin. When mixed with water, the chemicals produce a volatile oil, a tiny drop of which may cause skin blisters or a burn.

This oil is the basis of the renowned mustard plaster that doctors in past generations prescribed, and mothers had the task of applying, for bad chest colds and bronchial conditions. The plaster consisted of a mixture of powdered mustard, flour, and water spread between two soft pieces of cloth such as flannel, which were placed on the chest. If the plaster was left on too long or if the preparation was too strong, the skin blistered.

The plaster was effective because the mustard seed oil is a counterirritant—an agent that, when applied externally to an inflamed area, causes the blood vessels to dilate. The resulting increased blood supply to the area carries away the toxic products that produced the original inflammation.

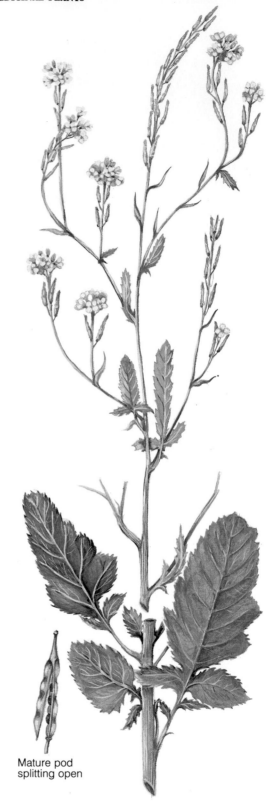

Mature pod
splitting open

X A powerful irritant, mustard oil should be used sparingly, in diluted form, and only externally, for short exposure periods.
Habitat: Roadsides and other waste places.
Range: A native of Europe, black mustard now grows wild throughout most of North America.
Identification: An annual herb, growing up to 6 feet tall. The leaves are pinnately divided at the base and toothed. The upper leaves are smaller and narrower than the lower ones. Yellow flowers (May–July) produce pods (June–October) containing the tiny brown to black seeds.
Uses: Ancient Greek physicians prescribed mustard plasters for lung congestion; Anglo-Saxons used them for bronchial problems. Research shows that black mustard seeds are an effective external agent for curing below-surface inflammations. The seeds are also the flavcring in table mustard. The greens are a nutritious food, either cooked or added to salads.

Black Poplar

Populus nigra L.

Balm of Gilead, Balsam Poplar
WILLOW FAMILY
Salicaceae

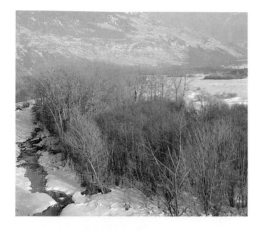

Well supplied with salicin, a substance closely related to the active agent in modern aspirin, the buds, young bark, and leaves of the black poplar have been used since antiquity, apparently with good effect, in preparations for coughs, asthma, rheumatism, earache, and inflammations of all kinds. The buds have been an ingredient in skin salves for burns, boils, and hemorrhoids and in liniments for rheumatic pains. Modern medical knowledge indicates that patients may benefit from the salves and liniments too, because salicin, like the acetylsalicylic acid in aspirin, is absorbed when applied externally. The buds also have antiseptic properties that may help healing.

The black poplar is closely related to the Lombardy poplar, *P. nigra* var. *italica*, which is commonly cultivated in North America. Another related species is *P. balsamifera*, or hackmatack, an aromatic native American species whose resins many American Indians recognized as an important source of medications for aches, pains, sprains, and severe burns, as well as heart trouble and tumors.

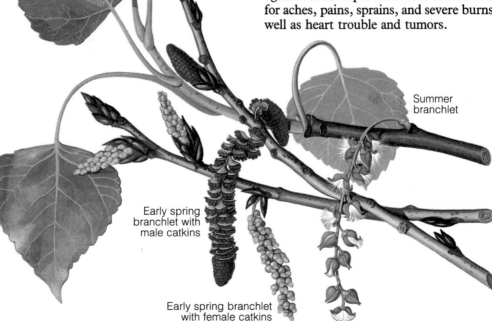

Summer branchlet

Early spring branchlet with male catkins

Early spring branchlet with female catkins

Habitat: Moist woodlands and shore areas.
Range: Introduced from Europe, black poplar is cultivated (and occasionally escapes) in Alaska, southern Canada, and the northern United States.
Identification: A fast-growing, slender deciduous tree 80–100 feet tall. Its smooth gray bark darkens and turns rough with age. Triangular, toothed leaves, 2–3 inches wide, taper to a sharp point. Male and female flowers are on separate trees. The buds (March–April) grow in sticky pointed clusters.

Catkins (clusters) of open male flowers (April–May) are red; the females yellowish green. Female catkins, 3–3½ inches long, bear cottony seeds.
Uses: In modern herbal medicine, black poplar buds are used to prepare a salve for relieving the pain of skin abrasions and hemorrhoids. Evidence exists that the salicin in poplar buds acts much like aspirin when taken internally or applied externally for the relief of pain and inflammation and that the buds have antiseptic and expectorant properties.

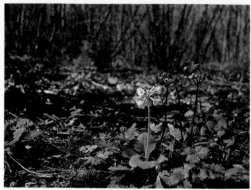

Black Snakeroot

Sanicula marilandica L.

American Sanicle, Black Sanicle, Sanicle

CARROT FAMILY

Umbelliferae

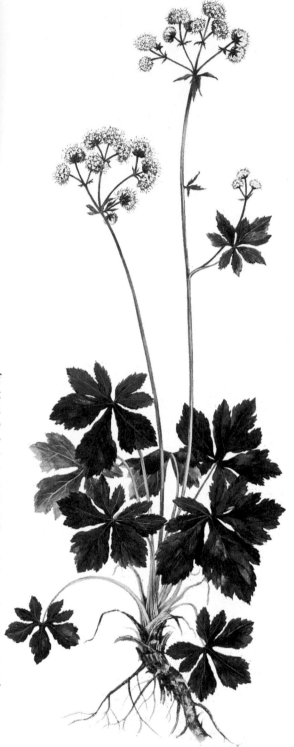

When European settlers made a poultice of the crushed roots of *S. marilandica* to draw out snakebite venom, they were expanding upon the long list of curative properties attributed to black snakeroot's European cousin *S. europaea*, or sanicle, which was considered a cure-all. English herbalists, for example, used sanicle to treat internal bleeding, chronic cough, tumors, stomach ulcers, varicose veins, pains in the bowels, gonorrhea, kidney problems, and "laxes of the belly." It was claimed to be equally good for chapped hands, hemorrhoids, and dysentery. John Gerard, the famed 16th-century English herbalist, had high praise for the mixing of sanicle in "vulnerary potions, or wound drinks, which make whole and sound all inward wounds and outward hurts."

North American Indians, quite independently, also developed uses for snakeroot. In particular, they used it to treat fever, sore throat, skin conditions, St. Vitus' dance (a type of chorea that results in temporary loss of muscular control) and St. Anthony's fire (erysipelas, a painful infection of the skin produced by streptococcus bacteria).

X Do not confuse black snakeroot with such poisonous members of the carrot family as water hemlock and poison hemlock.

Habitat: Meadows, thickets, and shady, moist, woodland soils.

Range: Native to North America, black snakeroot is distributed from Newfoundland south to Florida, and west to Washington and British Columbia.

Identification: A perennial herb with a thick rhizome and almost leafless flower stalks that grow erect, 1–4 feet tall. Basal leaves are long-stalked with five oval to elliptical, unequally toothed, often deeply cleft leaflets. Flower clusters (June–July), each with 12–25 greenish-white blossoms, are followed by fruits covered with hooked bristles.

Uses: Pharmacological studies reveal that black snakeroot contains some tannin, which causes an astringent action that may account for the use of snakeroot preparations as gargles for sore throat.

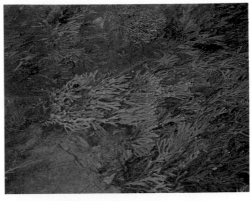

Bladderwrack

Fucus vesiculosus L.

Bladder Fucus, Kelpware, Rockweed, Seawrack
KELP FAMILY
Fucaceae

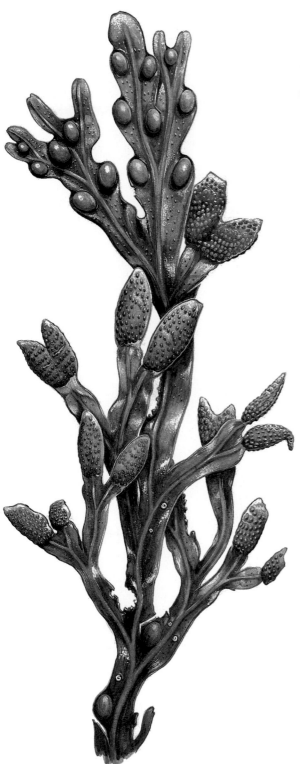

A type of seaweed found along both coasts of North America and the Atlantic shores of Europe, bladderwrack has been used medicinally since antiquity. Perhaps its most remarkable application was in the 18th century, when a British physician prescribed it as a treatment for goiter, an enlargement of the thyroid gland. No one knows whether the doctor had scientific knowledge of the plant's action or was just lucky in his recommendation, but there is a pharmacological basis for his prescription: bladderwrack, like other seaweeds, contains iodine, subsequently found to be essential for the healthy functioning of the thyroid.

Iodine pills and extracts gained particular favor as treatments for obesity, perhaps because of their ability to stimulate a sluggish thyroid gland. These treatments remained in favor well into the 20th century. Other, sometimes justifiable claims made for bladderwrack were that the fresh seaweed rubbed on the skin softens it and stimulates blood circulation, that a syrup prepared from the dried seaweed eases throat irritation, and that a liniment prepared from the juice of the plant's bladders is good for rheumatism. Bladderwrack and other seaweeds have been replaced in medicine by cheaper, more reliable sources of iodine.

Habitat: Submerged rocks along seacoasts.
Range: Atlantic and Pacific coasts of North America; Atlantic coast of Europe.
Identification: A light yellow to brownish-green perennial seaweed, bladderwrack grows about halfway between the high- and low-water marks. It has a branched, ribbonlike plant body that reaches 2–3 feet high when held afloat by water during high tide. The plant anchors itself to rocks by means of a rootlike suction disc at the base. Air-filled oval bladders, ½ inch in diameter, usually occur along the body's midrib and keep the plant afloat. Each branch ends in a fruiting structure.
Uses: Research has proved bladderwrack's efficacy in treating iodine deficiency, but its use is not recommended because of difficulty in controlling dosages. The mucilage in bladderwrack softens the skin and the mucous membranes—a fact that probably accounts for its use on the skin and in treating throat irritations.

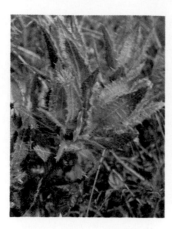

Blessed Thistle

Cnicus benedictus L.

Holy Thistle, Spotted Thistle
COMPOSITE FAMILY
Compositae

Monks once grew blessed thistle as a cure for smallpox, according to one source, and some say that is how the plant got its name. Early botanists gave the herb the scientific name *benedictus* in honor of St. Benedict, who founded the religious order that bears his name. That both the common and scientific names for the plant should honor monks is appropriate, because in medieval times monasteries were the repositories of such medical knowledge as existed in Europe.

Early herbalists believed the herb was a cure-all. They noted that the plant could both prevent and cure headache, provoke sweat, help memory, strengthen the heart and stomach, and cure external problems such as festering sores, boils, and the itch. Shakespeare knew of the plant's virtues, remarking: "Get you some of this distilled Carduus Benedictus, and lay it to your heart: it is the only thing for a qualm. . . . plain holy-thistle."

Nineteenth-century herbalists prescribed an infusion, or tea, made from the plant tops as a treatment for fevers and for liver and respiratory ailments.

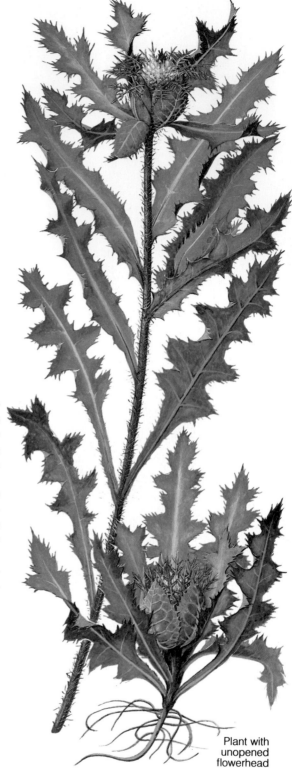

Plant with
unopened
flowerhead

Habitat: A rare plant, found in waste places and roadsides.
Range: Introduced from Europe, blessed thistle is now naturalized in many parts of North America.
Identification: An annual herb, growing to about 2 feet tall. The brown stem is hairy and erect. The lance-shaped leaves have spiny edges and may be either lobed or cleft (deeply cut). The plant produces numerous yellow flowers (May–August) arranged in a head at the tip of a branch or stem.

Uses: In herbal medicine today, blessed thistle is used as a contraceptive and to treat cancer as well as infections, heart and liver ailments, and fevers. Experimental evidence points to its effectiveness as a treatment for infections but does not support its use for fevers or cancer. Its effect on the heart and liver and its efficacy as a contraceptive have not been studied.

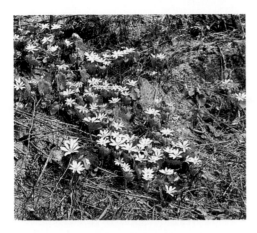

Bloodroot

Sanguinaria canadensis L.

Indian Paint, Red Puccoon,
Redroot, Tetterwort
POPPY FAMILY

Papaveraceae

Referring to the plant by its Indian name, *puccoon,* Capt. John Smith in 1612 recalled his experience with bloodroot in Jamestown, Virginia, noting: "this they use for swellings, aches, annointing their joints, painting their heads and garments." But that, Smith confessed, was not all they painted. He added, "they set a woman fresh painted red" to be a bedfellow of one of the colonists. Such was the Indians' fascination with bloodroot juice.

The properties of this native American plant, the settlers discovered, were more medicinal than decorative. As they learned from the Indians (who used the blood-red juice as a treatment for sore throats and cancer and an infusion of the rhizome for rheumatism), bloodroot is a powerful herb. Both the powdered rhizome and the juice from it are extremely caustic, chemically capable of corroding and destroying tissue. Therefore bloodroot came to be prescribed as a cure for surface cancers, fungal growths such as ringworm, and nose polyps. Folk healers also recommended bloodroot as an emetic (to induce vomiting), as an expectorant for bronchitis, as a laxative, and even as a stimulant for the digestive organs.

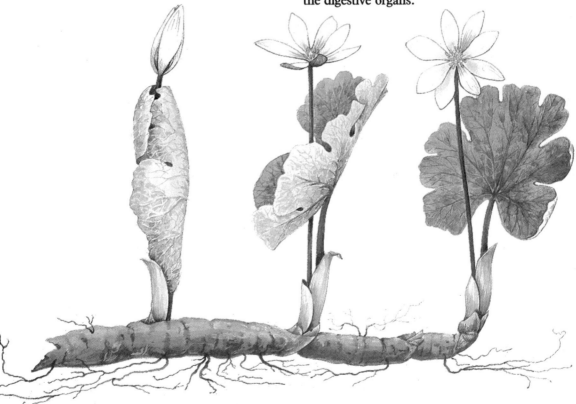

✗ The U.S. Food and Drug Adminstration lists bloodroot as "unsafe"; do not use it.
Habitat: Wet banks, fields, woods.
Range: Native to North America from Quebec south to Florida and Texas and west to Kansas. Bloodroot is an endangered or threatened species in some states.
Identification: A low-growing perennial, bloodroot has an orange-red rhizome (underground stem) from which solitary blooms emerge. Each bloom is enveloped in a single leaf that enlarges after flowering and is pale green and lobed. White flowers (March–May) usually have eight petals.
Uses: Research indicates that the red juice in the rhizome is an escharotic, a caustic substance that produces a mass of dead tissue after application. Bloodroot's effectiveness in specifically treating ringworm and eczema is probable, but has not been proved, nor has its use as an expectorant (since the plant may be toxic when taken internally).

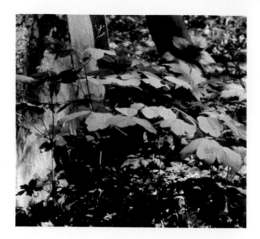

Blue Cohosh

Caulophyllum thalictroides (L.) Michx.

Blue Ginseng, Papoose Root,
Squawroot, Yellow Ginseng
BARBERRY FAMILY

Berberidaceae

In early spring, in the moist, rich recesses of the forest, the smooth, bluish stem and large, single, unfolding leaf of the blue cohosh stand out vividly against the surrounding bareness. As the plant develops, it blends in with the rest of the forest growth, until in late summer the deep blue "berries" (which are actually seeds) attract the eye.

The knotty, branching rhizome and roots of this native American plant were sought out by many Indian tribes. They harvested the underground parts in late fall and ground them into a powder, which they used as a remedy for rheumatism, colic, bronchitis, and menstrual cramps. But they especially prized blue cohosh as a parturient (an aid in childbirth). For a week or two before the expected date of delivery, pregnant women drank an infusion of the powdered roots in warm water to induce rapid and relatively painless labor. (It was not taken earlier in pregnancy, because it might have brought on a miscarriage.) Early settlers also used the roots as a parturient and dubbed the plant squawroot and papoose root.

The herbalists who gathered and prepared blue cohosh learned to treat it with caution, because they found that it tends to irritate the skin and mucous membranes, especially when it is powdered.

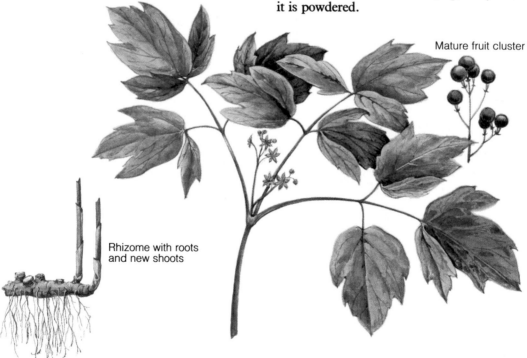

Mature fruit cluster

Rhizome with roots
and new shoots

X Blue cohosh "berries" (actually seeds) are poisonous. The plant is an irritant to the skin, the root to the mucous membranes.
Habitat: Deep, loamy, moist woodlands.
Range: New Brunswick and Ontario to Manitoba, south to South Carolina, Tennessee, and Missouri.
Identification: A perennial herb, blue cohosh in early spring sends up a bluish stem with a single large unfolding leaf. Three more stalks develop from the leaf, and these in turn divide into threes,

with each division bearing a single small, oval, notched leaflet. Clustered greenish-yellow flowers (April–May) are followed by handsome, berrylike blue seeds.
Uses: Herbalists today use the roots to treat rheumatism and bronchitis. Good experimental data exist to verify their effectiveness in treating rheumatism, and there is some evidence that the roots may have antispasmodic properties.

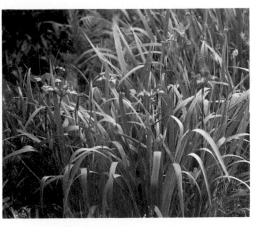

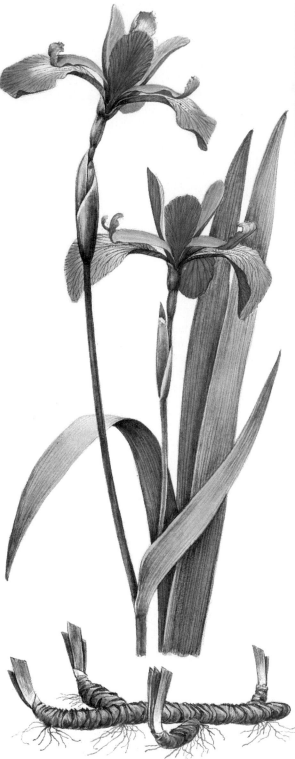

Rhizome with roots and leafy stems

Blue Flag

Iris versicolor L.

Liver Lily, Poison Flag, Water Flag
IRIS FAMILY
Iridaceae

Named in honor of the Greek goddess of the rainbow, the many-hued irises are among the most colorful of flowers and have long been a mainstay in perennial gardens. Blue flag is one of many wild irises native to eastern North America. It was so named by early settlers because of its close resemblance to a common European species, the yellow flag, which was the model for the fleur-de-lis, the emblem of French royalty.

Blue flag has also been known as the liver lily, because its dried and powdered rhizomes were traditionally believed to be an excellent remedy for impurities of the blood and diseases of the liver. Its many other uses in folk medicine included the treatment of skin diseases, rheumatism, and even syphilis. No one, however, prized blue flag more than American Indians, some of whom regarded it as a virtual panacea. One of their uses for it, not adopted by the white man, was as a poultice for treating sores and bruises. Certain tribes are said to have planted blue flag near their villages to ensure a convenient supply.

The rhizomes of blue flag can be dangerously toxic, as is indicated by one of its other names, poison flag.

X The rhizomes are poisonous and should not be taken internally. Blue flag when not in bloom can be mistaken for sweet flag.
Habitat: Marshes, wet meadows, and banks of lakes and streams.
Range: Labrador to Manitoba, south to Virginia, Ohio, Wisconsin, and Minnesota.
Identification: A perennial herb growing 2–3 feet high, with flattened stems; narrow, sword-shaped leaves; and thick, fleshy rhizomes. The flowers (May–July) are violet-blue, with yellow, green, or white markings on the three outer "petals" (actually showy sepals).
Uses: A potent diuretic, cathartic, and emetic, blue flag was used to treat a wide range of disorders, including diseases of the blood and liver, skin diseases, and rheumatism. Nowadays the plant is popular with gardeners as a flower for brightening wet sites.

Boneset

Eupatorium perfoliatum L.

Agueweed, Crosswort, Feverwort,
Indian Sage, Thoroughwort
COMPOSITE FAMILY

Compositae

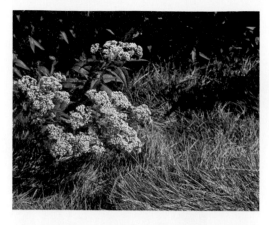

Legendary among North American Indians and early settlers for its capacity to cause profuse perspiration and to loosen the bowels, boneset was used to treat fevers associated with a number of illnesses, including colds and influenza as well as malaria and similar recurrent illnesses. The herb was usually taken as a hot tea made from the leaves and flowers. Boneset's genus name, *Eupatorium,* may be traced to an ancient king, Mithridates Eupator, who first used a species of this genus medicinally. The name boneset was bestowed on it because the plant was effective in treating a type of disease called breakbone fever, which was prevalent in the 19th century. Boneset was also classified as a diuretic. For nearly a century the plant was included in the *U.S. Pharma-copeia,* and it was listed in the *National Formulary* from 1926 to 1950—works that are standard references for pharmacists.

A related species, *E. purpureum,* more commonly known as joe-pye weed, generally shares the medicinal properties attributed to boneset. Identifiable by its purple flowers, joe-pye weed was named in honor of an Indian medicine man who was famous throughout New England for using it to cure typhus. Most herbal authorities, however, consider the species inferior to boneset in treating fever.

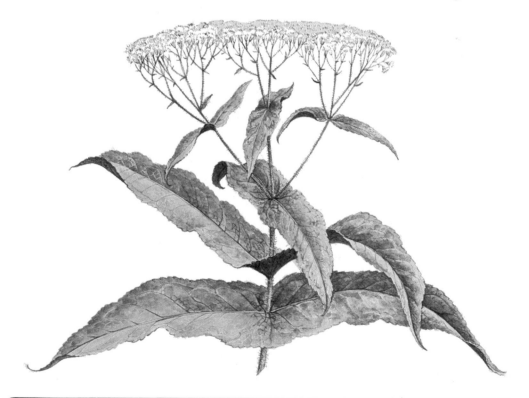

Habitat: Prairies, wet shores, swamp edges, and low woods.

Range: A native of North America, boneset is found from Quebec to Manitoba and south to Florida and Texas.

Identification: A hairy perennial herb growing 2–5 feet tall. Lance-shaped, wrinkled-looking, toothed leaves grow in opposite pairs and are joined at their bases around the stem, making it appear that the stem is growing through the leaves. Whitish flowerheads (July–October) are borne in flat-topped clusters at the top of the stem.

Uses: Since Indian times boneset has been thought of as a fever remedy. Pharmacologists have no experimental evidence, however, to corroborate that the plant is therapeutic either as an antipyretic (a fever-reducing agent) or as a diaphoretic (a medicine that causes perspiration and hence helps to break a fever).

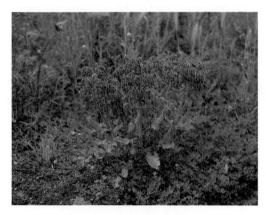

Borage

Borago officinalis L.

Bee Bread, Common Bugloss, Starflower
BORAGE FAMILY
Boraginaceae

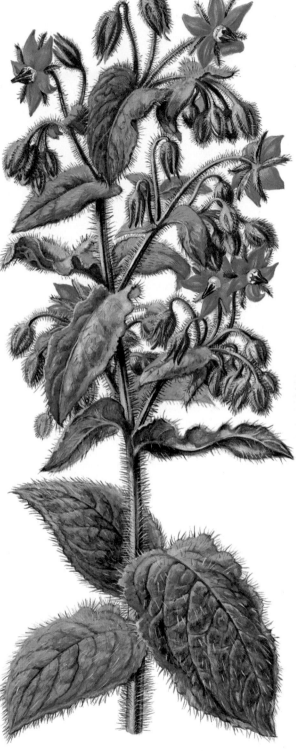

The Roman naturalist Pliny extolled borage for its power to make men merry and joyful, and well into medieval times, borage leaves and flowers steeped in wine were a popular remedy for melancholy. Competitors in jousts and tournaments drank borage tea to strengthen their spirits. "I, Borage, bring always courage" was a familiar rhyme for centuries. Today it seems more likely that the chief effect of borage in lifting spirits lies in the pleasure brought by its bright blue flowers, which are a traditional motif in embroidery designs.

Easy to cultivate, borage was planted in gardens throughout Europe, and from there settlers brought it to America. Bees like borage and make an excellent honey from it.

In the late 1600's doubt crept into the public mind about how useful borage was as a medicinal plant. However, the plant was used to flavor wine drinks, while the candied flowers were popular sweets. Borage is still used in salads and cooked as a green. The blossoms garnish summer drinks, and the leaves flavor cordials. The fresh leaves and flowers have a subtle cucumber flavor when steeped in water. Although borage has been consumed for centuries without apparent ill effect, current research suggests that it can be harmful in large doses.

X May be harmful in large doses.
Habitat: Rubbish heaps, roadsides, and other waste areas.
Range: Introduced from Europe, borage is naturalized throughout much of eastern North America to Tennessee and Illinois.
Identification: An annual growing to 2 feet high. Prickly hairs cover the entire plant. Large oval leaves with wavy edges grow alternately along branched stems that are hollow and succulent. Star-shaped blue flowers (April–September) bloom in drooping clusters.
Uses: Borage contains mucilaginous substances, which account for its mild medicinal properties. It has been used for kidney and bladder ailments, to soothe sore throats, to help reduce fevers, and as a poultice to soothe skin inflammations. Studies indicate its use as an anti-inflammatory and demulcent (soothing the mucous membranes) may be valid.

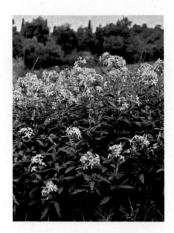

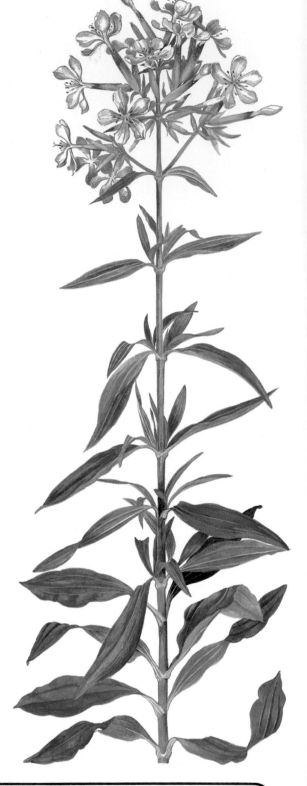

Bouncing Bet

Saponaria officinalis L.

Bruisewort, Fuller's-herb, Lady's-washbowl,
Latherwort, Old-maid's-pink, Soapwort
PINK FAMILY

Caryophyllaceae

Many of this plant's old folk names, such as
latherwort and soapwort, come from its best-
known characteristic—the ability to form a
soaplike lather. Popularly called bouncing Bet
in America, the plant is rich in saponins, which
are natural cleaning agents.

The early American colonists, who brought
bouncing Bet with them from England, used
the lather to clean everything from handmade
lace to pewter vessels. New England textile
workers cleaned and thickened newly woven
cloth with it—a process called fulling, which
accounts for another of its names, fuller's-
herb. The Pennsylvania Dutch had yet another use for the lather—to give beer a foamy
head—and commercially produced saponins
are still used for this purpose.

Bouncing Bet also has a long history as a
medicinal plant, taken internally as a diuretic,
laxative, and expectorant and administered
externally for the treatment of skin eruptions
such as psoriasis, eczema, acne, and boils. A
decoction, or extract, of the crushed roots is
still a popular home remedy for poison ivy—
effective probably because it thoroughly
cleanses the skin.

X Internal use may cause severe vomiting and
diarrhea.

Habitat: Pastures, roadsides, along railroads and
city streets, in old gardens.

Range: Native to Eurasia, bouncing Bet now
grows wild throughout the United States and
southern Canada.

Identification: A perennial with a single upright
stem rising to 2 feet or more, bouncing Bet grows in
clumps. Oval opposite leaves have pointed tips
and smooth edges. Five-petaled flowers (July–
September), whitish pink to rose, about 1 inch
across, grow in thick clusters at the top of the stem.

Uses: Once used internally as diuretic, expectorant, and laxative and externally to treat skin
eruptions, bouncing Bet has no medicinal value
attributed to it by pharmacologists or even by most
herbalists. But the leaves and rhizomes boiled in
pure water make a highly effective soapy lather for
cleaning and brightening delicate fabrics.

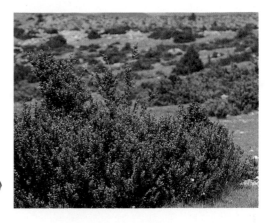

Boxwood

Buxus sempervirens L.

Box, Boxtree

BOXWOOD FAMILY

Buxaceae

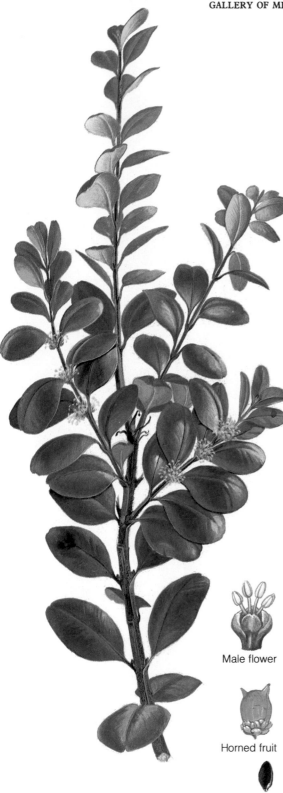

Male flower

Horned fruit

Seed

An Old World shrub or small tree, with dense, richly colored evergreen foliage, boxwood has been cultivated in North America since colonial days. It is especially favored for hedges and borders in formal gardens. William Penn, for one, chose it to edge the gardens on his great estate, Pennsbury Manor, and superb specimens can still be seen in the restored gardens at Colonial Williamsburg.

Medicinally the plant was believed to have many virtues. An old Swedish account tells of a peasant who had turned prematurely bald; treated with a boxwood extract, he magically regained a luxuriant head of hair—but unfortunately, dense hair sprouted all over his face and neck as well. Although the plant was once considered effective as a treatment for epilepsy, leprosy, toothaches, and other disorders, herbalists and pharmacologists today agree that boxwood has little if any medicinal value.

Its wood, however, continues to be prized just as it has been for centuries. Used since ancient times to make decorative boxes (hence its common name), it has also been employed in the manufacture of flutes and other musical instruments, chess pieces, and other fine wooden objects, as well as in inlay work.

X The leaves contain poisonous substances and have caused animal deaths.
Habitat: Well-drained soil.
Range: Hardy from southern New England southward and westward.
Identification: An evergreen shrub or small tree growing 4–15 feet high. Small elliptical to roundish leaves, about 1 inch long, grow in opposite pairs and are dark green above and pale green on the undersides. Clusters of small inconspicuous yellow-green flowers (April–June) produce horned capsules that burst open at maturity and release shiny black seeds.
Uses: Herbal lore attributes many healing virtues to boxwood, but it is virtually unused for medicinal purposes today. In modern times its value lies mainly in its dense, durable, finely grained wood. In addition to its traditional use in fashioning decorative boxes, it is used for inlay and other ornamental woodwork.

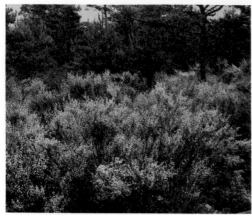

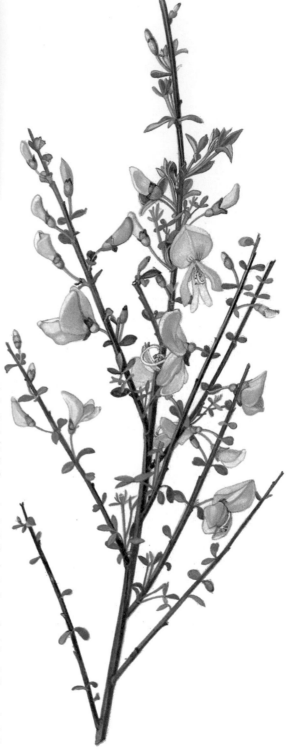

Broom

Cytisus scoparius (L.) Link

Broom Tops, Genista,
Irish Broom, Scotch Broom

PEA FAMILY

Leguminosae

In the Middle Ages, broom lent its name and its twigs and branches to the tool that housewives used for sweeping. The plant could ward off witches, it was said, but to use it in full bloom invited bad luck. An old English saying was quite specific: "If you sweep the house with blossomed broom in May, you are sure to sweep the head of the house away."

Broom also has a heraldic history. According to one tradition, Geoffrey, count of Anjou (1129–1149), adopted broom as a badge and affixed it to his helmet, perhaps so that his troops could easily follow him into battle. A century later, a new order of knighthood, founded by Louis IX of France, chose broom as its emblem of humility.

Broom had medicinal value too. In the 16th century it was recommended as a diuretic and as a purgative—once a common treatment for a host of ailments. Reportedly, no less a person than Henry VIII, king of England, drank the distilled water of the flowers when he was ill. Although some modern herbals list broom as a diuretic and cathartic (strong laxative), official medicine recommends against its use because the tops of the broom plant contain poisons.

✗ The U.S. Food and Drug Administration lists broom tops as "unsafe."

Habitat: Sandy coastal areas and roadsides, barrens, open woods.

Range: A native of Europe, broom has become naturalized in North America and is found from Nova Scotia south to Georgia and west to the Pacific Coast.

Identification: A stiffly branched shrub growing to 10 feet. The lower leaves are usually compound, consisting of three leaflets; the upper ones are often undivided. Bright yellow pealike flowers (April–June), about ¾ inch wide, bloom singly or in pairs along the branches and are followed by brown, hairy seedpods 2–3 inches long.

Uses: Broom has long been held in herbal medicine to be a diuretic and cathartic (strong laxative). Scientists have found that the plant has a diuretic effect but also that it contains toxic substances.

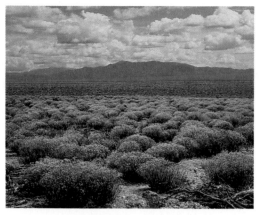

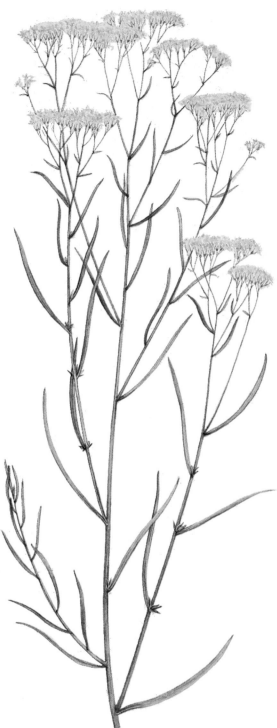

Broom Snakeroot

Gutierrezia sarothrae (Pursh) Britt. and Rusby

Broomweed, Matchbrush, Matchweed, Sheepweed, Snakeweed, Turpentine Weed
COMPOSITE FAMILY
Compositae

American Indians tied together the stems of the pretty yellow-flowered broom snakeroot and used them for brooms, and that is how this herb got its name. Because the plant has also been used to treat rattlesnake bite in sheep, it acquired another common name, snakeweed. To make this antidote, the leaves of the plant are ground, boiled, and made into a poultice that is placed directly on the wound.

Although broom snakeroot is not among the highly significant native American medicinal plants, Navajo Indians advocated it for a few purposes. After childbirth the women drank a tea made from the whole plant to help expel the placenta. The Navajos also chewed the plant and applied it as a poultice to ease bee, ant, and wasp stings. Hopi Indians prescribed a broom snakeroot tea to relieve upset stomach. Preparations of the plant have also been used to treat rheumatism and malaria.

The plant's prominence on grazing land indicates that the land has been overgrazed, because animals do not like it and will eat it only after they have consumed all other forage.

Habitat: Deserts, dry plains and hills, and among pine and juniper trees.
Range: A native of North America, broom snakeroot is found in Canada and the United States from Manitoba south to Texas and west to California.
Identification: A much branched, perennial, shrubby herb growing 1–3 feet tall, with stiff and brittle stems and branches. Lateral shoots arise from the axils of the slender principal leaves, which measure up to 3 inches long and are dotted with resinous glands. Yellow flowerheads (May–November), ⅛ inch across, are clustered at the tips of the branches. The plant has a resinous odor.
Uses: Broom snakeroot was used by western Indians in poultices for treating insect bites. A poultice of the boiled leaves is reported to be an antidote for rattlesnake bite in sheep. None of the medicinal values claimed for the plant have been experimentally verified.

121

Buckbean

Menyanthes trifoliata L.

Bogbean, Marsh Trefoil, Water Shamrock
BUCKBEAN FAMILY
Menyanthaceae

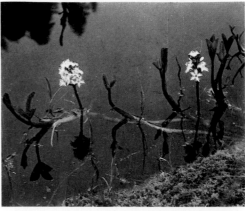

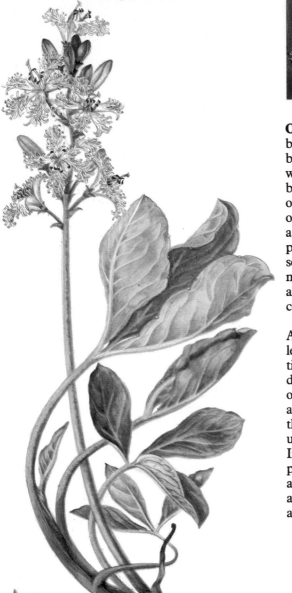

Only bees have an easy time finding buckbean, because it grows in often inaccessible bogs and marshes and in cold water. People who are fortunate enough to come upon buckbean in the wild will not confuse it with any other herb, for it is among the most beautiful of water plants. In bud buckbean flowers have a delicate whitish-pink color, and when the petals are fully open they are covered with a soft white fluff, or fringe. Man has long admired the buckbean for its beauty, and he has also used it as an herbal remedy—the leaves contain strong-tasting bitters.

Buckbean is native to Europe and North America. Early European physicians used the leaves as a cathartic and a remedy for constipation, fevers, rheumatism, scurvy, scabies, and dropsy (edema, or an abnormal accumulation of fluid). Buckbean also earned a reputation as a tonic and appetite stimulant. Colonists found the buckbean growing wild in America and used it much as they had in Europe. Some Indian tribes boiled the roots and stems of the plant to make a decoction for spitting blood and other internal problems. The herb was also employed to treat skin diseases, jaundice, and intestinal worms.

X Large doses of the whole plant may cause vomiting and diarrhea.
Habitat: Marshes, bogs, ponds.
Range: Native to Europe and to North America from Labrador to Alaska, south to West Virginia, and as far west as Wyoming. The species is rare or endangered in some states.
Identification: A perennial aquatic herb, buckbean has a thick, creeping underground stem, about 4 inches long, that sends out 2- to 12-inch stalks bearing leaves divided into three oval or oblong leaflets 2–3 inches long. The flowers (April–September) range in color from white to pink to rose and are covered with a thick fringe of white hairs. The fruit resembles a bean.
Uses: Research by pharmacologists indicates but does not prove conclusively that buckbean may have cathartic properties. The same studies show that buckbean's traditional use as an appetite stimulant is medically valid.

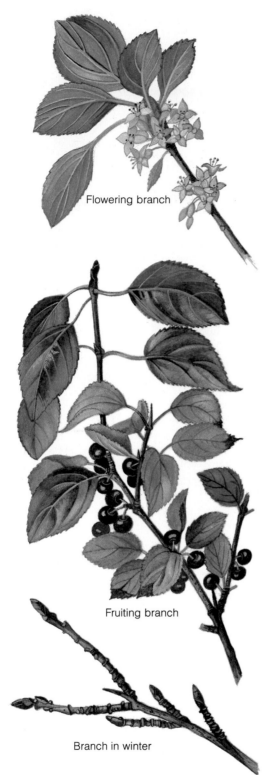

Flowering branch

Fruiting branch

Branch in winter

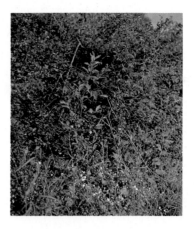

Buckthorn

Rhamnus cathartica L.

Common Buckthorn, European Buckthorn, Purging Buckthorn

BUCKTHORN FAMILY

Rhamnaceae

As the species name *cathartica* indicates, buckthorn was long known to be a cathartic, or powerful laxative. The berries are the part of the plant used for this purpose, and they are extremely unpleasant tasting. To make them more palatable, the 16th-century herbalist John Gerard offered a recipe: "It is better to break them and boil them in fat flesh broth without salt, and to give the broth to drink." Gerard added that they would then "purge with . . . fewer gripings." In 1650 a syrup of buckthorn was listed in a British pharmacopeia, and it too included ingredients, such as cinnamon, nutmeg, and aniseed, to cut the bitter taste. In the 19th century children in need of a laxative were given buckthorn syrup laced with ginger and sugar.

Nicholas Culpeper, the 17th-century herbalist, had quite different ideas about buckthorn's medicinal virtues. He said that a poultice of the bruised leaves would help stop the bleeding from a wound and that an application of the bruised leaves would get rid of warts.

The fruits, or berries, of buckthorn are recommended in modern herbals as a laxative, and are listed in the *National Formulary,* a reference work for pharmacists.

Habitat: Fencerows, open woods, pastures.
Range: Introduced from Europe, buckthorn is cultivated and has become naturalized in North America from Quebec to Minnesota, south to Virginia and Missouri.
Identification: A shrub or small tree growing up to 25 feet tall. Its slender branches are tipped with sharp spines. Opposite, elliptical or oval, pointed, sharp-toothed leaves, about 1–3 inches long, are dark green and smooth with visible lateral veins. Clusters of greenish flowers (May–June) produce berrylike fruits that contain three or four seeds and turn black when ripe.
Uses: For centuries buckthorn's purgative action has served herbalists when a strong laxative is needed. Pharmacological evidence supports this medicinal use.

123

Bugleweed

Ajuga reptans L.

Bugle, Carpenter's-herb, Common Bugle,
Middle Comfrey, Sicklewort
MINT FAMILY
Labiatae

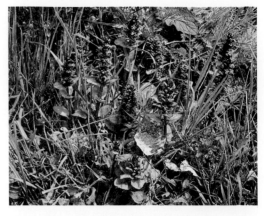

Opinion varies as to the value of bugleweed. Compare the old saw that promises, "He that has bugle and sanicle thumbs his nose at the surgeon," with the view of a modern French herbalist that this is the "most resolutely [medicinally] inactive of plants." It is generally agreed, however, that bugleweed is more than just a pretty flower. As another of its names, carpenter's-herb, suggests, it does have some ability to stop bleeding and to heal cuts, as do all plants that contain tannin. Bugleweed has also been given to stop lung and other internal hemorrhaging, and herbalists have recommended it for coughs, ulcers, rheumatism, and liver disorders, and to prevent hallucinations after excessive alcohol consumption. Some herbalists believe that bugleweed is mildly narcotic and sedative and may slow the heart rate in the way that digitalis does. Bugleweed's properties other than wound healing have never been thoroughly researched, however.

Bugleweed's species name, *reptans*, refers to the reptilelike creeping of the plant's runners.

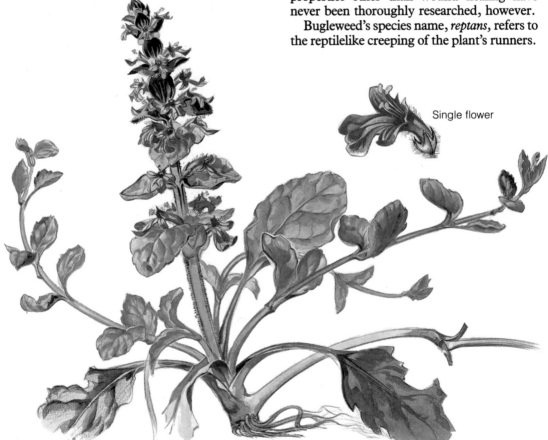

Single flower

Habitat: Roadsides, fields, lawns.
Range: Introduced from Europe, bugleweed has escaped cultivation and now grows wild from Newfoundland south to Pennsylvania and Ohio, and occasionally west of the Cascade Range.
Identification: A perennial herb growing up to 12 inches tall. Its creeping runners produce rosettes of leaves; the whole structure forms a carpetlike mat. The lower leaves are spatula-shaped and often have wavy edges, while the upper leaves are toothed and elliptical or oval. Small blue to purple flowers (May–July), ½ inch across, are borne in dense terminal spikes.
Uses: Bugleweed's use in folk medicine for healing external wounds is probably valid, because the plant contains tannin, an astringent substance that helps to stop bleeding. Many gardeners cultivate bugleweed as a ground cover and in rock gardens. The plant is also used as a black dye for wool.

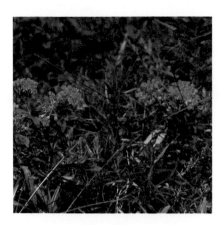

Butterfly Weed

Asclepias tuberosa L.

Canada Root, Pleurisy Root, Silkweed,
Swallowwort, Tuber Root, Wind Root
MILKWEED FAMILY
Asclepiadaceae

Those brilliant splashes of pumpkin-orange color in fields and along roadsides during the heat of midsummer are not mirages: they are members of the milkweed family, generally known as butterfly weed. The name is an apt one, because monarchs, swallowtails, and other butterflies are especially attracted to the plant when it is in flower.

Butterfly weed favors open, dry fields and can be abundant, particularly in the southern United States. Like all other milkweeds, butterfly weed produces pods, which open in autumn to reveal rows of silky seeds that drift with the wind. Unlike most milkweeds, however, this species does not have a milky sap.

Butterfly weed is a native of North America. It was long in use by Indians and pioneers. Powdered and mixed into a paste, the root was spread on sores. The Indians of several regions brewed a tea from the leaves to induce vomiting in certain rituals. Both settlers and Indians made a tea from the root to induce perspiration and expectoration in severe respiratory ailments, including pleurisy, whooping cough, and pneumonia. Stronger doses were given as an emetic and purgative. In the 19th century the *U.S. Pharmacopeia* listed the plant.

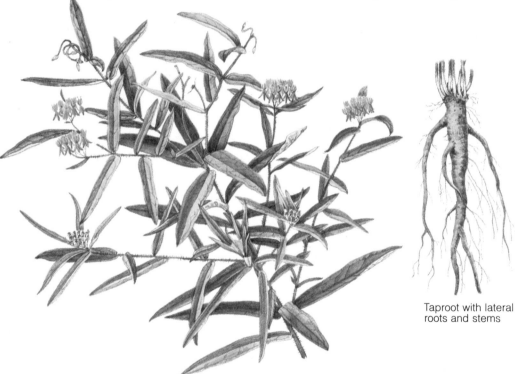

Taproot with lateral
roots and stems

X Poisonous if taken in large doses.
Habitat: Fields and other dry, open places.
Range: Maine to Minnesota and Colorado, south to Florida and Arizona.
Identification: A perennial herb with several stems, growing to 3 feet and branching at the top. Leaves with dark green upper surfaces and pale green undersides grow alternately from the stems and are shaped like spear points. Richly colored orange flowers (June–September) bloom in clusters 3–5 inches across and are followed by long (4- to 5-inch) narrow pods that open to release silky hairs that carry the seeds about on the wind. A large, deep, tuberous root acts as a storage tank in dry spells.
Uses: Because butterfly weed contains toxic cardiac glycosides, its use is no longer recommended, but it can be planted from seed or transplanted as a showy ornamental. But note that the species is rare or protected in some states.

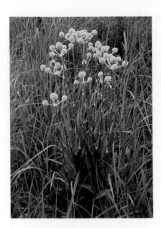

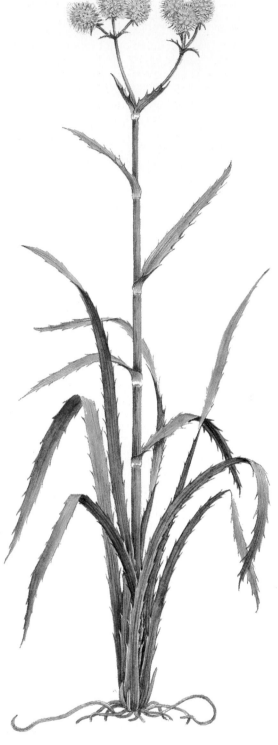

Button Snakeroot

Eryngium yuccifolium Michx.

Rattlesnake Master

CARROT FAMILY

Umbelliferae

According to James Adair, an 18th-century Indian trader who spent some years in what is now northern Mississippi and Alabama, a bitter tea brewed from button snakeroot figured in ceremonial use among his hosts, the Chickasaws. Adair also relates that he once saw a Chickasaw shaman chew some snakeroot, blow it on his hands, and then take up a rattlesnake without damage. There is no evidence, however, that button snakeroot was ever in wide use to treat snakebite, apart from its common names and a statement by the American physician and botanist Charles Millspaugh (1854–1923) that the Indians valued the plant as an "alexiteric," or antidote. There is better evidence that the Indians used the root in the treatment of venereal disease. White settlers readily tried this remedy, as they did so many other purported remedies for this virtually incurable category of diseases. They also employed it as a diuretic, as a stimulant, and as a treatment for impotence. It was reportedly effective in expelling worms, and large doses served to induce vomiting. By the 20th century the plant had fallen into disuse.

X Do not confuse button snakeroot with such poisonous members of the carrot family as water hemlock and poison hemlock.

Habitat: Open woodlands, thickets, prairies.

Range: A native of North America, button snakeroot grows wild from southern New England to the Midwest and along the Atlantic seaboard south to Florida, and then west to Texas.

Identification: A stiff and erect perennial herb growing up to 5 feet tall. Its long, narrow, spiny-edged leaves are only about 1–4 inches wide but up to 30 inches long. Tiny greenish-white flowers (July–August) are clustered in globular or button-like heads, about ½–1 inch across.

Uses: There is no scientific evidence to support any of button snakeroot's traditional uses either by the Indians or by the 19th-century physicians who experimented with the plant. Experimental evidence seems to indicate that the plant may have some effect in treating inflammations and malaria.

A relative of such aromatic trees as sassafras and camphor, the tall, densely leaved California laurel fills the air with a spicy fragrance during flowering time. The leaves contain a volatile oil and when crushed emit an even stronger smell—variously described as resembling either camphor or bay rum—that can be pleasant in small doses but highly irritating in larger concentrations. Indeed, the nickname pepperwood probably comes from the leaves' ability to cause sneezing and headaches. Indian tribes in California and southwest Oregon, where the tree is native, strewed the leaves around their lodgings to keep away fleas and other biting insects. To ward off colds they fumigated their homes by burning the boughs.

Medicinally, Indians used the leaves to relieve pain, possibly including the headache brought on by exposure to the tree's foliage. One method of treatment was to bind the leaves around the head; another was to place a leaf in a nostril. A tea from the leaves served as another remedy for headache and as a treatment for stomach disorders. For rheumatism the Indians and early settlers favored a hot bath in which they had steeped laurel leaves. Other settlers used the plant differently to treat rheumatism; they blended the oil from the leaves with lard and rubbed the mixture on the body. Settlers also used the leaf as a culinary herb.

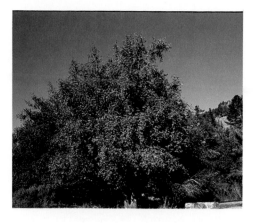

California Laurel

Umbellularia californica Nutt.

Bay Laurel, Oregon Myrtle,
Pacific Myrtle, Pepperwood
LAUREL FAMILY
Lauraceae

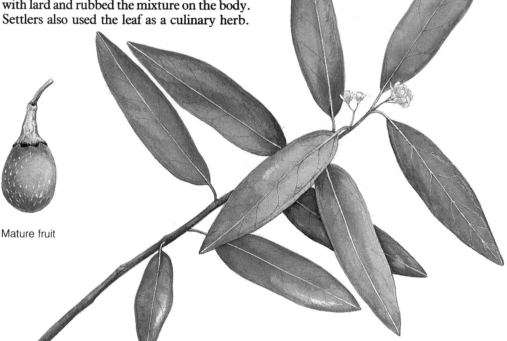

Mature fruit

Habitat: A variety of soils in coastal, hilly, and mountainous lands.
Range: Native to the United States, California laurel is found on the coast of California, in the western Sierra Nevada, and in southwest Oregon.
Identification: A small to large evergreen tree, growing up to 90 feet tall. The bark is thin and dark brown. The smooth lance-shaped leaves are alternate with a pointed tip; the upper sides are shiny green, while the undersides are paler. Tiny yellow flowers (December–May) are borne in clusters. In late summer and early fall they produce yellowish-green olivelike fruits that turn purple when ripe.
Uses: Like the Indians, some modern herbalists use the plant as a pain reliever for headaches and rheumatism. No research has been done to prove or disprove the efficacy of these uses. Cooks substitute dried California laurel leaves for bay leaves, but the former have a stronger flavor. The wood is used in furniture and other fine wood products.

127

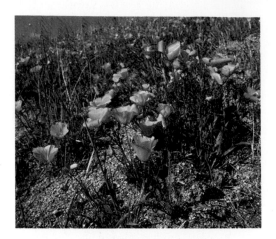

California Poppy

Eschscholzia californica Cham.
POPPY FAMILY

Papaveraceae

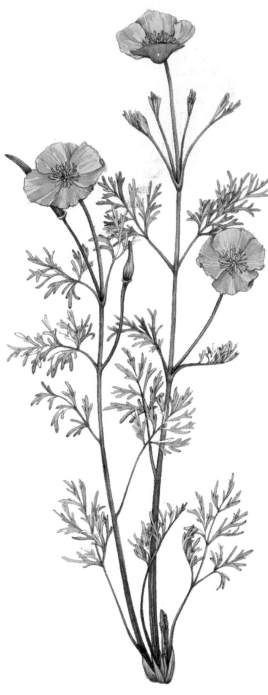

Like a golden blanket, orange and yellow poppy blossoms once covered the mountains of coastal California, so impressing Spanish explorers that they named the region the Land of Fire. Indeed, before development dimmed their luster, the flowered hills shone so brightly that sailors far out at sea used them as beacons to shape their course. Today this poppy is California's state flower.

Like many other members of the poppy family, the California poppy contains sedative alkaloids in its sap. The local Indians used the plant as a painkiller, especially for toothache; as a remedy for insomnia and headache; and as a poultice for sores and ulcers. Indian women employed it to charm unresponsive lovers, though this was considered a crime and, if detected, would result in the woman's expulsion from the tribe. Today some Californians of Spanish heritage cook the plant in olive oil to make a hair tonic that, they say, makes the hair grow thick and shiny. *Dormidera,* "the drowsy one," is the name they give this flower that, like any true Californian, worships the sun, closing up tightly at dark.

Habitat: Coastal dunes, grassy hillsides, valleys.
Range: Native to western North America, California poppy grows west of the mountains from southern California north to southern Washington, and on Vancouver Island.
Identification: A perennial herb, with spreading stems, growing up to 2 feet tall. The leaves are divided many times into fine greenish-gray segments. Conspicuous flowers (February–September) range in color from a brilliant yellow to a deep orange and have four petals and many stamens.
Uses: West Coast Indians used the California poppy chiefly as a pain reliever for toothache. The plant was also prescribed as a sedative for headache and insomnia, and it is still mentioned today as a gentle sedative and analgesic (an agent that allays pain).

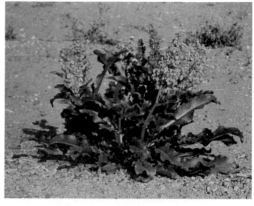

Cañaigre

Rumex hymenosepalus Torr.

Tanner's-dock, Wild Pieplant,
Wild Rhubarb

BUCKWHEAT FAMILY

Polygonaceae

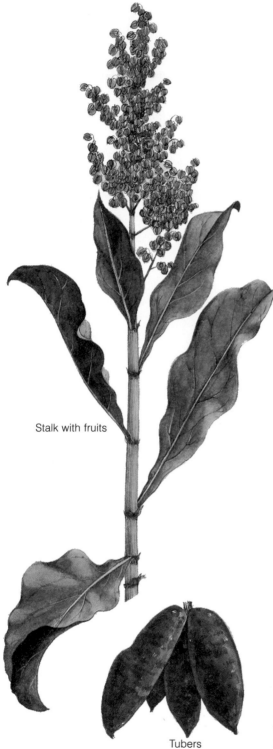

Stalk with fruits

Tubers

Products labeled "wild red American ginseng" and "wild red desert ginseng" have appeared on the American herbal tea market in recent years. Despite their labels, they are not the fabled cure-all ginseng but cañaigre, an herb that is in no way related to ginseng. This is not to say that cañaigre is without value. On the contrary, it contains tannin in large enough amounts to make it useful for tanning leather. American Indians recognized this property centuries ago, using the roots to soften their buckskins—a function that probably led to another of its common names, tanner's-dock (*Rumex* is known as the dock genus).

Herbalists have traditionally relied upon cañaigre as an astringent. They used its large tuberous roots to make a tea for treating diarrhea and a gargle for easing sore throat. One herbal suggests using the boiled root extract to stop bleeding from minor scrapes and cuts. The Indians also have used the roots of cañaigre, a native of the western United States, as a source of dye. The Navajos favor it especially for a yellow hue that they use in dyeing wool. Its stalks are an excellent substitute for rhubarb—a fact that explains the other common names, wild rhubarb and wild pieplant.

Habitat: Sandy, somewhat dry soils.
Range: Native to the western regions of the United States, cañaigre is distributed from Wyoming and Utah south to Mexico and from Oklahoma and Texas west to California.
Identification: A perennial herb growing up to 3 feet tall. The thick oblong to lance-shaped leaves are wavy-edged, with a conspicuous central vein, and grow as long as 1 foot. Greenish flowers (December—May) ripen into a thick, showy cluster of pink to reddish fruits. The dark reddish-brown tuberous roots resemble sweet potatoes.
Uses: The use of cañaigre root in folk medicine has been as an astringent, prepared as a tea for diarrhea and as a gargle for sore throat. These uses are probably effective, owing to the plant's high tannin content.

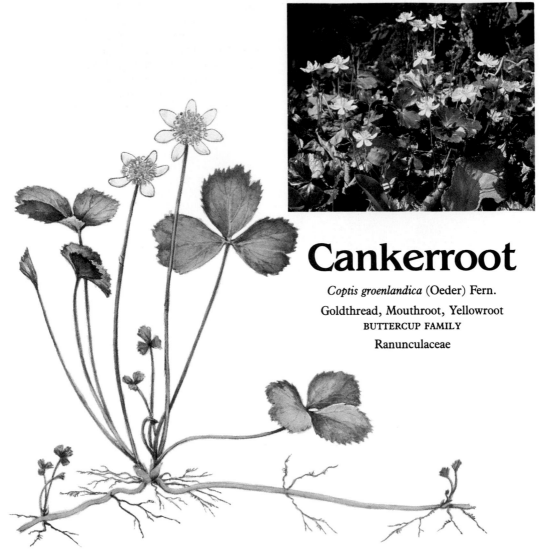

Cankerroot

Coptis groenlandica (Oeder) Fern.

Goldthread, Mouthroot, Yellowroot
BUTTERCUP FAMILY
Ranunculaceae

Growing in mountain bogs, forests, moist thickets, and swamps, the little-noted cankerroot bears solitary star-shaped flowers that sit on skinny, leafless stalks. There is just one bloom per stalk, rising out of clusters of tiny evergreen leaves. The shallow root system, which looks like a mass of gold threads, has earned the plant another of its popular names, goldthread.

Indians and early settlers made a brew from the plant's bitter-tasting rhizome as a gargle for sore throats and for ulcerated mouths (hence its common name cankerroot). The Penobscots are reported to have used it for "smoker's mouth." Cankerroot also enjoyed popularity as a rural remedy for inflammation of the mucous membranes of the eyes and as a topical anesthetic spread on the gums of teething infants. The plant was listed in the *U.S. Pharmacopeia* from 1820 to 1882. At the turn of the century the price of cankerroot reached about $1 per pound not only because it was difficult to gather the plant's threadlike roots but because they weighed very little after drying. A decoction of equal parts of cankerroot and goldenseal has acquired the reputation of eliminating the craving for alcoholic beverages. Today cankerroot is often cultivated as a ground cover in woody areas and around the edges of a bog garden.

Habitat: Mountain bogs, woods, moist thickets, and swamps.
Range: From Greenland to Alaska, south to North Carolina, Indiana, and Iowa.
Identification: A small perennial that grows 4–6 inches tall. Its leaves resemble those of the strawberry plant. Each leaf consists of three leaflets at the end of the leafstalk. Solitary white flowers (May–July) occur on slender, leafless stalks. The rhizome sends out many roots that are distinguishable by their bright yellow color.
Uses: The roots and rhizomes of cankerroot, chewed raw or boiled, have been used to treat canker sores, fever blisters, and other mouth irritations and to treat indigestion and sore throats. A medicinal brew from the roots has been used as an eyewash. The effectiveness of all these uses is due to the presence of the alkaloid berberine, a mild sedative, in the plant.

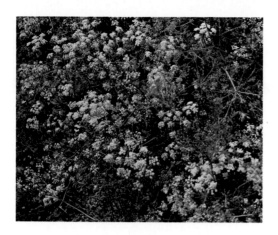

Caraway

Carum carvi L.

Caraway Seed
CARROT FAMILY
Umbelliferae

One of the most popular herbs today, caraway has long been prized for the excellence of its aromatic dried seeds (actually fruits) as a condiment and an aid to digestion. It gives rye bread and various cheeses their characteristic flavors and is the base for a well-known digestive liqueur, *Kümmel* (German for "caraway"). Bakers scatter the seeds over cakes, and cooks often add them to cabbage and sauerkraut not just for taste but for their gas-relieving properties. Caraway oil, extracted from the seeds, used to be given in very small amounts to relieve gassy indigestion or colic. In this use it is effective, but according to some sources, heavy doses may cause liver damage.

Like so many other favorite herbs, caraway acquired its own folklore. In Europe, popular belief held that caraway would prevent the theft of any item that contained it. This virtue gave it power as a love potion: feed your lover caraway and he or she cannot be stolen from you. In the same spirit, country people fed caraway to their chickens, geese, and pigeons to keep them from straying. Some pigeon keepers still place caraway dough in their lofts to keep the flock intact.

Leafy stem

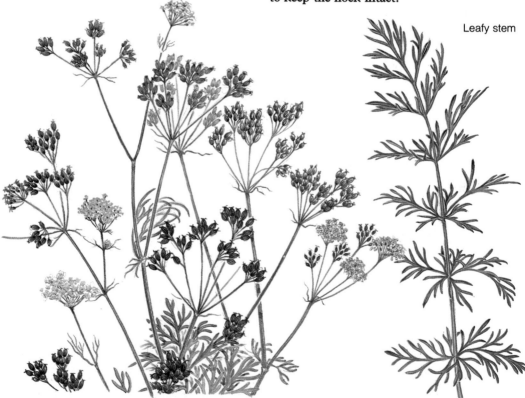

Habitat: Meadows, woods, rocky areas.
Range: Native to Eurasia and Africa, caraway now grows wild in many parts of North America.
Identification: A biennial with an erect, furrowed, branching stem growing to 1½−2 feet high. Feathery leaves grow from the stem in opposite pairs or in threes. The branches of the stems end in clusters of tiny white flowers (June−July); the flowerheads resemble those of carrots in bloom. The seeds are long, ribbed, and brownish.

Uses: The seeds have widespread culinary use as a flavoring in breads, cakes, cheeses, and liqueurs. An infusion made from caraway seed oil was once mixed with water or poured over a sugar cube as a remedy for indigestion. Research substantiates the use of caraway seeds for relieving gas pains and suggests that they may also have antispasmodic properties.

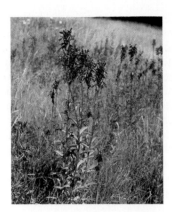

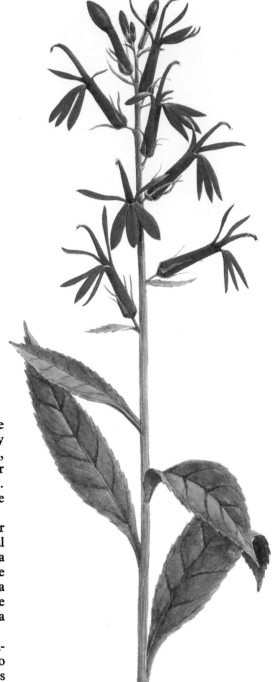

Cardinal Flower

Lobelia cardinalis L.

Cardinal Lobelia, Red Cardinal,
Red Lobelia

LOBELIA FAMILY

Lobeliaceae

In late summer, all across the country, one may see two members of the lobelia family blooming along muddy streams, lakeshores, and marshy riverbanks. The cardinal flower flaunts crimson red blossoms in showy spikes. The other member, often called great blue lobelia, sports purplish-blue flowers.

Both plants are now esteemed more for their beauty as wildflowers than for their medicinal properties, but in the early days of America this was not true. Cherokee Indians in the South employed the cardinal flower's root as a cure for syphilis, while Iroquois Indians in the North swore by great blue lobelia's root as a remedy for the same disease.

Sir William Johnson, superintendent of Indian affairs in North America from 1756 to 1774 and a friend of the Iroquois, sent samples of the blue flower to England, hoping to provide Europeans with a long-sought cure for the fatal disease. But the English trials of the plant had negative results, and European physicians had to discount it as a cure for syphilis. Nevertheless, the Swedish botanist Carolus Linnaeus labeled the plant *Lobelia siphilitica*.

Although Indians and settlers used the cardinal flower as an emetic (to induce vomiting) and an expectorant, as well as a treatment for venereal disease, herbalists never valued it as much as they did its potent (and poisonous) cousin *Lobelia inflata*, or Indian tobacco.

Habitat: Moist pasture lands, lakeshores, marshy and muddy banks of streams and rivers.
Range: Native to North America, both plants are found from southern Canada to Texas. Cardinal flower is a protected species in some states.
Identification: Both plants are perennials, and grow 2–4 feet tall with stiff, erect stems. The leaves are lance-shaped and toothed. The flowers of both plants grow in long spiky clusters. Cardinal flower (July–September) is intense crimson red, and great blue lobelia (August–September) is deep blue to purple.
Uses: North American Indians used both plants to treat venereal disease. Great blue lobelia's effectiveness against the disease was tested but not substantiated when the plant was introduced into traditional Western medicine around 1800. Neither physicians nor herbalists ascribe any medicinal value to either plant today.

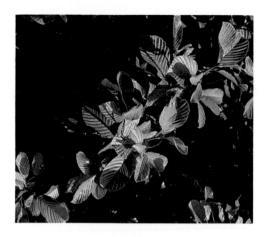

Spanish priests in California, who noted that American Indians used the bark medicinally, gave this tree the name cascara sagrada, meaning "sacred bark." The Indians stripped the bark from the tree in early spring or autumn, dried it, and then aged it for at least a year. To prepare the medicine, they steeped the bark in boiling water; they drank the cooled liquid to relieve constipation. A century elapsed between the time the Spaniards took note of the plant's medicinal use in California and its acceptance by American physicians in 1877. It has been listed in the *U.S. Pharmacopeia* since 1894. Cascara bark has been called the world's most widely used laxative. It is still marketed.

Cascara sagrada acts by irritating the intestines to produce wavelike contractions of the muscles of the intestinal wall. Properly diluted, it is especially useful as a mild laxative for elderly people or those in delicate health. Honey produced from cascara flowers also has a slight laxative effect. Two related European species, *R. frangula* (alder buckthorn) and *R. cathartica* (buckthorn), have similar laxative effects, but cascara sagrada is milder and also safer to use.

Cascara Sagrada

Rhamnus purshiana DC.

Cascara Buckthorn, Chittembark, Sacred Bark
BUCKTHORN FAMILY

Rhamnaceae

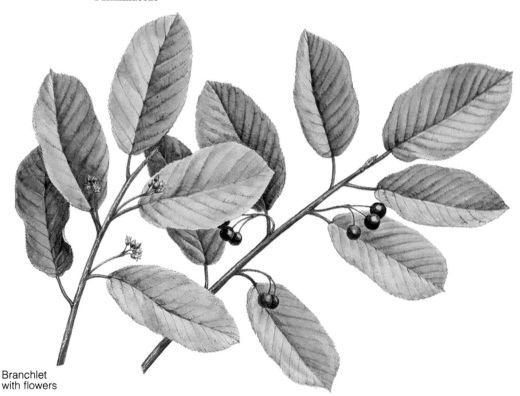

Branchlet with flowers

X The fresh bark causes nausea; long-term use of the laxative may induce chronic diarrhea.

Habitat: Forested mountain slopes, canyons, and bottomlands.

Range: Pacific Northwest from British Columbia to northern California.

Identification: A deciduous tree growing 20–30 feet tall, with a trunk averaging 1½ feet in diameter, cascara sagrada has slender branches and a reddish-brown bark. Its green or yellow-green leaves are elliptical, finely toothed, and rounded at the base, with either blunt or sharp ends; the leaves are crowded at the tips of branchlets. Greenish-white flowers (May–June), borne in clusters in the axils of the leaves, develop into round black fruits (September), each with two or three smooth seeds.

Uses: Cascara sagrada is a key ingredient of many commercial laxatives. It can also be used in small doses as a tonic to promote digestion.

133

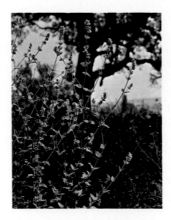

Catnip

Nepeta cataria L.

Catmint, Cat's-play

MINT FAMILY

Labiatae

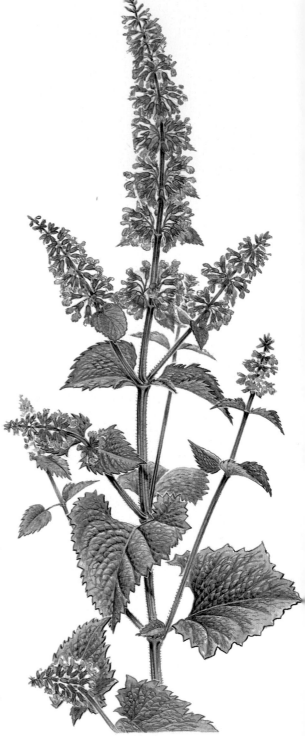

The excited joy that catnip inspires in cats is caused by an oil the plant secretes to ward off insects that otherwise would eat its leaves. This defense mechanism goes awry when cats discover catnip. In their ecstatic rolling and rubbing against the plant, they may destroy it entirely, for they quickly learn that the more they demolish the plant, the more pleasurable oil is released. Cat owners often rub catnip on places where a cat will do no harm in sharpening its claws.

In recent years widely publicized reports stated that catnip has exciting effects on human beings—that it is a mild hallucinogen when smoked or taken in a strong infusion. The reports are incorrect. Only members of the cat family ever get high from catnip.

Catnip is native to Europe and was for many centuries a popular garden herb, used in cooking and for a range of medicinal purposes, from the easing of menstrual cramps to the relief of insomnia and the prevention of nightmares. Upon its introduction from Europe to North America, it escaped from gardens and spread across the continent so rapidly that native Indians included it in their inventory of useful plants and did not associate it with the coming of the Europeans.

Habitat: Roadsides and other waste areas and dry fields.

Range: Throughout North America.

Identification: A perennial herb, growing upright to 3 feet high. The branching square stems and toothed, heart-shaped opposite leaves are covered with downy gray hairs, giving the whole plant a grayish-green appearance. Clusters of white or pale lavender tubular flowers (June–October) with purplish spots grow at the ends of the main stem and of the branches. The plant has a minty smell.

Uses: Chewing catnip leaves has long been a folk remedy for toothache. Catnip tea has also been used to relieve intestinal cramps, infant's colic, and gas pains; and the juice from the leaves was used to stimulate menstrual flow. Some evidence exists that catnip acts as an antispasmodic and a carminative, relieving flatulence. There is good experimental evidence in nonfeline animals for its use as a mild sedative for the relief of insomnia.

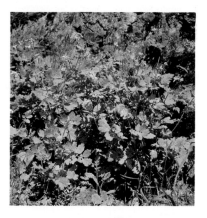

Celandine

Chelidonium majus L.

Swallowwort, Tetterwort

POPPY FAMILY

Papaveraceae

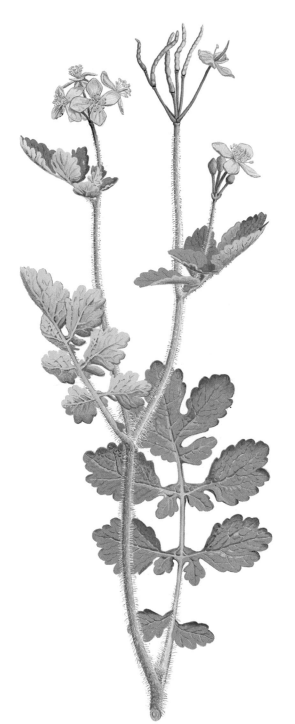

Queen Elizabeth I, whose teeth were euphemistically described as "black pearls," was said to have once avoided a painful tooth extraction by dropping the acrid juice of celandine into the hollow of a decaying tooth and easily removing the tooth with her fingers.

The name celandine comes from *chelidon*, the Greek word for swallow. The belief that the plant flourished with the swallows' spring arrival and withered with their fall departure derived from classical antiquity, when the plant was accordingly called *chelidonium*—equivalent to the common name swallowwort ("swallow herb"). Another legend held that the swallows used the juice of the herb to strengthen the eyesight of their fledgings. By extension, the plant's juice was used for eyedrops to treat cataracts in humans, but this use was discontinued long ago.

Herbalists, following the doctrine of signatures, took the bright orange color of the juice as a divine sign that it was a remedy for jaundice and liver ailments. The juice was also employed to remove warts and soften calluses. The name tetterwort comes from the use of the juice in folk medicine to treat skin problems such as pimples and blisters, disorders that were formerly called tetters.

X The juice can cause severe irritation of the mucous membranes and is also a central nervous system depressant. Skin irritation results from handling crushed parts of the plant.
Habitat: Damp rich soil on the edges of forests, paths, and walls and among rocks and bushes.
Range: Northeastern Canada and United States, south to Georgia, Tennessee, and Missouri.
Identification: A perennial herb with branching stems that grow to 2½ feet high and swell at the nodes. Smooth, deeply divided leaves with lobed leaflets spread alternately along the lower stem. The flowers (April–September) are bright yellow. When any part of the plant is broken, it exudes an acrid, sticky orange juice with an unpleasant smell.
Uses: The juice has a strong skin-irritating effect, and was used in folk medicine to remove warts and treat such skin diseases as eczema and ringworm. Today the plant is mainly used in the production of a yellow dye for wool.

135

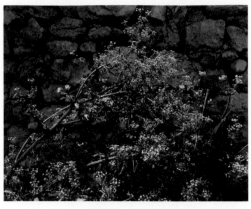

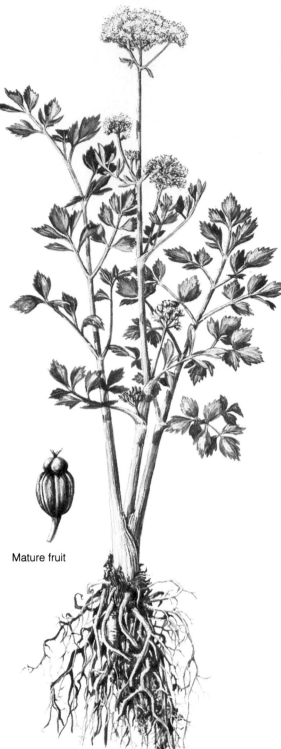

Mature fruit

Celery

Apium graveolens L.

Marsh Parsley, Smallage, Wild Celery
CARROT FAMILY
Umbelliferae

Tough and well-nigh inedible, with an acrid, nasty taste, wild celery is not a green one would want to add to a salad. It is, however, an herb that herbalists use medicinally. Wild celery has long been known as a remedy for the homely complaints of flatulence and rheumatism, and herbalists have also occasionally recommended wild celery root for jaundice, urinary blockage, dropsy, and hysteria. It is possibly a mild sedative as well. According to the 17th-century herbalist Nicholas Culpeper, the leaves when "eaten in the spring, sweeten and purify the blood and help the scurvy."

The Latin name *Apium* may be derived from a prehistoric Indo-European word for water; if that is true, it is entirely appropriate in view of celery's long-observed preference for wet soils and salt marshes.

In the 17th century, Italian gardeners developed from the wild plant not only the familiar stalk celery (*Apium graveolens* var. *dulce*)—an essential ingredient for soups, sauces, and stocks—but also celeriac (*A. graveolens* var. *rapaceum*), a plant much grown in Europe for its edible root. Introduced into the New World as a vegetable, celery has escaped from cultivation in some places and may be found growing wild.

Habitat: Wet and salty soils, swamps, marshes.
Range: Native to southern Europe, celery is cultivated in North America and has occasionally escaped from gardens.
Identification: A biennial herb, growing 1–2 feet tall. The green stems ("stalks") are ribbed and tough. Fleshy green leafstalks bear dark green, highly segmented leaves with toothed leaflets. (In cultivation, celery is blanched to produce the edible white stem.) Small whitish flowers (June– July) are borne in flat clusters, followed by smooth gray fruits (the "seeds").
Uses: Pharmacologists confirm that celery seed is a carminative, effective for the relief of gas pains, and their research suggests celery seed may also have a sedative action. Stalks of cultivated celery are eaten raw or cooked; leaves and seeds are used as flavoring for soups and stews. The seeds mixed with salt make celery salt. Celery seed oil is the flavoring agent in "celery tonic."

Chaparral

Larrea tridentata (DC.) Cov.

Creosote Bush, Greasewood, Hediondilla

CALTROP FAMILY

Zygophyllaceae

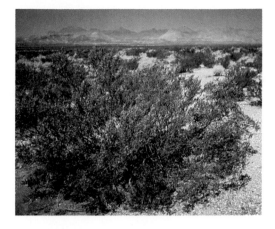

Generally acknowledged as the most adaptable plant in desert regions in the United States, chaparral, or creosote bush as it is often called, endures long periods without rainfall. When rain does come, the shrub's thick leaves become sticky and emit a tarry or creosotelike smell. By some accounts, this aroma accounts for the Mexican name *hediondilla*, meaning "little stinker." The genus name honors the 18th-century Spaniard Juan Antonio Hernández de Larrea, a patron of science.

In the desert and semidesert regions of the southwestern United States, where the plant is indigenous, chaparral is sometimes found in gardens of native plants or used to ornament the landscape. Near Los Angeles, in the Johnson Valley, is an unusual specimen of this species known as the King Clone—a 25- by 70-foot bush some 12,000 years old. The large elliptical plant began as a single creosote bush after the last ice age and has grown outward over the centuries.

Chaparral has had limited medicinal use. Some Indians prepared a decoction (extract) from the leaves that they used to purge the body and to heal sores. In the past *L. tridentata* was considered synonymous with the Argentinian species *L. divaricata*, but most botanists now think of *L. tridentata* as a separate species.

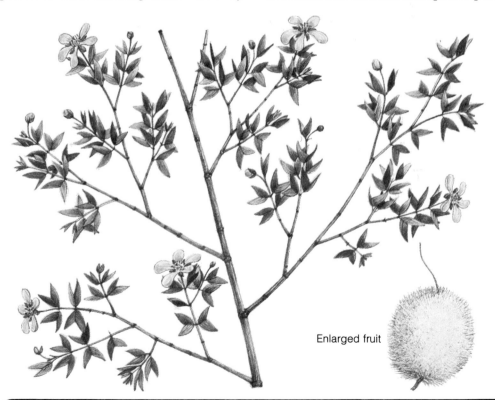

Enlarged fruit

Habitat: Scrub deserts.

Range: Native to the southwestern United States, chaparral is found growing wild from Texas to California and south to Mexico.

Identification: A resinous, many-branched evergreen shrub growing 3–9 feet tall. Its branches are distinguished by black rings at the nodes. The leaves grow in opposite pairs; each leaf consists of two olive-green leaflets, ⅜ inch long. Yellow flowers (normally January–May, but may occur throughout the year in warmer climates) have five petals, and are followed by showy globular fruits (seed balls) that are covered with fuzzy white hairs.

Uses: Chaparral is an ingredient in an herbal tea recommended today by some folk healers as an antitussive (to relieve or prevent coughing), an antiarthritic (to ease symptoms of arthritis), and a cancer remedy, but researchers cannot substantiate these claims.

137

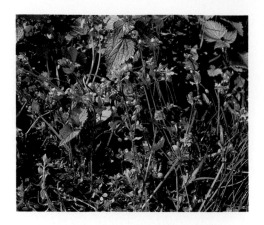

Chickweed

Stellaria media (L.) Cyrillo

Mouse-ear, Satinflower, Starweed,
Tongue Grass, White Bird's-eye, Winterweed
PINK FAMILY

Caryophyllaceae

How the humble herb chickweed could stir up such a storm of controversy is difficult to imagine. But some herbalists swear by this extremely common weed as a remedy for both internal and external inflammations and for colds, coughs, tumors, hemorrhoids, sore eyes, and rheumatism, while others in the field dismiss chickweed as nearly worthless—distinguished only by its promiscuity as a weed. Even in the animal kingdom, opinions about chickweed vary. Chickens, hogs, and rabbits dote on its succulent, pale green foliage and tiny seeds, but it is said that sheep disdain it and even goats will not touch it.

In truth, chickweed is neither a wonder cure nor a simple pest. It does contain nutrients and has long been prescribed by herbalists as a tonic to restore the strength of the frail and sickly. Capable of producing five generations of offspring in a single season, chickweed invades lawns and fields to the dismay of gardeners and farmers but the delight of cooks, who relish it as an herb and an almost year-round source of salad greens.

Completely ignored by ancient herbalists, chickweed received its Latin name, *Stellaria*, from the Swedish botanist Linnaeus, who noted the starlike shape of the delicate white flowers. The flowers open on sunny days, but they may close on rainy or cloudy days.

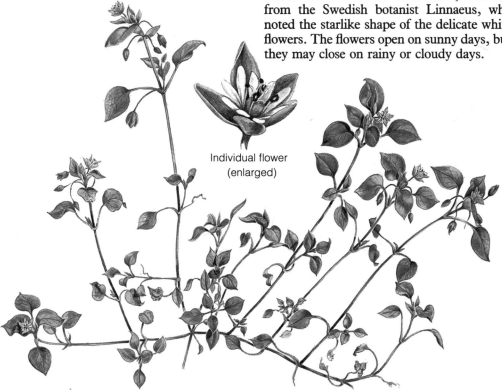

Individual flower
(enlarged)

Habitat: Gardens, lawns, meadows, pastures, fields, waste places.
Range: Native to Europe, but found throughout the temperate regions of North America.
Identification: An annual herb, chickweed grows 12–15 inches high; its sprawling, tangled stems reach up to 2½ feet in length. From each stem node grow pairs of oval leaves that vary in size. White flowers (February–December) ¼ inch across, with usually five two-parted petals that are shorter than the sepals, are followed by oval seed-bearing capsules.
Uses: Historically herbalists have used chickweed to treat both internal and external inflammations. They still prescribe it today for that purpose although its effectiveness has not been scientifically proved. Claims have also been made for chickweed as an antitussive (a medicine that relieves coughing), but again, these too have not been proved. An herbal chickweed tea is commercially available.

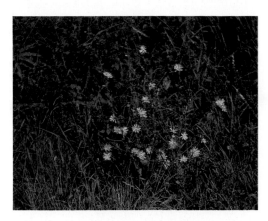

Chicory

Cichorium intybus L.

Blue-sailors, Coffeeweed, Succory
COMPOSITE FAMILY
Compositae

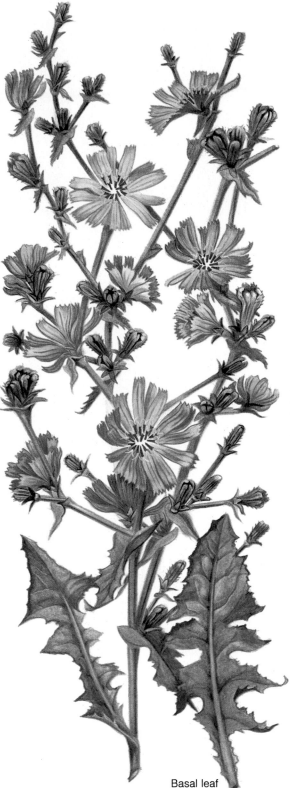

Basal leaf

Because chicory's sky-blue flowers can be counted on to open and close at precisely the same time every day, the Swedish botanist Carolus Linnaeus included this beautiful weed in the floral clock he planted at Uppsala. Chicory had been known to the ancients, who used it both as a food and medicinally. The Romans prescribed it for liver ailments. In later centuries herbalists recommended preparations made from the roots as tonics, laxatives, and diuretics, and poultices made from the bruised leaves for swellings and inflammations. At one time herbalists looked upon chicory's milky sap as a divine sign that the juice provided a remedy for nursing mothers who had trouble producing milk.

Today chicory, both wild and cultivated, is used principally as a food. Young chicory leaves can be gathered in spring for a salad; older leaves can be cooked but have a bitter taste. Belgian endive is actually a variety of *Cichorium intybus*. The roots are dug up, replanted in a dark cellar, and left to grow until small pale leaf heads reach a height of a few inches. The dried, roasted, and ground root is often blended with coffee; it gives the brew a pleasantly bitter taste while reducing its stimulating effect, since chicory has no caffeine.

Habitat: Fields and waste areas, such as roadsides and vacant city lots.

Range: Introduced from Europe, chicory is naturalized throughout most of the United States and southern Canada. It will grow in almost any soil. It grows more profusely in humid areas.

Identification: A perennial herb, with blue flowerheads (July–November) arranged at the bases of the few small leaves found on the rough, stiff stem. The stem grows from a rosette of leaves on the ground and can reach a height of 6 feet, but most are closer to 3 feet. The plant is inconspicuous until the showy flowers bloom. A long, tough taproot enables chicory to grow wild in areas hostile to other plants.

Uses: Ground chicory roots for blending with coffee are available in specialty food stores. Chicory is also sold as a bitter, tangy seasoning for soups and stews.

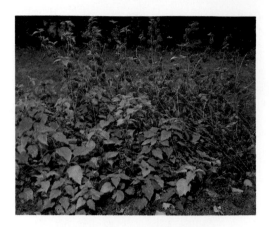

Chinese Lantern

Physalis alkekengi L.

Bladder Cherry, Ground Cherry,
Strawberry Tomato, Winter Cherry
NIGHTSHADE FAMILY

Solanaceae

In autumn, after the small whitish petals of the Chinese lantern disappear, the hitherto inconspicuous outer whorl of green sepals (the calyx) begins to expand and change color. Soon the calyx becomes a pretty scarlet pod, resembling a Chinese paper lantern, inside of which is found a red berry.

The plant is also known as bladder cherry because the pod also resembles a bladder. Old-time herbalists, following the doctrine of signatures (according to which a plant's resemblance to a human part was a sign of its usefulness in treating that part), concluded that Chinese lantern was a remedy for kidney and bladder stones. In fact, the plant's botanical name, *Physalis*, is the Greek word for bladder. In England the Gerard and Culpeper herbals in the 16th and 17th centuries extolled the fruits' virtues as a diuretic, both to expel bladder stones and to promote urine flow. (One patient testified that he prevented gout attacks by eating eight fruits at each change of the moon.) By the end of the 18th century, however, doctors seldom prescribed the fruits.

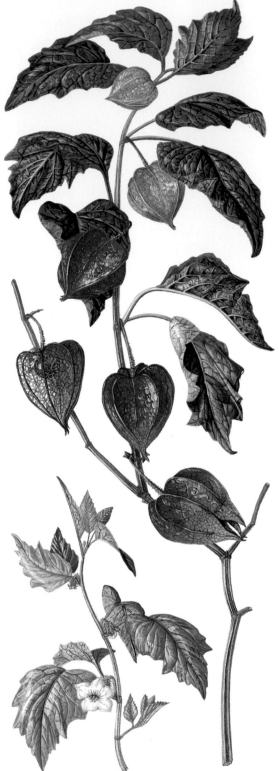

Twig with flowers

X Unripe fruits may be toxic, and the ripe fruits eaten in large quantities may cause diarrhea.
Habitat: Woodlands, old fields, other waste areas.
Range: Native to Asia, Chinese lantern was introduced into gardens in the United States and has escaped cultivation in some places.
Identification: A perennial plant with upright, branched stems growing to about 2 feet tall. Oval, pointed leaves, 2–3 inches long, are toothed and heavily veined and grow in pairs. Whitish petals (June–August) drop off as the calyx, or "lantern," expands. When mature (August–September), the lantern contains a red fruit resembling a cherry.
Uses: Although modern herbals occasionally mention Chinese lantern fruits as a diuretic, there is no scientific evidence to validate this use. Hikers, in particular, appreciate the fresh fruit, which can also be made into jellies and jams. The dainty pods, or lanterns, are often dried and used in autumn and winter floral arrangements.

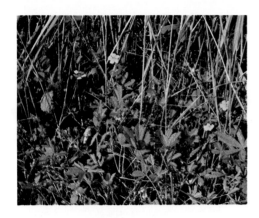

Cinquefoil

Potentilla reptans L.

Five-fingers, Five-leaf, Sunkfield
ROSE FAMILY
Rosaceae

A pretty and dainty species, easy to identify, cinquefoil gets its name from an Old French word meaning "five-leaf." The stem creeps along the ground very much like that of a strawberry plant, produces roots, and sends up stalks that bear either a solitary yellow flower or a leaf divided into five or seven distinctive leaflets. The Latin name *Potentilla* refers to the medicinal potency of the plant.

Medieval knights vied to emblazon cinquefoil's five-fingered leaf, symbol of the five senses of man, on their shields, because the right to use the heraldic device was given only to those who achieved self-mastery. Witches were said to be afraid of the herb, sweethearts used it in love potions and divinations, and fishermen added it to their nets to bring in heavier catches.

Cinquefoil's medicinal value was recognized by a Greek naturalist and student of Aristotle's, Theophrastus, who was the first to describe it. Through the ages herbalists have recommended a decoction of the root as a remedy for fever, an analgesic for toothache, a gargle for mouth sores, and generally as a disinfectant and astringent. The bark of the root was also applied to stop nosebleeds, and a leaf or root tea was recommended for diarrhea.

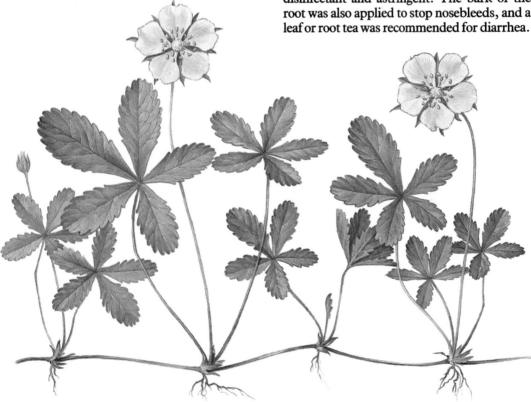

Habitat: Roadsides, pastures, edges of woods.
Range: Introduced from Europe, cinquefoil now grows wild in eastern North America from Nova Scotia to Ontario and south to Virginia.
Identification: A creeping perennial herb, cinquefoil has stem runners that can reach up to 5 feet in length. Toothed leaves with hairy veins grow on long stalks and are divided into five or seven leaflets. Bright yellow flowers (May–August) are borne singly on leafless stalks.

Uses: Historically cinquefoil has been employed as an astringent, an antihemorrhagic agent, and a remedy for fevers. Even though early users did not know it, the tannic acid in the plant accounts for its effectiveness as an astringent in stopping bleeding. Its ability to cure fevers, however, has been found questionable as the result of pharmacological investigation.

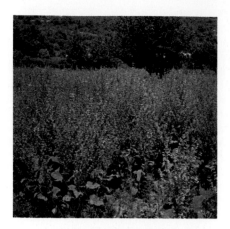

Clary

Salvia sclarea L.

Clary Sage, Clear Eye, Muscatel Sage
MINT FAMILY
Labiatae

A tall, stately herb both cultivated and found in the wild, clary bears large, opposite, velvety, oval leaves, measuring up to 9 inches long, at the base of its imposing 3-foot-tall stem. Whorls of white, pale blue, or lilac flowers cap this handsome plant.

Although it graces many gardens, clary is also well known for its medicinal and other practical properties. For centuries, herbalists thought (as its common name clear eye suggests) that the seeds of clary had ophthalmic value. A moistened seed becomes so mucilaginous, or sticky, that when a solution of it is placed under the eyelid it will clear the eye of any grit or other foreign substances. A mucilage made from the seeds was also used to help draw thorns and splinters from the skin. Herbalists once recommended the powdered root to provoke sneezing and thereby rid the head and brain of "rheum and corruption."

Clary's chief importance, however, is as a fixative in perfumes, to which it adds a lavenderlike scent. It has also been employed as a flavoring in alcoholic beverages: vintners still use it sometimes in making muscatel and other wines, and brewers used to count on it as a strengthener of beer.

Habitat: Sandy and dry soil; along roadsides.
Range: Native to parts of the Mediterranean region and Middle East, clary has become naturalized in Kansas, Idaho, Washington, and Oregon.
Identification: A biennial or sometimes perennial herb, clary grows up to 3 feet tall. The stem is square. Large, oval, velvety leaves are arranged in pairs and are finely toothed. White, pale blue, or lilac flowers (May–September) with pink or lilac bracts produce blackish-brown seeds.

Uses: A solution of clary seed has long been used to rid the eyes of foreign matter. An infusion of the leaves probably helps upset stomachs, as modern herbal healers believe, but there is no evidence to support claims that it alleviates kidney complaints. Clary is chiefly known for its aromatic oil, which is used in the manufacture of perfumes, soaps, and cosmetics. Chefs sometimes add clary to omelets and soups.

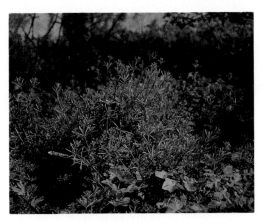

Cleavers

Galium aparine L.

Bedstraw, Catchweed, Goose Grass
MADDER FAMILY
Rubiaceae

As a member of the madder family, cleavers is a relative of coffee. Cleavers seeds, lightly roasted, make a caffeine-free coffee substitute. Herbalists, today as in the past, have claimed medicinal virtues for the plant, too. They prescribe a tea made from the entire plant for kidney stones and bladder problems. Used as a wash, or lotion, the tea is said to fade freckles and sunburn as well as to treat psoriasis. The roots have been used, too. Dried and powdered, they are sprinkled on wounds to halt bleeding and promote healing. Old-time herbalists concocted a soup consisting of cleavers, mutton, and sometimes oatmeal as an aid to dieting, perhaps because cleavers was believed to be a powerful diuretic. The shoots, rich in vitamin C, were once given as a spring tonic and a cure for scurvy.

Cleavers can be hard to spot. It hides in thickets and woods, clinging in dense mats to nearby plants by means of bristles on its stem and leaves. Its white flowers produce bristly fruits that hitch a ride on passing animals. These clinging habits have earned the plant the names cleavers and catchweed. Many farm animals, including geese, relish the plant—a fact that accounts for the name goose grass.

Mature fruit with
bristles (much enlarged)

Habitat: Moist, rich loamy soils in woods, hedgerows, and thickets.
Range: A native of Eurasia and North America, cleavers grows throughout the United States.
Identification: A weak-stemmed sprawling annual that forms dense, prickly mats over nearby plants. The square bristly stem, 1–5 feet high, bears whorls of prickly lance-shaped leaves. Small white flowers (May–June) produce tiny bristled fruits about ⅛ inch across.

Uses: Cleavers is known to modern herbalists as a remedy for vitamin C deficiency as well as for urinary and skin problems, but research has not substantiated its value as a diuretic or claims that it combats psoriasis. The seeds can be roasted and made into an ersatz coffee, and the dried plant is used as a tea substitute in some parts of the world. The cooked shoots and young plants make a nourishing vegetable dish. A red dye can be extracted from the root.

143

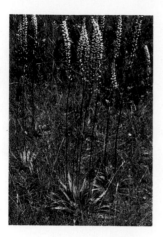

Colicroot

Aletris farinosa L.

Ague Grass, Ague Root, Aletris, Aloeroot,
Crow Corn, Devil's-bit, Star Grass
LILY FAMILY
Liliaceae

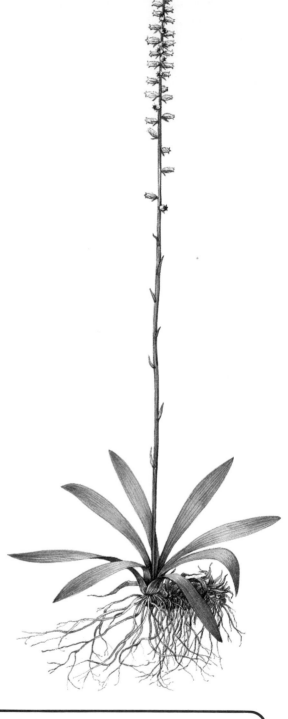

Colicroot enjoys a degree of medicinal celebrity to the present day. It was listed as a therapeutic herb in the *U.S. Pharmacopeia* in the 19th century and in the *National Formulary* until 1947, when the plant lost medicinal standing for lack of conclusive scientific data regarding its usefulness. Current research suggests, however, that colicroot may offer some relief for intestinal muscle spasms, the cause of some colic.

The Indians in North America were the first to experiment with colicroot, which is native to the eastern United States. For stomachaches, colic, dysentery, and menstrual disorders they took a bitter-tasting tea made from the plant's roots or leaves. The settlers of Appalachia adopted these uses, adding a few of their own. They applied a poultice of the leaves for the relief of aching backs and sore breasts. Sometimes they used a potent drink of dried and powdered colicroot mixed with whiskey or brandy, which surely reduced the pain by one means or the other.

Colicroot is a member of the lily family. Its single stalk grows from a basal rosette of shiny leaves, hence the nickname star grass.

Habitat: Sandy, acid, consistently damp soils, as in bogs, open woods, coastal barrens.
Range: Southern Ontario and Maine west to Minnesota, south to the Gulf of Mexico. The species is endangered or threatened in part of its range.
Identification: A perennial herb. Its single stalk grows 1–3 feet high from the center of a rosette of pale green, lilylike leaves 2–7 inches long. Tiny white urn-shaped flowers (May–August), ¼–½ inch long, form a spike along the upper part of the leafless stalk. The fruits are leathery egg-shaped capsules containing many seeds. The "root" is actually a rhizome, or underground stem.
Uses: Modern herbalists use the rhizome and rootlets for digestive complaints. Recent research by pharmacologists indicates, but does not definitely prove, that the plant may have antispasmodic properties. Experimental evidence suggests that the use of the plant for dysmenorrhea (menstrual cramps) may be valid.

Colorado Four-o'clock

Mirabilis multiflora (Torr.) A. Gray

Desert Four-o'clock, Maravilla,
Wild Four-o'clock
FOUR-O'CLOCK FAMILY
Nyctaginaceae

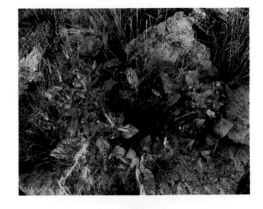

"Many-flowered marvel" is what the Latin name means, and it fits. The plant stays inconspicuous throughout the day, until about four in the afternoon. Then dozens of spectacular flowers open, covering the plant with a magenta blanket. Low mounds of these beauties are visible from a mile away. The flowers stay open all night, then close in the bright sun of morning. Look for Colorado four-o'clocks at elevations of 2,500 feet to 7,500 feet above sea level and in sandy and alkaline soils. These night bloomers are often pollinated by the night-flying sphinx moth, which uncoils its long proboscis to suck nectar from deep within the funnel-shaped flower.

The plant has sturdy roots that can be more than a foot in circumference and can sink 4 feet into the ground. The roots yield a starchy, acrid-tasting substance that somewhat numbs the mouth and tastes peppery after a few seconds. Hopi shamans are said to have chewed the root to induce a visionary trance. According to one source, the root, whether chewed or boiled as a tea, appears to act as an appetite suppressant and is used for that purpose. A paste made of the powdered roots is applied to inflamed joints and tendons as a local anesthestic.

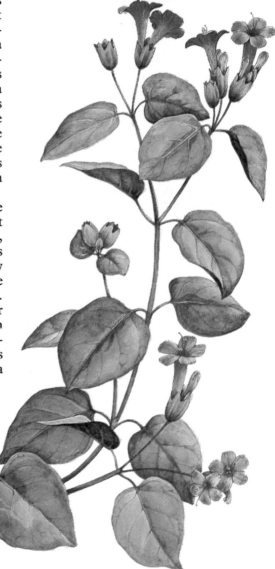

Habitat: Dry roadsides, rocky hillsides, streambanks, plains, piñon and juniper forests.
Range: A native of the United States, Colorado four-o'clock is found in Colorado, Texas, Utah, Arizona, New Mexico, and California.
Identification: A many-branched erect perennial herb growing up to 3 feet tall. Brilliant deep pink or magenta funnel-shaped blossoms (April–September), about 1 inch across, are borne in the leaf axils and are surrounded by cups of five-lobed bracts. Dark green, heart-shaped, opposite leaves are up to 4 inches across.
Uses: Colorado four-o'clock has been used as an appetite suppressant and vision-inducing drug. There are no scientific data available to account for any of the physiological effects that have been attributed to it.

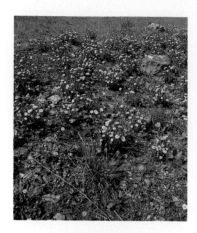

Coltsfoot

Tussilago farfara L.

Coughwort, Son-before-the-father

COMPOSITE FAMILY

Compositae

People thought this plant's leaf was shaped like a colt's hoof—hence the name coltsfoot. Its universal use as a cough remedy earned it the ancient Roman name *tussilago*, "cough dispeller," and another of its English names, coughwort (*wort* is an old English word for herb). One of the very earliest of spring wildflowers to blossom, the plant does not open its distinctive, stout leaves until its bright yellow flowers have bloomed—hence the alternative name son-before-the-father.

From ancient times, people have used coltsfoot as a cough and asthma remedy. The herb has been a main ingredient in cough syrups and asthma teas; the smoke has been inhaled to relieve bronchial congestion since Greek and Roman times; and after the introduction of smoking from America to Europe, coltsfoot became the basic part of the herbal smoking mixtures to which asthmatics resorted for several hundred years—up to the modern discovery of antihistamines and other more effective drugs. Herbalists also applied crushed coltsfoot leaves to burns and skin ailments.

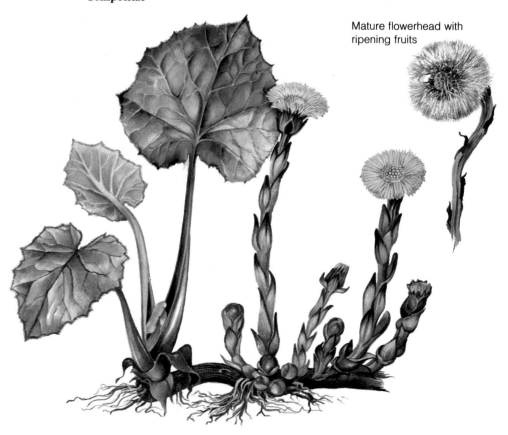

Mature flowerhead with ripening fruits

X Laboratory tests on rodents indicate that coltsfoot may cause cancer if taken in large doses or repeated small doses. Do not use coltsfoot internally.
Habitat: Damp clayey ground.
Range: Introduced to North America from Europe, coltsfoot now grows wild from Newfoundland south to New Jersey and west to Minnesota.
Identification: A perennial growing 4–20 inches high. Yellow dandelionlike flowerheads (February–June), 1 inch across, have an overall bristly appearance. The flower stalks bear brown-tipped scales. The leaves are broadly heart-shaped and somewhat toothed, with downy white hairs on the underside; they have an aromatic smell and appear only after the flowers are in bloom.
Uses: The efficacy of extracts of coltsfoot leaves and flowers, long included in cough syrups, asthma teas, and herbal smoking mixtures for asthmatics, is probably due to the mucilage in the plant, which soothes inflamed mucous membranes.

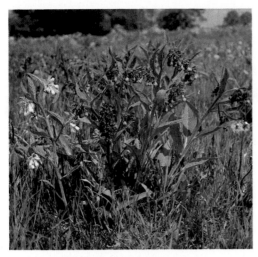

Comfrey

Symphytum officinale L.

Ass-ear, Blackwort, Bruisewort,
Healing Herb, Knitback, Knitbone
BORAGE FAMILY
Boraginaceae

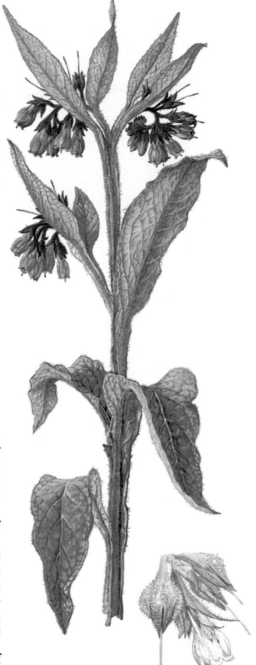

Flower and fruits inside calyxes

Since Greek and Roman antiquity the versatile comfrey has been used in a great variety of ways—as an external application for wounds and fractures, and as a remedy for numerous internal problems, including bleeding. Introduced into North America by early settlers, the plant now grows wild in the eastern part of the continent and is also cultivated.

The name comfrey probably comes from the Latin *conferva*, "knitting together," from the plant's reputed power to make broken bones heal more quickly. Its botanical name, *Symphytum*, means "grown together," and several of the plant's local names in English likewise refer to its mending properties.

Some question exists as to the wisdom of using comfrey internally. First, when it is not in bloom it can be confused with foxglove, a deadly poisonous plant. Second, it may be carcinogenic if taken internally over an extended period. However, a preparation of the roots or leaves shredded and pounded into a gluey mass is safe when applied to external injuries. The healing process is accelerated, stubborn sores disappear, and broken bones—held in place by the preparation when it dries—heal much more quickly. Comfrey leaves have at times been used as fodder for livestock. Containing almost 35 percent protein, they are highly nutritious.

X There is evidence that comfrey may cause cancer if taken internally over a long period of time.
Habitat: Wet places.
Range: Newfoundland south to Georgia, west to Ontario and Louisiana.
Identification: A large, conspicuous perennial growing to 3 feet high. Narrowly oval, alternate dark green leaves grow on an erect stem that branches at the top. The lower leaves may be 10 inches long, the upper ones smaller. Both stem and leaves are hairy and rough. Downy, pale yellow to purplish bell-shaped flowers (May–September) bloom continuously in drooping clusters.
Uses: A poultice of the crushed leaves accelerates healing of surface wounds and sores and broken bones. Comfrey contains a substance called allantoin used in ointments for psoriasis and other skin problems. Comfrey tea, said to ease bronchial and intestinal disorders, may not be safe when taken over a long period of time.

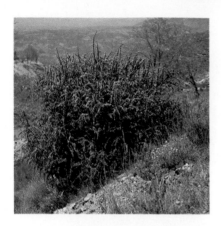

Common Barberry

Berberis vulgaris L.

Barberry, Berberry, European Barberry,
Jaundice Berry

BARBERRY FAMILY

Berberidaceae

The yellow wood of common barberry most likely was a sign to physicians long ago that the plant was useful for jaundice, a condition (usually caused by liver disease or gallstones) in which the skin turns yellowish. They concluded this on the basis of a theory called the doctrine of signatures, which held that a plant's appearance or other characteristics were a divine sign of the type of disease or injury it would cure.

The root bark and stem bark of the plant contain tannin and a substance known as berberine, which may account for the plant's effectiveness in treating diarrhea. Common barberry's employment for bloodshot eyes appears valid, for modern pharmaceutical products use the berberine it contains in eye preparations. In ancient Egypt a syrup made of common barberry mixed with fennel seed was used against plagues. Modern research indicates that this remedy was probably effective because the plant has antibacterial properties that would help ward off infectious diseases.

The berries have been used in cooking, and the wood is favored for marquetry work.

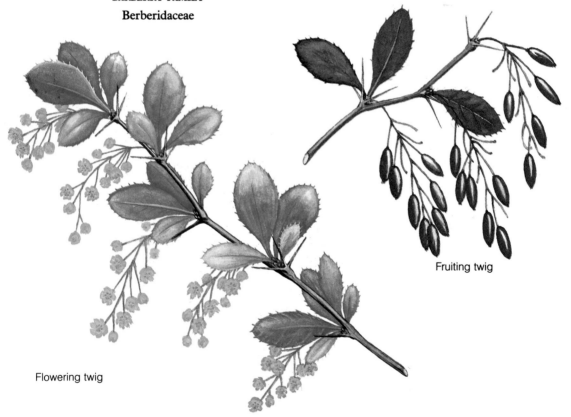

Fruiting twig

Flowering twig

Habitat: Thickets, pastures, waste places.
Range: Introduced from Europe, common barberry now grows wild in North America from Nova Scotia south to Delaware and Pennsylvania, and west to Missouri, Minnesota, and Iowa.
Identification: A bushy, deciduous, upright shrub growing up to 10 feet tall. Oval to oblong, spiny-toothed leaves are pale green above, grayish green below. Small yellow flowers (May–June) bloom in drooping clusters and are followed by clusters of oval orange-red to scarlet-red fruits.

Uses: Researchers investigating common barberry's traditional use for liver and gallbladder ailments find that preparations from the plant may improve liver function by stimulating the production of bile by the liver. Scientists have found, however, that barberry is more likely effective as an antiseptic and antidiarrheal agent. Berberine salts, derived from common barberry and other plants, are used in eyedrops and eyewashes.

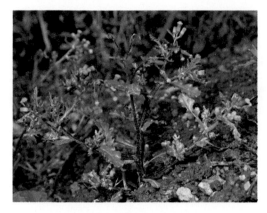

Common Groundsel

Senecio vulgaris L.

Grundy-swallow, Ground Glutton
COMPOSITE FAMILY
Compositae

A familiar weed that grows quickly and spreads rapidly in gardens and fields, common groundsel probably gets its name from an Old English word meaning "ground swallower," a reference to the plant's rampant growth. The scientific name is derived from the Latin *senecio*, "old man," and refers to the tufts of white hair on the seeds.

History records common groundsel's use as an herbal remedy almost 2,000 years ago, although the toothache remedy that the Roman naturalist and writer Pliny mentioned in the first century A.D. consists as much of mumbo jumbo as of medicine: "If a line is traced round it with an iron tool before it is dug up, and if one touches a painful tooth with the plant three times, spitting after each touch, and replaces it into its original ground so as to keep it alive, it is said that the tooth will never cause pain thereafter."

According to later herbal tradition, groundsel mixed with wine relieved stomach pain. Groundsel tea has also been recommended as a purgative for various intestinal complaints, and at times it was administered for painful menstruation. The weed also figures among the ingredients of some modern-day herbal lotions for the eyes and for chapped hands. However, the herb contains toxic substances that, if taken internally in large or prolonged doses, may cause cancer.

X There is evidence that groundsel may cause liver cancer if taken internally over a long period of time.

Habitat: Fields and gardens, or wherever the soil has been upturned.

Range: Accidentally introduced from Europe, common groundsel has become naturalized in most parts of Canada and the United States.

Identification: A low-growing annual weed with erect, green to purple stems 6–12 inches tall. Its narrow, oblong, green leaves have irregular, jagged lobes. Cylindrical yellow flowerheads (March–October), about ¼ inch long, bloom in clusters. The seeds (actually one-seeded fruits called achenes), crowned by downy tufts, are dispersed by the wind. One weed, if all its seeds were to grow, could produce up to a million other plants within a year.

Uses: Groundsel no longer figures importantly in herbal medicine. However, groundsel seeds are a popular food for canaries.

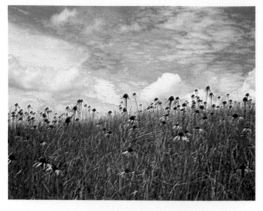

Coneflower

Echinacea angustifolia DC.

Black Sampson, Purple Coneflower
COMPOSITE FAMILY
Compositae

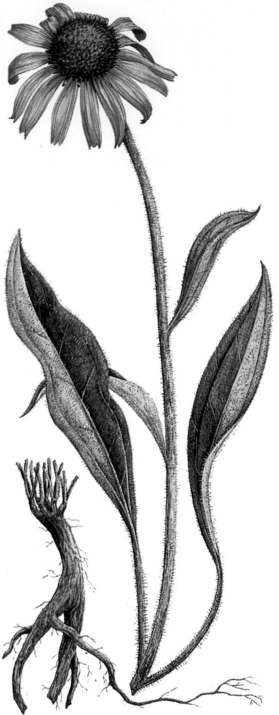

Rhizome with roots

Indians of the western plains held the coneflower in high regard. Magicians washed their hands with coneflower juice before plunging them into scalding water, and one Winnebago tribesman said he used the plant before placing a red-hot coal in his mouth. But the Indians chiefly employed the plant medicinally. They prescribed it for snakebite and other poisonous bites and stings, toothache, and enlarged glands such as those resulting from mumps. Inhaling the plant smoke was recommended as a headache remedy.

During the 19th century, coneflower's rhizome (underground stem) and roots captured the interest of some doctors, who used them as an antiseptic and as a "blood purifier"—an agent that was supposed to cleanse the body of toxic materials. The underground parts were said to be helpful in treating infections, carbuncles, boils, and abscesses. Coneflower was also specified as a drug that would help to restore health generally. The dried rhizome and roots have been used as an antibiotic, antiseptic, and sweat-producing agent.

The drug was included in the *National Formulary*, a pharmacists' reference book, from 1916 until 1946.

Habitat: Barrens, prairies, and other dry open places. **Range:** A North American native, coneflower grows from Saskatchewan south to Tennessee and Texas. **Identification:** A hairy perennial herb growing to about 2 feet tall. Narrow oblong to lance-shaped leaves have three veins along their length; the lower leaves have long stalks. Single long-stalked flowerheads (May–August) have drooping petallike purple-rose or white ray flowers, 1–1¾ inches long, and a center of brownish-orange disc flowers.

Uses: Scientists find that there may be some basis for the use of the plant as an external antiseptic. Extracts of the plant have also been shown to stimulate the immune system, and this action may account for the plant's value as an agent that helps restore normal body functions. Researchers have also investigated, but cannot substantiate, claims that the root works as an anti-inflammatory (an agent that reduces pain and swelling resulting from injury).

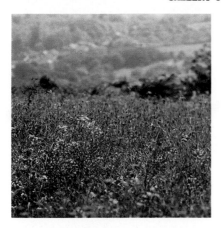

Cornflower

Centaurea cyanus L.

Bachelor's-button, Bluebottle, Hurtsickle
COMPOSITE FAMILY
Compositae

A favorite garden flower, cornflower is an easily cultivated annual that has many varieties and colors. The cornflower in herbal use is *Centaurea cyanus*—the familiar bright blue "bachelor's-button," as it is often called. Originally native to the Mediterranean, the plant was so completely naturalized in England— where it was common in grain fields—that farmers looked upon it as a weed, calling it "hurtsickle" because of its tough stem, which blunted their sickles. "Cornflower blue" is the color of incredibly blue eyes. People lucky enough to have such beautiful eyes are especially likely to enjoy the plant's beneficial effect on the eyesight, according to folklore—and a decoction of the dried flowers has been used to treat eye inflammations. In folk medicine the leaves or seeds steeped in wine were taken as a cure for pestilential fevers. Juice from the leaves was applied externally to wounds.

Since cornflowers retain their bright color when dry, they are often used in arrangements of dried flowers or in wreaths. Juice from the flowers mixed with alum water makes a blue ink, but the color is not fast as a dye for cloth.

The Latin name refers to a mythical centaur that the ancient Greeks worshiped as the father of medicine.

Habitat: Fields, roadsides, and waste grounds.
Range: A native of Europe and widely cultivated in North America, the cornflower has escaped from gardens and become naturalized.
Identification: An annual herb, with an erect, wiry, downy stem that grows 1–2 feet high and is branching. At the ends of the branches grow solitary, thistlelike, brilliant blue flowerheads. Long grayish-green leaves are alternate, lance-shaped, and downy like the stem.

Uses: Research concerning cornflower's medicinal value indicates that it may have some effect as an astringent, or substance that causes contraction of tissues and thus stops bleeding. This effect is a result of the tannin content of the plant. Pharmacologists find little evidence, however, to support its efficacy in treating fevers.

151

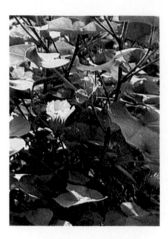

Cotton

Gossypium hirsutum L.

American Upland Cotton, Common Cotton,
Upland Cotton, Wild Cotton

MALLOW FAMILY

Malvaceae

Much of United States history once revolved around the cotton plant, because of its economic importance and its connection with the institution of slavery. According to archeologists, as long ago as 3500 B.C., Indians in the Tehuacán Valley of Mexico were probably cultivating *G. hirsutum*, a cotton species native to tropical America. As a cultivated crop, upland cotton, as this species is frequently called, now constitutes most of the world's cotton crop. Today oil from the seed is also an important product of the plant. It is used in the manufacture of shortening, margarine, and cooking and salad oils.

In addition to cotton's commercial uses, the plant has been considered a "female medicine" by Indian and other folk healers. To ease childbirth, Alabama and Koasati Indian women brewed a root tea and took it at delivery time. Modern herbalists continue this use, which they say is effective because of a substance in the root that increases the contractions of the uterus during birth. Herbalists also state that the root contains a substance that promotes normal menstruation.

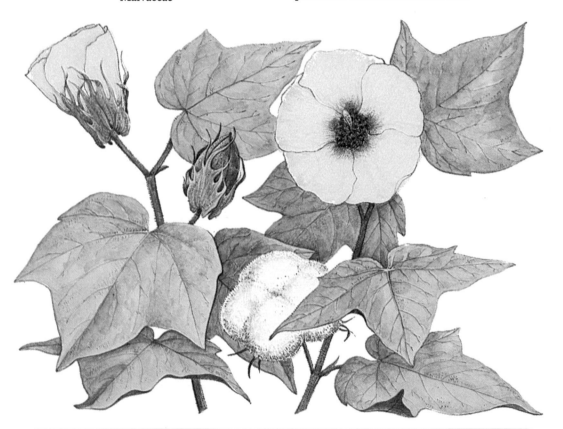

X Cotton seeds are toxic and may cause death. Cottonseed oil is not harmful because the toxic materials are removed in the purification process.
Habitat: Dunes, small coastal hills, railroad beds.
Range: Native to tropical America, cotton grows wild in southern Florida and the keys and is cultivated throughout the southern United States.
Identification: An annual herb or shrub 2–5 feet tall. Grayish-green alternate leaves, 2–6 inches long, are usually three-lobed. Cup-shaped flowers have large, showy, creamy white to yellow petals with a purple or red spot near the base. The fruit capsules (the boll) contain seeds covered with white hairs (the cotton fiber). The plant produces flowers and fruit throughout most of the year.
Uses: The root of cotton has been used as an aid in childbirth, and scientists state that this remedy may have worked. In modern folk medicine a root tea is sometimes given to induce a normal menstrual cycle. Studies show that this use may be valid.

Couch Grass

Agropyron repens (L.) Beauvois

Dog Grass, Quack Grass, Witchgrass

GRASS FAMILY

Gramineae

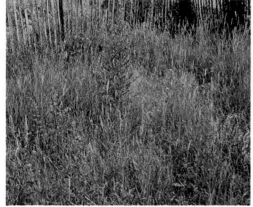

American gardeners and farmers bitterly regret that couch grass was ever introduced from Europe, for it is one of the most troublesome of weed grasses. Once established in a plot or field, it is practically impossible to eradicate. If even a single piece of its far-ranging rhizomes is left behind when the plant is rooted up, it will rapidly sprout anew. The plant's botanical name, *Agropyron repens*, means "creeping field-wheat." The tenacious grip that couch grass rhizomes have on the soil can at times be beneficial, however, since it also helps to prevent soil erosion.

Couch grass's thick networks of rhizomes have, in fact, proved to be its most valuable feature. Rich in carbohydrates, the rhizomes make a nourishing fodder for cattle. On occasion, they have also served for human consumption—either roasted as a coffee substitute or, in times of famine, dried and ground as a replacement for flour. In folk medicine, couch grass tea, brewed from the rhizomes, was used as a diuretic and recommended for a variety of urinary complaints, such as cystitis. Because the rhizomes have a high concentration of mucilage, they were believed to be soothing to the mucous membranes.

The name dog grass refers to the plant's popularity with dogs, who seek it out when they are sick and eat its foliage as an emetic.

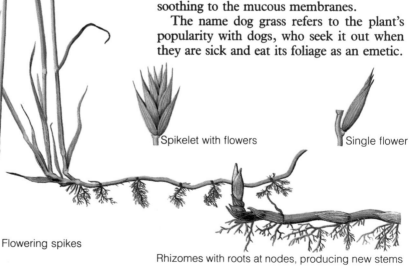

Spikelet with flowers

Single flower

Fruiting spikes   Flowering spikes

Rhizomes with roots at nodes, producing new stems

Habitat: Open cultivated fields, waste places, pastures, seashores.

Range: Introduced from Europe, couch grass is common in the central and northern United States, and through British Columbia to Alaska.

Identification: A coarse perennial grass growing 1–3 feet tall. When in flower (late May–September), it looks like rye or beardless wheat, with tiny purplish stamens in the flower spikes atop each stem. The yellow-white rhizomes are slender and very long with thin brown rootlets at the nodes.

Uses: Couch grass is known in pharmacology as triticum (the Latin name for wheat) because it contains the carbohydrate triticin. The plant has been useful as cattle fodder, a coffee substitute, and an emergency ration. Although couch grass tea may be recommended by herbalists for its soothing effects on the urinary tract, this use is questioned by scientists; moreover, the safety of drinking the tea has not been proved.

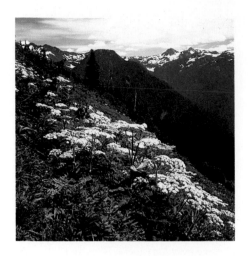

Cow Parsnip

Heracleum maximum Bartr.

Cow Cabbage, Masterwort
CARROT FAMILY
Umbelliferae

Tall and robust, cow parsnip is one of the largest members of the carrot family, which also includes cultivated parsnip, celery, parsley, dill, and other vegetables and herbs. Like them, it is most commonly used today as a food. Just as Indians once gathered and cooked the roots, so wild-food enthusiasts today boil them as a vegetable. The young stems can also be peeled and then cooked or eaten raw. And in a pinch ashes from the burned leaves can serve as a salt substitute—another trick Indians taught early settlers.

The Indians valued cow parsnip for more than food. One tribe used it in a charm that was supposed to drive off an evil spirit who stole the luck of deer hunters. Another tribe, more practically oriented, passed off the forked roots as the more valuable ginseng.

Medicinally, the Indians' uses for the plant were legion. They ate the cooked roots for intestinal disorders, employed the seeds in headache remedies, and stuffed raw pieces of the root into dental cavities to alleviate toothaches. Other cures were claimed, for everything from ear infections to epilepsy. Today herbalists use cow parsnip mainly in a poultice for boils and other skin problems.

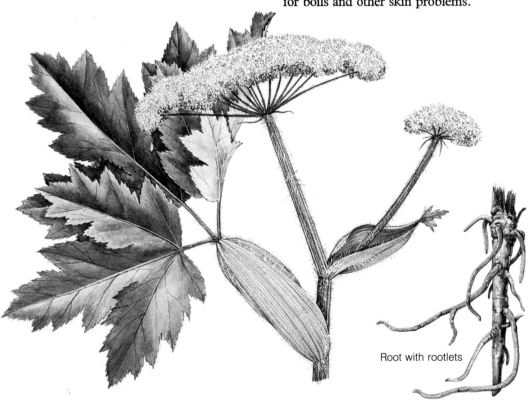

Root with rootlets

X Positive identification is essential in order not to confuse the plant with such poisonous members of the carrot family as water hemlock and poison hemlock.
Habitat: Rich, moist soil.
Range: Native to North America, cow parsnip is found from Labrador to Alaska, south to the mountains of Georgia and west to California.
Identification: A sturdy herbaceous perennial that sometimes grows to 10 feet. The hollow stem is grooved and covered with woolly hairs. The compound leaves consist of three oversized maplelike leaflets with white, woolly undersides; the leafstalks have large inflated sheaths at their bases. Flattened white or sometimes purplish flowerheads (April–September) can measure almost 1 foot in diameter.
Uses: Cow parsnip has not been studied experimentally in recent years; therefore, there is no scientific evidence to either prove or disprove its folk uses.

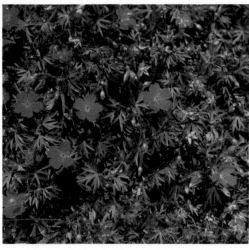

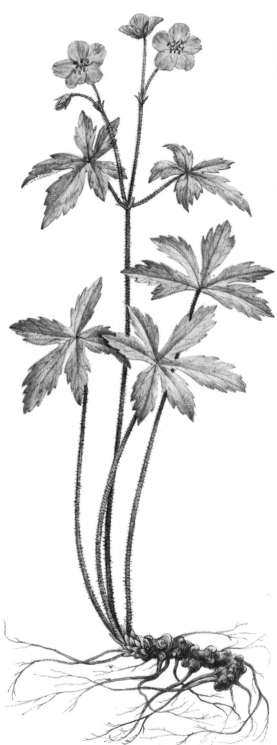

Cranesbill

Geranium maculatum L.

Alumroot, Dovefoot, Old-maid's-nightcap,
Shameface, Wild Geranium

GERANIUM FAMILY

Geraniaceae

"A very popular domestic remedy in many parts of the country," is what a 19th-century handbook for physicians says about cranesbill, or wild geranium, citing the widespread use of this astringent plant for diarrhea, dysentery, and hemorrhaging.

An herbal remedy that settlers picked up from North American Indians, the plant proved to be both effective and harmless. The Chippewas used the dried and powdered rhizome, or underground stem, on sores inside the mouth, especially of children. Other Indian peoples steeped the plant in water as an eyewash. Mixed with other herbs and water, the powdered rhizome was applied to sores and open wounds and, as a poultice, to swollen feet. The Indians also ate the young green leaves as food.

To this day herbalists recommend the plant for many of the same medicinal purposes. The fluid extract and powdered rhizome are both widely available in herbal stores. Cranesbill was listed in the *U.S. Pharmacopeia,* a reference for pharmacists, from 1820 to 1916.

Habitat: Woodlands, meadows, clearings.
Range: Native to North America, cranesbill is found growing in the wild from Maine to Manitoba, south to Georgia and Tennessee, and west to Missouri and Kansas.
Identification: A perennial herb, growing up to 2 feet tall with hairy stems. The leaves, which are arranged in opposite pairs, are usually divided into five toothed lobes. Five-petaled flowers (April–June) are pale pink to rosy purple and bloom in clusters at the end of each stem. The fruits bear a fanciful resemblance to cranes' bills.
Uses: Because of its tannin content, the rhizome (underground stem) of cranesbill acts as an external astringent (an agent that causes the skin and mucous membranes to constrict) and a hemostatic (an agent that stops bleeding). For the same reason it is probably effective when taken internally for diarrhea.

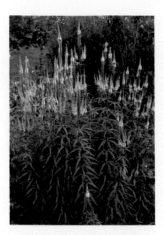

Culver's Root

Veronicastrum virginicum (L.) Farw.

Black Root, Bowman's Root, Brinton Root,
Culver's Physic, Physic Root

SNAPDRAGON FAMILY

Scrophulariaceae

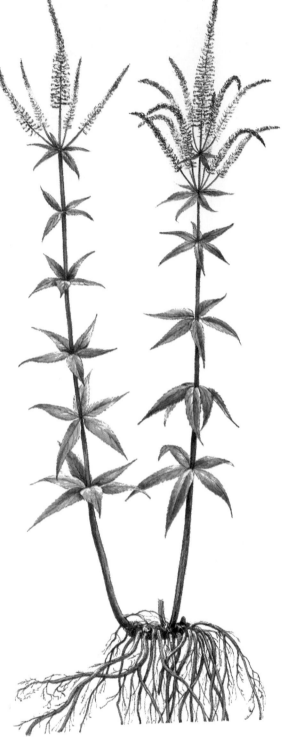

When Cotton Mather, the famous Puritan leader, sought a remedy for his daughter's tuberculosis in 1716, it was Culver's root that he asked for, and his request is the first recorded use of the name. Culver's root was well known to most early practitioners as a powerful laxative and emetic (a substance that causes vomiting). It was certainly a violent drug to use for a lung ailment, and Mather's daughter died soon afterward.

American Indians, who discovered the plant's therapeutic properties, employed it ritually too. For ceremonial purifications, the Seneca Indians induced vomiting by drinking a tea made from the plant's dried root. The Chippewas used the root as a "blood cleanser."

Another property that has been attributed to the root is its ability to increase the flow of bile from the liver. Herbalists employed dried Culver's root in the treatment of liver disorders and for chronic indigestion and other conditions thought to arise from liver dysfunction.

An almost identical twin to this native American plant grows half a world away, in eastern Asia.

Habitat: Meadows, woodlands, prairies, thickets.
Range: Native to North America, Culver's root grows wild from Manitoba to Vermont, south to Florida and Texas.
Identification: A perennial herb with slender stems growing up to 7 feet tall. Whorls of three or more narrow lance-shaped leaves circle the stem at its joints. Small white, pinkish, or blue flowers (June–September) cluster in spikes 3–8 inches long at the ends of the stems.

Uses: Dried Culver's root has been used in small amounts as a remedy for indigestion and diarrhea. Boiled in milk or steeped in hot water, the root was also taken as a powerful laxative. Scientists have not investigated the plant for its medicinal uses and therefore cannot confirm or refute claims made for it.

Cup Plant

Silphium perfoliatum L.

Carpenter Weed, Indian Cup, Ragged Cup
COMPOSITE FAMILY
Compositae

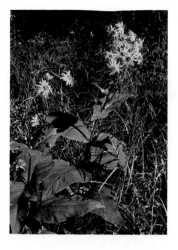

When American Indians wanted chewing gum, they did not go to the candy store; they just snapped off the top of a stalk of cup plant. From the broken stem would ooze a blob of resinous sap that would dry into a chewy, breath-freshening gum. In times of sickness, too, Indians turned to cup plant. They burned its long, crooked rhizome (underground stem) and inhaled the smoke to relieve a head cold or neuralgia, and they made potions from the root for liver problems, fever, or just general debility. The Chippewas used a root extract, or decoction, for hemorrhaging from the lungs, for back and chest pains, and to stop excessive menstrual bleeding. They also applied a moist compress made of dried and mashed root to wounds. Other Indian tribes used cup plant in similar ways.

Like many other medicinal plants, cup plant was held to have supernatural powers too. On the eve of a buffalo hunt or other important undertaking, Winnebago braves downed a decoction made from the rhizome to cleanse and purify themselves before they set off.

North American and European herbalists have long recommended the root tea for spleen ailments, to restore health, and as a tonic. The gum is said to be a stimulant and antispasmodic.

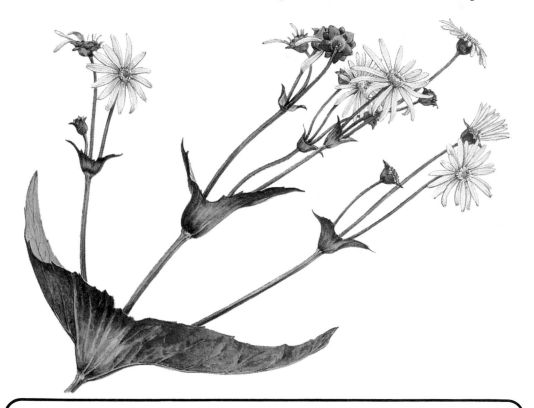

Habitat: Rich soils, especially of woodlands, prairies, riverbanks.
Range: A native of North America, cup plant flourishes from Ontario west to South Dakota and south to Georgia and Oklahoma, and is occasionally found in the Northeast.
Identification: A large perennial plant with a square stem reaching up to 8 feet in height. Its leaves grow in opposite pairs; the bases of the upper ones are fused, forming a cup around the stem. Yellow flowerheads (July–September), 2–3 inches across, are borne at the top of the stem and resemble small sunflowers.
Uses: Cup plant yields a resinous sap that hardens into a chewable, breath-freshening gum. Herbalists recommend the tea brewed from the plant's root as a tonic and as a restorative, or agent that generally helps restore a person's health. To date scientists have found no evidence for or against these uses.

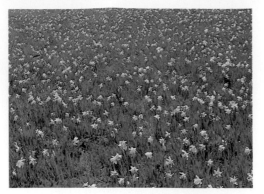

Daffodil

Narcissus pseudonarcissus L.

Lent Lily

AMARYLLIS FAMILY

Amaryllidaceae

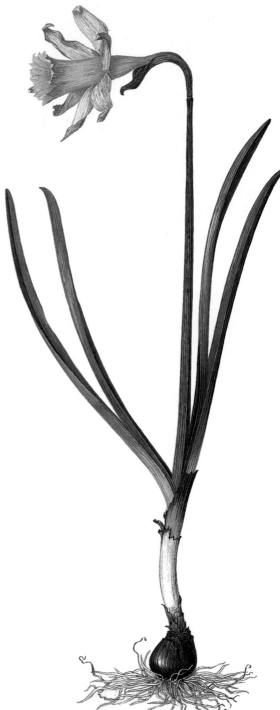

"I saw a crowd, a host, of golden daffodils"; so exclaimed William Wordsworth after beholding a "never-ending line" of the flowers that inspired his famous poem. Anyone who has seen them blooming can understand the poet's enthusiasm. But this lovely flower also has a darker side, as its botanical name, *Narcissus*, indicates. The word comes from the Greek *narke*, "numbness," and indeed, the bulb contains toxic alkaloids that can cause paralysis of the central nervous system, leading to death. Unaware of the daffodil's potential dangers, early physicians and apothecaries used the bulbs and flowers as an antispasmodic in the treatment of epilepsy and hysteria; they prescribed the flowers and roots when an agent to induce vomiting was needed. Herbals of more recent times recommend a tea or syrup made from the flowers for respiratory ailments, such as bronchial congestion.

Although gypsies regard the flower as unlucky, they used to hawk it in London in early spring, the daffodil's growing period; this may have earned it the name Lent lily. The more common name, daffodil, is a corruption of the Greek *asphodelos*—the flower that the Greeks thought bloomed in the afterlife.

X Daffodil bulbs, sometimes mistaken for onions, are toxic and may cause death. Symptoms include salivation, vomiting, nausea, and contraction of the pupils.

Habitat: Open woodlands, fields.

Range: Native to Europe, daffodils are naturalized locally throughout the United States, especially as survivors of abandoned gardens.

Identification: A bulbous perennial with narrow, flat, bluish-green leaves, ½–1 foot long. Each of the single yellow flowers (April–May) grows on a long stalk and has a distinctively long corona, or crown, that is commonly known as a trumpet.

Uses: Physicians and herbalists employed powdered daffodil flowers to induce vomiting, as in cases of poisoning. Because the daffodil bulb is extremely dangerous, herbalists no longer use it. The plant is still a favorite flower, inspiring countless verses and songs and beloved as a harbinger of spring.

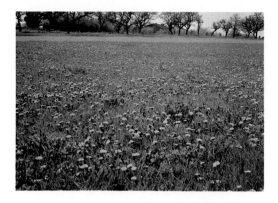

Dandelion

Taraxacum officinale Weber

Pissabed, Priest's-crown, Telltime

COMPOSITE FAMILY

Compositae

Much money is spent on herbicides to remove this cheery flower from lawns and gardens, but the dandelion holds its own, producing seeds with or without pollination and distributing them far and wide. In fact, the plant has many virtues. European settlers deliberately introduced it to the New World, where Native Americans quickly took it up. The Mohegans drank dandelion-leaf tea as a tonic, while other Indians prepared a tea from the roots for heartburn. Because the flowers have such a long blooming season, later settlers introduced the dandelion into the Midwest to provide food for bees.

Dandelion greens are edible, either as a salad or cooked, and furnish a rich source of vitamins A and C. The blossoms are made into wine, and the dried roots can be ground, roasted, and brewed into a coffeelike beverage. The brew from the roots has been drunk as a tonic and for the reputed diuretic effect that accounts for its common French name, *pissenlit,* or "piss-in-bed." Dried dandelion leaves make a tea that is mildly laxative. But the most notable medicinal use of the dandelion has been the treatment of liver ailments with a brew made from the roots.

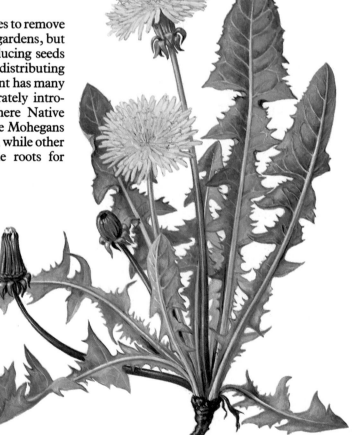

Fruit with parachute intact

Mature fruit

X Do not eat dandelions from lawns treated with herbicides.

Habitat: Meadows, roadsides, lawns.

Range: Throughout most of North America.

Identification: A perennial herb with a short stem hidden beneath a basal rosette of deeply toothed leaves. The plant has slender, hollow stalks that bear single heads of tiny, tongue-shaped yellow flowers (March–September). The flowerheads open wide in the morning and close in the evening.

When mature, these flowerheads turn into downy white balls of seeds (actually fruits), each with its own parachute that carries it away on the wind.

Uses: The flowers can be boiled to make a yellow dye, the roots a magenta one. A tea from the leaves is used as a tonic and to promote bowel regularity. Although a brew from the roots is given for liver, gallbladder, and other digestive ailments, only its use as a tonic is fairly well substantiated. Dandelion wine can be made from the blossoms.

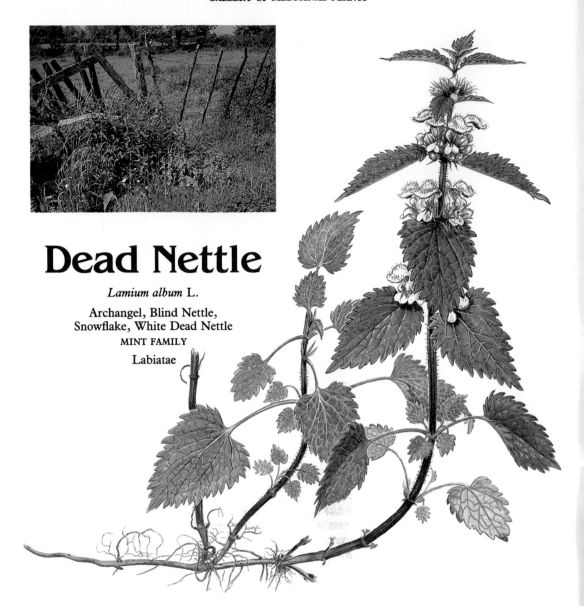

Dead Nettle

Lamium album L.

Archangel, Blind Nettle,
Snowflake, White Dead Nettle
MINT FAMILY
Labiatae

Because it looks so much like stinging nettle, hikers may give the harmless dead nettle a wide berth. Bumblebees, however, are not deceived. They throng to the flowers, for they know that the plant, like other members of the mint family, is an abundant source of nectar. This nettle is "dead" because it does not sting. In Britain it is known as archangel, probably because it first blooms about May 8, once a feast day of the Archangel Michael.

Though dead nettle never found a place in conventional medicine, it has long enjoyed popularity as a folk remedy. Rich in tannin,

the flowering plant has provided an astringent, anti-inflammatory dressing for cuts, wounds, and burns. When brewed as a tea, it has been used to halt internal bleeding. Dead nettle also is reported to cure diarrhea. The plant formerly enjoyed prestige in England as a reputed cure for scrofula (a type of tuberculosis of the lymph nodes), the so-called King's Evil, which was believed to respond to a monarch's touch. Dead nettle leaves mixed with axle grease were in fact already mentioned by the Roman naturalist Pliny in the first century A.D. as a folk remedy for the disease.

Habitat: Waste places, roadsides, gardens.
Range: Introduced from Europe, dead nettle now grows wild in North America from Quebec to Minnesota and south to Virginia.
Identification: A creeping perennial that spreads on rhizomes, dead nettle has stems reaching up to 2 feet in height. Long-stalked, oval, toothed leaves grow in opposite pairs. White flowers (May–October) grow in whorls in the axils of the leaves; the flowers have two lips, the upper one hooded and

hairy on the outside, the lower one having two to three lobes.
Uses: Dead nettle makes a nutritious vegetable or soup green. A tea from the flowering plant is a home remedy for diarrhea—a use that pharmacologists state may be effective because of the plant's tannin content. Scientific tests indicate that the plant may be effective as an emmenagogue, or agent that promotes menstruation. No other uses have been validated.

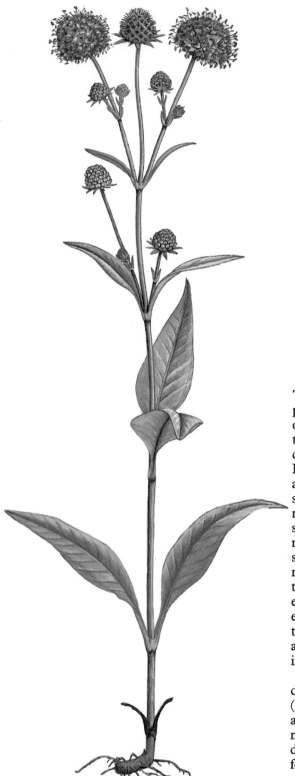

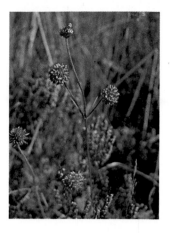

Devil's-bit

Succisa pratensis Moench

Devil's-bit Scabious, Ofbit, Scabious
TEASEL FAMILY
Dipsacaceae

The Devil gave his name to a number of plants in medieval times. The story behind this one is that Satan became so angry at the thought of the innumerable benefits people derived from the herb's root that he bit it off. From this the root got its gnashed appearance, and the plant its name. The common name scabious comes from the herb's once wide reputation for usefulness in treating certain skin diseases. In Medieval Latin *herba scabiosa* means "scabies plant." Not only scabies (a skin infection caused by itch mites) but external ulcers and wounds, thrush (a fungus infection known medically as moniliasis), worms, even plague, were reportedly treatable with extracts of devil's-bit root. Some herbalists to the present day recommend a tea of devil's-bit as a remedy for coughs and fevers, and for internal inflammations.

In herbal tradition, the plant is known as a diaphoretic, or medicine to produce sweating (in order to break a fever); and a demulcent, or agent that has a soothing effect on mucous membranes. One old-time remedy was to mix devil's-bit with rose honey and use it as a gargle for a swollen throat.

Habitat: Damp meadows, woods, marshes.
Range: Introduced from Europe, devil's-bit has escaped cultivation in scattered locations from Cape Breton Island in Canada south to Massachusetts.
Identification: A perennial herb growing up to 3 feet tall. The narrow elliptical to lance-shaped leaves, up to 1 foot long, are arranged in opposite pairs. The flowers (August–September) are violet-blue, or rarely pink or white, and are borne in round heads up to 1½ inches across at the top of the stem. In its first year of growth, the root is thick and tapered like a carrot; later, the bottom decays leaving a ragged stump, the "devil's bite" that gave the plant its name.
Uses: Herbalists still recommend tea brewed from devil's-bit root for coughs, fevers, and internal inflammations. A decoction (extract) also serves as a cleansing wash for itching skin and to heal wounds and sores. There is no scientific information available on the plant.

161

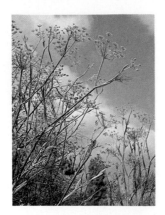

Dill

Anethum graveolens L.

Dillseed, Dillweed

CARROT FAMILY

Umbelliferae

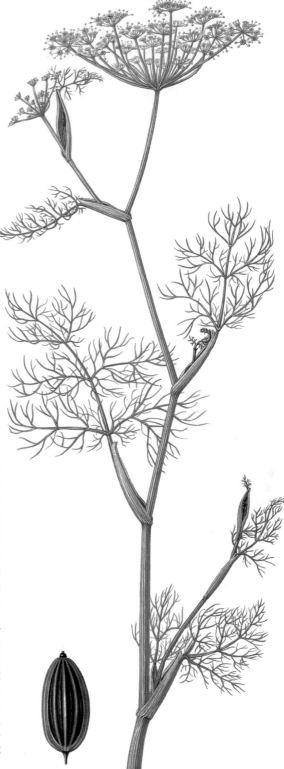

Mature fruit

Hang a bunch of dill over your door, says an old folk belief, and you will be protected against witches. Although such wonders are no longer required of the plant, other age-old uses of dill in cookery and medicine have persisted into modern times.

Apparently, dill has been used since the time of the Egyptians, who mentioned it some 5,000 years ago in their writings. The herb acquired its present name from the use of its oil (extracted from the seeds) in potions that soothed the colicky stomachs of infants. The Old Norse word *dilla*, from which *dill* is derived, means "to lull." Even now, some families use dill water, or gripe water, to relieve digestive discomfort. The oil is also used commercially for scenting soaps.

Dill is chiefly known today as a delightfully pungent, sharp-tasting culinary herb, whose fresh leaves add interest to salads and fish and whose seeds give dill pickles, a side dish that came to America from Germany, their characteristic flavor. Dillseeds also add flavor to stews, sauces, potato dishes, and breads. The leaves can be dried for use throughout the year; commercial herb dealers package them as dillweed. But the fresh leaves have more flavor.

Habitat: Roadsides and waste places; best cultivated in sunny, open areas.
Range: Native to Asia and naturalized in Europe and North America, dill grows in most regions of temperate North America.
Identification: A hardy annual or biennial reaching 2–3 feet or taller. From a single whitish-green stem grow leafstalks bearing finely divided light green leaves that create a feathery, misty look. The stem terminates in umbrellalike clusters made up of numerous light yellow flowers (July–August). Elliptical brown seeds (actually fruits) have prominent ribs.
Uses: Dill water, prepared from oil of dill, is a common folk remedy for infant colic, as well as for digestive disorders in older children. Experiments have validated these uses. The oil also scents perfumes and soaps. In the kitchen, dill is an essential pickling spice and is used to flavor sauces, salads, potatoes, fish, and bread.

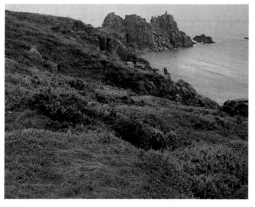

Dodder

Cuscuta epithymum Murr.

Love Vine

MORNING GLORY FAMILY

Convolvulaceae

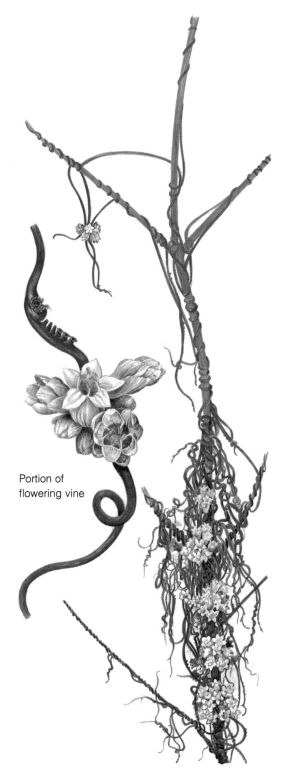

Portion of flowering vine

Love vine is another name for it, because when dodder meets a likely host, it twines its threadlike stem around the host, as a lover would embrace his beloved. There the resemblance to love ends. Dodder's suckers burrow into the host's stem to draw out nourishment, since dodder has no chlorophyll of its own and is obliged to live as a parasite—a relative rarity among flowering plants.

Clover and alfalfa are among dodder's favorite hosts in America, but in some countries the plant clings most happily to thyme, hence the species name *epithymum,* meaning "[growing] on thyme." In his *Materia Medica* (1749–1763) the Swedish botanist and classifier of plants Carolus Linnaeus pointed out that an infusion (tea) of any herb attaching itself to thyme will have the odor of thyme.

In the 1600's in England Nicholas Culpeper's family herbal favored using dodder that had grown upon thyme. Culpeper noted that such a plant was "most effectual for melancholy diseases . . . as well as for the trembling of the heart, faintings, and swoonings." He also pointed out that it was helpful in diseases of the spleen, in obstructions of the gallbladder, and in cases of jaundice, which often results from liver disease.

Habitat: In fields where clover, alfalfa, and other legumes grow.
Range: Introduced from Europe, dodder has been naturalized in scattered locations from Ontario south to Pennsylvania and west to Washington.
Identification: A leafless parasitic vine that attaches its reddish-orange threadlike stems to green plants by means of suckers to draw out nourishment. Pinkish-white flowers (July–September) have five sharp, spreading, triangular lobes and grow in dense clusters. The seeds may remain dormant for up to eight years. The plant is a nuisance to farmers growing alfalfa and clover.
Uses: Dodder has long been considered a remedy for kidney complaints, and today herbalists mention the plant for treating liver diseases and as a laxative. No scientific studies have been reported that would confirm the validity of these uses.

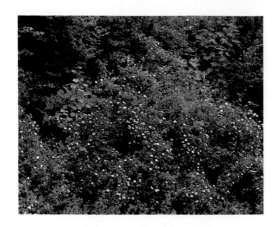

Dog Rose

Rosa canina L.

Dog Brier, Wild Brier
ROSE FAMILY
Rosaceae

Though its use in prescriptions goes back to Hippocrates, the dog rose came into full bloom as a medicinal plant only in World War II. With Great Britain unable to import fresh citrus fruits, the government organized the gathering of dog rose fruits, or hips, which were known to be rich in vitamin C. Processed into syrup, the rose hips helped to prevent scurvy in the isolated country.

Until that time the dog rose had been appreciated in modern times chiefly for its wild run of color through the countryside and for its ability to grow into impenetrable thickets. The abundant flowers, which bloom from May to July, are followed by scarlet hips, or fruits. By autumn, these are smooth-skinned and fleshy. The hips are processed into jellies, tonics, and pills, as well as syrups. The jelly is perhaps the most popular form.

The Roman naturalist Pliny attributed the name dog rose to a belief that the plant's root could cure the bite of a mad dog. Although the hips were once officially sanctioned as an astringent and refrigerant, or fever-allaying medicine, they are now valued medicinally almost exclusively as a rich source of vitamin C.

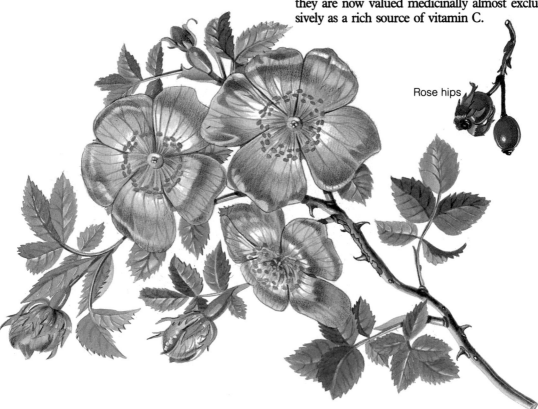

Rose hips

Habitat: Sunny roadsides, woodsides, hedges.
Range: Native to Europe, dog rose is naturalized in much of eastern North America.
Identification: A perennial shrub, growing usually as bushes or as thickets 6–10 feet tall, but known to reach 15 feet or more. The stems have hooked thorns. The leaves are pinnately divided into oval leaflets and are smoother and greener than those of garden roses. The flowers (May–July) are normally pale pink, borne on long stalks. The flask-shaped scarlet hips, ½–1 inch long, are compound fruits consisting of single-seeded fruits (achenes).
Uses: Rose hips can be eaten straight from the shrub and are said to be nutritious. More commonly, the hips are made into jelly or syrup as a vitamin C supplement or manufactured into pills or powder for the same purpose. Health food stores and some food stores sell rose hip tea. The leaves are sometimes applied as a poultice to heal wounds.

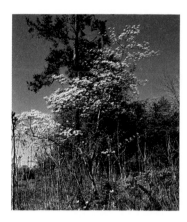

Dogwood

Cornus florida L.

Boxwood, Dog Tree, Flowering Dogwood,
Virginia Dogwood
DOGWOOD FAMILY

Cornaceae

So beloved by Virginians is the dogwood that they named it their state tree. One early native, George Washington, noted in his diary in 1785 that "a circle of dogwood" had been planted "close to the old cherry near the south garden house." Thomas Jefferson, another famous Virginian, known for his impeccable taste and appreciation of beautiful things, planted dogwood near his cherished home, Monticello.

In springtime, as the dogwood began to bloom, the beautiful creamy white petallike bracts signaled to the Indians that it was time to plant corn. The tree was a source of medicine for them, too. They simmered the bark in water and used the extract to relieve sore and aching muscles. They also made a tea of the bark to promote sweating and hence break a fever—a remedy that physicians and herbalists later adopted. During the blockade of southern ports in the Civil War, when cinchona bark, the source of quinine, was not obtainable for treating malaria, dogwood bark tea became a substitute.

Dogwood is also known for its extremely hard wood, which has been used for all kinds of objects, from shuttles for weaving to golf club heads.

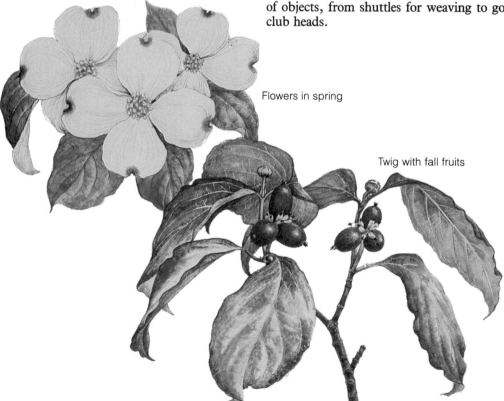

Flowers in spring

Twig with fall fruits

X The fresh bark is a harsh laxative.
Habitat: Well-drained soils, woods, old fields, roadsides.
Range: A native of North America, dogwood is found from southern Ontario and Maine south to Florida and Texas, and west to Kansas.
Identification: A shrub or small tree growing up to 30 feet tall. The prominently veined oval leaves are pointed and dark green above and paler green or whitish and often downy below. The true flowers (March–June) are tiny and greenish white, forming a central cluster surrounded by four showy, notched, creamy white bracts that look like petals. The flowers produce red fruits.
Uses: Once widely used to break a fever and as a substitute for quinine in treating intermittent, or recurring, fevers such as malaria, dogwood bark tea is now regarded chiefly as an appetite stimulant. There is no evidence that any of these uses are effective.

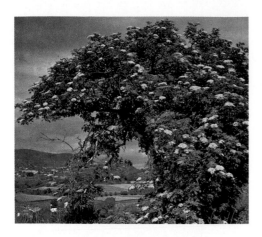

Elderberry

Sambucus nigra L.

Bourtree, European Elder, Pipe Tree
HONEYSUCKLE FAMILY

Caprifoliaceae

Elderberry wine is an old European tradition, but the elderberry, or elder, supplies much more than beverages: from the manufacture of musical pipes to the treatment of human ailments, the shrub has aided countless generations. Man apparently recognized it as a useful plant even in prehistoric times—evidence of its cultivation is found at Stone Age village sites in Switzerland and Italy. He also imbued it with myth and magic. Spirits were said to live in the shrub, and some people therefore refused to cut it down or burn it.

Medicinally, elderberry has been used for common ailments. A syrup from the berry juice was once a remedy for coughs, and cold sufferers comforted themselves with hot toddies of mulled elderberry wine. A tea made from the flowers was taken as a mild laxative or diuretic and to promote sweating. Elder flower water, a mild astringent used as a skin lotion, is still sold in some old-fashioned pharmacies.

The American, or common, elder (*S. canadensis*), a species native to North America, is similar in appearance and medicinal effects to its European relative. American Indians used it for some of the same purposes.

The wood once served to make shoemakers' pegs, butchers' skewers, and needles for weaving nets, as well as musical instruments.

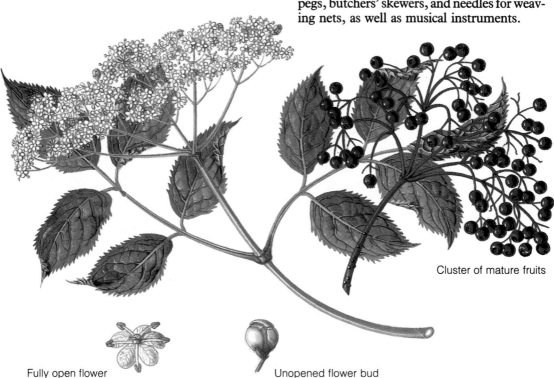

Cluster of mature fruits

Fully open flower

Unopened flower bud

X The leaves, bark, and roots of some elders, including American elder, contain poisonous alkaloids and should not be used internally.
Habitat: Wet areas next to rocks and walls.
Range: European elderberry was introduced into North America and has escaped cultivation locally.
Identification: A shrub or tree growing up to 30 feet tall. Leaves grow in opposite pairs and are pinnately compound. Leaflets are toothed and oval, usually five to seven per leaf. Small white flowers (June–July) sit in flat clusters; ripening berries turn purple-black (September).
Uses: The berries yield delicious wine and jam. Pharmacologists question the usefulness of elderberry flower tea as an expectorant, but find more likely its efficacy in promoting sweating. The bark and roots produce a black dye, the leaves a green dye, and the berries a purple coloring.

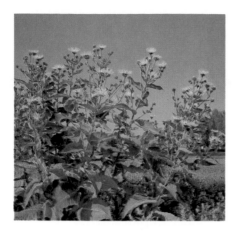

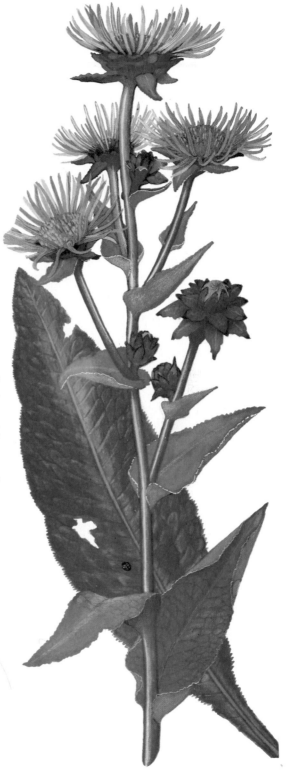

Elecampane

Inula helenium L.

Horseheal, Scabwort, Wild Sunflower

COMPOSITE FAMILY

Compositae

Elecampane entered folk medicine with the ancient Greeks and Romans, who used it in cold remedies because it was thought to promote sweating and help bring up phlegm. In the 19th century the roots were boiled in sugar water to make cough drops and asthma lozenges or just candy.

Elecampane was also thought to be good for the stomach. The Romans served it regularly as an aid to digestion. Later it was the main herbal ingredient in a medieval digestive wine called *potio Paulina*, or "drink of Paul," an allusion to St. Paul's biblical injunction to "use a little wine for thy stomach's sake."

Although its large radiant yellow blossoms make elecampane a strikingly beautiful garden flower, it seems likely that the European settlers of North America introduced the plant neither for their eyes' nor for their stomachs' sake, but because of its widely held reputation as an effective remedy for skin diseases on sheep and horses. The veterinary use is the origin of elecampane's other common names, scabwort and horseheal. The root was used to treat human ailments too, particularly respiratory diseases, and was at one time listed in the *U.S. Pharmacopeia*.

Habitat: Roadsides and damp pastures and fields.
Range: Eastern Quebec to Minnesota, south to Missouri and North Carolina.
Identification: A perennial herb, 3–6 feet tall, the plant has a stout, branched stem rising from a basal rosette of large, ovate, pointed leaves 1–1½ feet long and 3–4 inches across. Smaller leaves that grow along the stem clasp it. The foliage has velvety undersides. Bright yellow flowerheads (July–September), 4 inches across, look like small sunflowers. The root—large, heavy, and long—is yellow on the outside, white within, and gives off a strong odor of violets.
Uses: Elecampane root has long been used in traditional medicine for the treatment of asthma, chest colds, and stomach ulcers; and research indicates that the root is probably an antispasmodic and expectorant. The plant contains a substance that researchers also think may prove to be an antiseptic or antibiotic.

English Holly

Ilex aquifolium L.

Common Holly, European Holly, Mountain Holly
HOLLY FAMILY
Aquifoliaceae

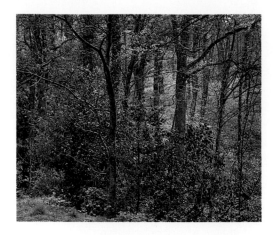

To **"deck the halls** with boughs of holly," as the old carol enjoins, is to observe a custom that early Christians most likely adopted from the Roman Saturnalia. The observances of this pagan festival, which began each year on December 17, influenced those of the Christian Yuletide. According to Roman folk belief, the holly's white flowers would turn water into ice. Hollies planted near houses would ward off lightning and witchcraft—a precaution still followed in parts of rural England. According to medieval legend, the holly first sprang up in Jesus' footsteps, with spiny leaves to symbolize the crown of thorns and red berries to recall the blood shed on the cross.

In times past, physicians and herbalists found many uses for holly. An infusion, or tea, of the leaves was believed to promote sweating and hence was given for malaria and other intermittent, or recurring, fevers. The juice of the berries, although highly toxic, was a common remedy for jaundice. Indians of the southern United States brewed a strong tea from the leaves of a native American holly, the yaupon (*I. vomitoria*). This tea, known as the "black drink," may have played a role in ritual purifications. Yaupon leaves contain caffeine, and pioneers sometimes used them as a substitute for imported tea.

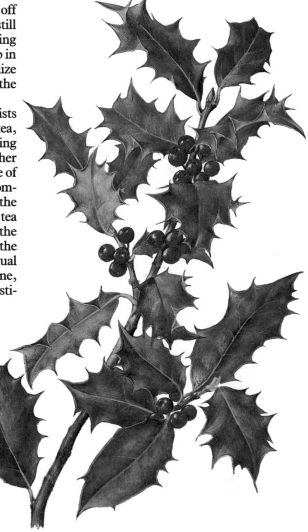

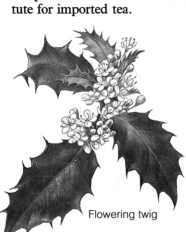

Flowering twig

X Raw holly berries are poisonous, causing vomiting and severe purging.
Habitat: Open, sunny areas.
Range: Introduced from Europe, English holly is cultivated throughout North America from New Jersey southward, west into Oklahoma and Arizona, and along the Pacific coast into British Columbia. An American species, the yaupon (*I. vomitoria*), grows wild from coastal North Carolina south into northern Florida and west to Texas.

Identification: An evergreen tree growing up to 70 feet tall, but averaging 6–15 feet in height when cultivated. It has glossy, leathery, spiny-edged, alternate leaves and small white flowers (June–July). Only female trees produce the berries.
Uses: Herbals list holly leaves as a fever-reducing agent, tonic, and sedative. Experimental evidence suggests that the leaves have sedative properties, but their effectiveness as a tonic and for treating fevers has not been validated.

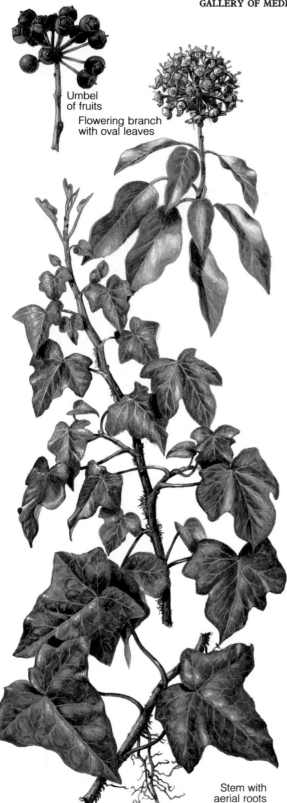

Umbel
of fruits

Flowering branch
with oval leaves

Stem with
aerial roots

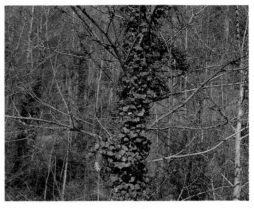

English Ivy

Hedera helix L.

True Ivy

GINSENG FAMILY

Araliaceae

No wonder ivy symbolizes so many different things to so many nations, for while it is called English ivy, it grows virtually everywhere in the Northern Hemisphere, creeping along in open woodlands and covering the walls of cottages and castles alike with its lush greenery. One old folk belief holds that if you put a piece of ivy under your pillow, you will see your truelove's face in your dreams; yet another warns that more ivy than holly in your Christmas decorations will bring bad luck during the year to come. The plant also had many associations with drink. It was sacred to Dionysus, the Greek god of wine. Revelers at ancient Athenian drinking parties wore ivy wreaths—the equivalent of modern party hats. In England, in Elizabethan times, a bush of ivy or a painting of one was a commonplace tavern sign.

The medicinal properties attributed to English ivy have been almost as varied as the traditions associated with it. Herbals once recommended that the resin of the bark (called ivy gum) be taken internally to stimulate menstruation and used externally as an antiseptic. The bark resin was sometimes used on dental cavities in the same manner as present-day toothache gels.

X The berries and large quantities of the whole plant may cause poisoning.
Habitat: Open woods, but the plant can grow almost anywhere.
Range: Native to Eurasia and North Africa, ivy has become naturalized in North America and is cultivated worldwide.
Identification: A climbing or creeping plant with a woody stem, English ivy can reach up to 100 feet with the aid of aerial roots on the undersides of the shoots. Dark glossy evergreen alternate leaves are triangular, three- to five-lobed, and veined. Umbels of yellow-green flowers (October) produce bitter black berries, which ripen the next year.
Uses: Poultices made from the leaves may be applied to cuts, sores, and skin eruptions. A tincture of the bark resin and a tea prepared from the fresh leaves were once given internally for a variety of problems but are no longer recommended.

169

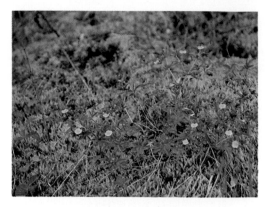

Erect Cinquefoil

Potentilla erecta (L.) Raeusch.

Bloodroot, Cinquefoil, Tormentil, Tormentilla
ROSE FAMILY

Rosaceae

Tormentil or tormentilla—the "torment" plant—is what medieval physicians once called erect cinquefoil, because they believed it would cure almost any pain. They attributed powerful medicinal properties to this modest herb with dainty four-petaled yellow flowers. Over the years, herbalists specified the plant for fevers, syphilis, measles, smallpox, and warts. Indeed, as late as the 17th century the English court apothecary and herbalist John Parkinson wrote that, when steeped overnight in wine and then distilled, erect cinquefoil would "expel any venom or poison, or the plague, or any fever or horror, or the shaking fit that happens."

Since then, the employment of erect cinquefoil has declined to the extent that folk healers now esteem it chiefly as an astringent, a fever-reducing agent, and an agent that stops the flow of blood. Its rhizome (underground stem) is the source of the tannin that accounts for the plant's astringent properties.

Because of its tannin content, erect cinquefoil has been used in the tanning of leathers, and the brownish-red rhizome has also been the source of a red dye.

Habitat: Wet meadows, damp woods, mossy places.
Range: A native of Eurasia, cinquefoil has become naturalized locally in Newfoundland and eastern Massachusetts.
Identification: A perennial herb reaching 20 inches high and growing from an underground stem (rhizome). The leaves have three oblong toothed leaflets surrounded by two smaller leaflike appendages (stipules). Yellow flowers (June–August), about ½ inch wide, have four petals.

Uses: Modern herbals cite a tea made from the rhizome as an antipyretic (fever-reducing agent), an external astringent, and an antihemorrhagic (an agent capable of stopping the flow of blood). Scientists who have studied these uses question the tea's efficacy in reducing fever. But they have evidence that it may help stop moderate external bleeding and that it most likely does act an an external astringent, causing the skin and capillaries to contract.

Mature flowering branch

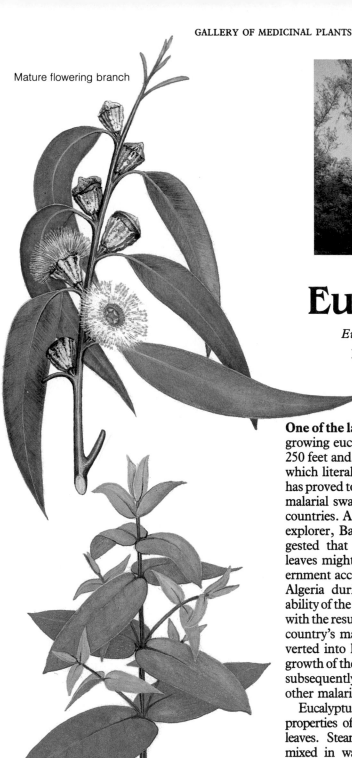

Juvenile branch

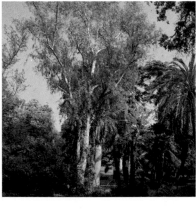

Eucalyptus

Eucalyptus globulus Labill.

Blue Gum, Fever Tree

MYRTLE FAMILY

Myrtaceae

One of the largest trees in the world, the fast-growing eucalyptus can reach heights of over 250 feet and send out a vast network of roots, which literally drain marshy areas. In fact, it has proved to be highly effective in eliminating malarial swamps in a number of hot, humid countries. A famed 19th-century botanist and explorer, Baron Ferdinand von Müller, suggested that the fragrant exhalations of the leaves might be antiseptic. The French government accordingly sent eucalyptus seeds to Algeria during the 1850's, and the drying ability of the roots was accidentally discovered, with the result that many of that North African country's marshy "fever districts" were converted into healthful, dry areas by the rapid growth of the trees. Eucalyptus plantings were subsequently used for the same purpose in other malarial regions worldwide.

Eucalyptus is known today for the medicinal properties of the aromatic oil contained in its leaves. Steam inhalations of the distilled oil mixed in water are a popular treatment for respiratory ailments, particularly bronchitis and asthma. The oil is also applied locally as a chest rub for lower respiratory infections and to treat chapped skin and dandruff.

Habitat: Thrives in areas with average temperatures above 60°F.
Range: Native to Australia but introduced in parts of India, Africa, Europe, and the Americas.
Identification: An evergreen growing to 300 feet tall with a straight, smooth, gray trunk and leathery leaves. Young leaves are opposite, heart-shaped, bluish green, and sticky; adult leaves are alternate, lance-shaped, green, and smooth. When crushed, the leaves emit a pungent aroma.

Uses: Eucalyptus is famous for its aroma and the antiseptic, germ-killing properties in the essential oil of its leaves and resin. Products combining eucalyptus and other ingredients are made for application on the chest for bronchial congestion and for preparing steam inhalations to alleviate coughs and asthma. The oil is an ingredient in some cough drops and syrups.

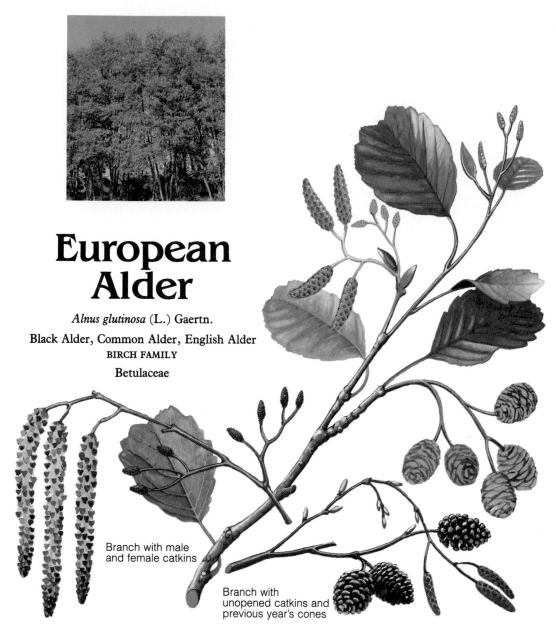

European Alder

Alnus glutinosa (L.) Gaertn.

Black Alder, Common Alder, English Alder
BIRCH FAMILY
Betulaceae

Branch with male
and female catkins

Branch with
unopened catkins and
previous year's cones

So indestructible is the wood of the European alder that it was used to make the piles on which the city of Amsterdam and Venice's famed Rialto section were raised. The tree's remarkable resistance to wet rot made it a prime choice for posts and pilings in the construction of bridges and sluice gates, for water conduits, and for wooden shoes.

Herbalists through the centuries have used brews made from the bark and leaves of the alder as an astringent and a quinine substitute,

and to fight inflammations and fevers. The leaves and branches also have a reputation as natural pesticides. The inner bark, boiled in vinegar and rubbed on the body, reportedly kills lice and scabies mites and dries up scabs.

The red, or Oregon, alder (*A. rubra*) looks like its European cousin, which now grows wild in parts of eastern North America, and has similar properties. Alders are also valued for the nitrogen-fixing bacteria that colonize their roots and thereby enrich the soil.

Habitat: Moist forests in cool climates.
Range: The European alder is now naturalized in parts of eastern North America. The red alder is native to the Pacific Coast from southern Alaska to northern California.
Identification: A deciduous tree, the European alder can reach 100 feet. The branches spread to a rounded crown. Broad, sharply toothed leaves, up to 4 inches long, are dark glossy green on top, pale and sticky below. Greenish-yellow male and reddish

female flowers (March) are borne in separate cone-like clusters (catkins). The fruits grow in roundish cones, green in summer and brown and woody in fall. The red alder resembles the European tree but has elliptical, bluntly toothed leaves.
Uses: Both species supply natural materials for dyers and tanners and wood for smoking meats and fish and for making pilings used in wet locations. The red alder is used for furniture. Medicinally, the trees have fallen into general disuse.

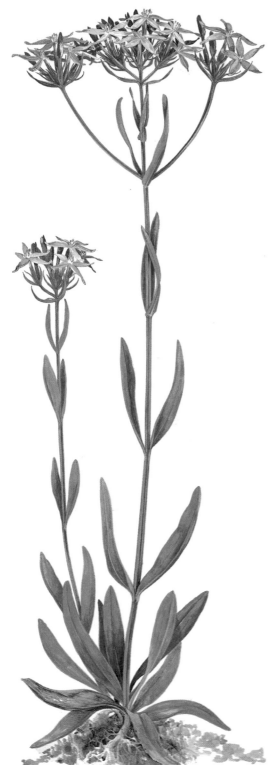

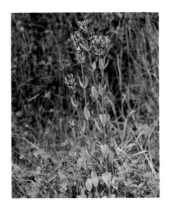

European Centaury

Centaurium umbellatum Gilib.

Bluebottle, Bluet, Cornflower

GENTIAN FAMILY

Gentianaceae

Humanity first learned the use of medicinal plants, said the storytellers of ancient Greece, from the centaur Chiron, half man, half horse. When he was wounded by a poisoned arrow, this sage monster cured himself with a pretty blue wildflower, and in his honor—so the story goes—the plant was named centaury.

Although pharmacologists find no basis for the use of centaury as an antidote, they have substantiated other traditional applications of this plant—its use to stimulate the appetite and to relieve gas pains. Centaury, they have discovered, contains a substance (called erythrocentaurin) that stimulates the flow of saliva and gastric juices and the secretion of bile by the liver. A tea brewed from centaury flowers will perk up a flagging appetite, aid digestion, ease an attack of heartburn, and may even mitigate the sufferings of jaundice in certain cases; it will, however, cause nausea if taken in excess. Because the chemicals in centaury are extremely bitter, herbalists recommend mixing the tea with sweeter herbs. Another method has been to take the herb in the form of vermouth, a popular aperitif wine in whose recipe it figures.

Habitat: Moist meadows, fields, waste places.
Range: Native to Europe, centaury is naturalized from Quebec to Michigan, south to Georgia and Indiana, and, in the West, from northwestern California north to Washington and east to Idaho.
Identification: An annual or biennial 4–20 inches tall. A branched stem rises from a basal rosette of leaves. Each branch bears pairs of lance-shaped leaves. Five-petaled rose-purple flowers (July–August) are borne in dense, flat-topped clusters.

Uses: A tea brewed from the dried flowering plant serves as an appetite stimulant and carminative (a substance that expels intestinal and stomach gas). Scientific studies have confirmed that both of these uses of the plant are valid. Centaury is an ingredient of vermouth. The plant was once recognized as a drug in the *National Formulary*, a reference book for pharmacists.

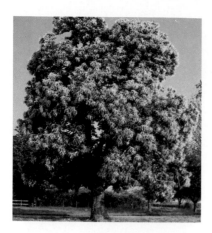

European Chestnut

Castanea sativa Mill.

Spanish Chestnut, Sweet Chestnut
BEECH FAMILY
Fagaceae

Nowadays, when the chestnut vendor appears on city streets, it is a sure sign that winter is arriving. Years ago, these sweet, shiny nuts supplied not just a hearty snack but a major source of food to the rural poor of southern Europe, where dense forests of the chestnut tree grew. Rich in starch, oils, and vitamins B_1, B_2, and C, the nuts can be eaten roasted or boiled, or they can be ground into a flour for thickening soups or baking cakes and breads. As the ancient Greek physician Dioscorides noted, this tree is also a particularly fruitful source of medicinal remedies. The leaves, twigs, bark, and even the flowering catkins and the spiky cases of the nuts are astringent, and so can be used to help control bleeding, to aid healing, and in cases of diarrhea. Chestnut leaves also furnish a tea that soothes irritated mucous membranes and hence relieves the symptoms of whooping cough or any cough due to irritation.

Colonists in North America must have been delighted to find a related species, *C. dentata*, or American chestnut, which had all the properties of *C. sativa*. But at the turn of the century, a deadly fungus blight struck the great American chestnut forests and devastated them, so that the species has become rare.

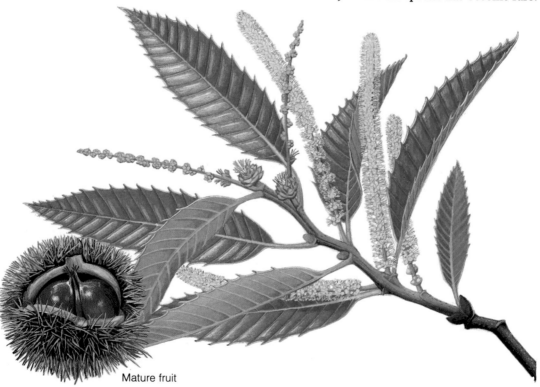

Mature fruit

Habitat: Well-drained soils.
Range: Native to southern Eurasia, European chestnut is mainly cultivated in North America.
Identification: A deciduous tree growing to 100 feet tall. The bark of older trees is dark brown and has a network of longitudinal to spiral ridges. The upper surfaces of the oval, toothed, pointed leaves are green and shiny, while the undersides are paler. Pale yellow male flowers (June) grow in upright catkins (clusters); green female flowers grow at the base of the male catkins or in separate round catkins. The nuts are enclosed in a woody, spiny bur that is brown when ripe.
Uses: All parts of the tree are rich in tannin, used medicinally as an astringent, a substance that causes the skin and mucous membranes to contract. Because the leaves also contain demulcents, or agents that soothe the mucous membranes, they have been made into a tea to soothe the irritations of coughs and colds.

Shakespeare made seven mentions of the cowslip—a flower so beloved by Englishmen that they considered it a favorite of the fairies. Alexander Pope praised the soothing capacity of wine made from its flowers. European cowslip was held in equal esteem by herbal practitioners. The 17th-century English herbalist Nicholas Culpeper claimed that any woman who used an ointment or the distilled water of cowslip would become more beautiful.

To this day, herbalists make a skin-cleansing lotion from the plant. Cowslip also was once in wide use as a sedative, and herbalists still make a soporific tea from its sweet-smelling yellow flowers, which are said to contain mildly narcotic juices. Over the centuries, the dried flowers and sometimes the rhizomes served as an expectorant, to loosen phlegm in chest colds, and they were formerly recommended in the treatment of arthritis and rheumatism. The plant also had a reputation for analgesic and antispasmodic properties.

One of the first flowers to bloom in spring, cowslip is also called keyflower and key of heaven because its flowers suggest a bunch of keys, the emblem of St. Peter.

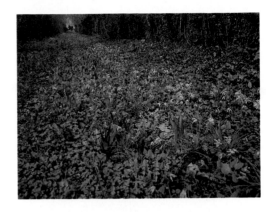

European Cowslip

Primula veris L.

Fairy Cup, Keyflower, Key of Heaven, Paigle
PRIMROSE FAMILY

Primulaceae

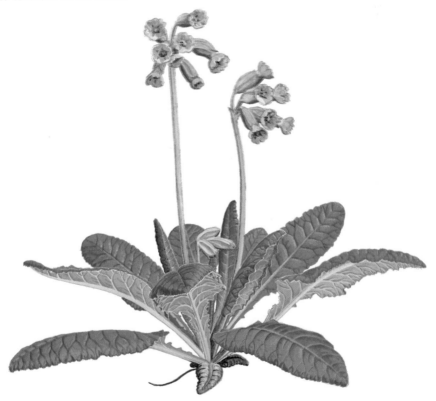

Habitat: Dry meadows, roadsides, woodland.
Range: Native to Eurasia, cowslip is now a common escape from gardens in temperate North America.
Identification: A perennial herb with oblong-oval, finely hairy leaves forming a basal rosette, European cowslip has pleasantly sweet-smelling yellow flowers (May–June) marked with orange dots; the flowers grow in a hanging cluster atop an unbranched, leafless flower stalk.

Uses: In herbal medicine, tea made of European cowslip has long served as a mild sedative to treat restlessness, headache, and insomnia. Herbalists recommend cowslip flower water as a skin lotion. People have at various times also used it as an expectorant, an antispasmodic, a mild painkiller, a laxative, and a diuretic. None of these uses have been verified scientifically.

175

European Mountain Ash

Sorbus aucuparia L.

Quickbeam, Rowan Tree
ROSE FAMILY
Rosaceae

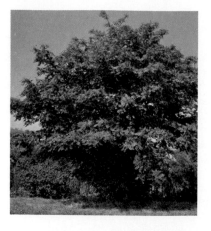

Although it is popular as an ornamental tree today, the European mountain ash was once in ill repute. Perhaps because the Celtic Druids had venerated the tree, it came to be associated with witchcraft in 15th- and 16th-century England, earning itself a reputation as a symbol of paganism and involvement with the supernatural. Herbalists refused even to comment on the tree. But birds always found its fruits irresistible, and hunters used to bait their traps with the fruits—hence the species name *aucuparia*, from the Latin "to go fowling."

Colonists imported the tree to the New World for its berries, which are similar in taste to cranberries. They not only supplied many delectable items—pies, jellies and jams, and a bittersweet wine—but had medicinal value too, primarily as an astringent. Herbalists to this day prescribe a fruit tea for diarrhea and hemorrhoids. Because of their vitamin C content, the berries were specified explicitly for scurvy, a vitamin C deficiency disease.

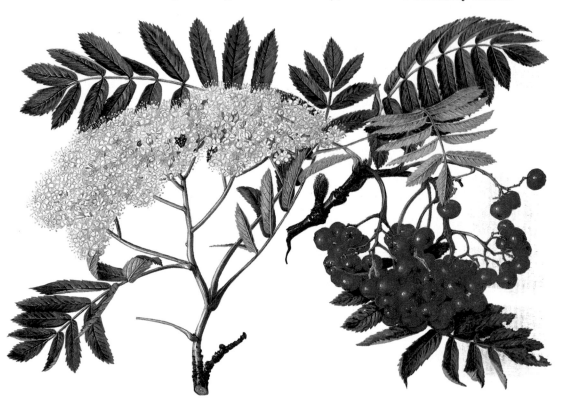

X The fruits are reported to contain a cancer-causing compound, parasorbic acid. There is some evidence that they may be toxic to children, but the poisonous elements are neutralized by cooking.
Habitat: Fields, bogs, near streams and swamps.
Range: Native to Europe, European mountain ash is naturalized in North America from Newfoundland to southwestern Alaska and British Columbia, and south to the northern United States.
Identification: A small deciduous tree occasionally reaching 60 feet tall. The leaves are alternate and pinnately divided, consisting of 11–17 oblong toothed leaflets, which are softly hairy below. Creamy white flowers (May) grow in large dense clusters, followed by bunches of round red berries.
Uses: The berries of European mountain ash have been processed for jams, pies, and wine, and are a source of vitamin C. In herbal medicine the berry tea is employed as an astringent in treating hemorrhoids and diarrhea.

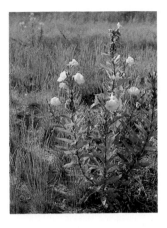

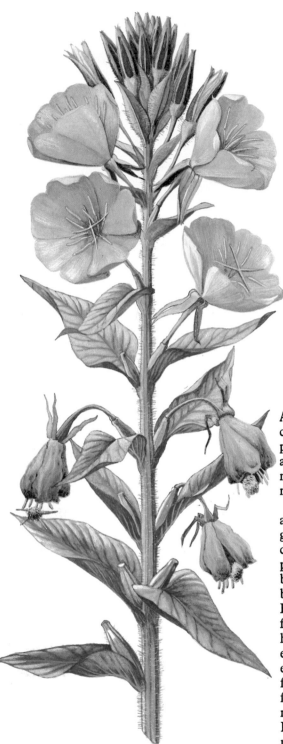

Evening Primrose

Oenothera biennis L.

Evening Star, King's-cure-all,
Night Willow Herb, Scabish, Tree Primrose
EVENING PRIMROSE FAMILY

Onagraceae

As daylight wanes, and the evening grows cool, the shiny yellow petals of the evening primose unfurl, and it exudes a perfume that attracts the nocturnal sphinx moth, which pollinates it. By daybreak the flowers have faded, and new blossoms open the next evening.

In recent years this pretty plant has become a focus of medical research. One line of investigation reveals that the plant may have an anticlotting factor that would make it useful in the prevention of heart attacks caused by thrombosis—the blocking of a blood vessel by a blood clot. And in 1982 the distinguished British medical journal the *Lancet* published findings that oil of evening primrose might help people suffering from atopic eczema, or eczema due to allergy. Another study indicated that the oil might help people suffering from other atopic diseases such as asthma and from migraine. Responding to varied claims made for the plant in the mid-1980's, the U.S. Food and Drug Administration declared that no drugs containing oil of evening primrose are approved for sale in the United States.

Habitat: Dry soils; meadows; old fields, roadsides, and other waste places.

Range: A North American native, evening primrose is found from Newfoundland to British Columbia, south to Texas and Florida, and west to North Dakota and Idaho.

Identification: An erect biennial herb, growing 3–6 feet tall from a rosette of basal leaves during the first year. A hairy stem bears alternate lance-shaped leaves. During the second year showy, yellow, four-petaled flowers (June–October), about 2 inches across, bloom in diminished light or in the dark.

Uses: In modern herbal medicine the plant mucilage is used in cough remedies to help inhibit coughing and in external preparations to soothe skin eruptions. It is also advocated as an astringent for healing wounds and as an antispasmodic. The seed oil has been shown to alleviate inflammations in experimental animal studies.

Eyebright

Euphrasia officinalis L.

Meadow Eyebright, Red Eyebright
SNAPDRAGON FAMILY
Scrophulariaceae

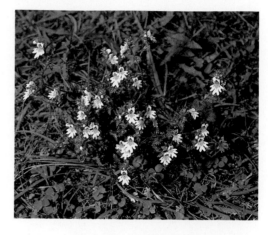

As its name suggests, eyebright is an herb with a long history of use in the treatment of eye diseases. Its botanical name, *Euphrasia*, comes from a Greek word meaning "good cheer," which is supposed to recall the gladness felt by those whose eyesight was preserved by this plant. The plant owes its use for pinkeye, or conjunctivitis, to its astringent and anti-inflammatory properties. Traditional herbalists also note that its flower often resembles a bloodshot eye, an indication to them that the plant is good for sore eyes. This harks back to the doctrine of signatures, according to which the appearance of a plant, or of some part of it, indicates its use in medicine.

Eyebright was introduced into medical literature in the works of the pioneering naturalist St. Hildegard (1098–1179). Its curative powers came to be so praised that the 17th-century herbalist Nicholas Culpeper claimed that if its use became general it would "half spoil the spectacle maker's trade."

A delicate, attractive plant, eyebright is difficult to transplant because of its semiparasitical nature. Eyebright attaches itself by underground suckers to the roots of neighboring grass plants and drains nutrients from them. To be cultivated, eyebright must be given nurse plants on whose roots it can feed.

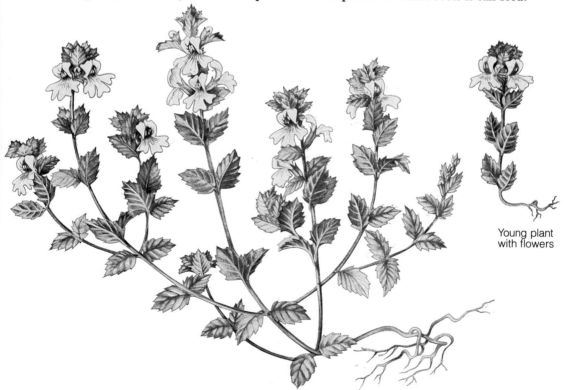

Young plant with flowers

Habitat: Disturbed ground and waste places.
Range: Cultivated in North America, eyebright has escaped from gardens and is found wild in the U.S. Northwest and in British Columbia.
Identification: A small, delicate annual, 2–8 inches high, eyebright has square, downy, branching stems. The leaves vary in shape, sometimes almost round, sometimes narrow and pointed, and are borne in opposite pairs. Tiny red or white flowers (June–August) have an upper two-lobed lip and a lower three-lobed lip and are borne in spikes from the axils of the upper leaves.
Uses: Eyebright is chiefly employed as an astringent and anti-inflammatory; its effectiveness for these purposes is most likely due to the tannin in the plant. An infusion of the flowering plant has long been used as a mild eyewash, and a tea made from the leaves, stems, and flowers as a treatment for throat irritations.

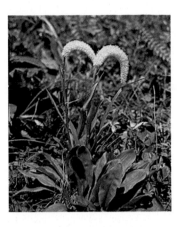

Fairywand

Chamaelirium luteum (L.) A. Gray

Blazing Star, Colicroot, Devil's-bit,
False Unicorn Root

LILY FAMILY

Liliaceae

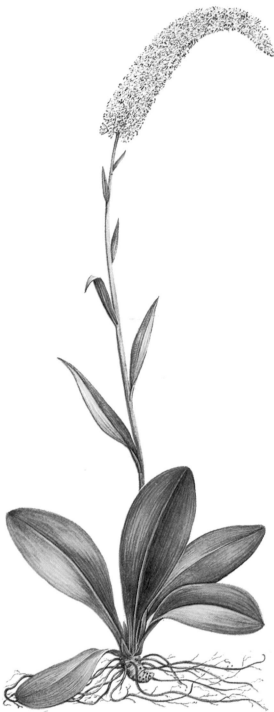

The first specimen of fairywand to be collected and described for classification by botanists happened to be a runt. As a result of this unfortunate mistake, fairywand received the genus name *Chamaelirium*, derived from Greek words meaning "ground lily," even though the genus is not low-growing and has no lilylike characteristics. The species name *luteum*, which means "yellow," was also a botanical misnomer, because the flowers are white—although the male plant does have yellow stamens that give the male flower spike a creamy cast. To complicate the nomenclature even further, fairywand is frequently referred to as devil's-bit, a name that really belongs to a European plant whose root was said to have been bitten off by the Devil—but the two plants are entirely different.

Fairywand, a native North American plant, was a good friend to pregnant Indian squaws, who chewed the root to prevent miscarriage. Medicine men relied on it for other uses, too. The powdered root's reputation won the plant a place in the pharmacopeia of the settlers, who employed it as a pain reliever, as a diuretic, and for uterine disorders, and modern herbals still prescribe fairywand for these purposes.

Habitat: Moist woods, meadows; thickets; bogs.
Range: A native of North America, fairywand is found from southern Ontario and Massachusetts south to Florida, and west to Illinois, Mississippi, and Arkansas.
Identification: A perennial herb, fairywand has a rosette of basal leaves and an aerial stem 1–4 feet tall growing from an underground stem (rhizome). The basal leaves are broad near their tips; the leaves on the upper stem are lance-shaped. Small flowers (June–July) are white on male plants and greenish white on the females.
Uses: Modern herbals perpetuate the use of fairywand as a diuretic, a uterine tonic (a substance that aids in childbirth by stimulating the muscles of the womb), an emmenagogue (an agent that promotes menstruation), and a substance to prevent vomiting due to pregnancy. Pharmacologists state, however, that they cannot support these claims with scientific evidence.

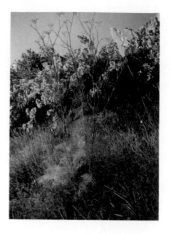

Fennel

Foeniculum vulgare Mill.

Sweet Fennel, Wild Fennel
CARROT FAMILY
Umbelliferae

The licorice-flavored fennel was in great demand during the Middle Ages. The rich relished the seed to add zest to fish and vegetable dishes, while the poor reserved it as an appetite suppressant to be eaten on fast days. Because fennel was supposed to be magically beneficent, householders hung it over their doors to repel evil spirits.

According to the Roman naturalist Pliny, snakes sought out fennel to sharpen their sight after shedding their skin, and ancient doctors, acting perhaps upon this observation, prescribed an extract of the root as a treatment for cataracts, and the whole plant as a remedy for blindness. Herbalists still recommend a tea made from crushed fennel seeds as an eyewash and also as a remedy for stomachache and cramps. Fennel is also reported to relieve flatulence, to help loosen phlegm, and to promote lactation.

Originally a Mediterranean plant, fennel was introduced into North America by Spanish priests, and it still grows wild around their old missions. It was also brought by the English to the early settlements in Virginia and may be seen today in the gardens of Colonial Williamsburg.

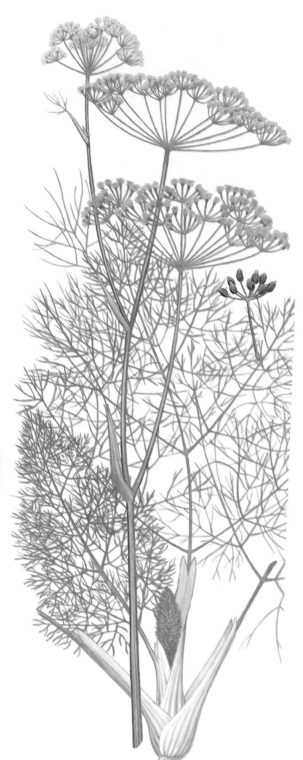

Young plant with juvenile leaves

Habitat: Dry fields and roadsides.
Range: Connecticut to Michigan, Nebraska, and the Southwest.
Identification: A graceful perennial herb, fennel grows 4–6 feet tall, with feathery, much divided leaves. Small yellow flowers (June–September) with five petals are borne in flat-topped, umbrella-like clusters. The flowers are followed by gray-green seeds (actually fruits) about ¼-inch long.
Uses: Fennel is basically used as a culinary herb.

Its seeds are added to fish and other dishes. The shoots and stalks of the cultivated variety are eaten both raw and cooked. Herbalists, as well as scientific evidence, attest to the plant's antispasmodic properties. A tea made from its crushed seeds is used to treat indigestion and cramps. In regions where fennel is plentiful, beekeepers grow it as a honey plant.

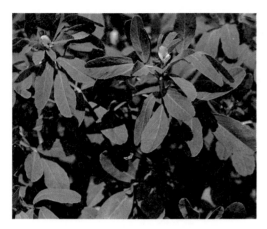

Fenugreek

Trigonella foenum-graecum L.

Bird's-foot, Greek Hayseed, Trigonella
PEA FAMILY
Leguminosae

"The Greatest Medical Discovery Since the Dawn of History"—so claimed the makers of Lydia E. Pinkham's Vegetable Compound, which was introduced to the American public in 1875 as a remedy for "female complaints." Fenugreek was one of its major ingredients. The compound also contained a comforting syrup that was about 18 percent alcohol.

Originating in the Mediterranean region and Asia, fenugreek is among the oldest of medicinal herbs. Its seeds were a favorite cure-all in ancient Egypt and India and later among the Greeks and Romans. Fenugreek tea was prescribed for tuberculosis, bronchitis, sore throat, and flagging sexual desire and as a general tonic. Poultices of fenugreek, prepared from pulverized seeds, were applied to relieve the pains of neuralgia, sciatica, swollen glands, wounds, skin irritations, and gout.

Modern wisdom is more specific about the herb's therapeutic effect. Fenugreek has value as a carminative, that is, as a substance that relieves intestinal gas. Its seeds also contain substances that soften the skin on application. Fenugreek is often used as one of the spices of curry, and its leaves are eaten in some parts of the world as a salad green.

Mature fruit (legume) splitting open

Seed

Habitat: Dry, loamy, moderately fertile soil.
Range: Introduced from Europe, fenugreek is a popular garden plant and often escapes.
Identification: An annual herb growing 1–3 feet high. Its leaves, arranged alternately on round stems, consist of three finely toothed oval leaflets ¾–2 inches long. Off-white flowers (April–May), about ½ inch long, grow singly or in pairs. The fruit is a beaked, beanlike, sometimes hairy pod, 3–6 inches long, with 10–20 aromatic seeds.

Uses: Fenugreek seeds yield a soothing mucilage that goes into poultices and ointments. Taken internally as a tea, they are also effective for relieving gas pains. In the Middle East fenugreek is used to treat diabetes; some experimental data suggest that extracts of the seeds do lower blood sugar levels. The seeds are an ingredient of Middle Eastern spice mixtures. They are often ground for use as animal fodder and are also the source of a yellow dye.

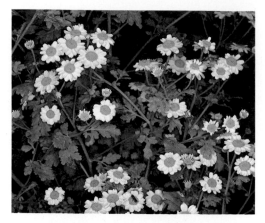

Feverfew

Chrysanthemum parthenium (L.) Bernh.

Bachelor's-button, Featherfew,
Featherfoil, Wild Chamomile
COMPOSITE FAMILY

Compositae

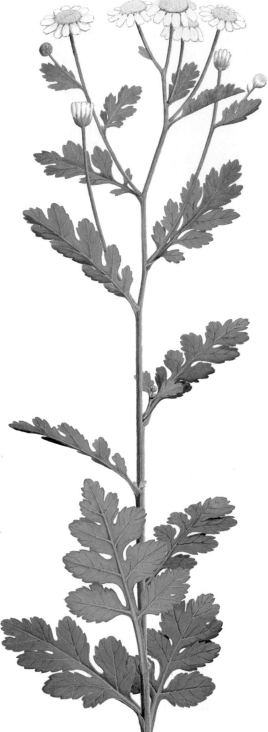

Yet another contender for the name chamomile, feverfew bears flowers similar to those of Roman chamomile. Aside from this single feature, however, feverfew has a quite distinct appearance. Unlike Roman chamomile, feverfew is an upright plant, growing to 2½ feet, and its foliage is bolder and coarser. The whole herb once had a reputation as a remedy for all sorts of fevers; indeed, the name feverfew is derived from *febrifuge*, a scientific term for a medicine that reduces fevers. Feverfew, which gives off a strong, lasting odor, was also planted around houses to purify the air.

The plant had many other uses in folk medicine. It received its Greek name *parthenion* ("girl") from its reputed power to promote menstruation and treat gynecological problems. A tea made from the whole plant or just the flowers was used as a stimulant or tonic for the stomach and to relieve indigestion. Feverfew flowers will keep bees away, and a tincture of the blossoms doubles as an insect repellent and a soothing balm for their bites.

Early settlers who imported feverfew called it featherfew. This name survives locally, a bit of Elizabethan English in modern America.

Habitat: Dry soils, waste places, roadsides.
Range: Introduced from Europe, feverfew is now a common garden escape in the Northeast, and is naturalized locally throughout the rest of the United States and southern Canada.
Identification: A hardy biennial or perennial, growing to 2½ feet. The stem is erect, hairy, and branching; the strongly aromatic leaves are alternate and divided into broad, lobed segments. Daisylike flowerheads (June–August), with white ray flowers surrounding nearly flat yellow centers (disc flowers), grow about 1 inch across.
Uses: A traditional remedy for reducing fevers, feverfew has also been used as a treatment for nervousness, hysteria, and low spirits. Herbalists recommend a tea made from the leaves to treat colds, indigestion, and diarrhea, and a tea from the flowers to promote menstrual flow. Sometimes used to flavor wines and pastries, the leaves are served with fried eggs in Italy.

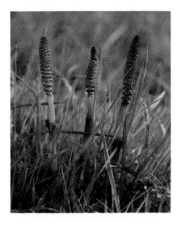

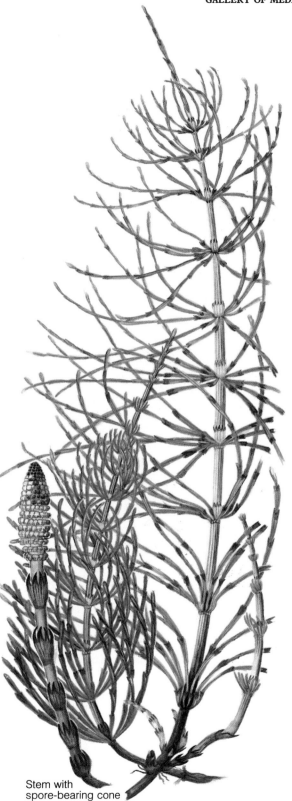

Stem with
spore-bearing cone

Field Horsetail

Equisetum arvense L.

Bottlebrush, Pewterwort, Scouring Rush
HORSETAIL FAMILY
Equisetaceae

Horsetails represent a venerable family of plants some 400 million years old. Before flowering plants evolved, forests of giant horsetails waved over Paleozoic landscapes. The tallest (*Equisetum giganteum*) of some 30 existing species of horsetail grows to a height of 32 feet in South America. A nonflowering plant, horsetail reproduces by means of microscopic spores. These are produced in spore cases underneath small scales atop a slender, pale brown shoot. When dry, the spores are released, to be spread by the wind.

After the spores have been released, the horsetail spike withers. From the same rootlike rhizomes there then appears the multibranched bushy stem from which the plant gets its name. Because the plant contains a large amount of abrasive silica, it once served as a scouring pad for kitchen utensils; resourceful campers still gather it for cleaning up after campfire meals.

Horsetail has long been used in folk medicine, externally to heal wounds, cuts, and sores, and internally to promote urination and to reduce bleeding in the genitourinary tract.

Habitat: Swamps and damp woods, fields, roadsides, embankments, and waste places.
Range: Temperate regions of North America. An endangered species in Texas.
Identification: The fertile shoot (March–May) is a single, jointed, brownish-pink stem about 8 inches tall with a spore-bearing conelike structure on top. It soon disappears and is followed by a green, bushy, jointed sterile stem with whorls of thin branches 1–2½ feet long.

Uses: Besides being used as an abrasive, horsetail has been an important remedy in folk medicine. A poultice of crushed sterile stems has been applied to wounds to stop bleeding. A liquid extract made by boiling the stems has been used as a mouthwash for oral infections, and there is evidence that horsetail has some antibiotic properties. This decoction is also said to increase urination (for which there is some evidence) and to reduce some kinds of internal bleeding.

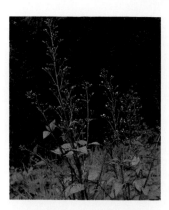

Figwort

Scrophularia nodosa L.

Carpenter's-square, Rose-noble,
Scrofula Plant, Square Stalk,
Stinking Christopher, Throatwort
SNAPDRAGON FAMILY

Scrophulariaceae

Although figwort has a taste and smell that are notably unpleasant, history records that when Cardinal Richelieu laid siege to the French city of La Rochelle for 14 months in 1627–1628, the Protestant garrison within was reduced to eating the herb. The French subsequently called it *l'herbe du siège*.

Figwort is an old medicinal herb, some of whose constitutents are only now being identified through biochemical analysis. Ancient pharmacists knew figwort as *ficaria major* and recommended it for treating hemorrhoids. Herbalists also called the plant scrophularia, after its use as a remedy for "scrofulous ailments," such as tuberculosis of the lymph glands and other diseases characterized by swellings and eruptions.

Like its close relative foxglove, figwort contains a cardioactive substance that strengthens the heart and slows its beat. Thus, its use as an internal medicine by other than a trained practitioner risks dangerous complications. Figwort also has strong, potentially injurious purgative and emetic properties.

Besides *S. nodosa*, several other *Scrophularia* species are called figwort—most notably *S. marilandica*, a native American species.

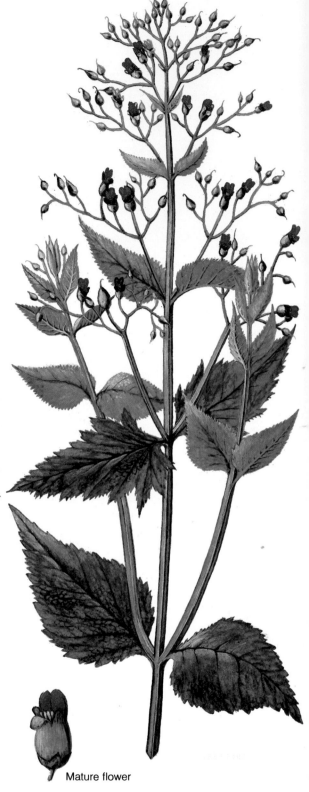

Mature flower

X Do not take internally.
Habitat: Rocky woods, thickets, roadsides.
Range: The Old World species, *S. nodosa*, is naturalized in places from Newfoundland to New England. The native American species, *S. marilandica*, is found from Maine south to Georgia, Alabama, and Louisiana, and west to Minnesota and Oklahoma.
Identification: A perennial shrub growing up to 10 feet in height. Square stems have opposite, toothed, oval leaves, 4–12 inches long, which taper to a point. Small reddish-brown flowers (June–September) are produced in loose clusters at the top of the plant. Egg-shaped capsules disperse seeds in autumn.
Uses: Figwort is not considered safe for internal use except under close medical supervision. Its effectiveness in the external treatment of skin disorders, wounds, ulcers, hemorrhoids, and eczema has not been established.

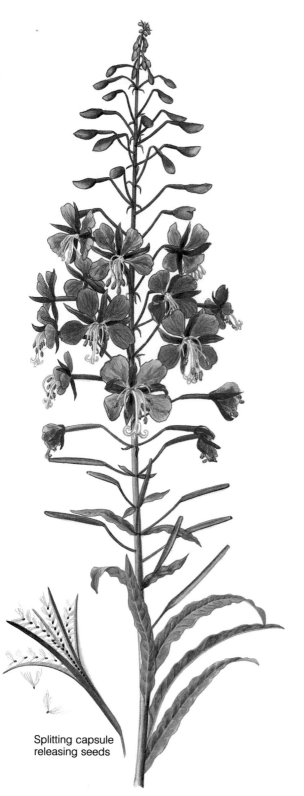

Splitting capsule
releasing seeds

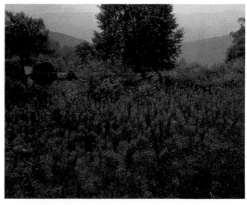

Fireweed

Epilobium angustifolium L.

Blooming Sally, Purple Firetop, Willow Herb

EVENING PRIMROSE FAMILY

Onagraceae

Anyone driving past the scene of a recent forest fire is likely to glimpse brilliant magenta blooms rising high above the blackened earth. The plant they see is fireweed, which gets its name from the fact that it thrives in burned-over or disturbed land. In fact, soon after bombs devastated London during World War II, fireweed sprang up in the heart of the city, where it had not been seen for generations. Newly excavated sites and ditches will often be filled with the plant, but fireweed also does well in rich, moist soil, and favors upland regions such as the Rocky Mountains.

A native of North America as well as Europe, fireweed was employed medicinally as an antispasmodic: its roots and leaves were made into an infusion to treat asthma, whooping cough, and hiccups. The dried leaves were also used as a demulcent (soothing to the mucous membranes) and an astringent.

Fireweed's greatest benefit to man, however, is as a food. Many Indian tribes ate the young shoots or cooked the pith of the stems as soup, and they and others used the leaves as a potherb. French Canadians esteem fireweed so highly they call it *asperge*, or "asparagus." Both the young flower stalks and the leaves can serve as salad ingredients.

Habitat: Burned-over areas, disturbed land, moist soil in mountainous areas.

Range: Alaska and Canada south to North Carolina and west to California.

Identification: A perennial herb with unbranched stems that grow 2–6 feet tall and bear magenta flowers on long spikes (July–September). The leaves are alternate, long (up to 6 inches), and willowlike, giving the plant another of its common names, willow herb. Tiny seeds produced inside long cylindrical capsules have tufts of white hairs enabling them to drift on the wind and sow themselves far away.

Uses: In folk medicine, fireweed's chief use has been as an antispasmodic to treat respiratory problems, but no scientific evidence supports this use. The plant's greatest use, now as in the past, is as a food. The dried leaves also make a tea; in England and Russia it has been a tea substitute for some time.

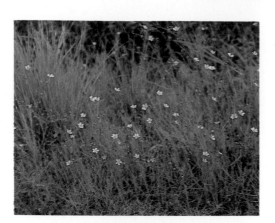

Flax

Linum usitatissimum L.

Linseed, Lint Bells

FLAX FAMILY

Linaceae

In medieval Europe many a person relied on the slender blue-flowered flax as a protection against witchcraft. The magical power attributed to this plant is not surprising in the light of its history, which is summarized in its scientific name, *Linum usitatissimum*, "most useful flax." Flax is one of the earliest plants for which man found uses other than as food. Archeologists have identified fibers spun from the plant among the remains of the prehistoric lake dwellers in Switzerland, possibly dating back some 10,000 years. The Egyptians used linen spun from the fiber for garments and to wrap the bodies of the pharaohs. The whiteness of linen symbolized purity, and the cloth became the fabric for the priestly garments of the Hebrews, Egyptians, and Greeks.

Flaxseed has also been used in medicine since antiquity—externally in liniments and salves and internally in cough syrups and in a tea taken to relieve coughs, colds, constipation, and urinary tract irritations.

Flax was introduced into North America by European colonists, who processed it for cloth. Its economic importance grew as flaxseed was used in a variety of products from flaxseed cakes, used for fattening cattle, to linseed oil, employed in making oilcloth and linoleum.

Mature fruit (seedpod)

Seed

X Immature seedpods can cause poisoning.
Habitat: Waste places and along railroad tracks.
Range: Introduced from Europe, flax is widely grown in the United States, primarily in the Northwest, and in Canada. It easily escapes cultivation.
Identification: An annual with an erect slender stem, 1–3 feet high, branching at the top. Small pale green alternate leaves grow on the stem and branches. Each branch is tipped with one or two delicate blue flowers (February–September).

Uses: A soothing mucilage obtained from the seed is used externally as a poultice for boils and burns, and internally as a demulcent, soothing inflamed or irritated mucous membranes, and as a laxative. The fibers are spun to make linen. Linseed oil, a drying agent in paints and varnishes and an element in the production of oilcloth and linoleum, is extracted from flaxseed. Flaxseed oil residue is made into a fattening agent for cattle.

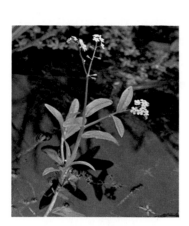

Forget-me-not

Myosotis scorpioides L.

Scorpion Grass
BORAGE FAMILY
Boraginaceae

Many legends surround the forget-me-not and its relatives, and in nearly all of them the flower figures as a symbol of loving remembrance. According to an old German tale, the name recalls the fate of a knight who, while picking the flower for his ladylove, accidentally fell into a river, shouting before he drowned, "Forget me not." Once, however, forget-me-not became the token of remorseless revenge. When King Richard II banished his cousin Henry from England in 1398, it is said that the exile adopted the flower as his badge. Henry's choice implied a threat, for the forget-me-not is also known as scorpion grass, because its coiled flower stalk looks like the curled tail of an angry scorpion. Henry ultimately returned to seize the throne and imprison Richard.

As a result of the plant's scorpionlike appearance, ancient herbalists thought it was an antidote for the bites of scorpions, snakes, and other venomous beasts—hence the species name *scorpioides*. Although almost forgotten in herbal medicine, the plant is still recommended as a poultice for insect stings, and a syrup made from it as an expectorant.

X There is evidence that forget-me-not may cause liver cancer if taken over a long period of time.
Habitat: Wet soils, streambanks.
Range: Native to Europe, forget-me-not is naturalized from Newfoundland to Ontario, south to Georgia, Tennessee, and Louisiana, and in the Pacific Coast states.
Identification: A perennial herb with angled stems growing to 2 feet tall. The stalkless, small, hairy leaves are alternate and lance-shaped. Dainty blue flowers (May–September), ¼–½ inch across, have yellow centers and are borne in clusters on long stalks that are coiled at the tips.
Uses: Forget-me-not was once used as an antidote for the bite of venomous animals. At least one herbal mentions it as a poultice for insect stings and as an expectorant in respiratory ailments. The plant has no scientifically verified medicinal uses. The pretty forget-me-not is a superlative addition to the flower garden.

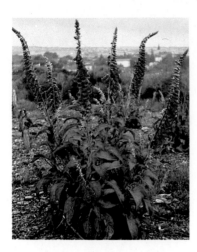

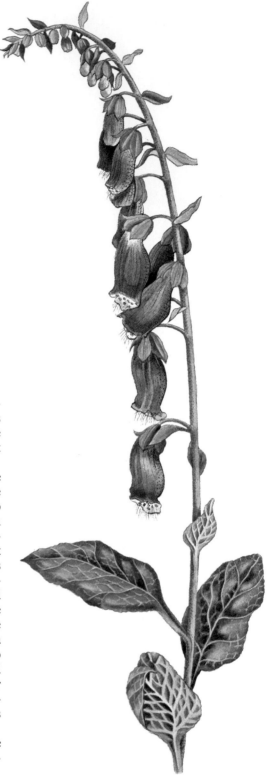

Foxglove

Digitalis purpurea L.

Deadmen's Bells, Witch's Bells
SNAPDRAGON FAMILY

Scrophulariaceae

Foxglove is among the loveliest, most famous, most important, and most dangerous medicinal plants. Its long green leaves are powdered into digitalis, the cardiac stimulant that keeps millions of heart patients alive.

This use was discovered in 1775 by the English physician William Withering. He heard of an old woman in Shropshire who practiced folk medicine with herbs gathered in the countryside. A patient afflicted with excessive fluid retention due to congestive heart failure, whom Withering expected to die, was cured by this healer. From the woman's mostly useless bag of weeds, Withering identified foxglove as the key element in treating the swelling, or edema, associated with congestive heart failure. He also learned that foxglove is a deadly poison, as likely to stop a heart as to keep it going. For 10 years he conducted precise experiments to determine the proper dosage of the new drug. The paper he published in 1785 to inform other physicians of his findings is a classic of medical literature.

The name foxglove is derived from the shape of the blossoms, which bear a resemblance to glove fingers.

✗ Extremely poisonous. A leaf chewed and swallowed may cause paralysis and sudden heart failure.

Habitat: Fields, moist clearings.

Range: Introduced from Europe to America in the 1700's, foxglove escaped from gardens to become naturalized in various parts of North America, particularly west of the Cascade Range.

Identification: A biennial, foxglove forms a rosette of long-stalked leaves in its first year; in the second, stems grow 2–5 feet tall. The leaves are lance-shaped to oval. Spires of white to pinkish-lavender to red thimble-shaped flowers (June–September) are speckled inside with red dots.

Uses: Prior to 1775 foxglove was used against all sorts of maladies, including epilepsy and tuberculosis. Doctors today prescribe digitalis to strengthen the heart and to regulate its beat. No synthetic drugs can duplicate the action of the glycosides in foxglove in treating heart failure.

Fringe Tree

Chionanthus virginicus L.

Graybeard, Old-man's-beard,
Poison Ash, Snowdrop Tree, Snowflower
OLIVE FAMILY

Oleaceae

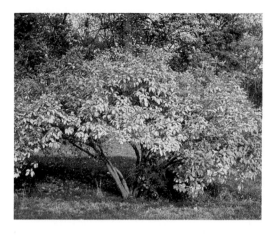

The Choctaw Indians of Louisiana used the native American fringe tree as an astringent. They boiled the bark in water and cleansed external wounds with the extract, and they mashed the bark to make a poultice to help close wounds. Dr. Charles Millspaugh, the American physician and botanist who was among the first to catalog American medicinal plants, noted in his well-known work *Medicinal Plants,* published in 1892, that "the previous use of the bark of this shrub as an astringent . . . has a great merit." He also mentioned that the root bark was successfully used as a tonic. And, he added, "this bark has often also proved itself a trustworthy diuretic." Modern herbals still cite the bark as a diuretic, and it has also been specified as a laxative.

The fringe tree has become increasingly popular with landscapers and gardeners. Found mostly in warmer climates, this true southerner wages a rebellion against the seasons. One of the last trees to acknowledge winter's end, the fringe tree does not leaf until late spring, and then it greets early summer with a mantle of white blossoms that look, from a distance, like a sheet of snow.

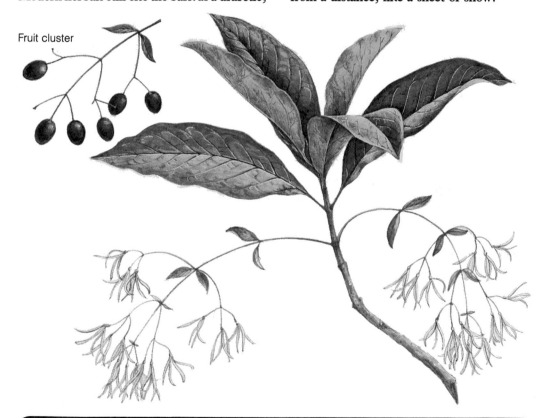

Fruit cluster

Habitat: Damp woods, thickets, streambanks, swamp borders.

Range: A native of the United States, fringe tree is found from New Jersey west to Oklahoma, south to Florida and Texas.

Identification: A deciduous tree or shrub growing up to 40 feet tall. The thin bark is covered with reddish-brown scales. Thick opposite leaves, 4–8 inches long, are elliptical to oval and dark green on top, pale green below. Fragrant white flowers (May–June), 4–6 inches long, have long white fringelike petals that give the tree its name. The fruits are fleshy, round, and dark blue.

Uses: Fringe tree bark has traditionally been employed as a tonic and astringent, and today herbalists mention it as a diuretic and laxative. But researchers note that none of these claims have been verified by scientific tests.

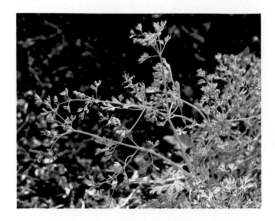

Fumitory

Fumaria officinalis L.

Earth-smoke, Hedge Fumitory, Wax Dolls

FUMITORY FAMILY

Fumariaceae

Like curls of smoke rising from the ground, fumitory's gray-green leaves have a ghostly appearance when seen from afar. The plant is a weed that has accompanied cultivation in Europe since at least Neolithic times. In the Greco-Roman world fumitory's name was *kapnos*, the Greek for smoke. According to the first-century A.D. naturalist Pliny, an ointment made from fumitory improved eyesight and prevented eyelashes that had been pulled out from growing again. Pliny's contemporary Dioscorides added that fumitory when taken internally worked as a diuretic. According to both authorities, the plant got the name smoke from its sharp-tasting juice, which causes the eyes to tear as they would from smoke.

In Shakespeare's day the plant was sold in apothecary shops under the Latin name *fumus terrae* ("earth-smoke"), and according to an herb book published at that time, an extract of the plant or a syrup made from its juice served to stimulate liver function, rid the body of impurities, and clear up certain skin infections. Some recent research suggests that fumitory contains substances that act on the heart and on blood pressure, but this remains unconfirmed. Folk belief credits fumitory with a special power to confer long life.

Fruit   Open flower

X Large doses cause stomachache and diarrhea.
Habitat: Cultivated ground and waste places such as rubbish heaps.
Range: Native to Europe, fumitory has escaped cultivation and now grows wild in scattered locations in North America from Newfoundland south to the Gulf states and inland.
Identification: An annual herb growing up to 30 inches tall, with slender stems and many limp branches. The gray-green leaves are divided into triangular toothed leaflets. At the ends of the branches bloom elongated clusters of small, tubular, pink-purple, crimson-tipped flowers (May–September).
Uses: Herbalists recommend fumitory as a diuretic, and for skin eruptions. Studies of the plant cast doubt on its effectiveness as a diuretic, but show that it may act to alleviate skin eruptions since the plant contains antibiotic substances.

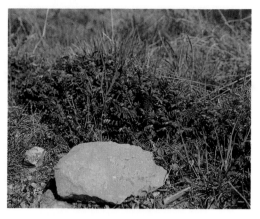

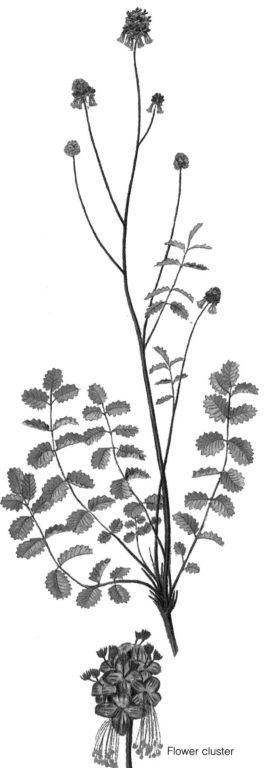

Flower cluster

Garden Burnet

Sanguisorba minor Scop.

Burnet, Salad Burnet

ROSE FAMILY

Rosaceae

On the night before a battle, soldiers fighting in the American Revolution dosed themselves with a tea made from garden burnet on the theory that if they suffered a wound in battle the next day, the garden burnet in their systems would keep them from bleeding to death. The plant's Latin name, *Sanguisorba*, translates loosely as "blood absorber."

In addition to its long traditional employment in checking the flow of blood, garden burnet has also been specified as a treatment for diarrhea and digestive disorders. In the 16th century garden burnet served the population of England as a remedy for rheumatism and gout, and in the 17th century it was recommended as a protection against the plague and other infectious diseases.

French and Italian cooks value the herb for its cucumberlike flavor and add the leaves to salads. The leaves have also been used in vinegars, cream cheeses, herbed butters, and iced drinks. Garden burnet's culinary uses are shared with its close relative greater burnet (*S. officinalis*), and both plants are frequently known as salad burnet.

Habitat: Roadsides, waste places, fields.
Range: Native to Eurasia, garden burnet was introduced into North America and has been naturalized in scattered locations from Nova Scotia to Ontario, south to Virginia and Tennessee.
Identification: A perennial herb with slender stems growing 10–30 inches tall and arising from a basal rosette of pinnately divided leaves. The toothed leaflets are oval and gray-green. The light green to yellowish-green flowers (May–July) grow in clusters; the female flowers on the upper part have protruding red stigmas that give the plant a red glow. The male flowers on the lower part have drooping yellow stamens.
Uses: Garden burnet was traditionally used to stanch the flow of blood, but today it is primarily enjoyed as a culinary herb in salads, vinegars, cheese, and butter. Scientists have not investigated the plant for its medicinal effects and so cannot confirm or refute claims made for it.

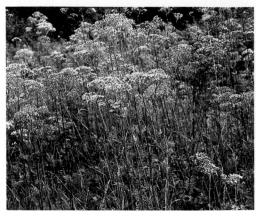

Garden Heliotrope

Valeriana officinalis L.

Allheal, English Valerian, German Valerian,
Great Wild Valerian, Vandalroot

VALERIAN FAMILY

Valerianaceae

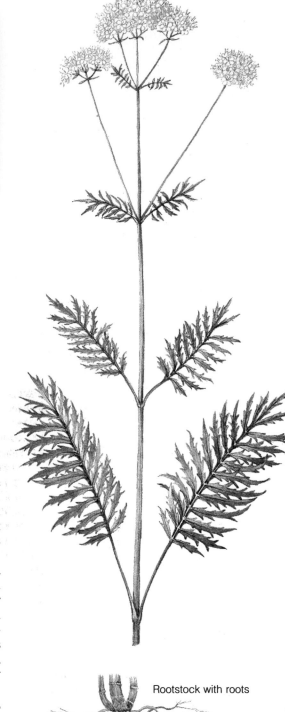

Rootstock with roots

Archenemies though they are, cats and rats reportedly share at least one passion: they both like the root of garden heliotrope. According to popular belief, the herb drives cats into a frenzy. Rat exterminators of long ago believed it made a foolproof bait for their traps. It is said that the legendary Pied Piper carried garden heliotrope roots in his pocket to lure the rats out of Hamelin.

Since ancient times people have believed garden heliotrope to be a cure for epilepsy and a host of other disorders—thus accounting for one of the plant's alternative names, allheal. In the 16th and 17th centuries, herbalists considered the herb a sedative for so-called nervous afflictions, such as "hysteric complaints"; an antispasmodic for convulsions; and a remedy for bad coughs and for constipation.

In Europe, garden heliotrope—or valerian, as it is called as a medicine—is the most common nonprescription herbal preparation sold as a sedative, but the U.S. Food and Drug Administration has not approved valerian's use as a drug in the United States.

Habitat: Roadside fields.
Range: Native to Europe, garden heliotrope is naturalized in North America from Quebec west to Minnesota, and south to New England, Ohio, and Pennsylvania.
Identification: A perennial herb, growing to 5 feet tall. The stem is erect. Opposite leaves are divided into 5–12 pairs of leaflets, which become smaller, narrower, and feathery toward the top of the stem. Tiny, sweet-scented, white to pale pink flowers (May–August) grow in long-stalked clusters at the end of the stem. Do not confuse the plant with borage family members called heliotropes.
Uses: For centuries the powdered rhizomes, or rootstock, and roots of garden heliotrope have been used as a sedative for "nervous" disorders and as an antispasmodic for intestinal pains. Pharmacological studies have validated these uses.

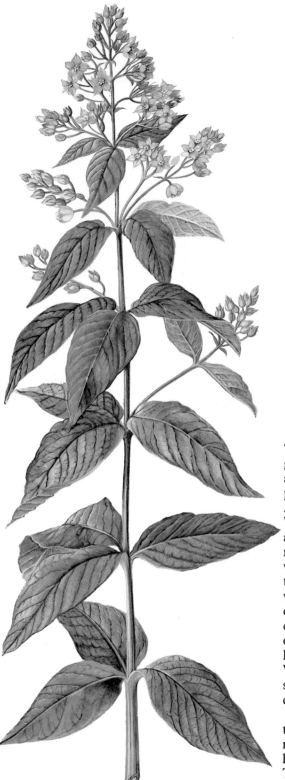

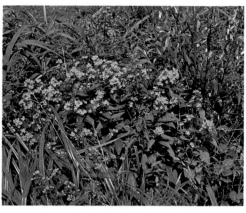

Garden Loosestrife

Lysimachia vulgaris L.

Loosestrife, Golden Loosestrife, Willow Herb,
Yellow Loosestrife, Yellow Rocket

PRIMROSE FAMILY

Primulaceae

The golden yellow flowering clusters of garden loosestrife are a common summer sight along roadsides and in marshes and other wet places throughout much of eastern North America. The plant is a native of the Old World, however, and has been part of European herbal medicine for some 2,000 years or more. The first-century A.D. Greek medical writer Dioscorides reported that the juice of the leaves administered as a drink or an enema was an effective treatment for persons who had dysentery or were vomiting blood. He also called loosestrife "a wound herb and stancher of blood," recommending it both for cases of heavy menstrual bleeding and for nosebleed. When the plant is burned, it gives off sharp-smelling fumes that Dioscorides said would drive off snakes and kill flies.

In present-day herbal tradition infusions, or teas, of the whole dried plant are still recommended for bleeding in the mouth and nose, to help heal cuts, and as a gargle for sore throat. The concentrated extract of the plant sometimes serves as a hair bleach.

Habitat: Roadsides, marshes, riverbanks.
Range: Introduced from Europe, garden loosestrife now grows wild from Quebec to Ontario and south to Maryland, Ohio, and Illinois.
Identification: A perennial herb reaching up to 5 feet in height, garden loosestrife produces stolons (runners) that send up erect, branched stems. Narrowly oval, pointed leaves grow in clusters of three or in opposite pairs and are almost stalkless. The yellow flowers (June–September) are borne in long-stalked clusters from the upper leaf axils.
Uses: Herbalists recommend a tea made from the plant as an astringent, which helps stop minor bleeding by causing the skin and capillaries to contract; as an expectorant, for bringing up phlegm; and as a gargle. Scientists have not investigated the plant for its medicinal value, and can neither confirm nor refute any of these claims. The rhizome (underground stem) yields a brown dye and the leaves or stalk a yellow one.

193

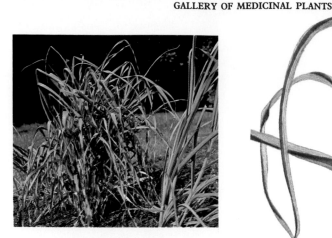

Garlic

Allium sativum L.

Poor-man's-treacle

LILY FAMILY

Liliaceae

An incongruous relative of the elegant lily, the plebeian garlic has nevertheless proved a good friend to mankind. Besides the savor it adds to food, garlic is said to have given strength to the pyramid builders, courage to the Roman legions, and fighting spirit to English gamecocks. It was also trusted as a charm against evil until modern times.

Whatever its purported magical powers, garlic's medicinal uses have been documented for centuries. It was always a popular remedy for colds, sore throats, and coughs—either eaten raw or taken as a syrup, which was made by boiling garlic cloves and water for half a day. Physicians and herbalists prescribed garlic as a diuretic and for intestinal disorders and rheumatism. When plagues ravaged Europe, people ate garlic daily as a protection against disease. Some say that garlic may have worked as a preventive simply by keeping others at a safe distance.

Colonists arriving in America discovered that the Indians knew about the healing powers of a native species of garlic (probably *A. canadense*) and relied on the plant to treat a variety of medical problems, from snakebite to intestinal worms. Taking a cue perhaps from their European forebears, New England set-

Harvested bulb

tlers strapped garlic cloves to the feet of smallpox victims as a cure for the disease.

Garlic may well have helped to cure many diseases because it is a potent antiseptic. It was used for that purpose in both World War I and World War II. Recent research has further revealed that garlic contains vitamins A, B_1 (thiamine), B_2 (riboflavin), and C.

Habitat: Roadsides, pastures, open woods.
Range: Introduced from Europe, garlic has been naturalized from New York to Indiana south to Tennessee and Missouri.
Identification: A perennial herb whose bulb, composed of small cloves, is identifiable by its pungent odor. The plant grows to 2 feet, with flat, long, pointed leaves. The flowers (June–July) range from pink to white. Garlic can be cultivated in gardens but requires a sunny, warm climate.

Uses: For centuries garlic has been favored not only as a culinary herb, but as a remedy for colds and other respiratory infections. Herbalists today also use it to relieve gas pains and to rid the body of intestinal worms. In 1858 Louis Pasteur verified garlic's antiseptic properties; garlic is also a proved antispasmodic. Research further indicates that it may be effective in lowering cholesterol levels in the blood, in reducing hypertension, and as an expectorant in respiratory ailments.

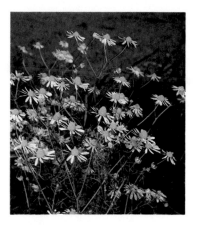

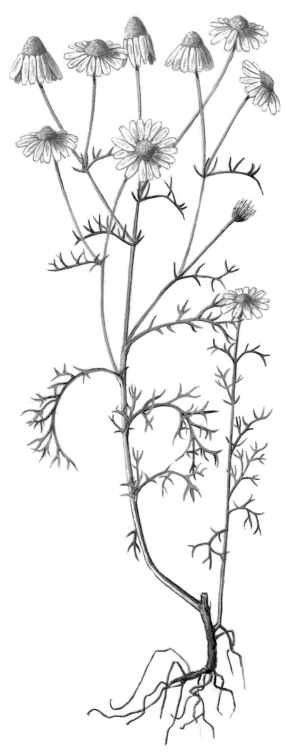

German Chamomile

Matricaria chamomilla L.

Hungarian Chamomile, Wild Chamomile
COMPOSITE FAMILY
Compositae

German people have long shown a fondness for the plant known as German chamomile. In fact, they have an expression for it: *Alles zu vertraut,* which translates as "completely trustworthy." Indeed, the plant is an extremely popular medicinal herb in many parts of Europe besides Germany, and it is used in North America too. Modern herbalists advocate a tea made from the flowerheads for muscular spasms and to relieve pain and swelling caused by arthritis or an injury. They also recommend the tea as a sedative.

According to one German herbalist, early Teutonic tribes discovered the plant in southern Europe and the Near East. They dedicated it to their sun-god because the flower center resembled the sun, and the white petals around it denoted the sun's forces to them.

Some people mistake German chamomile for Roman, or English, chamomile (*Anthemis nobilis*), since the plants are distantly related botanically. The Swedish botanist Carolus Linnaeus gave this plant the name *chamomilla* because that was already its common name.

Habitat: Roadsides and other waste places.
Range: Introduced from Europe, German chamomile is found from Newfoundland west to Minnesota and south to Pennsylvania.
Identification: An annual herb growing up to 20 inches tall, German chamomile has an erect, much branched, cyclindrical stem and light green leaves that are finely divided and almost feathery-looking. Single daisylike flowerheads (May–October), 1 inch across, grow on long stalks and have yellow centers and white petallike ray flowers. The blooms have an applelike smell.
Uses: A recent study among humans supports using German chamomile tea as a sedative. Extensive animal experiments reveal that the tea has potent anti-inflammatory properties, especially useful in allaying arthritis and other conditions characterized by pain, heat, redness, and swelling. Scientific evidence also shows that the tea is a valid antispasmodic for relieving cramps.

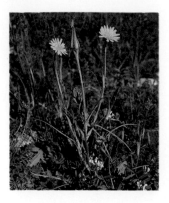

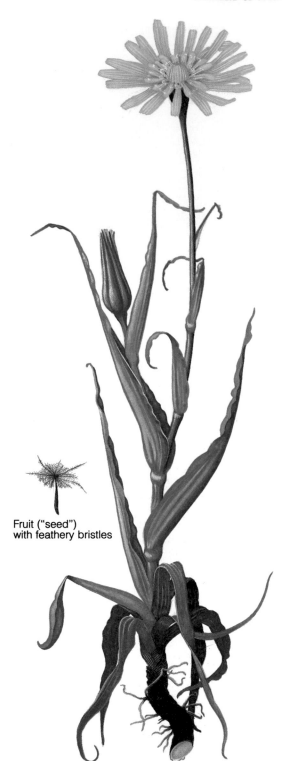

Fruit ("seed")
with feathery bristles

Goatsbeard

Tragopogon pratensis L.

Jack-go-to-bed-at-noon,
Meadow Salsify, Noonflower
COMPOSITE FAMILY

Compositae

The dirty-white seeds give goatsbeard its colorful name, as the 16th-century Italian botanist Pietro Mattioli explains: "From the top of the [seed] button hangs a frolicksome beard which is white and rather large." The plant is also known by the names Jack-go-to-bed-at-noon and noonflower because the flowers are open only in the morning.

Three species of *Tragopogon*—all of which are called salsify—are naturalized in North America. Many people know goatsbeard's purple-blossomed relative *T. porrifolius*, which is often cultivated and is known as oyster plant. *T. major*, another relative, is yellow-flowered like goatsbeard but is slightly larger. All three species have edible, nutritious taproots that many people claim taste more like parsnips than oysters. Because there is so little difference among the three, it seems sensible to throw whichever plant is available into the pot and call it salsify.

Although goatsbeard has fallen out of use medicinally, the plant was recommended in the Old World as a diuretic and for treating kidney stones and heartburn. Its use for heartburn was favored by the American Indians after settlers introduced the plant to them.

Habitat: Fields, roadsides, ditches, rocky banks.
Range: Introduced from Europe, goatsbeard has become naturalized in North America in Ontario and Quebec and south throughout most of the United States.
Identification: A biennial herb that grows up to 30 inches tall, goatsbeard has a smooth stem with narrow, grasslike leaves. The single yellow flowerhead (May–August) is less striking in appearance than the globular seed head (2–3 inches across) that develops after the flowers mature. The root is a brown and fleshy taproot.
Uses: Today the plant's use is strictly culinary. Cooks roast or boil the taproots as a vegetable, or they treat the stalks like asparagus and the crowns, or leaf bases, like artichokes and gently simmer them. They also use the tender leaves in salads or cook the leaves as a green vegetable.

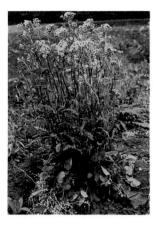

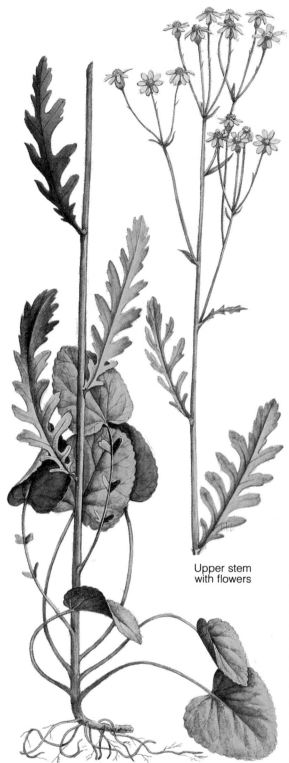

Upper stem
with flowers

Golden Ragwort

Senecio aureus L.

Cocashweed, Coughweed, False Valerian,
Golden Senecio, Liferoot, Squawroot

COMPOSITE FAMILY

Compositae

One of the largest genera of flowering plants, *Senecio* includes more than 2,000 species, several of which have been important in the garden or the dispensary. One of these is golden ragwort, a native North American species that has long been used to treat an assortment of gynecological complaints. Indian women found the plant helpful in childbirth, taking it to speed up a protracted labor. Similarly, 19th-century herbalists set great store by golden ragwort as a "female regulator," using it to treat a host of disorders from leukorrhea (vaginal discharge) and menstrual problems to various irregularities connected with menopause. Before the introduction of chemical substances into modern medicine, a case of tuberculosis was tantamount to a death sentence, and in the early stages of the disease golden ragwort was believed to afford relief. A teaspoonful of the fluid extract in water was supposed to have a tonic effect on those suffering from the disease. Herbalists also prescribed the plant for the treatment of urinary tract problems such as kidney stones.

X Do not use the plant internally for any purpose. It contains alkaloids that are toxic to the liver and that have produced cancer in laboratory animals.
Habitat: Moist soils and woods, streambanks.
Range: A native of North America, golden ragwort is found from Quebec west to North Dakota and south to Florida and Arkansas.
Identification: A perennial plant bearing slender, erect, flowering stems that grow to 4 feet tall from a horizontal underground stem. The lower leaves are long-stalked and oval to heart-shaped. The length of the leafstalks decreases on the upper stem, and at the same time the blades become divided. Yellow flowerheads (April–July), about 1 inch across, are borne at the tops of the stems and are followed by seeds tipped with silvery hairs.
Uses: Pharmacologists have investigated the plant's effectiveness as a diuretic—used in the treatment of kidney stones and other urinary problems—and find it questionable.

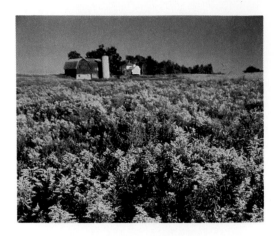

After the American colonists rebelled against British taxes by dumping a cargo of taxable tea into Boston Harbor, there was no tea around to drink until someone made a brew (aptly called Liberty Tea) from the leaves of the native American goldenrod. So goes one account of the more commonplace consequences of the Boston Tea Party. The tea was so tasty that it was later exported to China.

Indian medicine men recommended a tea of the leaves for intestinal disorders and of the leaves and flowering tops specifically for colic. They made another brew from the flowers to treat urinary disorders and dropsy (edema). A close relative, Canadian goldenrod (*S. canadensis*), was also a medicinal source for the Indians, who applied a tea from the leaves to bruises and wounds. Early physicians approved of the use of goldenrod leaves—as a diuretic, a carminative (to ease gas pains), and a diaphoretic (to promote sweating).

Goldenrod was once badly maligned as a cause of hay fever until it was shown that its pollen is not airborne but is carried by bees and other insects. It blossoms at the same time as ragweed, the real culprit, which has inconspicuous flowers.

Goldenrod

Solidago odora Ait.

Blue Mountain Tea, Sweet Goldenrod
COMPOSITE FAMILY
Compositae

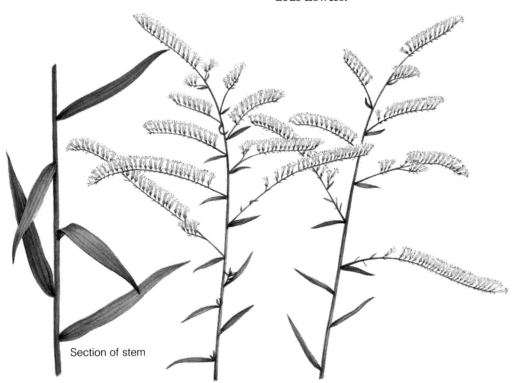

Section of stem

Habitat: Dry, open fields and woods.
Range: Native to the United States, goldenrod is found from New Hampshire and Massachusetts south to Florida, and west to Texas and Oklahoma.
Identification: A perennial herb growing 20–40 inches tall, goldenrod has extremely narrow, deep green, smooth-edged leaves, up to 5 inches long, that smell like anise when crushed. Tiny yellow flowerheads (July–September) form clusters on the upper ends of outwardly curving branches.

Canadian goldenrod (*S. canadensis*) is somewhat taller, with leaves that are more pointed, and broader flower clusters.
Uses: Herbals still recommend a goldenrod leaf tea to alleviate intestinal gas and to promote sweating in cases of fever. Pharmacologists state that its use as a carminative (for intestinal gas) is probably valid. The leaves are also used to make a beverage tea. Handicrafters often choose the yellow flowerheads as a source for yellow dye.

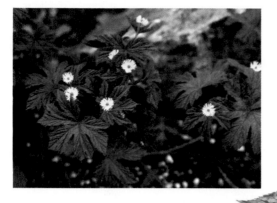

Goldenseal

Hydrastis canadensis L.

Eyeroot, Ground Raspberry,
Indian Dye, Yellow Indian Paint,
Yellow Puccoon, Yellowroot
BUTTERCUP FAMILY
Ranunculaceae

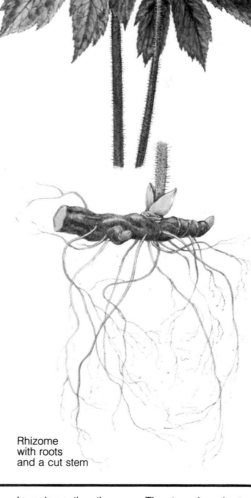

Rhizome
with roots
and a cut stem

Few wildflowers were as important to the American Indians as the versatile goldenseal. Its rhizomes and roots supplied them with a brilliant yellow dye for their weapons and clothing, a paint for their faces, and remedies for inflamed eyes, mouth ulcers, cancer, tuberculosis, and dropsy (edema). It may not have been effective for all of these, but its efficacy as an antiseptic and in stopping bleeding, even hemorrhaging, is unquestionable.

Pioneers quickly adopted goldenseal, and it became a mainstay of American folk medicine. The root is an ingredient of many herbal remedies because, in addition to possessing medicinal virtues of its own, it is said to enhance the potency of other herbs. Goldenseal has also found its way into modern medicine as a treatment for inflamed eyes. Drug manufacturers include an alkaloid extracted from the root in some eyedrops.

The name goldenseal comes from the yellow scars left on the rhizome by the stem that bursts forth every spring; these scars look like the imprint of an old-fashioned letter seal.

Once common in eastern North America, goldenseal has been almost exterminated in many places by commercial harvesting.

X Do not take goldenseal except under medical supervision. The alkaloids that cause this plant's drug action are poisonous in large doses.
Habitat: Rich, well-drained woodlands.
Range: Native to North America from Vermont to Minnesota and Nebraska, south to Georgia, Alabama, and Arkansas.
Identification: A perennial herb with a hairy stem 6–18 inches high. The blossoming stem bears two alternate hairy five- or seven-lobed leaves, the lower larger than the upper. The stem gives rise to a greenish-white solitary flower (April–May), ¼–½ inch wide, with no petals, just three tiny sepals. The fruit looks like a raspberry.
Uses: Goldenseal root is antiseptic and hemostatic (it stops bleeding). It is used in eyewashes and, brewed as tea, is taken for stomachaches. Formerly prescribed for morning sickness, goldenseal root is very poisonous in large doses. The tea has also been used as a douche for vaginal inflammations.

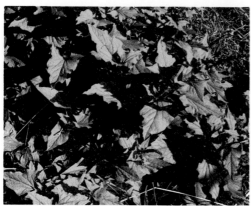

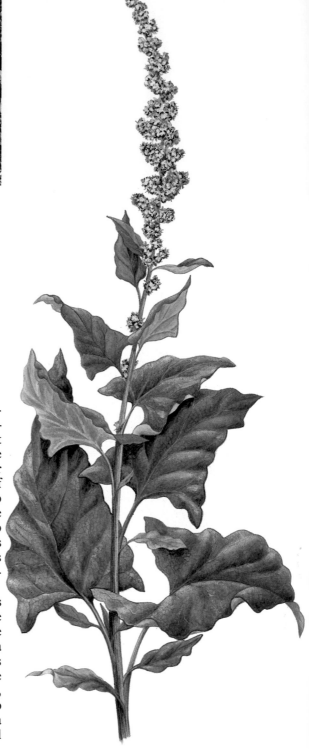

Good-King-Henry

Chenopodium bonus-henricus L.

Allgood, Fat Hen, Goosefoot,
Mercury, Smearwort, Wild Spinach
GOOSEFOOT FAMILY
Chenopodiaceae

Although it is now neglected, Good-King-Henry—a relative of spinach and Swiss chard—once enjoyed celebrity both as a medicinal plant and as a vegetable. Early herbalists in Europe prescribed a poultice of the leaves as a cleanser for sores. They also used it in the preparation of an ointment for painful joints. The plant was also recommended for indigestion and as a laxative and a diuretic. The leaves served as a potherb and a substitute for spinach, while the shoots were a replacement for asparagus. Rich in iron as well as vitamin C, the plant is a natural preventive against anemia.

The herb takes its name not from England's Henry VIII, as is often stated, but from some earlier tradition. One story has it that the Henry in question was *der gute Heinrich*, a Teutonic goblin. After helping housemaids with their work, the creature asked no more reward than a saucer of cream. The plant, which has a habit of springing up close to houses and barns, came to be regarded as a magical remedy for many complaints—a good King Henry of medicinal herbs.

Habitat: Roadsides, farmyards, pastures, and waste places.
Range: Native to Europe, Good-King-Henry is naturalized in scattered locations from Nova Scotia and Quebec west to Iowa, and south to New York and Pennsylvania.
Identification: A perennial dark green succulent herb with stout green stems that grow to 1 foot tall. Thickish leaves up to 6 inches long are shaped like an arrowhead or a goose's foot and have some-what wavy margins. Small greenish flowers (late May–September) are borne in dense, narrow, terminal clusters.
Uses: Good-King-Henry has been employed medicinally as a laxative, diuretic, and source of vitamin C, and to prevent and cure iron-deficiency anemia. Pharmacologists specializing in herbal medicine indicate that the plant is probably effective in these uses.

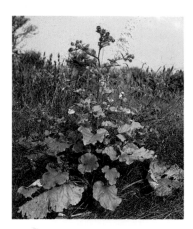

Great Burdock

Arctium lappa L.
Bur, Cockle Buttons
COMPOSITE FAMILY
Compositae

A tall coarse weed known for its burs, which attach themselves to passing animals and humans, great burdock is found in abundance in fields and waste areas along roadsides.

The pesky burs adorn large-leaved plants whose roots, seeds, leaves, and flowers have long been used for both medicine and food. In the Middle Ages great burdock leaves were pounded with wine to create a remedy for leprosy. The roots were considered effective in allaying high fevers, gout, and skin problems. Centuries later the Pennsylvania Dutch brewed a tea from the year-old root to use as a tonic. They thought it equally effective when applied externally as a treatment for dandruff and itchy scalp.

Young burdock leaves may be used as salad greens and flavorings for soups. The young roots and stems can be eaten after being boiled twice, with a change of water after the first boiling.

The related North American species, *Arctium minus,* is much the same as great burdock, except that (as the name *minus* suggests) it tends to be smaller.

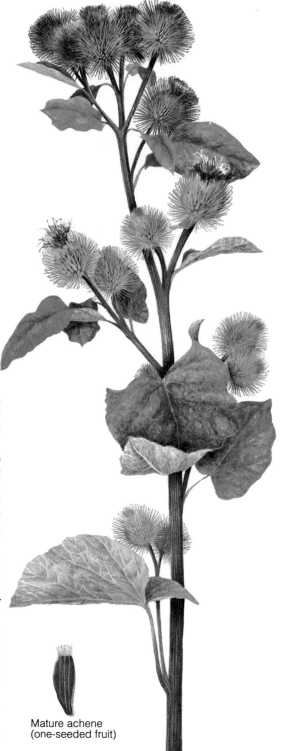

Mature achene
(one-seeded fruit)

Habitat: Fields, pastures, and weedy sites along roadsides.
Range: Originally from Europe, great burdock grows wild from Quebec to Michigan and south to Pennsylvania and Illinois.
Identification: A biennial growing to 6–8 feet tall, great burdock has large, wavy, heart-shaped alternate leaves and clusters of tubular purple flowers (July–September). The small, hooked burs that cling to passing animals contain the fruits, which are thus spread by the very animals that may later feed on the plants.
Uses: Boiled burdock root has been used for rheumatism, gout, lung disease, and as a mild laxative, a diuretic, and a perspiration inducer. A poultice of the crushed leaves is said to be effective against skin irritations and sores. Only burdock's properties as an external antiseptic have been scientifically proved.

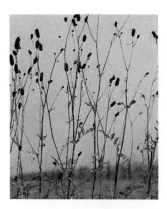

Greater Burnet

Sanguisorba officinalis L.

Burnet, Common Burnet, Italian Burnet,
Italian Pimpernel, Salad Burnet

ROSE FAMILY

Rosaceae

"It stancheth bleeding . . . as well inwardly taken, as outwardly applied," wrote the Elizabethan herbalist John Gerard of this plant, whose Latin name, *Sanguisorba*, means "blood absorber." Greater burnet's common name originally meant "brunette," referring to the dark color of its flowers. It is the tannin content that gives greater burnet its astringent and coagulant properties. Herbalists have also used a tea brewed from the leaves and stems to treat diarrhea and dysentery. The fresh peeled root of the plant is also said to make a soothing application for mild burns.

Greater burnet leaves have a cucumberlike taste and are a popular ingredient in salads. This culinary use overlaps with that of greater burnet's close relative garden burnet (*S. minor*), which has a long history of use as a seasoning for salads and beverages. Garden burnet is distinguished from greater burnet by its smaller size and its flowerheads, which are light to yellowish green with projecting red stigmas on the upper flowers that give the plant a red glimmer when seen at a distance. Both plants are also known as salad burnet.

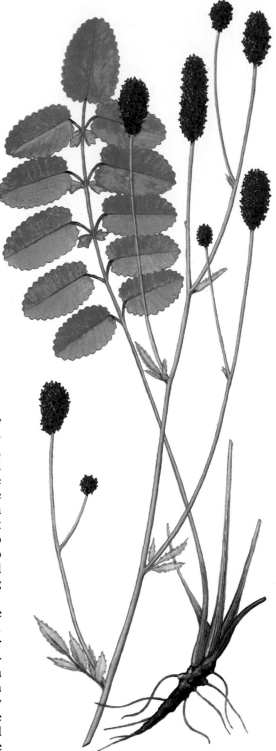

Rootstock with divided basal leaf

Habitat: Bogs, thickets, fields, roadsides.
Range: Introduced from Europe, greater burnet has become naturalized in parts of the eastern and central United States, and on the Pacific Coast from California to Alaska.
Identification: A perennial herb 1–3 feet tall, forming a basal rosette, about 1 foot across, of pinnately compound leaves. They are 10–15 inches long with 7–15 oval, toothed leaflets, each 1–2 inches long and whitish below. From the middle of the rosette several stems grow upright and bear dense, long-stalked, round to club-shaped clusters of tiny dark red flowers (June–October).
Uses: Herbalists use burnet tea to treat diarrhea and dysentery since its high tannin content makes it a strong astringent. Pharmacologists confirm this use. The young leaves sometimes serve as a salad green.

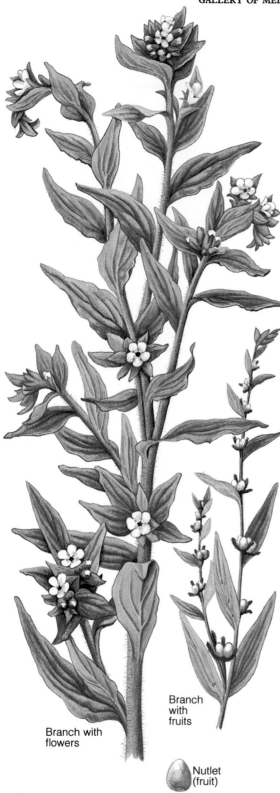

Branch with
fruits

Branch with
flowers

Nutlet
(fruit)

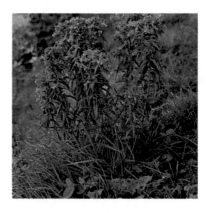

Gromwell

Lithospermum officinale L.

Pearl Plant, Stoneseed
BORAGE FAMILY
Boraginaceae

"No other plant is so obviously a born medicine," the Roman naturalist Pliny wrote of gromwell in the first century A.D. "Its very appearance is such," he went on, "that at once by a glance, even without being told, people can become aware of this property." The property in question was the plant's reputed ability to cure kidney stones and urine retention, and the fact that this was thought to be obvious from the plant's appearance is a classic example of the doctrine of signatures: gromwell has polished, stony, white nutlets that look like white pearls, and it grows in gravelly, pebbly soil. Therefore, Pliny states: "It is indisputable that a drachma by weight of these jewels taken in white wine breaks up and brings away stone . . . ."

A diuretic tea prepared from the nutlets was to figure in herbal medicine down to modern times. It migrated to North America with European settlers, who probably transmitted the medicinal lore to neighboring Indians. Some Mohawks were reportedly using it in fairly recent times. Indians also used the root bark of various native *Lithospermum* species for face and body paint and that of *L. ruderale* as a contraceptive. The roots yield a red dye, which settlers reportedly used for fabrics.

Habitat: Waste places, vacant lots, roadsides, pastures.

Range: Native to Europe and western Asia, gromwell was introduced to North America in colonial times and now grows wild from Quebec to Ontario and south to New Jersey and Illinois.

Identification: A perennial herb with red roots, growing up to 4 feet high on leafy stems, gromwell has lance-shaped leaves that are rough on top and soft below and have prominent veins. Creamy white five-petaled flowers (May–August) are borne in clusters on the upper portions of the stems. The flowers are followed by hard, lustrous, white fruits (nutlets, or "seeds").

Uses: Herbalists have traditionally prescribed the powdered fruits in hot water or wine as a diuretic, mainly to flush out kidney stones. Experiments have not confirmed its effectiveness as a diuretic. The dried leaves can be brewed as a beverage tea. Gromwell root yields a fast red dye.

203

Ground Ivy

Glechoma hederacea L.

Alehoof, Cat's-foot, Creeping Charlie, Field Balm,
Gill-over-the-ground, Haymaids, Hedgemaids

MINT FAMILY

Labiatae

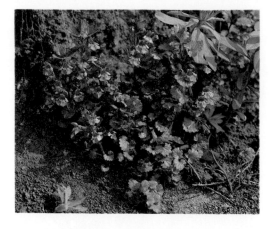

At one time ground ivy was highly favored. But today homeowners regard this violet-blue-flowered plant as a weed because it takes over lawns. Herbalists virtually ignore it, mainly prescribing it as a tea for persistent coughs. In the first century A.D. the Greek physician Dioscorides taught that a leaf tea was a remedy for sciatica; so, later, did the 16th-century English herbalist John Gerard, citing Dioscorides as his source. Gerard also mentioned that, boiled in a mutton broth, the plant was good for weak backs. But he reserved his highest praise for the plant's effectiveness in treating eye ailments, declaring that, mixed with celandine, daisies, sugar, and rose water, it removed "any grief whatsoever in the eyes . . . it is proved to be the best medicine in the world."

Ground ivy found its way to America and became a part of the pharmacopeia of the settlers. Because of its high vitamin C content,

herbalists and doctors found ground ivy helpful in treating scurvy. American physicians in the 19th century had a vast range of uses for the plant. They administered the sap or a tea to treat asthma, coughs, consumption, and ulcers in the lungs, and they recommended the plant for intestinal gas and fever as well. Doctors also prescribed the tea to treat painter's colic, or lead poisoning.

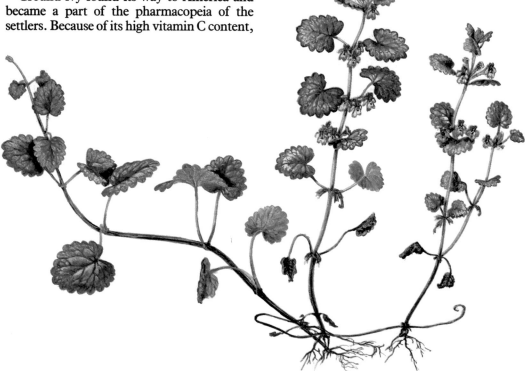

Habitat: Shaded areas, lawns, roadsides, woods.
Range: Native to Eurasia, ground ivy was introduced to North America and is naturalized from Newfoundland to Ontario, south to Georgia, and west to Kansas, and on the Pacific Coast.
Identification: A perennial evergreen ground creeper extending its trailing runners as much as 36 inches. It forms a dense mat wherever it grows. Small toothed leaves are bright green and heart-shaped. Violet-blue flowers (May–June) are borne in clusters of two to three. The plant's odor is mild and mintlike, but its taste is bitter.

Uses: Ground ivy has been chiefly employed to treat respiratory or lung ailments. The plant furnishes a tea (made from the leaves of the fresh flowering plant or from the whole plant) that some modern herbals recommend for the relief of coughing. Research involving animal experiments does not substantiate its use for coughs. Other claims made for the plant have not been tested.

Hart's-tongue Fern

Phyllitis scolopendrium (L.) Newm.

Hart's-tongue
FERN FAMILY
Polypodiaceae

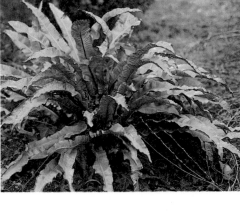

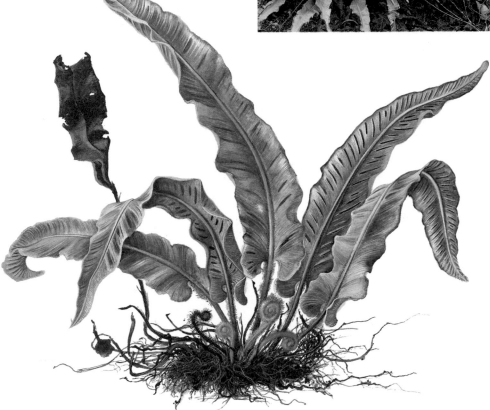

Because St. Patrick put a curse on ferns they have no flowers, says an old Irish legend; yet ferns were also an emblem of fertility in Ireland. Not only in Christian lore but since time immemorial ferns seem to have been subject to a taboo and closely associated with serpents. Snakes eat and control many plant pests and have had a symbolic place in medicine since ancient times. They were sacred to Aesculapius, the Greco-Roman god of medicine, whose rod, or caduceus, with a snake coiled round it, remains to this day the symbol of medicine. Old-time folk healers believed any plant that was a "snake plant" was powerful. In England, in Cornwall, they say that biting off the first fern seen in the spring will prevent toothache all the rest of the year.

Hart's-tongue fern's use was chiefly medicinal rather than magical. In 17th-century England it was taken for a variety of ailments from obstructions of the liver to passions of the heart. Today different preparations of the plant are also used for a range of disorders, from respiratory ailments to constipation.

Habitat: In and near damp, shady, cool caves, walls, wells, ravines, limestone cliffs.
Range: Introduced from Europe, hart's-tongue fern has escaped cultivation in parts of eastern North America from Ontario to Pennsylvania and west to Tennessee.
Identification: A fern with stalked undivided leaves (fronds) rising from a short rhizome (underground stem). The leafstalks are brownish and hairy. The fronds, about 1 foot long and 1½ inches wide, are wavy, lance-shaped, pointed, and heart-shaped at the base. The fruit dots, or clusters of spore cases, form dark brown, oblique lines on each side of the midrib on the underside of the frond.
Uses: Modern herbalists recommend hart's-tongue fern mainly as a diuretic, as an expectorant (to help bring up phlegm), and as a treatment for obstructions of the liver and spleen. There have been no scientific studies to confirm or deny these effects.

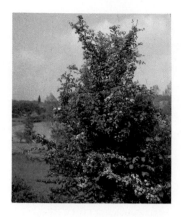

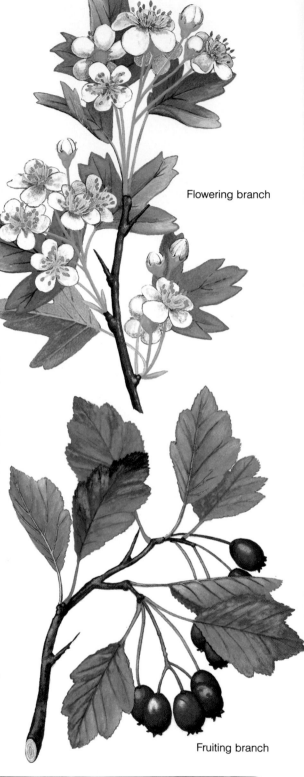

Flowering branch

Hawthorn

Crataegus monogyna Jacq.

English Hawthorn, Haw, Maybush, Whitethorn
ROSE FAMILY
Rosaceae

"Cleave to thy Crown, though it hang on a bush," says an old English proverb, alluding to the acccession of Henry VII, the first Tudor king, in 1485. It is said that, when his predecessor Richard III was slain in battle, Richard's battle crown was found by a hawthorn bush and placed on Henry's head, and thereafter the hawthorn became one of Henry's badges. In England the tree is also synonymous with the month when its flowers, praised by poets from Chaucer to Swinburne, begin to bloom. In France, hawthorn has a religious connotation: Norman peasants for years put sprigs of the tree in their caps to reflect the belief that Christ's crown of thorns was made of hawthorn.

Although hawthorn berries were known medicinally to the ancient Greeks, they apparently went out of fashion as a medicine until the 19th century, when an Irish physician included them in a secret remedy for heart disease. Years later the medicine was found to be made from hawthorn berries, which are still prescribed in folk medicine for a variety of heart-related problems—among them high blood pressure and overrapid heartbeat. They are also said to be effective for insomnia.

Fruiting branch

Habitat: Roadsides, fields, vacant lots, woods.
Range: Introduced to North America, the hawthorn grows wild from Quebec and Nova Scotia south to North Carolina and west to Oklahoma, and also in Oregon.
Identification: A deciduous shrub or tree with stout branches, growing up to 40 feet tall. The smooth leaves have three to seven lobes. The attractive white or pink flowers (May–June) are followed by oval red fruits each containing one seed.

Uses: Since the 19th century hawthorn leaves and fruits have been prescribed in herbals as a cardiac depressant (an agent that slows heartbeat in an enlarged or overactive heart) and as a hypotensive (an agent that diminishes blood pressure). Pharmacologists find evidence that these uses are probably valid, although they have not been positively proved effective. The hard wood of hawthorn has been used to make a variety of products, including walking sticks and boxes.

206

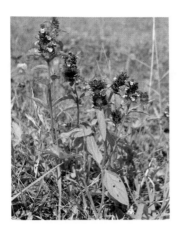

Heal-all

Prunella vulgaris L.

Allheal, Prunella, Self-heal
MINT FAMILY
Labiatae

Students of plant lore are at a loss to explain how heal-all got its name, for its medicinal applications were always limited. A member of the mint family, with the mint's square stem but not its aromatic fragrance, heal-all is easy to identify by the dense purple flower clusters at the top of the stem and branchlets. The flowers are set in rings around the spike, never all blooming simultaneously, so that the plant has an unfinished appearance. Seventeenth-century herbalists believed that because the flowers have the shape of a mouth, they were effective against mouth and throat infections.

Heal-all gained prominence when military physicians used it to treat a contagious fever that raged among the imperial armies in Germany in 1547 and 1566. Sore throat and a brown-coated tongue characterized the infection, and it became known as "the browns." This popular name was transferred, through medical Latin, to the plant used to remedy the disease—hence heal-all's botanical name of *Brunella* or *Prunella*.

Old-time doctors prescribed heal-all as an astringent. According to the 17th-century herbalist and physician Nicholas Culpeper, heal-all "stays the flux of blood from wounds and solders up their lips. It cleanses the foulness of sores and speedily heals them." Heal-all was also a popular gargle for sore throat.

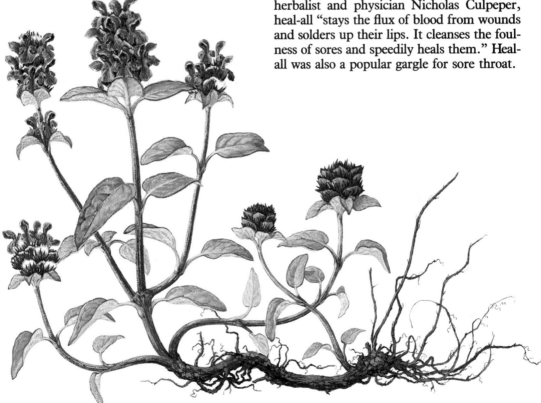

Habitat: Fields, lawns, pastures, preferably in damp spots. Heal-all usually appears in clumps, since it reproduces by runners as well as by seeds.
Range: Native to Eurasia, the plant is now naturalized throughout most of North America.
Identification: A perennial of the mint family (but without a minty fragrance), heal-all grows up to 28 inches tall. Several stems arise from one base, with long oval leaves growing from the nodes of the stem in opposite pairs. The flowers (April–November) grow in compact spikes at the tops of the stems. Each spike consists of clusters of small purple flowers, set in rings, which never bloom simultaneously on one plant.
Uses: Although heal-all was formerly much used as an astringent and often prescribed as a gargle for sore throat and to clean wounds, the plant has fallen into disuse medicinally and no scientific evidence exists to suggest that it is useful for any medicinal purpose.

Heather

Calluna vulgaris (L.) Hull

Scotch Heather

HEATH FAMILY

Ericaceae

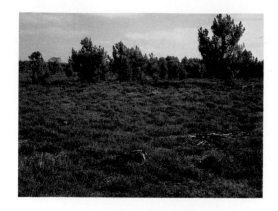

"No' a flow'r that man can gather . . . can beat the bonnie, bloomin' heather"; so goes one of the innumerable Scottish verses extolling heather. And proud the Scots may be, for this shrub that flourishes on the moors and heaths of their country, as in other temperate parts of the world, has served them well. They have used the wiry branched stems for roof thatch and brooms and boiled the tops and flowers to make a yellow dye for Scottish wools. Heather blossoms yield a coveted brownish honey that, it is said, is added to Scotland's famous Drambuie liqueur. The Scots regard white heather (*C. vulgaris* var. *alba*) as a good luck charm and tuck it into bridal bouquets.

Heather's many medicinal assets were recounted by the British herbalist John Parkinson, who wrote *Theatrum Botanicum* ("The Theater of Plants"), published in 1640. He cites its use by ancient physicians as an antidote "against the stings or bitings of . . . venomous creatures" and as a diuretic to be drunk for 30 mornings and evenings, with the result that it will "absolutely breake the [kidney] stone and drive it forth." Modern herbals mention heather as a diuretic, sedative, and antitussive (agent that suppresses coughing).

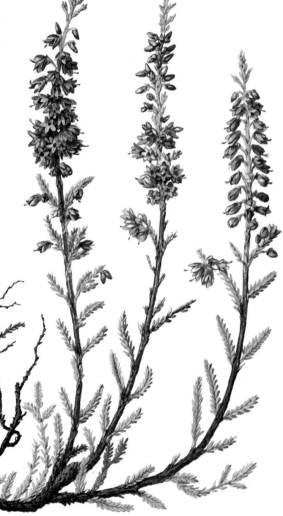

Habitat: Sandy and rocky soils on moors, dunes, and mountains; in bogs.

Range: Introduced from Europe, heather has become naturalized locally in North America and is found in coastal areas from Newfoundland to New Jersey and inland to West Virginia and Michigan.

Identification: An evergreen shrub with wiry branching stems growing 1–2 feet tall. Minute needlelike leaves, 1/16–1/8 inch long, are arranged in opposite pairs, crowded in four rows along short green twigs. Occasionally white but usually purplish-pink flowers (July–September) are somewhat bell-shaped.

Uses: Herbalists recommend a tea made of heather blossoms to suppress coughing fits and as a sedative for sleeplessness. There is laboratory evidence to validate these uses.

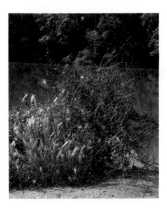

Hedge Mustard

Sisymbrium officinale (L.) Scop.

Scrambling Rocket, Singer's-plant
MUSTARD FAMILY
Cruciferae

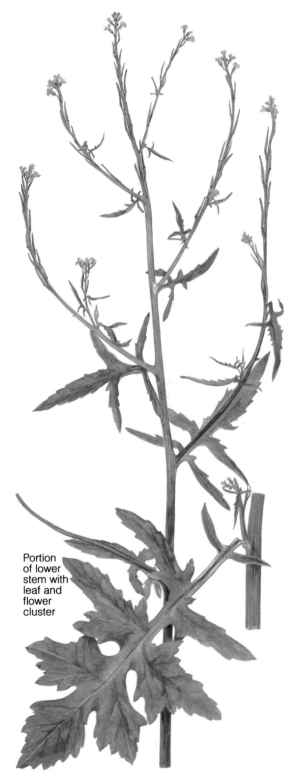

Portion
of lower
stem with
leaf and
flower
cluster

Actors, singers, and other performers who depend on their voice should keep hedge mustard on hand. Ever since the Roman naturalist Pliny declared it to be "extremely good for coughs, when given with honey," this plant has figured in herbals as a supreme remedy for laryngitis. In the 17th century, France's great classical dramatist and poet Jean Racine urged a fellow poet to use syrup of hedge mustard to cure voicelessness. A contemporary, the English physician Nicholas Culpeper, states the same in his *Herbal* (1681): "By use of the decoction [of hedge mustard] a lost voice has been recovered." Other ailments for which this plant has served as a remedy are colds, jaundice, pleurisy, sciatica, and canker sores. It also had a reputation as an antidote against poisons. Nearly all of these recommendations go straight back to Pliny's first-century A.D. classic, the famous *Natural History*.

After traveling to the New World with early European settlers, hedge mustard came to be used more as a food than as a medicine—wild food enthusiasts still recommend the peppery leaves, cooked or in salads. Beware of the seeds, however, for they can be poisonous.

X Hedge mustard seeds can be toxic, especially to heart patients, if ingested in quantity.
Habitat: Hedgerows, hayfields, waste places.
Range: Introduced from Europe, hedge mustard is now naturalized in North America.
Identification: An annual or biennial with many slender stems 1–3 feet tall, hedge mustard has deeply dissected leaves. Four-petaled yellow flowers (April–August), about 1 inch in diameter, grow in racemes, or long clusters. The fruit is an elongated capsule that contains tiny dark brown seeds.
Uses: Herbal tradition holds hedge mustard tea with honey to be sovereign for hoarseness and laryngitis. Why this should be so is a mystery. The plant contains mustard oil glycosides that should irritate rather than ease inflammation. The seeds also contain other glycosides whose effect, though much weaker, resembles that of the digitalis in foxglove: they can cause heart failure. The greens are edible raw or cooked.

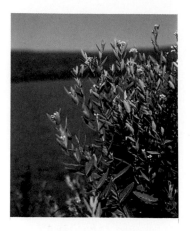

Hemp Dogbane

Apocynum cannabinum L.

American Hemp, Amyroot, Bitterroot,
Canadian Hemp, Dogbane, Indian Hemp,
Indian Physic, Rheumatism Weed

DOGBANE FAMILY

Apocynaceae

Seedpods

Rootstock with roots and cut stems

Among the vast array of useful native American plants is hemp dogbane. The stems of this unimpressive-looking weed furnish a tough fiber, from which American Indians wove fishing lines, baskets, and mats. From its roots they obtained a heart stimulant, cathartic, and diuretic. Early settlers learned these uses from the Indians, and official medicine employed hemp dogbane as a heart stimulant well into the 20th century. It was listed in the *U.S. Pharmacopeia* (1831–1916) and *National Formulary* (1916–1960). The plant has also served as a rheumatism medicine, and its mashed leaves used to be applied to wounds.

Hemp dogbane's cardioactive glycosides have proved poisonous in scientific experiments. A few cases of livestock poisoning have been reported, but animals are unlikely to seek out the plant since it contains a bitter sap. Although the literature cites no human fatalities, the glycosides in the plant make it dangerous except in a physician's hands.

The 1619 records of the Virginia House of

Burgesses show that settlers knew the plant and called it Indian hemp. This name has been in wide use ever since as a synonym for hemp dogbane—but hemp dogbane should not be confused with *Cannabis indica*, the hashish of India, which is also called Indian hemp.

X Do not use except under a physician's supervision.
Habitat: Thickets, fields, roadsides.
Range: A North American native, hemp dogbane is found in most parts of temperate Canada and the United States.
Identification: A perennial with branching stems, growing 3–5 feet tall. Hemp dogbane has oval to lance-shaped leaves in opposite pairs. Its inconspicuous greenish-white flowers (June–September) are clustered at the ends of branches. Slender pods, 5–

8 inches long, contain silky, tufted seeds. All parts of the plant produce a bitter, milky sap.
Uses: Medical science has validated hemp dogbane's effectiveness as a cardiac stimulant. In the Appalachian South, the roots, boiled in water or steeped in whiskey, were long taken as a physic for headache and constipation, but there is no evidence to substantiate this use.

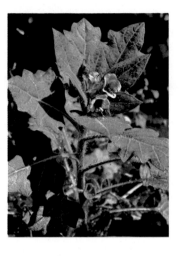

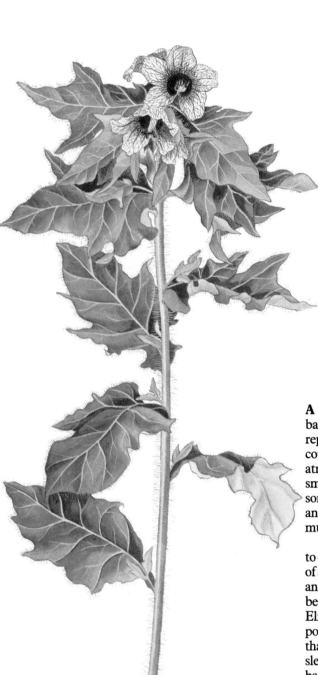

Henbane

Hyoscyamus niger L.

Black Henbane, Devil's-eye, Hog Bean,
Jupiter's Bean, Poison Tobacco,
Stinking Nightshade

NIGHTSHADE FAMILY

Solanaceae

A traditional witches' brew ingredient, henbane has suffered from a deservedly sinister reputation ever since ancient times. The narcotic alkaloids hyoscyamine, scopolamine, and atropine are derived from this ugly, foulsmelling weed. All parts of the plant are poisonous, and if eaten, even small amounts cause anything from dizziness to delirium. Too much brings slow and painful death.

In past times, henbane served as a sedative to ease pain and spasms, but the determination of a safe dose has always been a tricky business, and for long periods the drug seems to have been left alone by medical practitioners. To the Elizabethan herbalist John Gerard, henbane poisoning seemed akin to alcohol poisoning in that both caused stupor followed by comatose sleep. Externally, dressings of mashed henbane leaves reportedly ease the pains of rheumatism. Along similar lines, an Anglo-Saxon text gives this advice: "In case a man is not able to sleep, take henbane seed and juice of garden mint, shake them together, and smear the head therewith; it will be well with it."

X The U.S. Food and Drug Administration classifies henbane as "unsafe." It is an extremely dangerous poison; it can cause dizziness, stupor, blurry vision, delirium, convulsions, and, in large amounts, even death.
Habitat: Old fields, roadsides, waste places.
Range: Native to Eurasia, henbane is now naturalized in temperate North America.
Identification: Growing up to 2 feet tall, henbane has large, pale green, oval leaves with deeply toothed edges. Tiny hairs cover the stem and leaves. The flowers (July–August) are bell-shaped and 1¼ inch long, and have mustard-yellow petals with purplish-brown throats and veins. The seeds are enclosed in ½-inch-long capsules.
Uses: Henbane is a source of hyoscyamine, a narcotic sometimes used for sedation and relieving muscle spasms; scopolamine, also a narcotic and muscle relaxant; and atropine, an antispasmodic often used to dilate the pupils of the eyes.

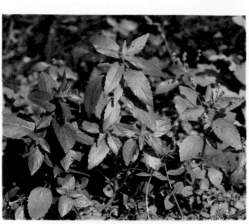

Male plant

Herb Mercury

Mercurialis annua L.

Annual Mercury, Boys-and-girls, Mercury
SPURGE FAMILY
Euphorbiaceae

Bizarre powers were attributed to herb mercury in times past. The pioneering 16th-century English herbalist John Gerard affirmed that hands washed in a mixture of the juices of herb mercury, hollyhocks, and purslane could be plunged into a bath of boiling lead with no ill effects. Although in the time of the Greek physician Hippocrates, who lived about the fourth century B.C., the herb was valued mainly as a laxative, a later Greek doctor, Dioscorides (first century A.D.), wrote that herb mercury might influence the sex of a couple's offspring: an extract of the male plant was thought to ensure a son, while the female plant might bring a daughter. Nicholas Culpeper, a 17th-century English herbalist, wrote that herb mercury would remove warts.

The medicinal assets of herb mercury and its relatives were, according to mythology, unearthed by Mercury, the messenger of the gods. In deference to this tale, the Swedish botanist Carolus Linnaeus gave the genus the name *Mercurialis*. Modern physicians and pharmacologists warn against any use of this plant because of evidence that, in large doses, it inflames the membranes lining the stomach and intestines.

Female plant

Open male flower   Open female flower

X Herb mercury is a strong laxative and may cause severe gastroenteritis.
Habitat: Waste places.
Range: A native of Europe, herb mercury has been naturalized in scattered locations from Quebec to Ontario, south to Florida and Texas.
Identification: A leafy-stemmed annual herb growing up to 20 inches tall. Light green lance-shaped to oval leaves have rounded teeth and are arranged in opposite pairs. The inconspicuous greenish-yellow male and female flowers (July–November) are borne in spikes in the leaf axils on separate plants.
Uses: Herb mercury was traditionally prescribed as a laxative and for external use to remove warts. Some herbal authorities mention its purgative, or strong laxative, effects, but present-day medical scientists warn against its use because of the dangers of an overdose, which may cause stomach and intestinal inflammation.

Herb Robert

Geranium robertianum L.

Bloodwort, Cranesbill, Felonwort,
Fox Geranium, Red Robin
GERANIUM FAMILY

Geraniaceae

The roster of the various names of herb Robert gives a vivid picture of the plant. It is a member of the geranium family, whose name derives from Greek *geranos*, "crane," because the seedpods are shaped like cranes' bills. The common name comes from Medieval Latin *herba Roberti*, but just which Robertus was meant remains a mystery. Leading candidates are St. Robert of Molesme (died 1110), a French monk; Robert, duke of Normandy (died 1134); or St. Rupert of Salzburg (died c. 718), a Bavarian ecclesiastic. St. Rupert was long invoked in cases of erysipelas, a painful skin disease, and some claim it was he who discovered the herb's power to stem bleeding—referred to in the alternative name bloodwort. Because of herb Robert's reputed efficacy in treating felons (inflammations near fingernails or toenails), it was called felonwort. The names fox geranium and red robin probably refer to the plant's reddish flowers.

Herb Robert's main usefulness is as an externally applied astringent for skin irritations and bruises. From medieval times onward, a compress made from the whole plant served to heal wounds and help stop bleeding. Today the plant's popularity has declined.

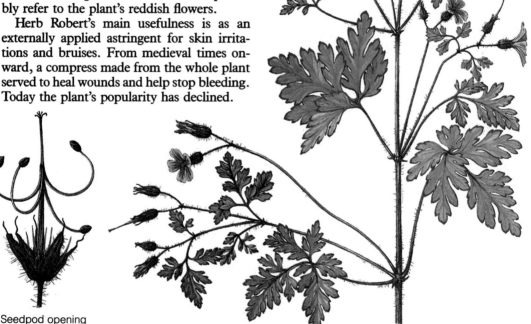

Seedpod opening
to release seeds

Habitat: Rocky woods, ditches, banks, clearings.
Range: Introduced from Europe, herb Robert grows wild in much of North America, from Newfoundland and Nova Scotia to Manitoba, south to Maryland, and west to Ohio, Indiana, and Illinois.
Identification: An annual herb growing up to 24 inches tall, with a reddish branched stem that is sticky and hairy. The leaves are palmately divided, with light green, purple-edged leaflets. Flowers (May–October) have five pink petals and five purple sepals. The seeds are ejected by a sudden opening of the pods, which are shaped like cranes' bills. Herb Robert has a strong disagreeable scent when handled.
Uses: Herb Robert is probably effective as an astringent, owing to its tannin content. Its astringency would account for its ability to stop bleeding and heal wounds and for its efficacy in treating diarrhea.

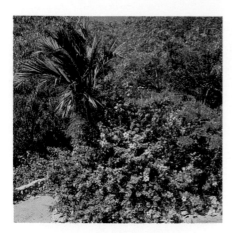

Hibiscus

Hibiscus rosa-sinensis L.

China Rose, Chinese Hibiscus, Chinese Rose,
Hawaiian Hibiscus, Rose-of-China
MALLOW FAMILY

Malvaceae

No less than 300 different species of hibiscus can be found around the world, thriving in tropical and subtropical regions. Because of its beauty, *H. rosa-sinensis* is one of the most widely cultivated of them. The plant flowers profusely in red, orange, or purplish-red shades. Although the brillantly hued, large blossoms rarely last for more than a day or two, new buds appear every morning, so that the hibiscus is in constant bloom.

H. rosa-sinensis has also been praised for its medicinal value. The flowers reportedly serve as an astringent, while the root contains some mucilage, which is known to have a soothing effect on the mucous membranes that line the respiratory and digestive tracts. Women in some parts of Asia have used the bark to bring about normal menstruation. The seeds were at one time believed to be effective for cramps and as a stimulant.

The hibiscus is also the source of a black dye that was used for varying purposes in the Far East, from blackening shoes to tinting women's hair and eyebrows. But the plant's greatest value lies in the beauty of its flowers and the tasty tea that can be brewed from its petals.

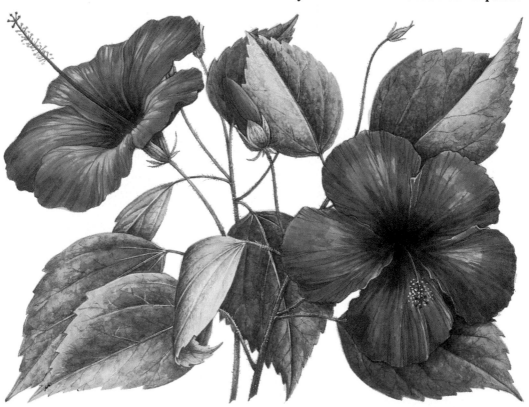

Habitat: Fields, roadsides, waste places.
Range: A native of tropical Asia, hibiscus grows in tropical and subtropical regions throughout the world. It is cultivated and found as a garden escape in certain parts of Florida.
Identification: An evergreen shrub or small tree growing 4–15 feet tall in cultivation but reaching 30 feet in the wild. Glossy green, roughly toothed leaves are pointed and oval, ¾–4½ inches long. Flowers (throughout the year) with five flaring petals, 4–6 inches wide, are usually red, but may be orange or purplish red. The filamentlike reproductive organs of the flower protrude conspicuously from the center.
Uses: Scientists find no evidence to substantiate any of hibiscus's medicinal uses. A tea can be made from the flowers and is available commmercially, but it offers no benefits besides affording a change of taste.

Highbush Cranberry

Viburnum opulus L.

Cramp Bark, Cranberry Bush, Cranberry Tree,
European Cranberry Bush, Guelder Rose,
Pembina, Pimbina, Snowball Tree, Whitten Tree

HONEYSUCKLE FAMILY

Caprifoliaceae

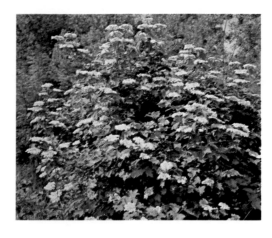

With its snowballs of white flowers, the highbush cranberry is a conspicuous and pleasant sight in many parts of northern Europe and North America, where it is both cultivated and quite commonly seen growing wild. A tea brewed from the bark has been in use as a household remedy for cramps ever since pioneering times in North America. American Indians had discovered the antispasmodic virtues of a closely related shrub, *V. trilobum*, and it was part of their repertory of drugs to ease the pain of childbirth, as well as menstrual and stomach cramps. They may indeed have been the original discoverers of both plants' medicinal properties. They also used the bark tea as a remedy for mumps and as a diuretic.

Though not a true cranberry, the highbush cranberry bears a similar fruit—bright red, tart, and rich in vitamin C. By boiling these berries with maple sap, the Indians prepared a jelly that they ate as a trail food. The alternative names pembina and pimbina are Cree for "berry growing by the water." The Indians smoked the bark as a substitute for tobacco. They also brewed a tea from the leaves.

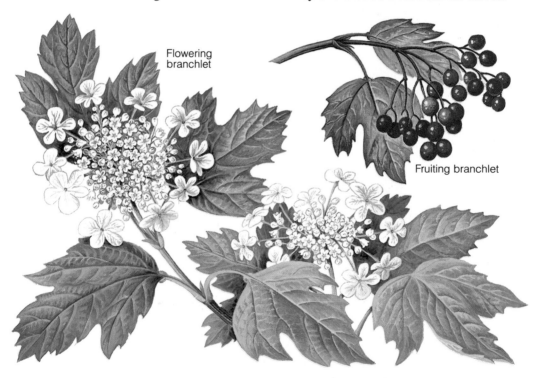

Flowering branchlet

Fruiting branchlet

X The uncooked berries are poisonous, causing severe gastrointestinal disturbance.
Habitat: Streambanks, low wetlands.
Range: Native to Eurasia and North Africa, highbush cranberry is naturalized throughout Canada and the northern United States.
Identification: A deciduous shrub growing up to 12 feet tall, highbush cranberry has an abundant foliage of opposite, maplelike leaves. Its flowers (May–June) are white, borne in flat-topped snowball clusters. The fruits are cranberry-red when mature. *V. trilobum*, a species native to North America, is considered by some authorities a variety of *V. opulus*.
Uses: Pharmacological research indicates that the traditional use of highbush cranberry bark as an antispasmodic for menstrual cramps is probably a valid one. Herbalists also recommend the bark for other types of cramps and for palpitations. The berries are edible after cooking.

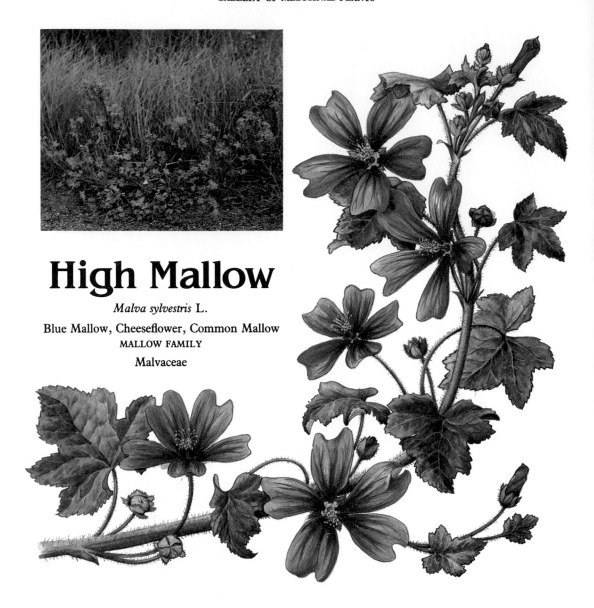

High Mallow

Malva sylvestris L.

Blue Mallow, Cheeseflower, Common Mallow
MALLOW FAMILY
Malvaceae

One high-living ancient Roman poet esteemed high mallow as a restorative to undo the aftereffects of orgies. His contemporary, the first-century A.D. naturalist Pliny, claimed that a drink made of mallow seed taken with wine cured nausea. In 16th-century Italy herbalists described high mallow as an *omnimorbia*, or cure-all, because the plant served a variety of medicinal purposes for them.

High mallow's early reputation as a cure-all no doubt stems from the fact that it contains a large amount of mucilage, particularly in its roots. Because of the presence of this gelatinous substance, folk healers prescribed high mallow for digestive and urinary tract inflammations. But the plant has been in even greater medicinal demand for its ability to soothe the mucous membranes lining the upper respiratory system (as in the case of colds). The mucilage in high mallow can also help inhibit coughing caused by irritation. American Indians and modern herbalists have recommended poultices made from the plant to relieve the pain of sores, insect stings, and swellings.

Habitat: Roadsides, abandoned lots, and other waste places.
Range: Introduced from Europe, high mallow now grows wild in some parts of North America from Quebec to North Dakota and the southwestern United States.
Identification: A hairy biennial or perennial herb growing up to 3 feet tall. Ascending downy stems bear long-stalked, downy alternate leaves that are heart-shaped or kidney-shaped and deeply lobed.

Flowers (May–August), about 2 inches across, have purplish-pink, veined petals. The fruits, called cheeses by some (hence the alternative name cheeseflower), resemble flattened discs.
Uses: Old-time and modern herbalists agree that high mallow is a helpful soothing agent for irritations caused by respiratory infections and a useful agent for soothing external inflammations such as sores and stings. Pharmacologists report that these medicinal uses of the plant may be valid.

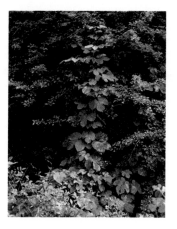

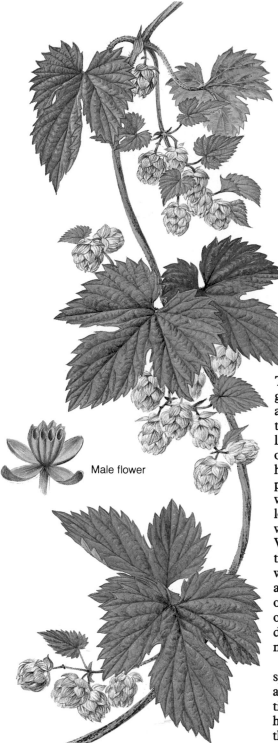

Male flower

Hop

Humulus lupulus L.

Common Hop
HEMP FAMILY
Cannabaceae

The plant associated with beer not only gives the beverage its pleasantly bitter taste but also preserves it. Hop bitters, responsible for these effects, are found only in the ripe cone-like fruits of the female plant. Although the use of hops in brewing was mentioned earlier, hops apparently were not commonly employed in beer making until about the 1300's, when the Dutch used them. The English looked upon the plant as an unwholesome weed that promoted melancholy, and Henry VI and Henry VIII prohibited its use during their reigns in the 15th and 16th centuries. It was not until the 17th century that hops gained acceptance in England, both as an ingredient of beer and as a medicinal herb, and even then one writer noted that the herb "preserves the drink, indeed, but repays the pleasure in tormenting diseases and a shorter life."

In America, where hops are also a native species, the Indians apparently had no qualms about their medicinal use. They made a sedative from the blossoms, and they also applied heated, dried flowers to relieve toothaches. In the late 19th century, doctors were recommending hops as a diuretic, tonic, and sedative. Herbals still cite the plant as a sedative.

Habitat: Thickets, roadsides, abandoned house sites, other waste places.
Range: Native to both North America and Europe, hops are distributed on the North American continent from New Brunswick west to Montana and south to Kentucky, and in New Mexico.
Identification: A perennial vine reaching up to 30 feet long. Opposite leaves commonly have three to five coarsely toothed lobes. Tiny male flowers (July–August) are greenish yellow; female ones are pale green, and are followed by greenish to greenish-pink fruiting cones (called strobiles), which are covered with yellow glands that contain the hop bitters.
Uses: Hops are universally known as a flavoring and preservative in beer. Herbalists value the plant for its sedative properties, and pharmacologists agree that the plant probably has a sedative effect.

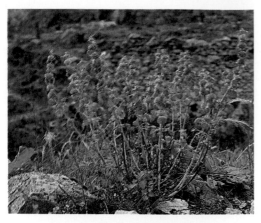

Horehound

Marrubium vulgare L.

Common Horehound, Hoarhound, Marrubium,
Marvel, White Horehound
MINT FAMILY
Labiatae

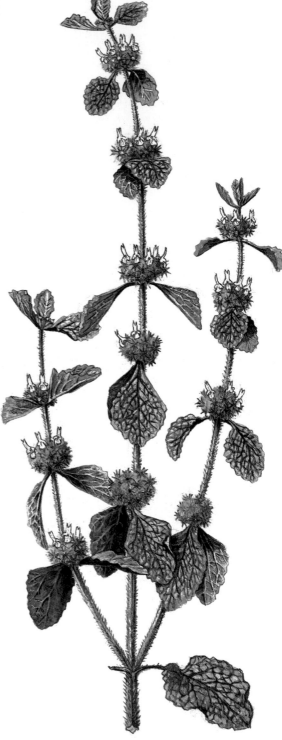

Horehound drops are hard to find nowadays,
perhaps because their musky, bittersweet flavor is an acquired taste. Yet for a long time this
confection served as more than a mere candy,
because horehound has a high mucilage content that soothes mucous membranes in the
throat and respiratory passages. Horehound
drops and syrup (made by mixing honey with a
decoction, or extract, of the boiled fresh or
dried plant) have been remedies for colds and
chest infections since ancient times.

Horehound acquired other medicinal uses
over the centuries. Some 400 years before the
birth of Christ, the famous Greek physician
Hippocrates mentioned it in a work on infertil-
ity in women. The Roman naturalist Pliny,
writing in the first century A.D., held horehound to be an herb of prime importance,
listing a score of uses for it, from a laxative to
an antidote for snakebite and other poisoning.
The celebrated 16th-century Italian physician
and botanist Pietro Mattioli prescribed a horehound salve to increase nursing mothers' milk
production. In North America during the 19th
century horehound was administered not only
for lung complaints but also for jaundice,
dyspepsia, and hysteria.

Habitat: Dry soils, fields, waste places.
Range: Introduced from Europe, horehound now
grows wild in North America.
Identification: An erect perennial with woolly,
whitish-gray, square stems up to 3 feet tall. Opposite, oval or round, toothed leaves are downy and
wrinkled; the lower leaves are long-stalked. Small
white flowers (June–September) are borne in
roundish clusters in the axils of the leaves.
Uses: The plant is a source of flavoring for candies, teas, and syrups used in folk medicine as
cold and cough remedies. Pharmacologists who
have studied the plant conclude that it is probably
effective as an expectorant (a substance that
helps bring up phlegm in respiratory passages).
Horehound is effective as an appetite stimulant
because bitters usually stimulate the stomach to
produce acids that cause a desire to eat. Horehound may be mildly sedative and laxative if it is
taken in quantity.

Horse Chestnut

Aesculus hippocastanum L.

Buckeye

BUCKEYE FAMILY

Hippocastanaceae

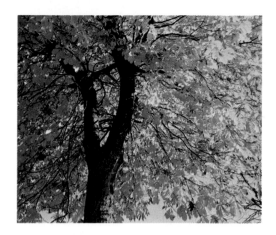

With its heavy foliage, which is graced with candelabras of white flowers in late spring or early summer, the fast-growing horse chestnut speaks of prosperous, settled people who can afford to enjoy beauty for its own sake.

The horse chestnut is a native of the Balkans. According to a Renaissance herbal writer, the Turks used the nuts to treat respiratory ailments in horses. The trees came to the West as ornamentals. They were still exotic in Austria during the 1500's and in England a hundred years later. By the 18th century, horse chestnuts were common throughout western Europe, and in 1763 the first North American horse chestnut was blooming in a Pennsylvania garden. The buckeye tree is a relative and a native of North America, but it is not as large or showy as the horse chestnut. Their nuts are similar in size and appearance.

Although the nuts are considered inedible by humans, people have at various times attempted to use them medicinally, and an extract from the nuts has joined the legion of hemorrhoid remedies. American Indians of the Northeast used a snuff made from horse chestnuts to relieve cold symptoms and carried the nuts to ward off rheumatism.

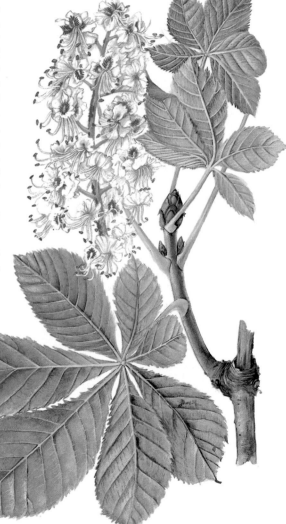

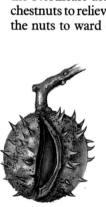

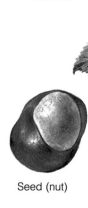

Seedpod splitting open

Seed (nut)

X There are reports that children have died from eating the nuts.

Habitat: Gardens, streets, parks.

Range: Native to southeastern Europe, the horse chestnut is cultivated in temperate North America.

Identification: A deciduous tree reaching a height of 100 feet. It has a smooth gray bark that becomes increasingly scaly with age. Long-stalked opposite leaves, dark green above and light below, are palmately compound with five to seven toothed and stalkless leaflets up to 9 inches long. Creamy white flowers (May–June) with yellow or red spots stand erect in terminal clusters 8–15 inches long. Prickly green seedpods mature in autumn, when they split open to release one to three seeds (the nuts).

Uses: Extracts, or decoctions, from the nuts and the bark of the horse chestnut tree have been used to treat hemorrhoids and varicose veins. Present-day scientific opinion is that the nuts may have anti-inflammatory properties.

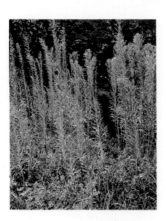

Horseweed

Erigeron canadensis L.

Butterweed, Canadian Fleabane, Colt's-tail,
Fleabane, Hogweed

COMPOSITE FAMILY

Compositae

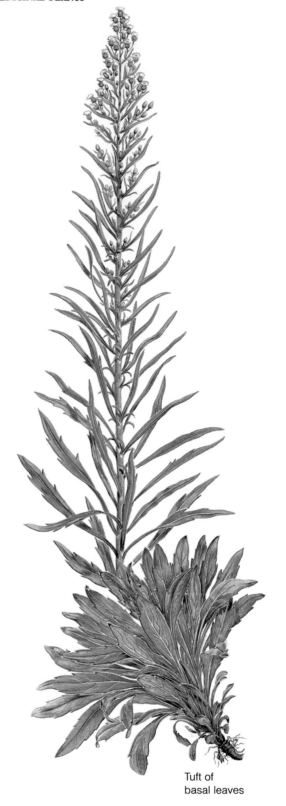

Tuft of
basal leaves

Strictly a North American weed at one time, horseweed (or fleabane, as it is often called) was introduced as a medicinal plant by American Indians to early settlers in the New World. Word of its attributes reached John Parkinson, herbalist to King Charles I of England. He described horseweed in 1640 as an American species. Thirteen years later in France, horseweed was listed in an inventory of plants found in Paris's Jardin des Plantes, or botanical gardens. To explain its presence, French botanists proposed that the seeds might have been imported from Canada with beaver skins or stuffed birds. Horseweed, it appears, has spread ever since, because it is now reported growing in many parts of the world.

North American Indians favored an extract from the boiled leaves (a decoction) to treat dysentery. Later, horseweed was used as a diuretic, as a tonic, and as an astringent to stop bleeding. Herbals still specify the plant for these uses. It is most likely called horseweed because of its large size in comparison to other related species. The plant may have been given the name fleabane because it produces a turpentinelike oil that repels fleas or because the plant's tiny seeds look like fleas.

Habitat: Pastures, roadsides, waste places.
Range: A North American native, horseweed is found throughout temperate North America.
Identification: An annual weed with an erect downy stem growing up to 7 feet tall and coming out of a tuft of basal leaves that later wilt. Dark green lance-shaped alternate leaves are sometimes toothed and have scattered coarse white hairs. Numerous small flowerheads (July–November) in loose clusters have tiny yellow central disc flowers and minute greenish-white to lavender petallike ray flowers. The flowers are followed by white-tufted, one-seeded dry fruits, or achenes.
Uses: The essential oil in the leaves of horseweed has traditionally been employed as a hemostatic, or agent that helps arrest the flow of blood. Pharmacologists believe that the plant may be effective in stopping external bleeding because of its tannin content. Scientific studies have validated the plant's use as an insecticide.

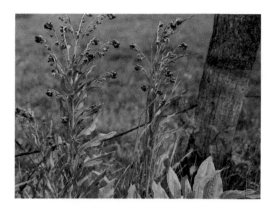

Hound's-tongue

Cynoglossum officinale L.

Dog Bur, Dog's-tongue, Gypsy Flower,
Sheep-lice, Woolmat

BORAGE FAMILY

Boraginaceae

Place a piece of hound's-tongue beneath your feet, and you can see whether it will keep dogs from barking at you, for according to tradition the herb used this way ties the animals' tongues. Because the plant's pointed leaves resemble a dog's tongue, there was also a belief—*not* recommended for testing—that the leaves could cure the bite of any dog.

Hound's-tongue is recognizable not only by its distinctive leaves, but also by its hairy stem and clusters of reddish-purple flowers. What is more, when the fresh leaves are rubbed, they give off an unpleasant odor.

Hound's-tongue was used medicinally by the Greeks and Romans. At one time the leaves were thought to be a narcotic and were mixed with opium, henbane, and other herbs. Various English herbalists prescribed a decoction of hound's-tongue for diarrhea, coughs, and shortness of breath, and preparations of the herb and root for hemorrhoids and burns. Modern herbalists recommend the plant for digestive problems and hemorrhoids. The plant is also made into a tea, said to be beneficial to a sore throat.

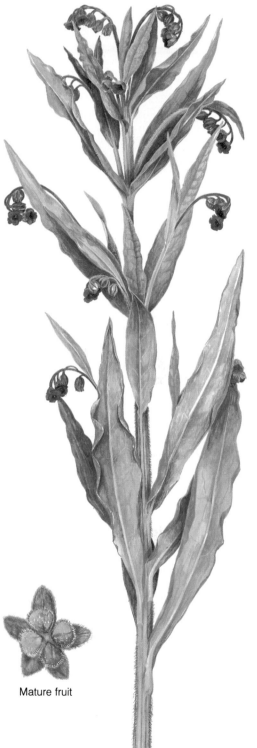

Mature fruit

X Mildly poisonous when taken internally. Handling hound's-tongue may cause dermatitis.
Habitat: Sandy and rocky roadsides and waste places, mountain forests.
Range: Naturalized from Quebec to British Columbia south to temperate areas of the northeast and north central United States, west to high elevations in New Mexico, Colorado, Arizona, and Utah.
Identification: Usually a biennial, with a hairy stem, 1–3 feet tall, and pointed alternate leaves.

Clusters of small, reddish-purple flowers (May–August) are followed by prickly fruits in the form of burs that will stick to any passersby. Do not confuse with comfrey, from which it may be distinguished by its larger mauve-purple flowers.
Uses: Scientific evidence does not back up the belief that hound's-tongue has sedative properties. Furthermore, it contains chemical substances that suggest it may cause adverse effects similar to those produced by comfrey.

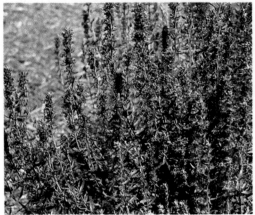

Hyssop

Hyssopus officinalis L.
MINT FAMILY
Labiatae

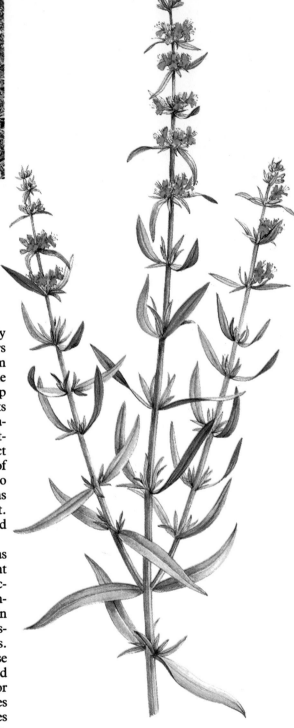

So powerful is the scent of hyssop that elderly women in Europe are said to press its flowers in their psalm books to keep themselves from falling asleep during church services. Like most members of the mint family, hyssop contains a highly aromatic volatile oil in its leaves, stems, and flowers. The strong fragrance attracts bees, which make a sweet-smelling honey from the nectar, and an extract of hyssop lends its aroma to a good number of colognes and liqueurs. Although hyssop is too pungent for most modern palates, the Romans liked its taste and made an herbal wine from it. Medieval monks also favored the herb, and spiced soups and sauces with it.

Medicinally, hyssop has been used mainly as a remedy for respiratory ailments. The ancient Greek physicians Hippocrates and Galen recommended it for bronchitis and other inflammations of the chest and throat. Herbalists in the 16th and 17th centuries prescribed a hyssop preparation as a remedy for bad coughs. Modern herbalists also use the plant in these ways. At one time or another, hyssop found other uses too: the hot vapors of a decoction for inflammations of the ear; the crushed leaves for cuts and bruises; infusions of the leaves applied externally for the pains of rheumatism.

Habitat: Dry fields and roadsides.
Range: Native to Eurasia, hyssop is naturalized in North America from Quebec to Montana as far south as North Carolina.
Identification: A perennial shrubby herb, growing to 2 feet tall, with slender, stiff stems. The opposite leaves are narrow and pointed. Blue to purplish-blue flowers (July–October) appear in small one-sided clusters along the upper part of the stems.
Uses: Through the centuries herbalists have prescribed a tea of hyssop flower tops as a treatment for respiratory problems. Today herbalists recommend the herb for easing coughs, hoarseness, and sore throat, and for loosening phlegm. Pharmacologists state that hyssop probably does act as a demulcent, a substance soothing to the mucous membranes, and this may explain its effectiveness in alleviating respiratory problems. Some organic vegetable gardeners maintain that hyssop drives away cabbage butterflies.

Iceland Moss

Cetraria islandica (L.) Ach.

Iceland Lichen
ICELAND MOSS FAMILY
Parmeliaceae

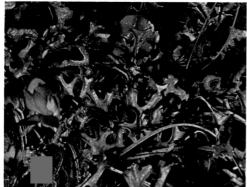

Here is another misnamed plant. Although Iceland moss is abundant in Iceland, it is not a moss at all, but a lichen. Like all lichens, it is made up of two types of plants, a fungus and an alga. The alga's cells are entangled in the threads of the fungus, and the plants live together in a mutually beneficial relationship known as symbiosis. While the green alga synthesizes, or makes food for itself and the fungus, the fungus absorbs and retains water that the alga uses in photosynthesis.

Centuries ago Iceland moss became known as a remedy for many kinds of respiratory ailments. The plant consists of large amounts of a starch called lichenin, and when boiled, it forms a mucilagelike substance that is especially soothing to irritated mucous membranes of the respiratory tract. Iceland moss also contains bitters, which stimulate the appetite. This, together with its food value, accounts for its use as a tonic for convalescents. Because of its high carbohydrate content, Iceland moss has sometimes served as a food, particularly in cold northern countries where the lichen flourishes. When used as a food, the boiled extract was sometimes flavored with wine, sugar, or lemon to make it more palatable.

Modern herbals still name Iceland moss as a tonic and a remedy for irritations of the respiratory tract.

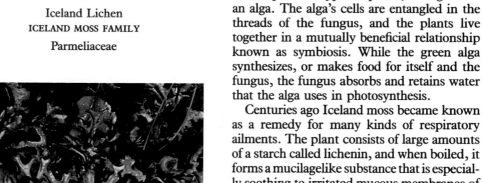

Portion of thallus (plant body)

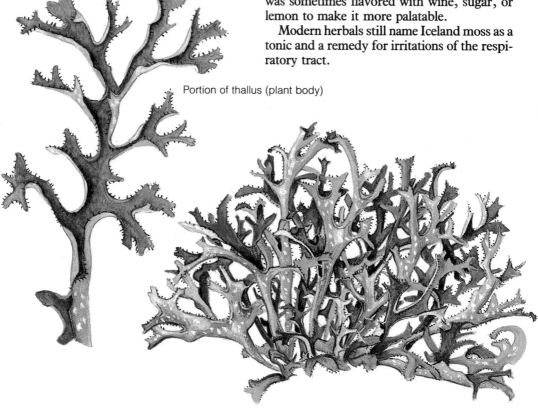

Habitat: Cold, humid mountain areas; woods; moors.
Range: Primarily an Arctic species, Iceland moss grows in North America as far south as Quebec and Ontario in the east, and in the west from Alaska to Oregon and Montana to New Mexico.
Identification: A lichen growing up to 4 inches tall. Its thallus, or plant body, is curled, erect, and highly branched, with spiny edges. The upper surface is brown; the lower (outer) surface is a lighter brown or gray-brown with white spots.

Uses: Today, as in the past, folk healers esteem Iceland moss as a demulcent, or agent that helps soothe irritated mucous membranes. They particularly advocate its use for chronic bronchitis and for the inflammation and discharge that accompany colds and sinusitis. Herbals also specify Iceland moss as a nutritive and useful for improving the appetite, especially in convalescence. Pharmacologists indicate that these uses are probably valid.

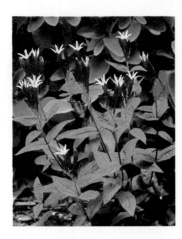

Indian Pink

Spigelia marilandica L.

American Wormroot, Maryland Pink, Pinkroot,
Starbloom, Worm Grass, Wormweed
LOGANIA FAMILY
Loganiaceae

Once abundant throughout the southern United States, the beautiful Indian pink was reported scarce as early as 1830 and came close to extinction in that region later in the century because of overharvesting. In earlier times native Indians had discovered that the plant's root was a remarkable cure for intestinal worms, especially roundworms, and this use was rapidly taken up not only by American pharmacists but by European medical people too. As demand for the root grew, the gathering and sale of Indian pink became an important source of income, particularly to the Creeks and Cherokees. Effective as Indian pink was, its popularity declined in the early decades of the 20th century, when doctors became alarmed at its occasional side effects, which included dizziness, rapid heartbeat, dimmed vision, and convulsions. There was also the problem of adulteration: when supplies began to fall short, greedy traders often stretched their stock with similar-looking but worthless plant materials. By the 1920's, the once-prized remedy had fallen into disuse.

Indian pink once grew as far north as Maryland. It now grows wild mainly in the Deep South, but fortunately because of its side-effects, the plant remains extant.

Root with stems and rootlets

X Do not take internally. An overdose can be fatal.
Habitat: Rich, deep soils at the edges of woods and in woodland clearings.
Range: South Carolina south to Florida, southern portions of the Mississippi Valley, and along the Gulf coast to Texas.
Identification: A perennial herb, 1–2 feet tall, with several smooth, four-sided, purplish-colored stems, each ending in a one-sided spike of 4–12 flowers. Stalkless opposite leaves, 2–4 inches long, are somewhat oval with a pointed tip. Flowers (May–July) are showy 2-inch-long funnels with flaring lobes, red outside and yellow inside.
Uses: Decoctions, or extracts, of the root expel intestinal worms, but are no longer used in official medicine because the plant contains the toxic alkaloid spigeline. Indian pink was listed in the *U.S. Pharmacopeia* from 1840 until 1926.

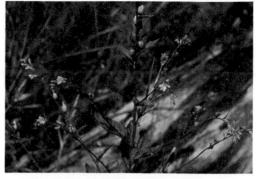

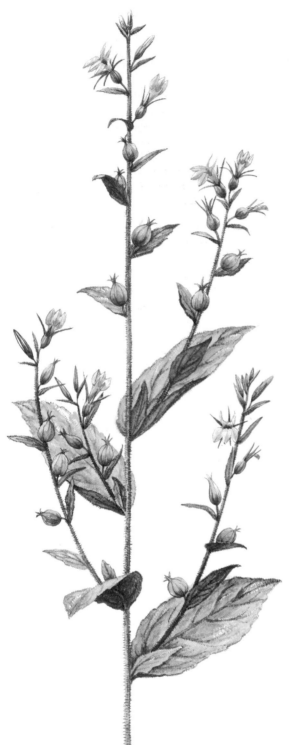

Indian Tobacco

Lobelia inflata L.

Asthma Weed, Bladderpod, Gagroot,
Pukeweed, Vomitroot, Wild Tobacco
LOBELIA FAMILY

Lobeliaceae

Beware of the harmless-looking, pretty blue-flowered plant commonly known as Indian tobacco—it is described as "poisonous" by the U.S. Food and Drug Administration.

American Indians first used the plant, smoking its leaves (hence its common name) to relieve asthma and other lung ailments. The American herbalist Samuel Thomson, who thought the plant was a cure-all, brought it into prominence early in the 19th century. He continued to advocate its use even after he was charged with poisoning one of his patients with it. Thomson and his followers administered Indian tobacco not only as a remedy for respiratory disorders but also for the relief of convulsions, to aid childbirth, and as an emetic.

Scientific analysis shows that *Lobelia inflata* contains an alkaloid, lobeline, and other substances thought to relax muscles: these account for its use in early American medicine.

In recent years Indian tobacco gained popularity as a euphoriant among members of the counterculture who smoked it or brewed it into tea. For whatever intended use, the plant should be avoided by laymen; overdoses can result in paralysis, coma, and even death.

X Indian tobacco has been declared poisonous by the U.S. Food and Drug Administration.
Habitat: Fields, roadsides, and open woods.
Range: Native to eastern North America, Indian tobacco now grows in much of the United States.
Identification: An annual or biennial growing to 1 foot or more, the plant has a fibrous root and an erect, hairy stem. The leaves are oval, alternate, finely serrated, veiny, and hairy. Dainty pale blue to lavender flowers (June–October) are followed by fruits that contain numerous brown seeds.
Uses: Historically employed as a respiratory aid, Indian tobacco contains lobeline, which research confirms is effective against asthma and probably works as an expectorant, too. Lobeline is an ingredient of some cough medicines today, and is also found in some over-the-counter preparations marketed to break the smoking habit.

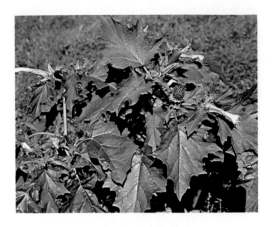

Jimsonweed

Datura stramonium L.

Apple-of-Peru, Devil's-apple, Jamestown Weed,
Mad Apple, Stinkweed, Thorn Apple
NIGHTSHADE FAMILY

Solanaceae

Although it has antispasmodic, painkilling, and narcotic properties, jimsonweed is a plant to be avoided. Every part of this weed, which is a member of the notorious nightshade family, is extremely poisonous and may cause death.

Jimsonweed was once a popular asthma remedy. Asthma sufferers inhaled the smoke of the burning plant leaves or smoked the dried leaves for relief. Because of its dangerous side effects, jimsonweed has been outlawed as an over-the-counter remedy, and it is rarely used in prescription medicines. The root and leaves were used externally in folk medicine to treat boils and cuts. The American physician and botanist Charles Millspaugh stated in his *Medicinal Plants* (1892) that jimsonweed was employed "as a narcotic, soothing drug" for epilepsy and neuralgia. He also noted that it was recommended as an ointment in burns and scalds.

According to many sources, the word jimsonweed is a corruption of the common name Jamestown weed. That name refers to an incident (about 1676) when soldiers, sent to quell a rebellion in the Jamestown colony, put some of the herb into their cook pot and spent the next 11 days in a state of incoherence.

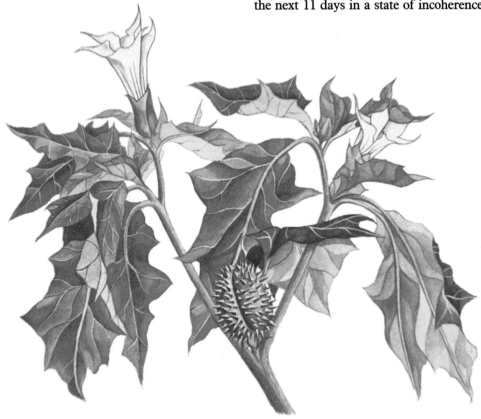

X U.S. Food and Drug Administration has declared jimsonweed poisonous. Symptoms include dry mouth, dilated pupils, reddening of the face and neck, abnormally rapid heartbeat, and delirium. Jimsonweed may be fatal in large doses.
Habitat: Rich soil, fields, barnyards, waste places.
Range: A native of Asia, jimsonweed has become naturalized in southern Canada and in the United States except in southern Texas and in most of the northwest and north central states.

Identification: An annual herb, growing up to 4 feet tall, with a foul odor. Unevenly toothed oval leaves are about 8 inches long. Showy, white, trumpet-shaped flowers (July–October) produce a spiny globular capsule that contains dark brown to black, kidney-shaped, flattened seeds.
Uses: Scientific tests have proved that jimsonweed has both antispasmodic and antiasthmatic properties, but the plant is dangerous to use because of its often fatal side effects.

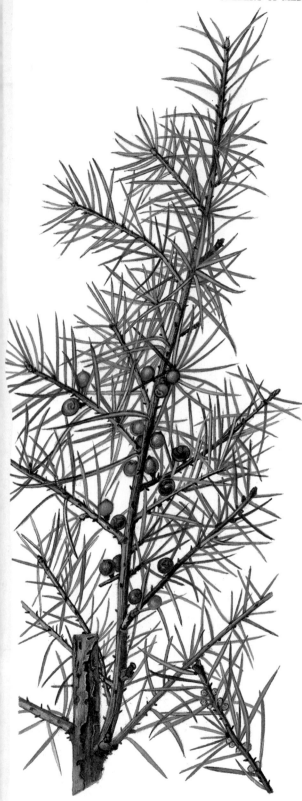

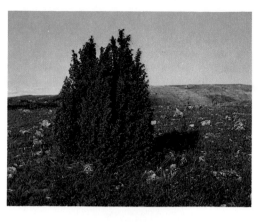

Juniper

Juniperus communis L.

Dwarf Juniper, Ground Juniper,
Hackmatack, Horse Savin

CYPRESS FAMILY

Cupressaceae

Once upon a time, parents burned juniper during childbirth in the belief that its smoke prevented the fairies from substituting a changeling for their newborn baby. In the Middle Ages people thought juniper smoke gave protection against contagious diseases such as the plague and leprosy.

Juniper remains closely linked to spirits to this day, but they are spirits of a different nature: the aromatic blue-black berrylike cones of this evergreen shrub or tree are the primary source of flavor in gin. Cooks use the berries to flavor game, stuffings, marinades, and stews.

Juniper has also served as a remedy for many medical complaints. The American Indians believed that a tea of juniper twigs cured stomachaches and colds. They applied hot packs of twigs and boiled berries to sores and aches, and used the berries as a diuretic, as a blood tonic, and for hemorrhaging. By the 17th century, juniper berries had become known in Europe and America as effective for relieving gas; as a remedy for scurvy, worms, and dropsy; and as an aid in childbirth. Juniper has recently been employed as a urinary antiseptic, particularly for treating cystitis.

X Should be avoided by pregnant women and persons with kidney disease.
Habitat: Dry, rocky soil in fields, pastures, and woods, and on mountain slopes.
Range: Native to both Europe and North America, juniper is found from Newfoundland to Alaska, south to Texas, and west to California. It is a rare or endangered species in some states.
Identification: Usually an evergreen shrub but sometimes a tree growing as tall as 30 feet. The bark is reddish brown to brown. Sharp, needlelike leaves (½–¾ inch long) spread at nearly right angles to the twigs. Near the end of branchlets appear small berrylike cones that turn blue-black when they mature in three years.
Uses: Medicinally, juniper has long been regarded as a diuretic and as a carminative (relieving intestinal gas). It is still used for these purposes today, but pharmacological research cannot substantiate its effectiveness in either role.

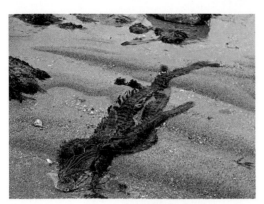

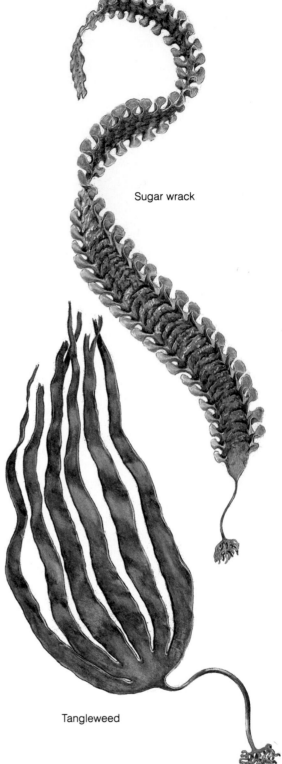

Sugar wrack

Kelp

Laminaria digitata (Huds.) Lamk.

Tangleweed

Laminaria saccharina (L.) Lamk.

Sugar Wrack

KELP FAMILY

Laminariaceae

Rich in micronutrients—vitamins, minerals, and trace elements—the brown seaweeds tangleweed and sugar wrack, also known as kelp, grow along the rocky coastlines of the colder northern oceans and are not visible until low tide. Powdered kelp may serve as a salt substitute in cooking. It has also been recommended as a soothing agent in the treatment of stomach ulcers and as a bulk laxative. The pharmaceutical industry has found a great number of uses for both species—from toothpaste to hand lotions and skin creams. The food packaging industry also benefits from these species; algin, a chemical substance manufactured from the plants, is a stabilizing ingredient in many industrially packaged foods.

Folk healers have made claims for the ability of kelp powder or tablets, concocted from various species, to treat a host of problems from overweight to arthritis, but pharmacologists have not been able to verify the claims. Kelps of various species also figure in American Indian medicinal lore. The Shinnecocks of Long Island would steep the seaweed and use the liquid to bathe sore parts and treat rheumatism.

Tangleweed

Habitat: Rocks below the high-tide line.
Range: From Nova Scotia northward on the Atlantic coast and from Washington to Alaska on the Pacific coast.
Identification: Tangleweed has a slender, horny stalk and a thick, shiny, brown-speckled, olive-green to brown thallus (body) divided into ribbon-like "fingers." Sugar wrack has a single, shiny, brown to dark olive-green blade up to 15 feet long, with ruffled edges and a tough, slender stalk. Both species are anchored to rocks by a rootlike organ called a holdfast.
Uses: Algin derived from kelp serves as a stabilizing agent in the pharmaceutical, cosmetic, and food industries. Algins are also demulcents (agents that soothe mucous membranes, such as those lining the respiratory tract) and emollients (skin-softening agents). Kelp preparations such as sodium alginate prevent the absorption of radioactive strontium from atomic fallout.

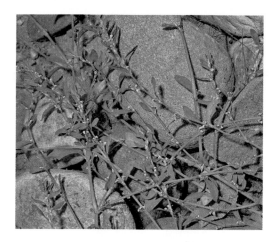

Knotweed

Polygonum aviculare L.

Armstrong, Cowgrass,
Knotgrass, Nine Joints, Pigweed
BUCKWHEAT FAMILY

Polygonaceae

Devotees of fine lawns despise the lowly knotweed: wherever grass grows thin and the soil becomes compacted, this weed can take over, forming a sturdy mat. Once established, knotweed is so hard to pull up that it acquired the name armstrong. Shakespeare in *A Midsummer-Night's Dream* referred to it as the "hindering knot-grass," echoing an Elizabethan belief that the juice stunted growth.

But the scorn is not wholly deserved, because knotweed has a history of beneficial uses too. One use for the juice has been as a styptic, recommended especially for stopping nosebleeds. Some herbalists prescribe a tea made from the dried plant as an external astringent for healing bleeding hemorrhoids and as an internal one for diarrhea. An extract of knotweed mixed with oak bark has been used as a substitute for quinine. In times past, American Indians believed it helped kidney problems.

Knotweed can hold its own as a food, too. Birds are happy with its seeds, and both pigs and cattle like it—hence the alternative names pigweed and cowgrass. In a pinch, humans too have used this weed (a member of the buckwheat family) for nourishment by pounding the seeds into meal.

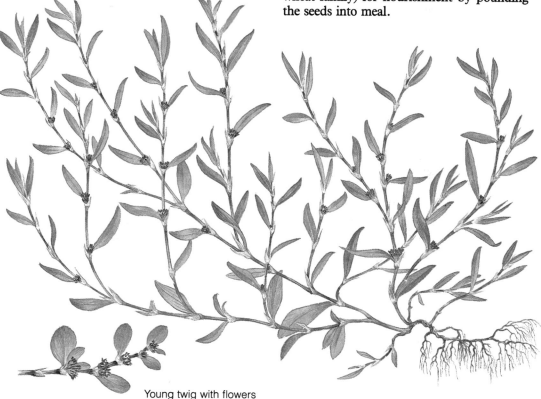

Young twig with flowers

X Cook knotweed before eating it; raw knotweed can cause intestinal disturbances. Do not confuse with smartweed, a relative with an acrid taste.
Habitat: Lawns, paths, roadsides, waste areas.
Range: Native to North America and also introduced from Europe, knotweed grows wild in Newfoundland, in Alaska, and throughout southern Canada and the United States.
Identification: An annual herb that usually grows prostrate, sending out straggly stems, 6–12 inches long, that form a thick mat. Narrow elliptical to oval leaves, ¼–½ inch long, issue alternately from joints, or "knots," on the stems. Tiny flower clusters (June–November), produced in the leaf axils, are pale green or pink to purple.
Uses: Scientific testing has not definitely proved knotweed's effectiveness externally as an astringent or internally as a remedy for diarrhea, but pharmacologists state that these uses may be valid owing to the plant's tannin content.

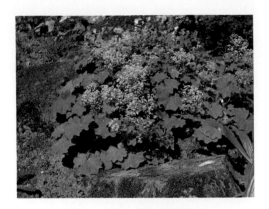

Lady's-mantle

Alchemilla vulgaris L.

Bear's-foot, Leontopodium,
Lion's-foot, Nine Hooks, Stellaria

ROSE FAMILY

Rosaceae

Lady's-mantle owes its scientific name and a certain pseudoscientific reputation to the fact that its leaves are efficient collectors of dew. The alchemists, to whom the name *Alchemilla* refers, believed that the dewdrops that gather on the leaves had magical powers to help them in their search for the philosopher's stone, with which they expected to turn base metals to gold. The name lady's-mantle refers to the plant's shapely, pleated leaves, which resemble a medieval lady's cloak—one suitable for the Virgin Mary, hence the plant's original common name, Our-Lady's-mantle.

Generations of folk healers have prized the plant for its astringent properties. They have used it externally and internally to stop bleeding (including excessive menstruation), to heal wounds, to relieve vomiting, and in a host of other cures. Early herbalists believed that the plant had such strong contractile powers that it could "restore" lost virginity and give new firmness to flabby breasts. Lady's-mantle is still used in herbal medicine, but its chief function is as a garden plant. The leaves usually have nine lobes, which account for the name nine hooks.

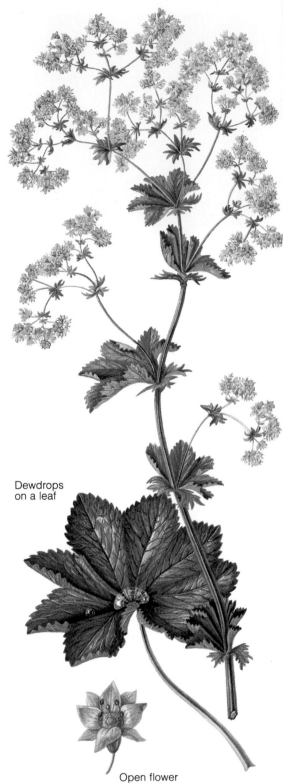

Dewdrops on a leaf

Open flower

Habitat: Cold wet slopes and rocky areas, banks of brooks and streams.

Range: A native of Europe, lady's-mantle is naturalized in the northeastern United States and maritime Canada.

Identification: A low-growing perennial herb with branched stems reaching up to 1½ feet in height. The stems are slender. The leaves are fan-shaped, having 7 to 11 (usually 9) pleated lobes with toothed margins. Tiny yellow-green petalless flowers (June–August) bloom in loose, divided clusters.

Uses: Old-time herbalists used lady's-mantle to stop bleeding, and to heal wounds and bruises. In folk medicine today, the dried herb is prescribed for diarrhea and dysentery, and for excessive menstruation as well as general bleeding. To some extent these uses may have arisen because lady's-mantle contains tannin, which is astringent and thus stops bleeding.

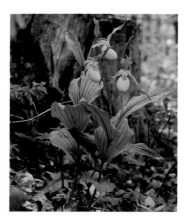

Lady's-slipper

Cypripedium calceolus L. var. *pubescens*

American Valerian, Moccasin Flower, Nerveroot,
Whippoorwill's-shoe, Yellow Indian Shoe
ORCHID FAMILY
Orchidaceae

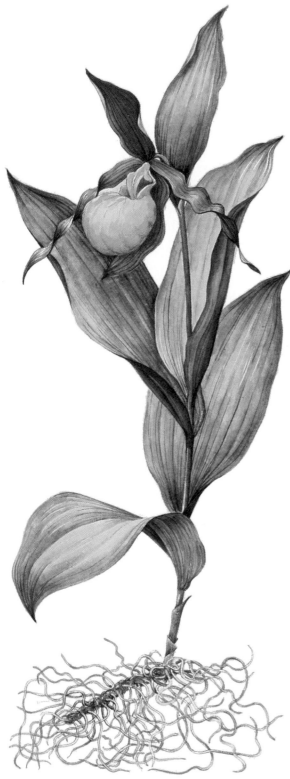

The bright yellow, moccasinlike lip of the flower makes lady's-slipper easy to recognize when it blooms in spring. Wildflower lovers seek out this beautiful orchid; but with the shrinking of American forested areas, they find that lady's-slipper, like many other native orchids, is increasingly rare.

The value of lady's-slipper is due to more than its decorative qualities, however, for it has a distinguished medicinal past. American Indians used a boiled extract of the roots for calming the nerves, and early settlers found that an extract was a good substitute for the garden heliotrope, or valerian, that women and children in particular had used as a sedative in Europe. They began to refer to the plant as American valerian. By the mid-19th century, American doctors were prescribing the root for such ailments as hysteria, delirium, irritability, headache, epilepsy, and neuralgia. It was reported that lady's-slipper was superior to opium for inducing sleep and that the plant was not narcotic. Today herbalists recommend it as a sedative and an antispasmodic.

X Large doses are dangerous—they may cause giddiness, headache, and hallucinations. People susceptible to dermatitis should not touch the plant.
Habitat: Dry to moist woodlands, bogs.
Range: Native to North America and Europe, lady's-slipper is found from Nova Scotia south to Alabama and west to Missouri and Minnesota.
Identification: A perennial herb growing 1–2 feet tall. The stems bear oval leaves up to 8 inches long. A solitary yellowish to purplish-brown flower (April–June) is borne at the tip of a long stalk. One of the petals is transformed into a yellow pouchlike structure (the "slipper").
Uses: Modern herbals list an extract of lady's-slipper root as a sedative, especially for nervousness, hysteria, and anxiety accompanied by insomnia. It is also mentioned as an agent that relieves muscle spasms. The plant's medicinal value has not been scientifically proved, but evidence exists that it is probably effective as a sedative and an antispasmodic.

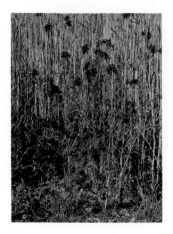

Larkspur

Delphinium ajacis L.

Rocket Larkspur
BUTTERCUP FAMILY
Ranunculaceae

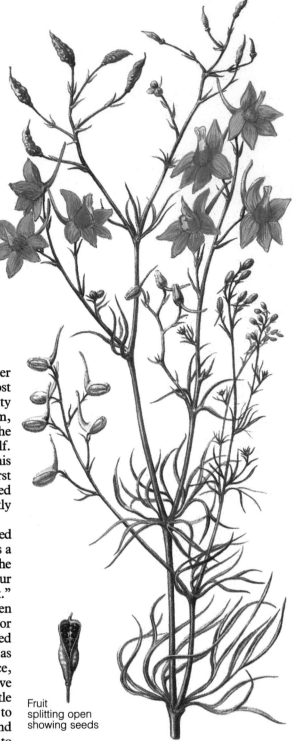

When Achilles was slain at Troy, his mother asked that her son's armor be given to the most deserving hero of the Greeks. The mighty Ajax, bravest next to Achilles, put in a claim, but the judges awarded the armor to the prudent Ulysses—and Ajax killed himself. According to legend, a flower sprang from his blood. It is said that the letters "AI," the first two letters of Ajax's name in Greek, appeared on the petals. The species was subsequently denoted *ajacis*.

Larkspur is distinguished by a spur, formed by the upper sepal of the flower, which bears a likeness to a bird's claw. The Greeks thought the flower resembled a dolphin. Hence larkspur received the name *Delphinium*, "dolphin plant."

Rocket larkspur, as this species is often called, is closely related to *D. consolida*, or forking larkspur. Both plants have been used to kill parasites that live on humans, such as lice or itch mites. According to one source, larkspur was held to be the most effective delousing agent in medieval days. At the Battle of Waterloo in 1815 the British issued it to Wellington's troops for that purpose. And Union troops are said to have used larkspur to kill body lice during the American Civil War.

Fruit
splitting open
showing seeds

X In the western United States, larkspur is second only to locoweeds in causing death to livestock that accidentally eat it while grazing.

Habitat: Wet places, waste places, fields.

Range: A native of Europe, larkspur has escaped cultivation in North America and is found from Nova Scotia to South Carolina, west to Montana and Texas, and along the Pacific coast.

Identification: An annual herb growing 1–3 feet tall. The leaves are finely divided into long narrow segments. The flowers (May–September), about 1½ inches wide, occur in long terminal clusters (racemes) and vary in color from clear blue to purple to pink and occasionally to white.

Uses: For centuries larkspur has served mankind as an agent that destroys human parasites such as lice, their eggs (nits), and itch mites. Herbals still specify larkspur for this purpose, and pharmacologists confirm that larkspur is a valid "pediculocide," or agent that kills body lice.

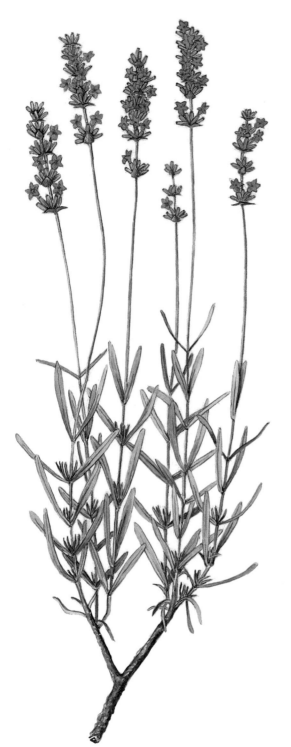

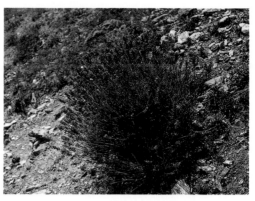

Lavender

Lavandula officinalis Chaix
MINT FAMILY
Labiatae

Lions and tigers in zoos grew docile from the scent of lavender water, the 20th-century herbalist Maud Grieve noted. Indeed, lavender has long been recognized as a sedative. In 16th-century England women and men had its spicy-smelling flowers quilted into their hats to "comfort the braines." Herbalists prescribed the essential oil, extracted from the flowering stalks, for head pains, apoplexy, and cramps. Most likely, it was lavender's reputation as a mild tranquilizer for easing tension that accounted for the hardworking Queen Elizabeth I's fondness for lavender conserve, an old-time medicinal preparation made by mixing the flowers and sugar.

Over the years physicians prescribed lavender water (made, for example, by steeping the flowers in wine) to dispel intestinal gas and as a gargle. Victorian ladies kept lavender water or oil handy to sniff in case they felt faint.

Lavender is best known, however, as a fragrance. Early Romans scented their bath water with lavender, and the plant's name probably comes from the Latin verb *lavare*, "to wash." But its use as a perfume began with the ancient Phoenicians and Egyptians and continues to this day. Lavender oil is a popular scent in toilet water, perfume, soap, and other toiletries. The flowers are often dried and made into sachets for linens and lingerie.

X Lavender oil may be poisonous; no more than two drops should be taken internally in undiluted form.
Habitat: Dry, well-drained soils in sunny locations.
Range: A native of the Mediterranean area, lavender is widely cultivated in gardens across much of the United States and occasionally escapes.
Identification: A perennial herb, lavender grows 2–3 feet tall. The opposite leaves are gray-green, narrow, and about 2 inches long. Purplish-blue flowers (July–September) are borne in clusters on spikes 2–3 inches long at the tops of the stems.
Uses: Lavender has long been used as a fragrance. Although the plant's chief medicinal value formerly was as a sedative, modern-day herbalists prescribe lavender oil in diluted form for intestinal gas, and scientific evidence indicates that this use is valid. There is not sufficient pharmacological proof, however, to support lavender's use as an antispasmodic. The dried flowers have been said to repel moths.

Lavender Cotton

Santolina chamaecyparissus L.

French Lavender, Santolina
COMPOSITE FAMILY
Compositae

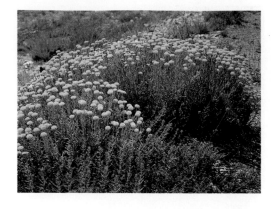

Not related to true lavender at all, the yellow-flowered lavender cotton plant was once a staple of physicians' medical supplies, for a medicine made from its seeds and flowers was believed to be successful in banishing ringworm (a fungus infection) and intestinal worms and other worm infestations. But the plant had other medicinal values as well—or so the ancients thought. The Roman naturalist Pliny asserted that, if it were quaffed in wine, it would cure snakebite, and for centuries the Arabs reportedly used it to bathe their eyes for relief from the desert dust. A 17th-century herbalist assured readers that lavender cotton "resists poison, putrefaction, and heals the biting of venomous beasts" besides thwarting the itch. Like most aromatic herbs, lavender cotton was valued as an insect repellent. The dried stems and leaves, which smell somewhat like chamomile, were used to repel moths.

In modern times lavender cotton is frequently seen as an ornamental shrub. This use dates from 16th-century England, when the plant was a necessary element in so-called knot gardens, formal plantings whose convoluted patterns resembled knots. Today gardeners employ it as a good edging plant.

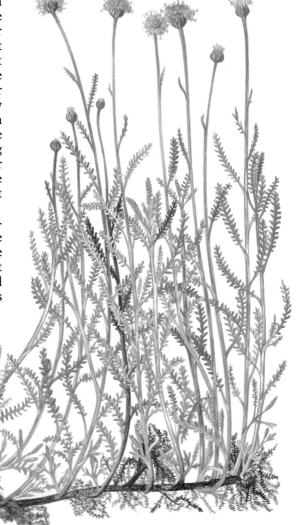

Flowerhead,
upper view

Habitat: Roadsides, dry streambanks.
Range: Native to Europe, lavender cotton is cultivated in North American gardens, from which it has sometimes escaped.
Identification: A shrubby perennial with a thick woody base, lavender cotton grows up to 2 feet tall and produces many branches. The densely hairy, aromatic, grayish leaves are ½–1½ inches long and divided into tiny comblike segments, which to some people resemble coral. Bright yellow, globular flowerheads (June–August) that look like buttons grow singly at the end of a long flower stalk.
Uses: Lavender cotton is seldom used for medicinal purposes today, although a few herbals still list it as an antiseptic, stimulant, and vermifuge (for combating worms). Research indicates that the plant has some antibiotic activity and therefore is probably useful as an antiseptic. Lavender cotton has sometimes been used as an ingredient in scented sachets placed in bureau drawers.

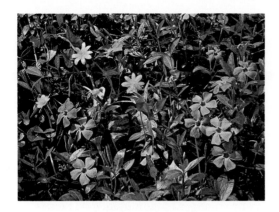

Lesser Periwinkle

Vinca minor L.

Common Periwinkle, Myrtle
DOGBANE FAMILY

Apocynaceae

The demure little lesser periwinkle hardly seems an object worthy of controversy, but the plant and its relative *V. major,* or greater periwinkle, have been a topic of some discussion. Although the plants have been cited as helpful in arresting bleeding, they are listed as "unsafe" by the U.S. Food and Drug Administration. Researchers studying the pharmacological aspects of plants have protested the agency's findings, stating that the plants should not be included on the dangerous plant list.

Probably because they wanted to ensure for themselves a supply of this useful herb, immigrants brought lesser periwinkle, or myrtle as it is frequently called, to the New World. Although greater periwinkle is classified as the principal medicinal species, the plants have been used interchangeably. In addition to its antihemorrhaging qualities, lesser periwinkle has been named as an astringent, as a remedy for "nervous disorders," and as a treatment for high blood pressure.

Like many plants, periwinkle once had ties with magic and superstition. Supposedly the plant could ward off evil spirits, and in some places it was held that no witch would dare enter a home where it hung at the entrance. In France the flower is sometimes referred to as *violette des sorciers,* or "violet of the sorcerers."

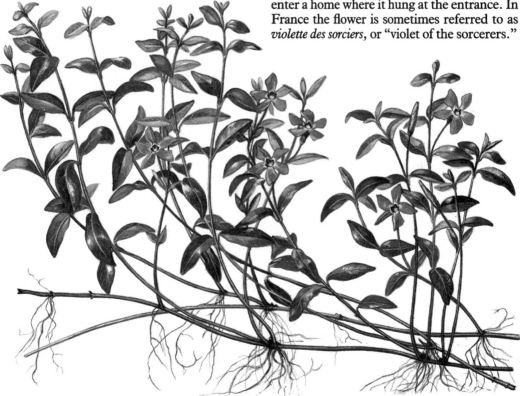

X Lesser periwinkle has been declared "unsafe" by the U.S. Food and Drug Administration.
Habitat: Shady areas, edges of woods, roadsides.
Range: Introduced from Europe, lesser periwinkle has escaped from gardens and grows wild in eastern North America from Ontario to Georgia.
Identification: A perennial evergreen herb with creeping stems reaching 30 inches long. The plants often form a thick mat. Glossy, dark green, oval to oblong leaves, 2 inches long, grow in pairs on short leafstalks. The single blue to violet or, rarely, white flowers (May–June) rise from the leaf axils and produce two small slender seedpods.
Uses: Over the years herbalists have classified lesser periwinkle as a hemostatic, or agent that stops the flow of blood. Pharmacologists have substantiated this claim and have also found that the plant contains substances that reduce blood pressure. The plant's pretty flowers and shiny leaves provide a most attractive ground cover in shady areas.

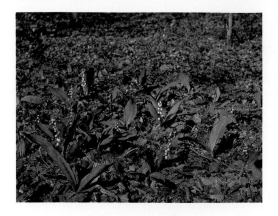

Lily of the Valley

Convallaria majalis L.

Ladder-to-heaven, Lily Convalle,
May Lily, Our-Lady's-tears

LILY FAMILY

Liliaceae

Although they are small and unspectacular, the lily of the valley's sweetly perfumed, bell-shaped blossoms are familiar to everyone and a universal favorite. Adapting easily to a wide range of growing conditions, the sturdy little plant thrives on neglect and, although not a native, it has escaped from many gardens to become a common feature of the North American countryside.

In its native Europe, the lily of the valley is the subject of many legends. Its chaste white flowers became a symbol of the Virgin Mary and, called Our-Lady's-tears, appeared in many paintings of the Virgin. The even, step-like arrangement of the flowers along the stalk inspired medieval monks to name the plant ladder-to-heaven, while its fragrance was said to attract nightingales.

Herbalists as far back as the 16th century recommended the blossoms steeped in water for easing gout and in wine for strengthening the memory and soothing inflamed eyes. These remedies, called golden water, were so highly valued that they were stored in gold or silver vessels. Another of the plant's age-old uses—for the treatment of heart ailments—is considered valid to this day. Like foxglove, the plant strengthens the heartbeat, although its effects are milder. Lily of the valley should never be used without strict medical supervision.

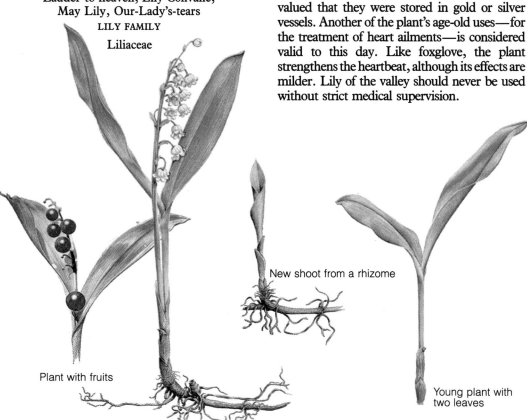

New shoot from a rhizome

Plant with fruits

Young plant with two leaves

X The U.S. Food and Drug Administration has classified the plant as poisonous.

Habitat: Shady gardens, open woods, thickets.

Range: A common garden plant, lily of the valley is naturalized locally in eastern North America.

Identification: A perennial herb that grows 5–12 inches tall from a creeping underground stem (rhizome). It has two or three oblong, pointed leaves. White, bell-shaped, very fragrant flowers (May–June) are borne on a single 4- to 10-inch upright stalk. The fruits are round red berries.

Uses: Popular for wedding bouquets, the flowers are also an ingredient of perfumes. All parts of the plant are used in various preparations for the treatment of heart disease. Pharmacological studies prove that the plant does have cardiotonic (heart-strengthening) properties. Investigations do not bear out claims that it is an expectorant and emmenagogue (inducing menstruation).

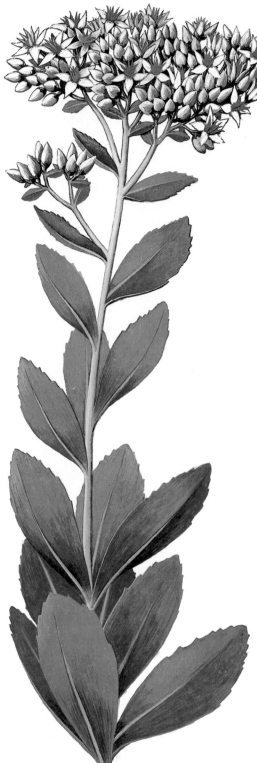

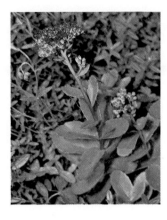

Live-forever

Sedum purpureum (L.) Link

Evergreen, Frog Plant, Garden Orpine,
Life-of-man, Livelong, Orpine,
Witches'-moneybags

ORPINE FAMILY

Crassulaceae

"This plant is very full of life," the 16th-century herbalist John Gerard remarked about live-forever, noting that one could set a stalk of it in clay and the stalk would stay green and even grow if watered. This resistance to drying and dying made the plant an object of superstition over the ages: Keeping it in the house ensured a healthy household. In Scandinavia live-forever was planted on the roof to ward off lightning. If it suddenly withered, superstition held that someone in the house would die.

From ancient times, the juice of live-forever's leaves served as a salve to treat certain skin diseases. The first-century A.D. Roman naturalist Pliny stated that the juice was also a good treatment for wounds and fistulas. In more recent herbal tradition, the plant has also enjoyed a reputation as an internal remedy for ulcers, lung disorders, and dysentery, and as an external astringent for the treatment of slow-healing wounds. The name live-forever is a translation of the plant's ancient Greek name *aeizoon*, "ever living."

Habitat: Roadsides, edges of fields, open woods.
Range: Native to Eurasia, live-forever has been naturalized in North America and grows wild from Newfoundland to Ontario and south to Maryland and Indiana.
Identification: A fleshy perennial growing up to 2 feet tall. The stem is erect and slightly branched. The leaves are stalkless, usually arranged alternately along the stem, but sometimes in whorls of three; they are fleshy, oval, and often unevenly toothed. Starlike five-petaled flowers (July–September) are usually pink to purple-red, and are borne in dense clusters atop the stem. Tuberous rhizomes and roots extend like a spider's legs and have swollen, transparent, water-storing nodes.
Uses: The fresh leaves of live-forever yield a juice that is used as an astringent to help heal wounds, but no scientific studies have been made to confirm or refute the effectiveness of this use.

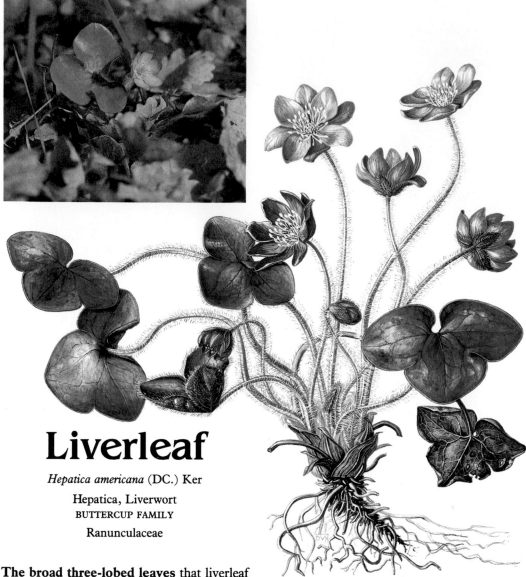

Liverleaf

Hepatica americana (DC.) Ker

Hepatica, Liverwort
BUTTERCUP FAMILY
Ranunculaceae

The broad three-lobed leaves that liverleaf bears on slender hairy stalks are its most persistent and noteworthy feature. Though winter mutes their normal green to a dull reddish brown, the leaves survive under the snow until a new crop emerges in spring.

The curious appearance of these leaves originally inspired the botanical and common names of the closely related European species *H. nobilis*. In both the shape and winter color of the leaves early European physicians saw a resemblance to the human liver. The Greeks called the plant *hepar*, meaning "liver," and they employed it as a remedy for disorders of

that organ. A dose of liverleaf, herbalists believed, would cure liver diseases or their supposed symptoms: cowardice, freckles, or indigestion. Liverleaf thus became a classic example of the doctrine of signatures, which had a great following among medieval physicians. According to the theory, a plant's outward appearance provided a divine sign, or signature, of its healing properties.

Settlers used a native American liverleaf, *H. americana*, to soothe the irritations of sore throat and coughs.

Habitat: Moist, shaded woodlands.
Range: A native of North America, liverleaf is found from Nova Scotia to Manitoba, southward to Florida, Alabama, and Missouri.
Identification: A perennial herb growing 4–6 inches tall, with hairy leafstalks and flower stalks. Solitary, long-stalked flowers (February–June), ½–1 inch across, emerge before the new dark green, leathery, three-lobed leaves. Delicate petallike sepals vary in color from bluish purple to pink

to white; numerous stamens arise around the flower's green to yellow domelike center, which consists of the pistils.
Uses: Although the European liverleaf was once highly reputed as a liver tonic and remedy, both it and the American species have fallen into disuse medicinally. *H. americana*'s chief employment is in the garden, where it serves as a handsome, shade-tolerant ground cover.

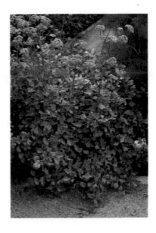

Lovage

Levisticum officinale W.D.J. Koch

Sea Parsley

CARROT FAMILY

Umbelliferae

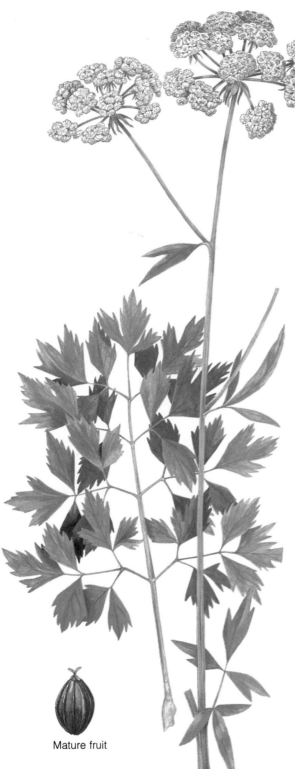

Mature fruit

With their strong aromatic flavor, the leaves and stems of lovage have been a soup and stew ingredient, and the stalks have been blanched as a vegetable, ever since classical antiquity. Like its relative celery, the plant relieves gas pains—a power attributed to it by writers from the ancient Greeks to present-day pharmacologists. New Englanders planted lovage for its roots, too, which they candied and used as a sweet and a breath lozenge. Nineteenth-century Shaker religious communities grew and sold lovage as part of their commercial enterprises. Herbalists have also recommended various preparations of the root to promote urine flow and bring on menstruation and as a skin wash, or lotion.

The name lovage goes back to a Latin word meaning "Ligurian," because the herb flourished in ancient times in Liguria, a region that includes the Italian Riviera. The name was garbled beyond recognition by the time it entered English, in Chaucer's day, as *love-ache*, or "love-parsley." Misled by the name, many people over the past 600 years have fancied a connection between lovage and love potions. There is none, except insofar as any breath sweetener encourages romance.

X Do not confuse lovage with such poisonous members of the carrot family as water hemlock, poison hemlock, and fool's parsley.

Habitat: Gardens, meadows, hedgerows.

Range: Introduced from Europe, lovage is cultivated and may escape cultivation from New Jersey to Virginia and west to Missouri and New Mexico.

Identification: A perennial herb 3–7 feet tall, lovage has dense clusters of tiny pale yellow flowers (May–July) arranged in umbels (umbrella-like clusters) atop a thick, hollow stem. The leaves are divided several times, with lobed or sharply toothed leaflets. The lower leaves may grow 2 feet long. The plant has a strong celerylike smell.

Uses: Lovage has proven value for relieving gas pains, and research indicates that it probably acts as a breath deodorizer too. Pharmacologists have not confirmed the value of lovage root tea as a diuretic or for bringing on menstruation.

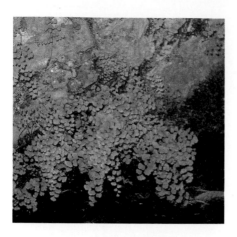

Maidenhair Fern

Adiantum capillus-veneris L.

Black Maidenhair Fern, Rock Fern,
Southern Maidenhair Fern, Venus'-hair Fern
FERN FAMILY
Polypodiaceae

A plant of great delicacy, maidenhair fern has a thin, polished, black main leafstalk and fanlike leaflets supported by stalks as fine as hair. The plant has a gossamer look that makes it in demand for dried flower arrangements. Maidenhair fern prefers a wet environment, usually growing in limestone soils dampened by waterfall spray. Water runs off its foliage with the result that, even after being immersed in water, it emerges with dry leaves—hence its scientific name, *Adiantum*, meaning "unwetted." The fern's association with hair gave rise to an old belief that drinking a tea made from the plant could keep hair from falling out. Unhappily, it has no such powers.

A tea from the fresh plant has been used as an expectorant in treating coughs since the time of the ancient Greeks. Later herbalists prescribed maidenhair fern for more serious respiratory conditions, such as pleurisy, but with less success, for it is not a potent plant. It was also employed to promote menstruation and as a mild diuretic.

A relative is the northern maidenhair (*A. pedatum*), which has a somewhat forked stalk, as opposed to the single stalk of *A. capillus-veneris*, also called southern maidenhair fern.

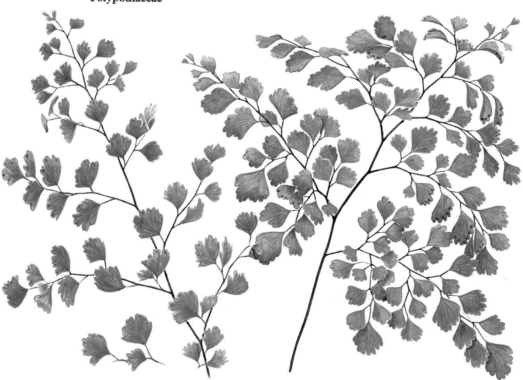

Habitat: Rich, moist soil near springs, especially in canyons and caves and on shaded slopes.
Range: Native to warm temperate and subtropical regions, maidenhair is found across the southern United States as far north as Virginia and Colorado.
Identification: A perennial fern 12–15 inches high, with slender, dark brown to shiny black leafstalks arising from a rhizome (underground stem). The pinnately compound leaves consist of lobed or notched, fan-shaped, pale green leaflets, arranged alternately along the leafstalks. The spore cases (June–August) are found in brown creases at the outer edges of the leaflets.
Uses: Although maidenhair fern was long used as an expectorant, an emmenagogue (to promote menstruation), and a diuretic, pharmacologists find no evidence for any of its medicinal uses. Herbalists today favor a rinse made from the plant to give body and sheen to the hair. No evidence exists to support this use either.

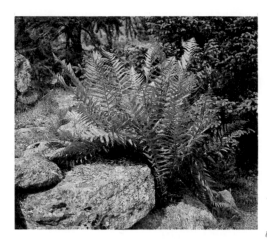

Male Fern

Dryopteris filix-mas (L.) Schott

Bear's-paw, Knotty Brake,
Shield Fern, Sweet Brake

FERN FAMILY

Polypodiaceae

One of the most potent remedies for tapeworm ever recorded in the annals of medicine, male fern was listed in the *U.S. Pharmacopeia* as late as 1965. From Greek antiquity down to the present day, male fern has been recommended for expelling tapeworms. Tapeworms know no social boundaries—even Louis XVI of France paid a kingly sum for a formula containing this drug.

The fern probably got the name bear's-paw from the rough, hairy appearance of the brown rhizomes. The genus name *Dryopteris* means "oak-fern" in Greek, because the plant often grows in oak forests. Botanists gave the plant its species name, *filix-mas* ("male fern"), because of its vigorous nature. (Another species, *Athyrium filix-femina*, or lady fern, got its name for its delicate appearance.) It was not until the mid-1800's that botanists learned that ferns are neither "male" nor "female"; fern spores form small structures that produce both male and female cells. Because the spores cannot be seen by the naked eye, they were once believed to confer invisibility. Shakespeare alludes to this belief in *Henry IV*: "We have the receipt of fern-seed, we walk invisible."

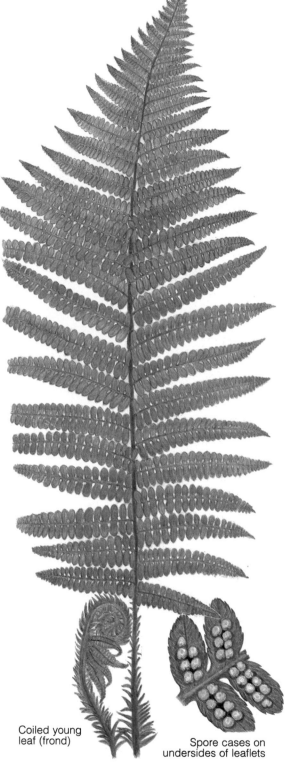

Coiled young leaf (frond)

Spore cases on undersides of leaflets

Habitat: Dry terrain in rich woods, rocky slopes.
Range: Native to northern temperate regions, male fern grows from the east to the west coast of Canada, south to Vermont, Texas, and California.
Identification: Growing from a creeping underground stem (rhizome), male fern has feathery leaves (fronds) 15–30 inches tall or taller; its shoots and the lower portion of the leafstalks have hairy scales. On the underside of each finely toothed leaflet are spore cases (June–August), marked with kidney-shaped or roundish shields.
Uses: To get rid of tapeworm, herbalists prescribe a tea of the rhizome. The rhizome contains a substance called an oleoresin that paralyzes the worm and causes it to release its grip on the intestines. Before taking oleoresin of male fern as a taeniafuge (tapeworm expeller), a person is placed on a fat-free diet for two to three days. After the dose is administered, a saline (salty) laxative is given to expel the worm from the body.

241

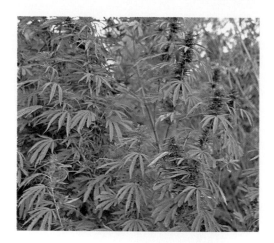

Marijuana

Cannabis sativa L.

Bhang, Ganja, Grass, Hashish,
Hemp, Mary Jane, Pot, Reefer

HEMP FAMILY

Cannabaceae

Although often abused, marijuana is one of the world's oldest economic plants. Besides providing the material, hemp, for a lucrative cordage and cloth industry, it has been a valuable medicinal drug. The ancient pharmacopeias of China, going back more than 2,000 years, listed marijuana, and the plant found favor around the world for its ability to ease pain, induce sleep, and soothe a variety of nervous disorders. Usually the leaves or seeds were taken, but in medieval Europe physicians prescribed the root to alleviate the agonies of gout and other painful diseases. Mixed with oil and butter, the root also made a salve for burns caused by that new import from the Orient, gunpowder. Today marijuana is under investigation as a treatment for asthma and certain types of glaucoma and as a means of controlling epileptic seizures and the nausea caused by radiation therapy and cancer chemotherapy.

Although marijuana's use as an intoxicant is not only widespread but socially acceptable in much of Africa and Asia, it has serious drawbacks. The extent to which marijuana can be physically or psychologically damaging remains a subject of discussion, but there is no dispute that it can be harmful, with a real danger of psychological, if not physical, dependence. Possession of the plant is illegal.

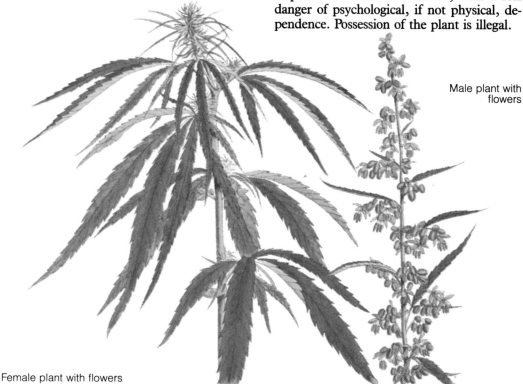

Male plant with flowers

Female plant with flowers

X Do not use except under a doctor's supervision. Smoking or eating marijuana may have physically and psychologically injurious effects.
Habitat: Abandoned lands, ditches, streambanks.
Range: Native to the Caucasus, northern India, and Iran, marijuana is now a common weed throughout much of North America, where it has escaped from cultivation for hemp fiber.
Identification: A vigorous annual with an erect stem 3–10 feet tall. The leaves are hairy and divided, with five to seven long, toothed leaflets. The male and female flowers (June–October) are small and greenish, and borne on separate plants.
Uses: The plant contains tetrahydrocannabinols (THC's), which induce euphoria and exhilaration, dull pain, and act as a sedative and antispasmodic. The fiber is used for rope, twine, and coarse cloth, while the seeds are an ingredient of many commercial birdseeds. Painters use hempseed oil to mix colors and as a varnish.

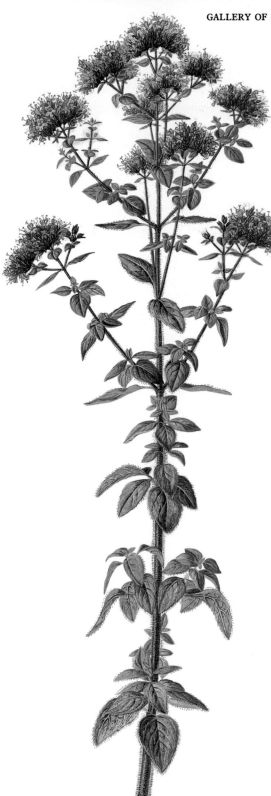

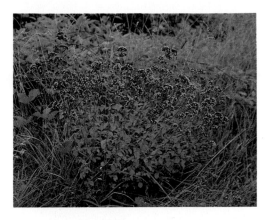

Marjoram

Origanum vulgare L.

Common Marjoram, Oregano, Wild Marjoram
MINT FAMILY
Labiatae

A pleasant, minty-smelling plant, marjoram, or wild marjoram, can be added to fish and meat dishes for its thymelike taste. Do not confuse it with *O. heracleoticum*, a more pungent herb that is packaged as oregano or Greek oregano, or with another common kitchen herb, sweet marjoram (*Majorana hortensis*).

Both the botanical name *Origanum* and the alternative common name oregano derive from the Greek words *oros* ("mountain") and *ganos* ("joy"), or "joy of the mountain." Its vivid purplish flowers so gaily adorn the hilly Mediterranean landscape that the plant became a symbol of happiness. When the Greeks saw the herb spring up on a grave, they believed it meant that the deceased was happy in the afterlife. At both Greek and Roman marriages, the wedding couple wore wild marjoram wreaths to symbolize the joyful event.

In medieval times the herbalists prescribed the herb's oil for toothache. In the 16th and 17th centuries herbalists recommended the plant for internal use to aid digestion, as a diuretic, and as an antidote for venomous bites; and for external use to relieve itching.

Habitat: Old fields, woods, roadsides,
Range: A native of southern Europe, wild marjoram is naturalized in North America from Ontario and Quebec south to North Carolina and west to Oregon and California.
Identification: A perennial herb growing 1–3 feet tall. The erect purplish-brown stem and flower stalks are hairy. The small oval leaves are without teeth and can be hairy. Purplish-red flowers (June–October), about ¼ inch across, occur in heads about 1 inch across at the tops of the stems and branchlets.
Uses: Herbalists have long valued wild marjoram as an effective remedy for stomach disorders, and the herb continues to be recommended today for this purpose and as a diuretic as well. It probably has some effect as a carminative (an agent that expels stomach and intestinal gas), but its usefulness as a diuretic has not been confirmed.

243

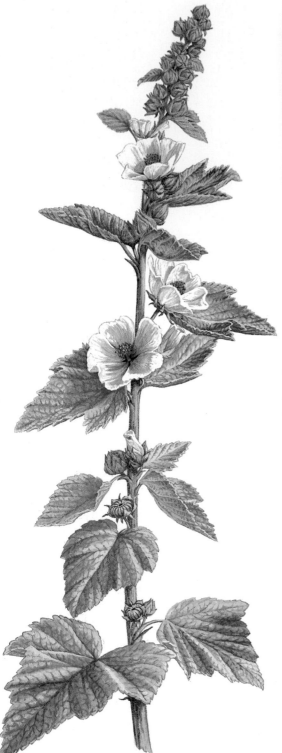

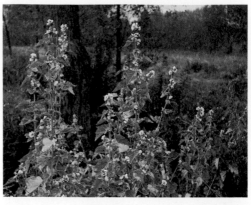

Marshmallow

Althaea officinalis L.

Althaea, Mortification Root, Sweetweed
MALLOW FAMILY
Malvaceae

Although the emperor Charlemagne (742–814) so highly esteemed marshmallow that he ordered its cultivation, the plant would be almost forgotten today if its name were not attached to the popular candy. Its fresh young tops are still eaten in France as a spring tonic, but it is used nowadays generally as a last resort, especially in times of famine. Some Middle Eastern peoples boil marshmallow and then fry it with onions and butter. A confection made from the herb was the inspiration for the candy called marshmallow, but the commercial product contains no trace of the plant.

Medicinally the whole plant, and especially its roots and leaves, are rich in mucilage and therefore good for soothing internal and external inflammations. The name *Althaea* derives from a Greek verb meaning "to heal," and the plant has been the basis for countless medicines since ancient times. Some druggists still sell marshmallow root. The peeled root, boiled and mixed with honey and orange juice, makes a pleasant-tasting, reportedly effective cough syrup. A poultice of the roots was once a home remedy for bruises, sprains, or muscle aches, and the plant's reputed ability to prevent infection earned it the name mortification root.

Habitat: Edges of salt and freshwater marshes.
Range: Introduced from Europe, marshmallow now grows wild in scattered locations in North America from Quebec to Virginia and west to Michigan and Arkansas.
Identification: An upright perennial growing to 4 feet tall, marshmallow has oval to heart-shaped, usually lobed and toothed velvety leaves. Lavender to pinkish-white flowers (July–October) are large, with five petals.

Uses: The mucilage extracted from marshmallow root by boiling is used to soothe the skin and mucous membranes. Scientific studies have established that marshmallow preparations do have a softening and soothing effect when applied to the skin and that an extract from the boiled plant makes a gargle for sore throat.

Marsh Marigold

Caltha palustris L.

American Cowslip, Cowslip, Kingcup, May Blob

BUTTERCUP FAMILY

Ranunculaceae

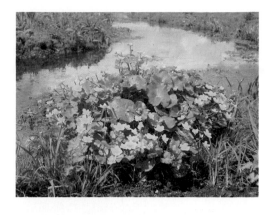

Although it does grow in marshes and other wet places, marsh marigold is not a marigold as its most popular common name implies. Nor is it a cowslip. A New World cousin, likewise called marsh marigold, grows in marshes of western North American mountains. This native species, *C. leptosepala*, is called elkslip in some regions because it is a favored food of elk. It has white flowers but otherwise resembles the yellow marsh marigold.

Human beings eat the raw leaves of either plant at their peril. The leaves contain helleborin, which not only has a burning taste but is also toxic. Cooking removes this poison and also makes the plant more palatable. Commonly, two boilings with a change of water between are necessary to make the taste acceptable. The immature plant's closed buds can be pickled, preferably after boiling, and some wild-food gourmets say that they compare favorably with capers. The flowers have also served to color butter. The plant has certain uses in folk medicine, in external applications for rheumatic pains and to make warts drop off.

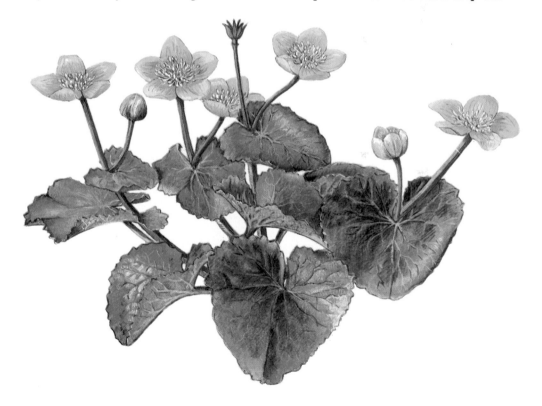

X Do not eat the raw leaves; they can cause violent gastritis and are toxic to the heart. External application of the leaves can cause blistering.
Habitat: Marshes, swamps, wet meadows.
Range: Introduced from Europe, marsh marigold is naturalized from Labrador to Alaska, south to South Carolina and Nebraska. The native species is found in western North American mountains.
Identification: A semisucculent perennial growing 10–30 inches tall. Smooth, round, kidney- or heart-shaped, toothed leaves are clustered at the base and scattered along the hollow branching stem. Shiny yellow flowers (April–August), 1–2 inches across, have five to nine petallike sepals.
Uses: All parts of marsh marigold contain an irritating juice, and poultices of the dried leaves have served to produce skin irritations that were thought to ease rheumatic pains. A drop of the caustic juice squeezed from a leaf or the stem may irritate warts away. The plant is edible after boiling.

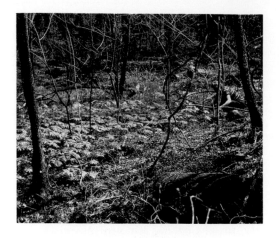

Mayapple

Podophyllum peltatum L.

Devil's-apple, Hog Apple,
Indian Apple, Mandrake,
Umbrella Plant, Wild Lemon

BARBERRY FAMILY

Berberidaceae

The umbrellalike leaves of the mayapple are a common sight in woodlands, where the plant is native. It was well known to North American Indians, who valued it for its powerful laxative effect, as a treatment for intestinal worms, as a cure for warts, and even as an insecticide for use on their crops. Apparently the Indians recognized mayapple's toxic qualities; it is said that they sometimes ate the roots and shoots to commit suicide.

Indians also ate the mayapple's fruits (the only part of the plant that is not poisonous), as many people do to this day. Some, however, say they are insipid. One 19th-century botanist dismissed them as "somewhat mawkish, beloved of pigs, raccoons, and small boys."

The plant's creeping rhizome, pencil-thin and up to 6 feet long, is the part that is used for medicinal purposes. Gathered in autumn as the plants are dying down, the rhizomes are dried and crushed into a powder. Although the remedy has traditionally been used to treat conditions ranging from liver ailments to cancers, mayapple remains best known as a laxative. But its purgative action is so strong that the U.S. Food and Drug Administration lists this use of the plant as "unsafe."

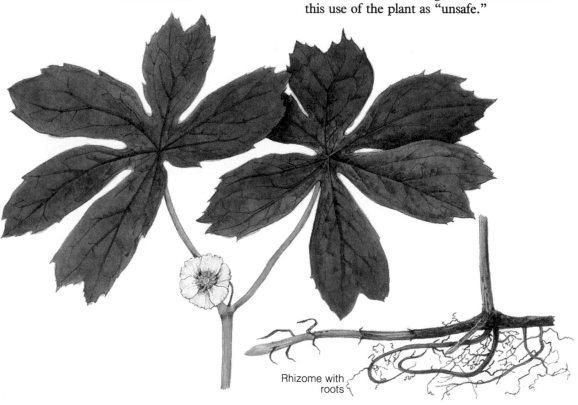

Rhizome with
roots

X All parts except the ripe fruits are poisonous.
Habitat: Well-drained soils in rich, moist woodlands and clearings.
Range: From Quebec to Minnesota south to Florida and Texas.
Identification: A perennial herb 6–18 inches high, usually found growing in patches. The single, forked stem is topped by two deeply lobed, umbrellalike leaves. A solitary waxy white flower (May), 1½ inches across, dangles at the fork of the stem.

The fruit, a pulpy lemon-yellow oval berry, ripens in July–August. Nonflowering plants have an unforked stem and a single leaf.
Uses: Fully ripe fruits can be eaten raw in moderation. The powdered rhizomes have a potent laxative effect. The rhizomes also contain potent anticancer substances, and a derivative of one of these is used to treat human cancers. But extracts of the rhizomes are much too poisonous to be used for self-medication. Mayapple is listed in the *U.S. Pharmacopeia*.

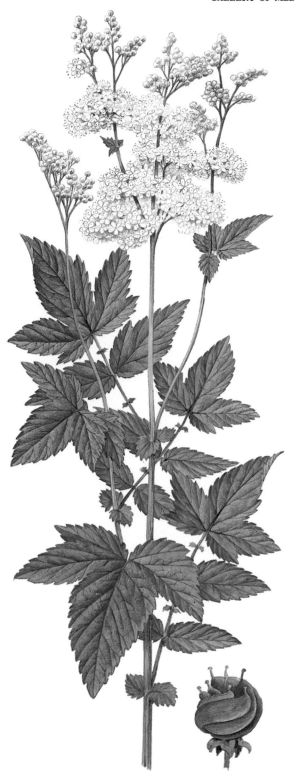

Mature fruit

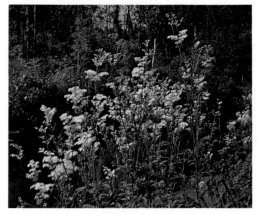

Meadowsweet

Filipendula ulmaria (L.) Maxim.

Bridewort, Queen-of-the-meadow

ROSE FAMILY

Rosaceae

Every time you reach for an aspirin, you owe a debt to meadowsweet, for it was reportedly from this herb that salicylic acid was first obtained, in 1835. Salicylates found in the flowers are the basis of meadowsweet's longstanding reputation as a remedy for flu, rheumatism, arthritis, and fevers. At least part of the relief procured from these blossoms may have been psychological, however—a result of their sweet, almondlike odor. Because of its aroma, Queen Elizabeth I favored the herb above all others for strewing on the floors of her chambers. Its leaf has a pleasant taste, too.

Apt though it may seem, the name meadowsweet is actually a corruption of an older name, *meadsweet*, which like *meadwort* (its oldest English name, going back to Anglo-Saxon times) probably refers to the plant's use as a flavoring for mead, or honey liquor.

According to some herbalists, meadowsweet may well be the best plant remedy for hyperacidity and heartburn, and also helps control peptic ulcers and gastritis. Likewise, herbalists recommend the plant for certain urinary infections. Meadowsweet has a high tannin content, which gives it an astringent action and may make it effective in treating diarrhea.

Habitat: Wet soils, marshes, moist woods.
Range: Introduced from Europe, meadowsweet now grows wild from Newfoundland south to West Virginia and west to Ohio.
Identification: A stout perennial growing up to 6 feet tall, meadowsweet has a creeping underground stem (rhizome) with fleshy nodules. The leaves are pinnately compound with oval, toothed, green leaflets that are gray-white, hairy, and prominently veined below. The terminal leaflet has three lobes. Tiny, fragrant, cream-white, five-petaled flowers (June–August) grow in terminal clusters.
Uses: Herbalists recommend meadowsweet for fever, flu symptoms, and rheumatic pains. The plant contains salicylates, which are useful in treating all of these complaints. Herbal preparations for these and a number of other ailments include a tea brewed from the flowers, a root tea, and a root extract, all of which are astringent.

247

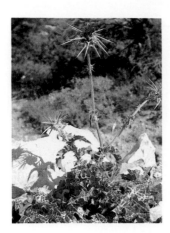

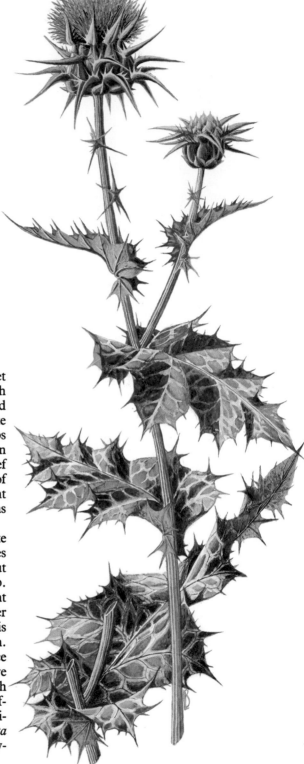

Milk Thistle

Silybum marianum (L.) Gaertn.

Marian Thistle
COMPOSITE FAMILY
Compositae

Like athletes in training, European wet nurses once kept to a special diet, which included milk thistle. The plant increased lactation, they believed, because the white veins that mottled its leaves represented drops of the Virgin Mary's milk, fallen there when she nursed the baby Jesus. This homely belief imposed no hardship apart from the chore of removing the spines; without them, the plant makes a wholesome and delicious food that has long been popular in France.

Apart from its imaginary power to promote lactation, one of the several medicinal virtues traditionally ascribed to milk thistle turns out to have a factual basis. The first-century A.D. Roman naturalist Pliny stated that the plant was "excellent for carrying off bile." In other words, it restores impaired liver function. This has been demonstrated by modern research. The plant contains the chemical substance silymarin, which has a dramatic regenerative effect on the liver. By stimulating the growth of new liver cells, the substance promotes self-repair in a damaged liver. It supplies an antidote to the death cap mushroom (*Amanita phalloides*), which kills its victims by destroying liver cells.

Habitat: Fields, roadsides, waste places.
Range: Native to the Mediterranean region, milk thistle is naturalized in North America mainly on the Pacific Coast, from British Columbia to California, and in the East from Ontario to Alabama.
Identification: A annual or biennial herb growing up to 6 feet tall, milk thistle has coarse, lobed, prickly-edged leaves streaked with conspicuous white veins. Crimson to reddish-violet flowers (May–June) are borne in solitary heads, 2 inches across, surrounded by prominent, spiny bracts.
Uses: The fruit is the source of silymarin, a liver-regenerative drug used in the treatment of hepatitis and cirrhosis and in death cap mushroom poisoning and other forms of liver poisoning. Herbalists say the whole plant is good for both appetite and digestion. Milk thistle is used as a salad green and cooked vegetable.

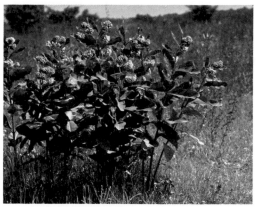

Milkweed

Asclepias syriaca L.

Common Milkweed, Common Silkweed,
Cottonweed, Silky Swallowwort,
Virginia Silk, Wild Cotton

MILKWEED FAMILY

Asclepiadaceae

Milkweed is a native of America, where the Indians discovered its medicinal properties and taught them to the first English settlers of Virginia, as reported in John Gerard's *Herball* (1597). The plant's name refers to its milky white sap, or latex, which the Indians used for skin ailments and which is still used in folk medicine as a treatment for warts, ringworm, poison ivy, and other skin problems. Some tribes used extracts from the boiled roots for conditions as various as bowel and kidney disorders, rheumatism, worms, dropsy (edema), asthma, and venereal diseases.

In the 1800's, American physicians also valued both the sap and the root of milkweed for their medicinal properties, particularly in treating respiratory diseases. They prescribed a tea made from powdered milkweed roots as an asthma remedy and a sedative.

Milkweed is found in many parts of North America. It will thrive in any sunny, open space, from a country meadow to an empty city lot. Milkweed was once cultivated for the silky down from its giant seedpods, which was used to stuff beds, pillows, and—during World War II—life jackets.

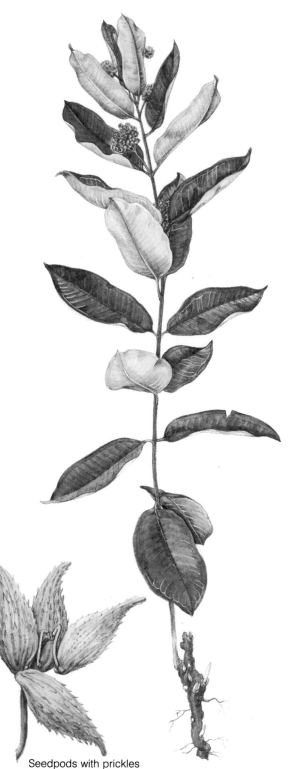

Seedpods with prickles

X Milkweed roots are poisonous.
Habitat: Thickets, roadsides, meadows, dry and cultivated fields, vacant urban lots.
Range: New Brunswick to Saskatchewan; New England south to Georgia and Tennessee and west to Iowa and Kansas.
Identification: A perennial with a stout, un-branched stem growing to 3–6 feet. The large, leathery leaves are opposite, 4–8 inches long, smooth above, densely downy below. Conspicu-ous, nodding clusters of fragrant, usually purplish flowers (June–August) are followed by fleshy, grayish-green seedpods, 2–5 inches long, filled with seeds bearing down. All parts of the plant ooze milky latex when bruised or cut.
Uses: The young shoots, flowers, and pods may be boiled as vegetables. The latex is a traditional remedy for skin problems. The roots were formerly used to treat many ailments, including respiratory and intestinal diseases, but are poisonous.

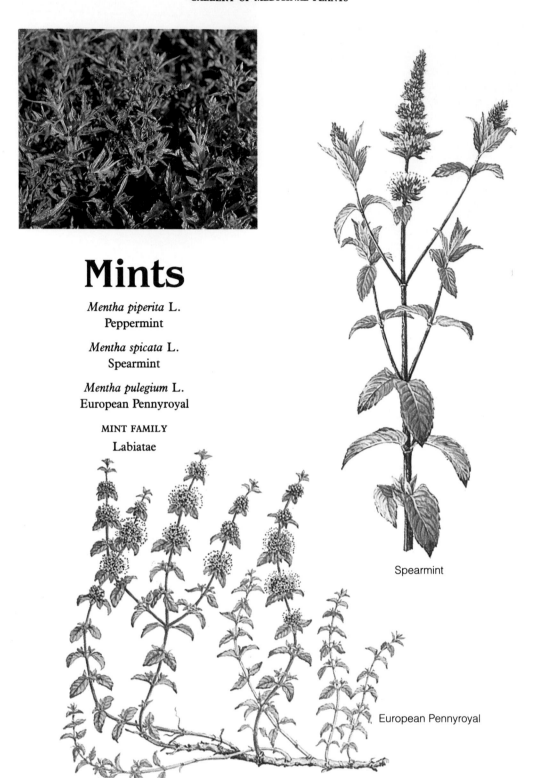

Mints

Mentha piperita L.
Peppermint

Mentha spicata L.
Spearmint

Mentha pulegium L.
European Pennyroyal

MINT FAMILY
Labiatae

Spearmint

European Pennyroyal

X European pennyroyal taken internally in large doses has produced convulsions and coma.
Habitat: Damp shade; moist, rich soil.
Range: Native to Europe, peppermint, spearmint, and European pennyroyal are cultivated throughout most of temperate North America and have escaped locally.
Identification: These perennial herbs, all with square stems, spread by means of runners and flower from June to October.

Peppermint, 3 feet tall, has toothed, oblong to oval, stalked leaves, up to 2 inches long. Lilac-pink flowers grow in dense club-shaped spikes.

Spearmint, growing to 3 feet tall, has sharply toothed, lance-shaped leaves, up to 2½ inches long, which are either stalkless or on short stalks. Lilac to pink to white flowers occur in whorls in slender spikes at the end of the stem or branches.

European pennyroyal is approximately 1½ feet in height and has smooth-edged or slightly

With more than 25 species and perhaps hundreds of varieties and hybrids, mints are a complex plant group to classify. The different species share many common characteristics and chemical properties. Even botanists frequently find it hard to determine how to name a given specimen. The best-known species in North America are peppermint and spearmint, which are highly valued for commercial use. Peppermint's volatile oil, which contains menthol, is employed in the manufacture of medicines, candies, liqueurs, cigarettes, and other products. Spearmint's pleasant but less potent flavor comes from its leaves and oil and has made it an important commodity in the food industry. Not only is spearmint an ingredient in mint sauces and jellies, but it is used to flavor chewing gum and candy, liqueurs, and baked goods; it is packaged as dried flakes for household use; and the fresh product is bought by restaurants and bars to flavor lamb and vegetable dishes and to garnish iced teas, mint juleps, and other drinks. Growers in the United States plant about 67,000 acres of peppermint and some 28,000 acres of spearmint annually.

Medicinal interest in mints dates from the first century A.D., when it was recorded by the Roman naturalist Pliny. In Elizabethan times more than 40 ailments were reported to be remedied by mints, a fact that may have prompted John Josselyn, a 17th-century visitor to New England, to note that mint was included in a list of plants being taken to the New World. The foremost use of mints today in both home remedies and in pharmaceutical preparations is to relieve the stomach and intestinal gas that is often caused by certain foods. The many varieties of after-dinner mint candies and liqueurs attest to mint's competence in this role. The utilization of menthol, derived from peppermint, in upper respiratory ailments and as a soothing rub for sore muscles is easily verified by a trip to the corner pharmacy, where the labels of many respiratory preparations and rubs indicate the presence of this oil. The oil in spearmint is largely responsible for scenting toiletry goods.

Many of the mints' past uses continue in one form or another to the present time. Because of their strong smell, mints were scattered about to rid houses and public places of foul odors and to repel vermin. Today the plants' deodor-

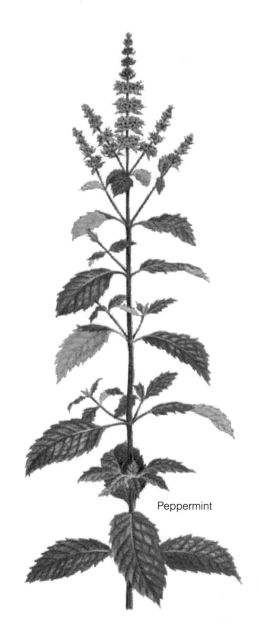

Peppermint

ant properties have been capitalized on in mint-flavored mouthwashes and toothpastes manufactured to sweeten the breath.

European pennyroyal has a strong odor that is offensive to insects. Its oil, if taken orally, is highly poisonous—more than half an ounce may cause severe liver damage.

---

toothed, hairy, oval leaves, up to 1½ inches long, on short stalks. Lilac to pink flowers grow in round whorls in the leaf axils at the top of the stems or branches.
Uses: Peppermint's menthol is added to many medications for its therapeutic effects, particularly to ease the discomfort of gas.

Spearmint, also cited as a carminative (an agent that relieves gas pains), is widely used in cooking, especially in lamb dishes and to enhance bever-

ages such as mint juleps, punches, and iced teas.

European pennyroyal has been used to ward off insects, as a carminative, and as an emmenagogue (an agent that induces menstruation).

Scientists confirm the use of peppermint and spearmint as carminatives and the employment of European pennyroyal as an insect repellent, but they cannot verify pennyroyal's usefulness as a carminative or as an emmenagogue. Spearmint and peppermint make refreshing herbal teas.

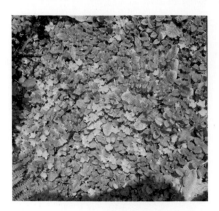

Moneywort

Lysimachia nummularia L.

Creeping Jenny, Meadow Runagates,
Twopenny Grass, Wandering Jenny,
Wandering Sailor
PRIMROSE FAMILY

Primulaceae

So extraordinary are the wound-healing virtues of moneywort that even snakes know of them! Injured serpents, the story goes, seek out the plant to curl up on its leaves and thereby heal themselves. Moneywort's serpentine way of creeping along the ground may account for this old folk belief.

Ever since medieval times, moneywort has served for the treatment of wounds and sores. In the early 1700's the pioneering Dutch physician Hermann Boerhaave recommended the dried and powdered plant for the treatment of scurvy and bleeding wounds. In this he was in line with predecessors such as the Englishmen Nicholas Culpeper and John Gerard. The latter had gone so far as to declare of moneywort, in his *Herball* (1597): "There is not a better wound herb." Gerard also stated that the plant's juice boiled with wine and honey was good for any internal bleeding. Herbalists have also recommended a decoction, or extract, brewed from the whole plant for external application on wounds, cuts, and sores, and a syrup made from it was at one time given for whooping cough. The plant's shiny, coinlike leaves inspired its common name and its species name, *nummularia*, which comes from a Latin word for money.

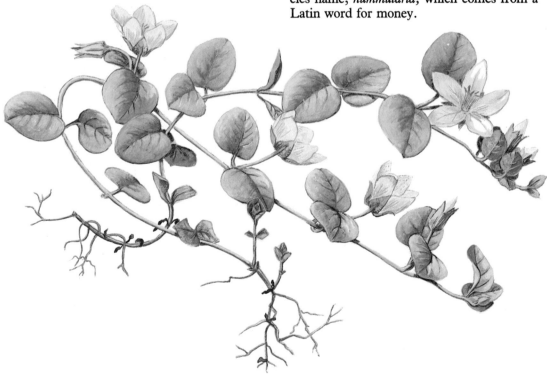

Habitat: Moist places, shores, roadsides, meadows, grasslands.

Range: Introduced from Europe, moneywort now grows wild in North America from Newfoundland south to Georgia, west to Missouri and Kansas, and on the Pacific Coast.

Identification: A creeping perennial with trailing stems up to 5 feet long. Glossy rounded leaves grow in opposite pairs. Golden yellow flowers (June–August), ¾–1¼ inches across, have five petals, often marked with dark spots, and grow singly at the axils of the leaves.

Uses: There is no modern evidence to support moneywort's traditional use to stop internal bleeding or as a whooping cough remedy. However, pharmacologists agree that it has a mildly astringent action and would therefore be effective in helping to heal minor external wounds.

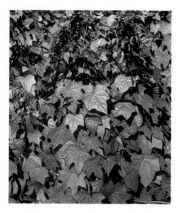

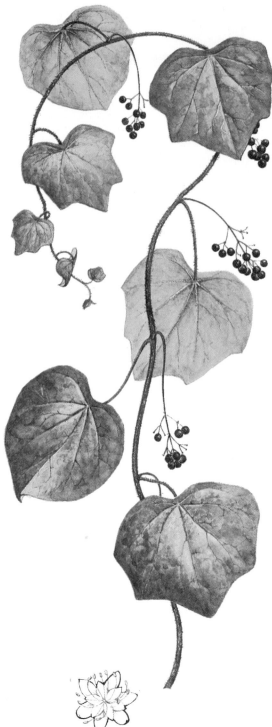

Open male flower

Moonseed

Menispermum canadense L.

Canada Moonseed, Texas Sarsaparilla,
Vine Maple, Yellow Parilla

MOONSEED FAMILY

Menispermaceae

Like the moon, moonseed has its bright and dark sides. On the bright side, this North American vine's roots furnished 19th-century medicine with a drug that was not only an effective diuretic and laxative but also reportedly useful in treating a wide range of ailments, from tuberculosis of the lymph glands in the neck to certain rheumatic and arthritic diseases. The plant contains berberine and related alkaloids long employed in the treatment of various chronic illnesses. American Indians had already arrived at some similar uses empirically and passed the lore along to settlers in pioneering times. Moonseed was an official drug in the *U.S. Pharmacopeia* at the turn of the century. The root extract once served as a substitute for sarsaparilla in soft drinks.

On the the dark side, this plant produces poisonous blue-black berries that can easily be mistaken for wild grapes, and there have been accidental deaths. Excessive doses bring on an increased pulse rate and violent vomiting and purging. The berries give the plant both its common and botanical names. Each berry contains one seed shaped like a crescent moon—hence the name *Menispermum*, from Greek words meaning "moon" and "seed."

X The berries may cause death by inducing an extremely rapid pulse rate and severe vomiting and purging.
Habitat: Banks of streams, moist woods.
Range: Native to North America from Manitoba to Quebec and through the eastern United States south to Georgia and west to Oklahoma.
Identification: A deciduous perennial climbing vine growing up to 12 feet tall. The yellow root is long and round. The leaves are broad and lobed, with long slender stalks, and are shaped like shields. Small greenish-yellow flowers (June–July) appear in clusters, soon followed by the poisonous blue-black one-seeded berries.
Uses: A tea prepared from the root or a root extract long served in herbal medicine as a diuretic, laxative, appetite stimulant, and what was called an alterative, or drug that favorably alters the course of an ailment. Herbalists today recommend the same tea as a tonic, diuretic, and laxative.

253

Mormon Tea

Ephedra nevadensis Wats.

Brigham Tea, Desert Tea, Joint Fir,
Mexican Tea, Popotillo, Squaw Tea

EPHEDRA FAMILY

Gnetaceae

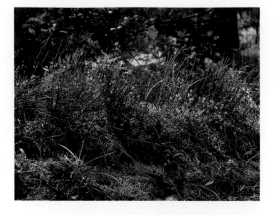

A stunted, weather-beaten shrub, Mormon tea has furnished a refreshing beverage for residents of Mexico and the American Southwest since Aztec times. By one account the name refers to the early Mormon settlers, who abstained from regular tea and coffee, but drank the beverage made from this plant. The tea is brewed from the powdered twigs.

There are in fact several North American ephedras known as Mormon tea; the commonest are *E. nevadensis*, pictured here, and *E. trifurca*. The Indians used one species of Mormon tea or another for colds, fever, and headache; as a remedy for syphilis; and for various other internal troubles. The dried and powdered twigs were used in poultices for burns and ointments for sores. A preparation from the scales on the leaves was applied to help stop bleeding. The plant has also enjoyed a reputation as a diuretic, and this home use remains popular among Indians and Spanish-speaking people on both sides of the Rio Grande. It is

also used for rheumatic and arthritic pains.

Mormon tea is related to the Chinese plant mahuang (*E. sinica*), which contains the drug ephedrine—a bronchial dilator, decongestant, and central nervous system stimulant much used in modern medicine. The American species has no ephedrine, however.

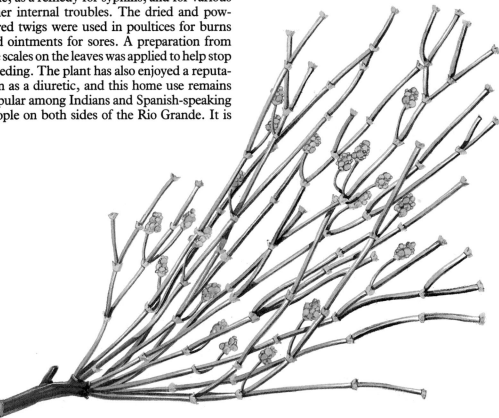

Habitat: Deserts, dry mountainsides.
Range: Native to the U.S. Southwest and Mexico.
Identification: A profusely branched broomlike shrub growing up to 4 feet tall, with slender, jointed stems. Scaly leaves grow in opposite pairs or whorls of three and are fused for half their length. Male and female yellow-green flowers (March–April) are borne in separate conelike structures and followed by small brown to black seeds.
Uses: A tea brewed from twigs of the plant is to this

day a popular thirst quencher and folk remedy; however, none of its uses in folk medicine have been validated by research. Although no ephedrine is found in the American ephedras, proponents of Mormon tea maintain that it works as a decongestant and asthma remedy, like its ephedrine-rich Chinese relative, mahuang. In the desert, people chew a piece of the twig to relieve the pain of sunburned lips.

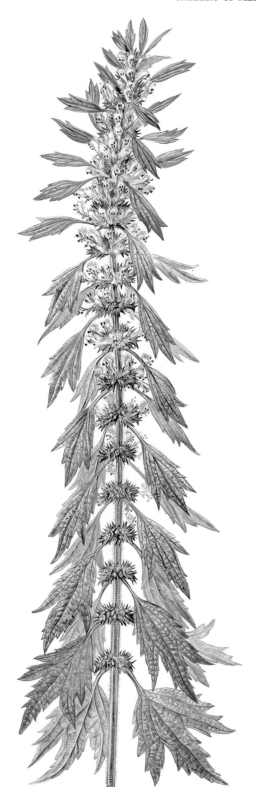

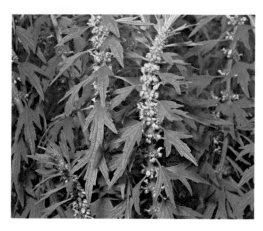

Motherwort

Leonurus cardiaca L.

Lion's-ear, Lion's-tail,
Lion's-tart, Throwwort
MINT FAMILY
Labiatae

Many "commend it against the infirmities of the heart: it is judged to be so forceable that it is thought it took this name *cardiaca*, of the effect," the 16th-century herbalist John Gerard observed of motherwort. Since ancient times people have used motherwort in the way that its botanical name, *cardiaca*, indicates— as a sedative for cardiac complaints. In Europe even today some herbalists prescribe motherwort conserve, a mixture of the fresh young plant tops and sugar, for heart palpitations.

The Greeks long ago proclaimed the plant's sedative powers. They valued motherwort not only as a remedy for heart disease but also as a pain reliever during childbirth, a fact that accounts for its common name. English colonists brought the plant to America for these uses, which had spread throughout Europe over the centuries, and as a medicine for menstrual cramps. Belief in the plant's tranquilizing powers also led to its use as a treatment for convulsions and nervous disorders.

In other lands, motherwort found more exotic uses. The Japanese once drank a beverage from the flowers to prolong life, and the Russians used motherwort in the treatment of rabies.

X Persons prone to dermatitis should avoid handling motherwort.
Habitat: Vacant lots and other waste places.
Range: Native to Europe, motherwort is naturalized in North America from Nova Scotia to Montana and south to Texas and North Carolina.
Identification: A perennial herb growing to 5 feet tall. The leaves are shaggy-looking and to some resemble a lion's tail—hence one of the plant's alternative names. Each leaf has three lance-shaped lobes. The tiny flowers (June–September) are pink, white, or purple and grow in clusters.
Uses: Motherwort has long been specified for female disorders and as a childbirth aid. Today it is used as an emmenagogue (to promote menstruation). Pharmacologists state that this use of the plant may be valid, but they question motherwort's effectiveness either as an antispasmodic or as a sedative and hence its effectiveness as a heart medicine.

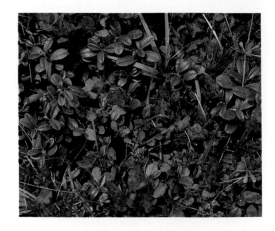

Mountain Cranberry

Vaccinium vitis-idaea L.

Cowberry, Foxberry, Lingberry
HEATH FAMILY

Ericaceae

Not to be confused with the American cranberry (*V. macrocarpon*), from which comes the popular Thanksgiving sauce, the mountain cranberry is a dwarf shrub with smaller fruits and lives in a still harsher environment. Although the American cranberry is raised in lowland bogs, the mountain type, true to its name, is found on high northern slopes and sometimes in Arctic peat bogs. For gourmets there is an added plus: the American cranberry is an ordinary supermarket item, but *Vaccinium vitis-idaea* is something of a delicacy. In Canada and parts of Europe, however (especially in Scandinavia, where they are called lingonberries), the berries are standard fare and are made into a jelly.

Mountain cranberry leaves, as several herbals indicate, have antiseptic and diuretic medicinal properties. A French legend hints at even greater powers, verging on the magical: a young girl who had lost her arms steeped a copious supply of the berries in water, and then plunged into the mixture. Thereupon—so the story goes—her arms miraculously grew back, and she emerged as good as new.

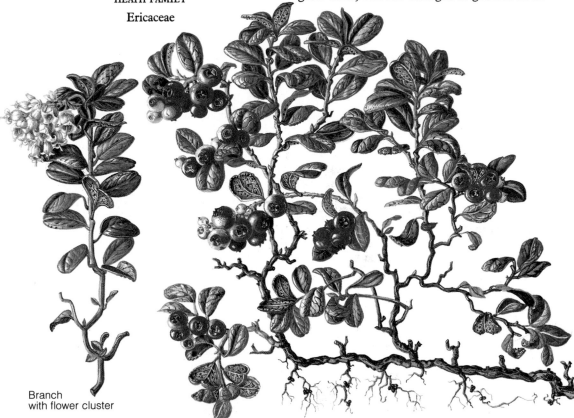

Branch
with flower cluster

Habitat: Rocky, dry, acid soil in upland forests, especially pine; peat bogs and tundra.

Range: Native to northern climates, mountain cranberry is found in North America from Arctic and subarctic regions to southern Canada, New England, and northern Minnesota.

Identification: An evergreen shrub growing to 8 inches tall. The slender stems bear tiny (¼- to ½-inch-long), leathery alternate leaves with minute black bristles below. Tiny white to pinkish-red flowers (June–July) are bell-shaped and produce dark red berries that are edible when cooked.

Uses: Some people substitute mountain cranberries for American cranberries in sauces and jelly. Medicinally, the plant leaves are used as an antiseptic and a diuretic. Pharmacologists find that the plant's use as an antiseptic is valid, but question its effectiveness as a diuretic.

Mouse-ear

Hieracium pilosella L.

Felon Herb, Hawkweed, Mouse-ear Hawkweed, Pilosella

COMPOSITE FAMILY

Compositae

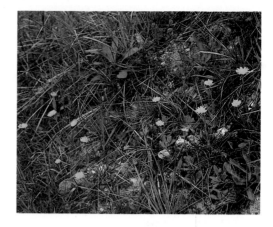

Though it is a lowly dwarf of a weed that shows up in carpetlike patches over dry pastures and waste areas throughout the Northern Hemisphere, mouse-ear belongs to a genus whose botanical name has fierce connotations. *Hieracium* means "hawkweed," and the plant is so called because the ancients fancied that hawks would tear open the plant and wet their eyes with its juice to improve their vision, so that they could swoop down on their prey with deadlier accuracy. Of all the hawkweeds, the humble mouse-ear enjoyed the longest-lasting reputation as a remedy for a number of common ills. A tea brewed from its small hairy oblong leaves—like a mouse's ears—reputedly cured liver ailments, intestinal inflammations, and diarrhea, and was also recommended for asthma and other respiratory troubles. In addition, mouse-ear figured in herbal medicine as a fever-reducing agent, and a powder made from it was used to stem nosebleeds.

Mouse-ear's alternative name felon herb has nothing to do with criminals. It derives from an old sense of *felon* meaning "boil, inflammation on a finger or toe." External application of the tea, which is an astringent, doubtless served in such cases. Even today, mouse-ear tea is an occasional home remedy for fever, bronchial complaints, and diarrhea.

Habitat: Pastures, fields, waste places.
Range: Native to Europe, mouse-ear now grows as a weed from Newfoundland to Minnesota, south to North Carolina, and west to the Pacific Coast.
Identification: A perennial growing 3–15 inches high, mouse-ear grows carpetlike on creeping runners, each of which forms a basal rosette of oval leaves. The leaves are green with white hairs above and gray-green or white with softer hairs below. Bright yellow to orange-yellow flowerheads (May–September), resembling dandelions, are borne singly on leafless stalks.
Uses: Herbalists claim that mouse-ear has expectorant, tonic, astringent, and antibiotic properties. A tea brewed from the whole plant is used both internally and externally, and may be used as a gargle and skin wash, or lotion. However, very little research is available to substantiate these uses.

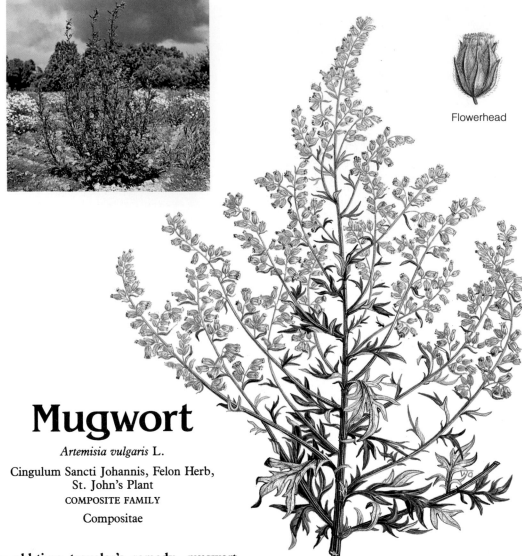

Flowerhead

Mugwort

Artemisia vulgaris L.

Cingulum Sancti Johannis, Felon Herb,
St. John's Plant

COMPOSITE FAMILY

Compositae

An old-time traveler's remedy, mugwort protected medieval pilgrims not only from fatigue but also from sunstroke and wild beasts or demons encountered along the road. John the Baptist wore a *cingulum,* or belt, woven from it in the wilderness, according to legend. Wayfarers once put it in their shoes to keep from becoming footsore. Even today, one modern herbal recommends steeping mugwort in water to make a bath for tired feet.

Just as useful for the stay-at-home, mugwort earned a place in the kitchen, the clothes closet, and the medicine chest. Used in England long ago as a tea substitute and in the making of beer, this aromatic herb continues to figure as a poultry stuffing in various eastern European cuisines. Mugwort leaves laid in clothing protect it against moths, and a pillow stuffed with the herb was formerly believed to reveal a sleeper's future to him or her in a dream. Mugwort also enjoyed the endorsement of Hippocrates and Dioscorides as a specific to ease and hasten childbirth, and some homeopathic doctors prescribe it as a mild sedative for women during menopause. The plant was also listed in old herbals as a remedy for palsy and epilepsy.

Habitat: Roadsides, vacant lots, riverbanks.
Range: Introduced from Europe, mugwort now grows wild in Canada from Newfoundland to Ontario and in the United States from New England south to Georgia and west to Minnesota, and along the Pacific coast.
Identification: An aromatic, many-branched, shrubby perennial, 1¼–6½ feet tall, mugwort has angular, grooved, red-brown stems and deeply cut leaves that are dark green above and white below. Yellow to red-brown flowerheads (July–September) are borne in long loose clusters.
Uses: According to herbalist tradition, mugwort leaves increase menstrual flow and facilitate childbirth; studies of the former use have shown it to be of questionable value. The leaves have also been used as a stimulant in folk medicine—also a practice of doubtful value, according to pharmacologists. Mugwort leaves are a natural insect repellent and are sometimes used as a culinary herb.

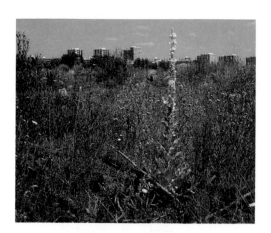

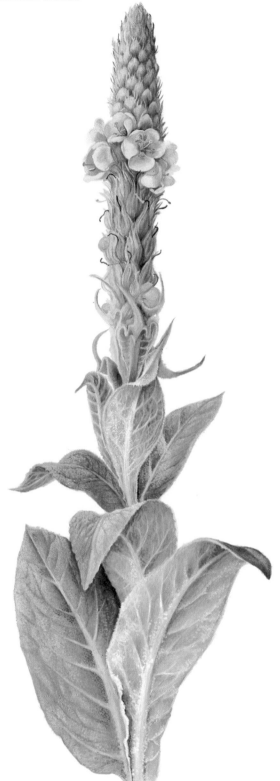

Mullein

Verbascum thapsus L.

Bunny's Ears, Flannelleaf, Jacob's-staff
SNAPDRAGON FAMILY

Scrophulariaceae

Since antiquity mankind has used the velvety mullein (rhymes with sullen) plant for many purposes. From Roman times the stem—stripped of the leaves and flowers and dipped in tallow—was carried as a torch in religious processions. In folklore, mullein torches were said both to repel witches and to be used by them. By a similar paradox, one belief held that wearing mullein leaves insured conception, while another declared that a leaf placed in a shoe would protect against it. Whichever questionable belief prevailed, woolly mullein leaves stuffed in shoes were known to keep thinly shod feet warm in winter.

Mullein also has an ancient history as a medicine and a cosmetic. The Greek physician Dioscorides prescribed it for respiratory ailments—a therapeutic use that continues to this day. Smoking mullein leaves is an old folk remedy for coughs and asthma. Preparations from the leaves were applied to soften the skin. Women, lacking rouge, sometimes rubbed their cheeks with the rough leaf to make them glow, and mullein therefore was dubbed Quaker rouge. In another cosmetic use, the yellow dye from the flowers has served as a hair rinse since Roman times.

Habitat: Fields, pastures, roadsides.
Range: Naturalized from Europe in temperate regions of North America.
Identification: A biennial plant, growing to 8 feet tall. A rosette of leaves appears on the ground the first year; a tall spike of flowers rises the next. Both leaves and stems are velvety. Five-petaled yellow flowers (June–September), ¼ to 1 inch across, bloom randomly along the stalk.
Uses: Large concentrations of mucilage in mullein make it a demulcent (a substance that soothes mucous membranes) and an expectorant and thus effective in the treatment of some respiratory ailments. Mullein leaf or flower tea was given for chest colds, bronchitis, and asthma. Mullein has also been used to relieve inflammations; extracts of mullein show strong anti-inflammatory activity in laboratory tests. Oil from the flowers is also said to be good for earaches.

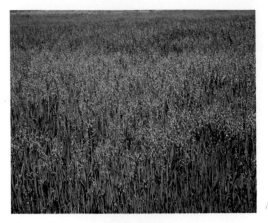

Oats

Avena sativa L.

Common Oats, Groats
GRASS FAMILY
Gramineae

In his dictionary of the English language, Dr. Samuel Johnson disparaged oats by referring to it as "a grain, which in England is generally given to horses, but in Scotland supports the people." Johnson may have found the Scots' appetite coarse, but in fact it showed their good sense, because oats is an exceptionally nourishing, wholesome food and also supplies fiber in the diet. Indeed, old-time physicians used to recommend a diet of oatmeal gruel for convalescents because it is so easily digested. Doctors also used to prescribe a solution of wine and oats as a restorative for those with "a deficiency of nervous power," such as "overworked lawyers, public speakers, and writers." Modern folk healers still mention oats for nervous exhaustion and also advocate it as an antispasmodic and an antidepressant.

Many modern doctors prescribe oatmeal, in an external pack, for psoriasis and other skin disorders. For those concerned with aging skin, a facial pack of oatmeal is a common treatment for staving off wrinkles—and far less expensive than commercial treatments.

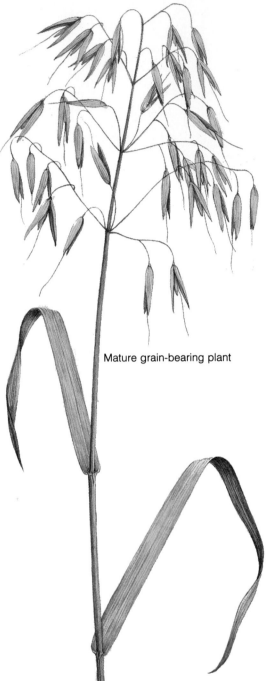

Mature grain-bearing plant

Habitat: Fields, waste places.
Range: Introduced from Europe, oats is cultivated throughout temperate regions of North America. It often escapes cultivation and grows wild.
Identification: An annual grass growing up to 4 feet tall, with a hollow jointed stem. Pale green leaves are narrow, flat, lance-shaped, and rough. Pale green flowers (April–June) are borne in loose terminal clusters, with each spikelet consisting of two florets. The fruit, or grain, is grooved and downy.

Uses: Oats has traditionally been considered an easily digestible food for convalescing patients. Nutritionists recommend oatmeal for its bran content, which supplies fiber. Pharmacologists have found that the use of oats as an antidepressant may have some validity. Medical science has established that oat preparations, which are available commercially, help to heal skin disorders.

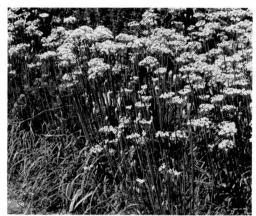

Onion

Allium cepa L.

Common Onion
LILY FAMILY
Liliaceae

According to the Greek historian Herodotus, nine tons of gold was spent buying onions to feed the builders of the pyramids, so popular was this vegetable in ancient Egypt. Indeed, much to the amusement of the conquering Romans, the Egyptians even offered the bulb as a sacrifice. In the later Middle Ages the onion—probably because of its strong smell—was used as a charm against evil spirits and the plague. Sulfur compounds give onions (and garlic) their sharp flavor and aroma, which folk healers thought were indications that the juice of the plant could prevent infection. Some modern herbals state that applications of onion will remove warts and prevent acne. They recommend an onion syrup as an expectorant. Onions are also held to be diuretic and to reduce high blood pressure. Certainly the onion is a superlative tonic, since it is rich in vitamins, including B_1 (thiamine), B_2 (riboflavin), and C.

The onion and its relatives have been known in North America for centuries, and were a favorite spring food of the Indians. Frontiersmen knew that a sure way to locate Indian encampments in spring was to follow the heavy onion scent that clung to the area.

Habitat: Prefers rich garden soil.
Range: Probably a native of southwest Asia, *A. cepa* is now cultivated worldwide and may have escaped cultivation in some places.
Identification: A perennial herb arising from a bulb. The plant can grow as high as 4 feet and has four to six hollow cylindrical leaves. The greenish-white flowers (June–July) grow in globular, solitary umbels, ¼–1 inch across, on a long hollow cylindrical stalk.

Uses: Like garlic, onion has been used medicinally for centuries as an external antiseptic. Studies conducted indicate that onion may be helpful in allaying intestinal gas pains; in reducing hypertension, high blood sugar (as in diabetes), and the cholesterol and fat content of the blood; and in relieving pain and inflammation. Both raw and cooked, onion is a popular vegetable throughout the world.

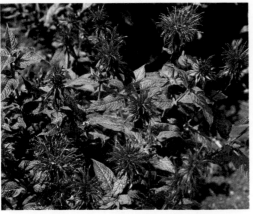

Oswego Tea

Monarda didyma L.

Bee Balm, Indian Plume, Scarlet Bergamot
MINT FAMILY
Labiatae

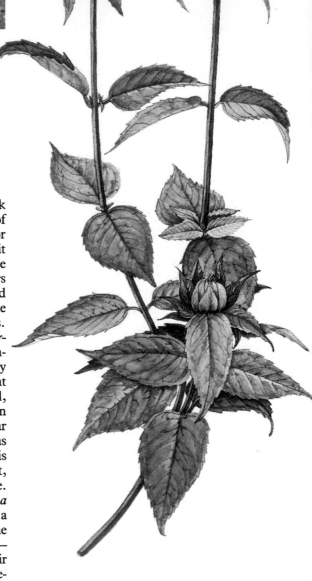

The Oswego Indians of western New York made tea from the dried aromatic leaves of *Monarda didyma* and shared their fondness for it with colonial settlers—who went on to use it as a substitute when imported tea became scarce after the Boston Tea Party. The Shakers thought the tea effective in treating colds and sore throats, while other settlers steamed the plant and inhaled the fumes to clear sinuses.

Closely related to *Monarda didyma* is *Monarda fistulosa*. The two species often share common names. However, *M. didyma* is the only one correctly called Oswego tea. It has bright red flowers and grows best in rich, moist soil, especially in deciduous forests. It is also known as scarlet bergamot because its scent is similar to that of the bergamot orange. *M. fistulosa* has lavender or sometimes white flowers and is seen in drier, sunnier areas. Apart from that, the two species are very similar in appearance. Both species are highly aromatic. *M. didyma* has a citrus smell, while *M. fistulosa* gives off a spicy, minty odor. From colonial days to the present both species—and several hybrids— have been garden flowers popular for their color and ability to attract butterflies, bumblebees, and hummingbirds.

Habitat: *M. didyma* prefers moist soil and woods while *M. fistulosa* favors dry, open places.
Range: Native to eastern North America, with *M. fistulosa* extending farther west, as far as Texas and British Columbia. *M. didyma* is an endangered or threatened species in some states.
Identification: Both *M. didyma* and *M. fistulosa* are perennial herbs whose opposite leaves emit a strong scent when disturbed. Square stems grow 2–5 feet tall. *M. didyma* has dark green leaves, 4– 6 inches long; *M. fistulosa*, gray-green leaves, about 2½ inches long. Roundish flowerheads (June–August) are crimson to bright red in *M. didyma*, lavender to white (July–August) in *M. fistulosa*.
Uses: Both species are cultivated as ornamentals, and the dried leaves are used for making tea and potpourris. The aromatic oil of Oswego tea is sometimes used in perfumery. Neither plant is officially recommended for medicinal use today.

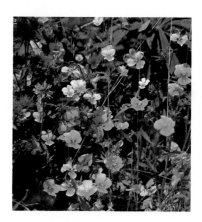

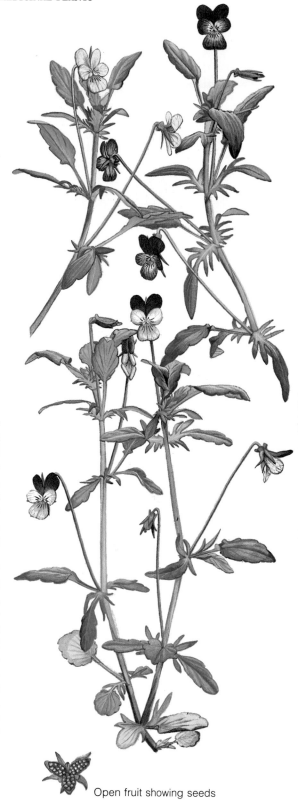

Pansy

Viola tricolor L.

Field Pansy, Heartsease, Johnny-jump-up,
Ladies'-delight, Wild Pansy

VIOLET FAMILY

Violaceae

"That's for thoughts," Shakespeare's Ophelia says of pansies, because their name comes from French *pensée*, "thought." In traditional "flower language," pansy's three colors—purple, white, and yellow—stand for memories, loving thoughts, and souvenirs, all of which ease the hearts of separated lovers. Pansy therefore is also called by the name heartsease, and its juice once served as an ingredient in love potions.

The flowers or whole flowering plant, either fresh or dried, yield a bitter tea that was employed to remedy a wide variety of ills. John Gerard's *Herball* (1597) quotes medical opinion that pansy tea is effective for infantile convulsions, goes on to commend it for "chest and lung inflammations," and also speaks of its effectiveness externally for scabs, itching, and ulcers. This external use caused pansy to be listed for a time in the *U.S. Pharmacopeia*, and has continued in herbal medicine. The tea also served in folk medicine as a fever-reducing remedy, a diuretic, a laxative, a sedative, an expectorant, a gargle, and a "blood purifier," or agent that rids the body of toxic substances.

Open fruit showing seeds

Habitat: Fields, wastelands, and forest edges.
Range: Introduced from Europe, pansy has escaped from gardens in temperate North America.
Identification: An annual growing to more than 15 inches tall, pansy produces many seeds sprouting so readily that it reappears like a perennial. Its flowers (May–September), ½–1 inch long, display patterns of purple, white, and yellow.
Uses: A tea or extract brewed from dried pansy flowers, from the whole flowering plant, or from the root long served in the treatment of skin ailments. It was applied externally as a lotion or taken internally to rid the body of toxic products that were thought to cause skin problems. Like its cousin *V. odorata,* it was used as an expectorant, for loosening phlegm. Pansy has also been thought to be a demulcent (a substance that soothes mucous membranes, as of the respiratory tract). There is no scientific evidence regarding the validity of any claims made for pansy's healing properties.

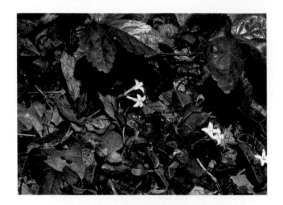

Partridge-berry

Mitchella repens L.

Deerberry, One-berry,
Squaw Vine, Winter Clover
MADDER FAMILY

Rubiaceae

Partridgeberry brightens the drab forest floor in fall and winter, its mats of evergreen leaves and scarlet fruits hugging the ground. Landscapers often transplant this cheerful creeper to residential yards, where it is used in rock gardens and as ornamental ground cover under shrubs, thriving especially in acid soil.

The twin white flowers that adorn the ends of partridgeberry stems merge to form a single fruit, as the name one-berry indicates. The low fat content of the fruits makes them resistant to rotting, so that they stay intact on the branches late into winter and are available to nourish wildlife when other foods are lacking.

The delectable-looking but nearly tasteless fruits are said to be favored by ruffed grouse, birds similar to European partridges—hence the name partridgeberry. Another common name suggests that this creeping plant supplies food for deer.

Partridgeberry is a native American plant, and the name squaw vine comes from its use among the Indians. During the final weeks of pregnancy women drank a tea made from the leaves to ease childbirth, and nursing mothers applied a lotion made from the leaves to their breasts to relieve soreness. English colonists also used the tea as an aid in childbirth and as a remedy for menstrual cramps.

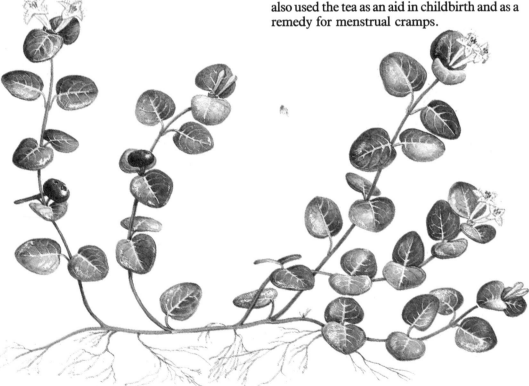

Habitat: Forests.
Range: Native to North America, partridgeberry is distributed from Newfoundland to Minnesota, as far south as Florida and Texas.
Identification: A creeping, evergreen perennial. Its round shiny leaves have white markings and grow in opposite pairs. White flowers (May–July), ¼ inch wide with four to five fringed petals, are borne in pairs at the ends of branches growing to 3 feet long. Conspicuous red berrylike fruits remain on the plant in fall and winter and throughout most of the remaining seasons of the year.
Uses: Partridgeberry plants contain tannin, which accounts for its traditional use as an astringent. Although the plant is used as an emmenagogue (to promote menstruation) and an ecbolic (to facilitate childbirth by increasing uterine contractions), scientific studies do not bear out the effectiveness of these uses.

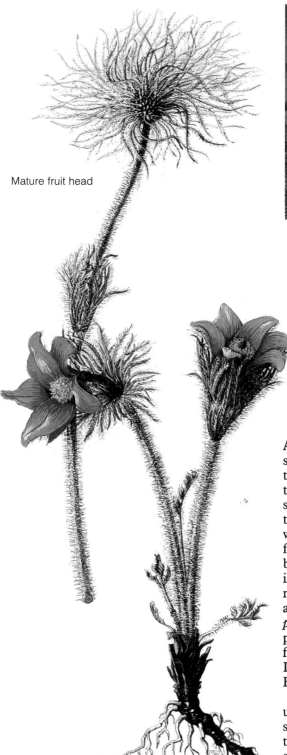

Mature fruit head

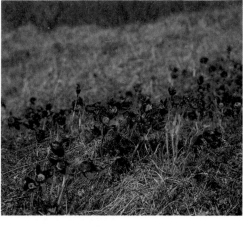

Pasque-flower

Anemone patens L.

Hartshorn Plant, Prairie Smoke,
Twinflower, Wild Crocus

BUTTERCUP FAMILY

Ranunculaceae

A harbinger of spring, the pasqueflower was so named because it blooms at Eastertime throughout much of its range. In some parts of the Midwest and West it is called prairie smoke, for after the flower has bloomed and the fruit head ripens, the long hairy threads to which the fruits are attached turn silky and feathery. When these feathery tails are blown by wind gusts, the resulting effect gives the illusion of smoke crossing the prairie. The name wild crocus also denotes the plant's role as a herald of spring. The Latin species name *patens* alludes to the spreading fashion of the plant's petallike sepals. Because the pasqueflower usually produces two flower stems, the Dakota Sioux Indians gave it a name that in English means "twinflower."

Some Indians, it is reported, found practical uses for the pasqueflower. They stuffed the sepals up the nose to help halt bleeding, and they crushed the leaves and applied them externally to relieve rheumatism.

Pasqueflower is South Dakota's state flower.

X A volatile oil in the plant irritates the skin and mucous membranes and may cause blistering.
Habitat: Prairies, woods, moist meadows, exposed slopes.
Range: Native to North America, pasqueflower grows from Alaska south through western Canada and the midwestern and western United States.
Identification: An erect perennial herb with usually two hairy stems growing up to 16 inches tall. It has silky-haired basal leaves, palmately divided into lobes, each of which is again cut into long segments. A golden yellow cluster of stamens, about ½ inch across at the center of the flower (March–July), is surrounded by five to seven white to blue or lavender petallike sepals. This cluster is followed by a fruiting head with feathery styles (tails), each of which is attached to a fruitlet.
Uses: North American Indians seem to have used the plant medicinally to a small extent, but it appears to be seldom if ever used today.

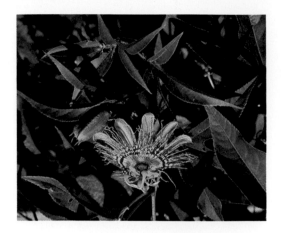

Passion-flower

Passiflora incarnata L.

Apricot Vine, Maypop, Passion Vine,
Purple Passionflower, Wild Passionflower
PASSIONFLOWER FAMILY

Passifloraceae

Exploring the New World in the 16th century, Spanish explorers were startled by the beauty of an exotic climbing vine whose white to pale lavender flowers seemed to symbolize the elements of the Crucifixion. The fringed corona, or crown, they felt, represented Christ's crown of thorns; the three stigmas, which receive the pollen, were the nails piercing the Savior's hands and feet; the five stamens were His wounds; the ten sepals and petals stood for the Apostles (leaving out Peter, who denied Christ, and Judas, who betrayed Him); and some said they saw the cross itself in the flower's center. The Spaniards accordingly named the plant passionflower. They also discovered that it grew throughout what is now the southeastern United States.

The flamboyant plant, a vine that can climb to the tops of many trees to present its blossoms to the sun, turned out to be a source of medicine for native Indians, who made a poultice of its leaves to help heal bruises and other injuries. Early physicians prescribed the fruit juice for bathing sore eyes. Since the late 19th century, herbalists have noted its power as a sedative. Today passionflower is still employed medicinally—its dried fruits and flower tops are ingredients of many sedatives.

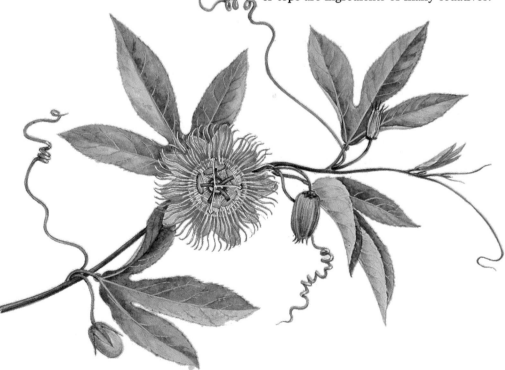

Habitat: Along hedgerows and edges of woods, in thickets, and over open ground.
Range: Native to the southeastern United States, passionflower is found from Maryland south to Florida and west to Texas and Oklahoma.
Identification: A perennial woody vine with a trailing stem up to 30 feet long. The leaves are deeply divided into three lobes that taper to sharp points. White to pale lavender flowers (June–September), about 2 inches across, produce oval yellow berries that are about 2 inches long and edible when ripe.
Uses: The plant and flower are used in herbal medicine as a sedative and painkiller, and to help relieve dysmenorrhea (painful menstruation). Research indicates—but is far from conclusive—that the plant may have these effects.

Pipsissewa

Chimaphila umbellata (L.) Bart.

Ground Holly, Prince's-pine, Wintergreen
WINTERGREEN FAMILY
Pyrolaceae

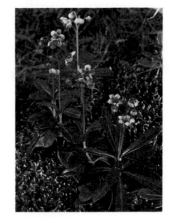

"It-breaks-into-small-pieces" is what the Cree name *pipsisikweu* means, because the pipsissewa's leathery evergreen leaves contain a substance that was supposed to dissolve kidney stones. (It does not, in fact.) Pipsissewa served Indians in a variety of other remedies, too. The Mohegans and Penobscots steeped it in warm water and applied the infusion externally to heal blisters. The Thompson Indians of British Columbia pulverized the plant and applied it in wet dressings to reduce swelling of the legs and feet. The Catawbas dubbed the plant fireflower and extracted a backache remedy from it. The Chippewas used a decoction of the root as eyedrops for sore eyes.

Taken internally, pipsissewa was popular both with Indians and with the pioneers who had picked up its use from them, especially for rheumatism and kidney problems. It served as an astringent and diuretic in folk medicine from the days of Daniel Boone on through the Civil War and afterwards, and was early adopted by official medicine. From 1820 to 1916 pipsissewa was listed in the *U.S. Pharmacopeia*. Until the early 20th century, pipsissewa tonic was a staple home remedy in many rural North American households, and the plant is still to be found as one of the traditional ingredients of root beer.

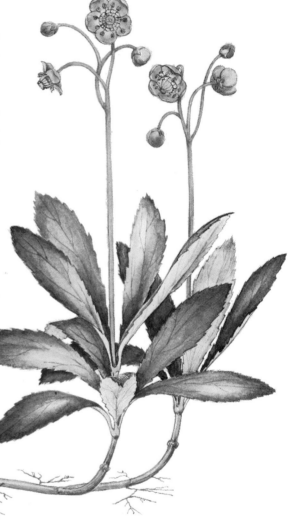

Habitat: Dry woodlands, sandy soils.
Range: Pipsissewa grows wild throughout most of temperate Canada and the United States, with the exception of the southernmost states.
Identification: A small evergreen perennial that grows 3–10 inches tall, pipsissewa has shiny, bright green, toothed leaves arranged in whorls along the stem. Small white to pink flowers (July–August) are clustered at the end of an erect stalk. When bruised, the plant's leaves have a peculiar taste that is astringent and sweetish and at the same time pleasantly bitter.
Uses: Long listed as a tonic and diuretic, pipsissewa is still sometimes prescribed by herbalists for rheumatic, kidney, and urinary tract complaints. Scientists who have investigated the plant question pipsissewa's effectiveness as a diuretic; however, they find that it most likely has value as a mild urinary antiseptic. Pipsissewa extract is a flavoring in candy and soft drinks, particularly root beers.

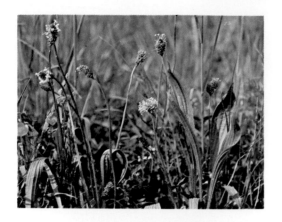

Plantains

Plantago major L.
Common Plantain

Plantago lanceolata L.
English Plantain

Plantago media L.
Hoary Plantain

PLANTAIN FAMILY
Plantaginaceae

"Carts creaked over you, queens rode over you, brides bridled over you, bulls breathed over you: all these you withstood, so may you withstand poison and infection . . . ." Thus an old Anglo-Saxon magical poem speaks of plantain, calling it the "mother of herbs." The leaves in the *Plantago* genus contain tannin and thus are astringent, or able to draw tissues together. They also help to stop bleeding. In Old World tradition plantains figured as a remedy for cuts, sores, burns, snake and insect bites, and inflammations. A tea brewed from the seeds, which have a high mucilage content, was a widespread folk remedy for diarrhea, dysentery, and bleeding from mucous membranes.

Plantains came to the New World with the settlers. A report from Virginia, dated 1687, states that the Indians there called the plant Englishman's-foot. Over the ensuing years Indians of North America put plantains to some of the same uses the plants had had in the Old World. Some tribes in the Northeast used a leaf tea as a wash for sore eyes. In modern times a leaf tea made from *P. major* has been cited as a diuretic, but there is no evidence that this use is valid.

These plantain species should not be confused with the cooking banana called plantain, whose name is a corruption of the Spanish word *plátano*, "plane tree" or "banana tree."

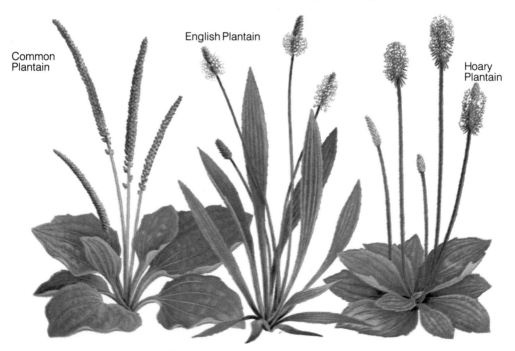

Common Plantain

English Plantain

Hoary Plantain

Habitat: Fields, roadsides, waste places, lawns.
Range: Native to Eurasia, *P. major* and *P. lanceolata* are naturalized throughout temperate North America and *P. media* in eastern Canada and the northeastern United States west to Michigan.
Identification: *P. major*, an annual or perennial reaching 1–2 feet tall, has a rosette of broad, oval, long-stalked leaves and bears spikes of greenish-white to greenish-brown flowers (April–October). *P. lanceolata*, a perennial of similar height, has narrow, lance-shaped, finely toothed leaves and greenish-white flowers (April–October) in short spikes. *P. media*, a perennial, also 1–2 feet tall, resembling *P. major*, has stalkless, narrower oval leaves and much shorter spikes of greenish-pink flowers (June–September).
Uses: Plantains have similar medicinal properties, which are due to their high mucilage and tannin content. The soothing effect afforded by the seeds is the most important medicinal quality of these herbs.

Polypody

Polypodium vulgare L.

Female Fern, Rock Brake,
Sweet Fern, Wood Licorice

FERN FAMILY

Polypodiaceae

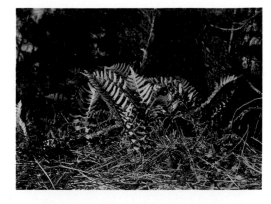

A thousand times sweeter than sugar, the licorice-flavored rhizome, or underground stem, of polypody has been prized since ancient times, not so much for its sweetness as for its medicinal powers. From Greco-Roman antiquity physicians prescribed preparations derived from this lovely evergreen fern as a mild laxative, purgative, and remedy for coughs and chest complaints. For all these uses, "rheum-purging polypod," as the Elizabethan poet Michael Drayton styled it, enjoyed a good reputation down to modern times. Herbalists also recommended preparations of the dried and powdered rhizome for internal use to expel tapeworms and for external use as a liniment.

Because polypody is often found clinging to oak trees, herbalists believed it absorbed the vigor of that mighty tree, and as late as the 18th century, they would use only "polypody of the oak." Even the fern spores were thought to have supernatural powers: anyone who carried them, people said, became invisible. The name polypody comes from a Greek word meaning "many-footed," and alludes to the appearance of the plant's branching rhizomes, which may be fancied to look like many feet.

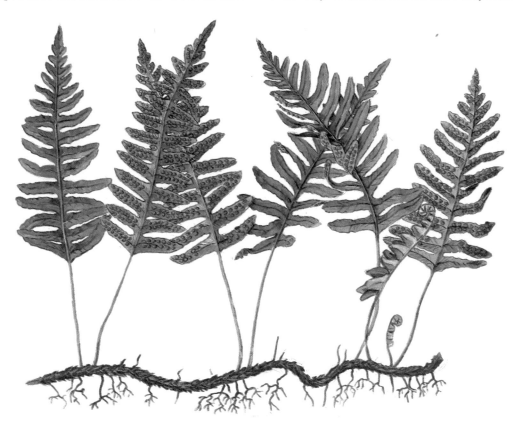

Habitat: Gardens and lawns.
Range: Native to Eurasia, polypody is cultivated throughout temperate North America.
Identification: A perennial evergreen fern with a brown creeping rhizome (underground stem), polypody has long-stalked, pinnately divided, smooth green leaves (fronds) growing up to 12 inches tall. Its spores are borne on the lower surface of the frond in rounded spore capsules called sori, which look like golden dots.

Uses: In herbal medicine a tea brewed from the rhizome is taken as an appetite stimulant and for coughs. A stronger brew has a laxative effect, and a very strong brew is recommended for tapeworm. All of these effects have been verified in animal experiments. Polypody is also popular as an ornamental plant for rock gardens.

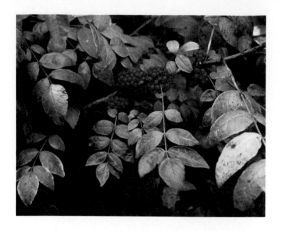

Prickly Ash

Zanthoxylum americanum Mill.

Angelica Tree, Northern Prickly Ash,
Suterberry, Toothache Tree

RUE FAMILY

Rutaceae

When American Indians had a toothache, they often sought relief from prickly ash, also known as the toothache tree. They either chewed the bark or used it in pulverized form. Constantine Rafinesque, a European naturalist studying medicinal plants in America in 1830, pointed out that it did not work for him: "I have ascertained on myself, the burning sensation which it produces on the mouth, merely mitigating the other pain, which returns afterwards." But the Indians had other uses for the tree, which they shared with settlers. They made a poultice of the bark mixed with bear grease for external sores and used the liquid obtained from boiling the bark to treat a range of illnesses, from gonorrhea to sore throat to rheumatism. Dr. Jacob Bigelow, author of the three-volume *American Medical Botany* (1817–1820), wrote of the plant: "Many physicians place great reliance on its powers in rheumatic complaints so that apothecaries generally give it a place in their shops." Today herbalists still specify prickly ash bark and berries as a remedy for rheumatism.

The closely related southern prickly ash tree (*Z. clava-herculis*), also known as Hercules' club, reportedly has many of the same medicinal properties as *Z. americanum*.

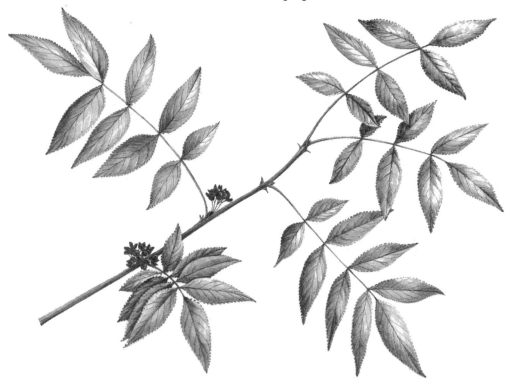

Habitat: Rich woodlands, riverbanks.
Range: A native of North America, prickly ash is found from southern Quebec and Ontario south to Georgia and Oklahoma, and west to North Dakota and Nebraska.
Identification: A deciduous, often shrubby tree growing 4–20 feet tall, with a thin, smooth, brown or gray bark. The twigs usually bear a pair of spines under each leafstalk. Pinnately divided leaves, 3–5 inches long, have 5 to 11 finely toothed leaflets, about 1 inch long, which are dark green above, paler below. Small greenish-white to greenish-yellow flowers (April–June) are followed by round, reddish, capsulelike fruits.
Uses: Modern herbals specify the bark and berries of prickly ash as a treatment for rheumatism and as a stimulant for blood circulation. Researchers, however, question the validity of the medicinal claims made for the plant.

Prickly Lettuce

Lactuca scariola L.

Compass Plant, Horse Thistle,
Wild Lettuce, Wild Opium
COMPOSITE FAMILY
Compositae

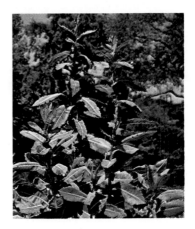

The Roman emperor Augustus reportedly built a statue of the physician who had prescribed lettuce for him, in the belief that the plant had cured him of a serious illness. Although the species responsible for the cure was not specified, it was probably prickly lettuce. Since ancient times, this ancestor of all lettuce plants has been so greatly valued as a sedative and pain reliever that it was considered an opium substitute into the 19th century. Like opium, the milklike juice (latex) of prickly lettuce solidifies and turns brown when exposed to air; this substance, which looks and smells like opium, is called lactucarium.

Over the centuries prickly lettuce enjoyed great versatility as a medicinal plant. The Romans put it on their banquet menus to prevent inebriation. New mothers once drank a tea brewed from the leaves to promote lactation. The plant sap has also been prescribed in herbals as a diuretic and as a soothing lotion for chapped skin. Also called compass plant because its leaves turn to follow the sun during the day, prickly lettuce is bitter to some people's tastes, but horses delight in it.

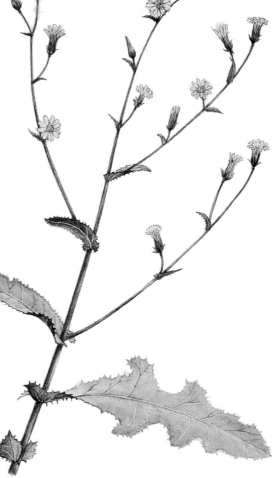

Habitat: Dumps, roadsides, other waste places.
Range: Introduced from Europe, prickly lettuce grows as a weed from Quebec to British Columbia, and south throughout most of the United States.
Identification: An annual or biennial herb growing up to 6 feet tall. Its erect slender stems and large prickly-edged leaves give off a milky juice when cut. Heads of tiny yellow flowers (June–September) are borne in long loose clusters at the ends of the stems. The fruits (seeds) bear tufts of white hairs.

Uses: Prickly lettuce long enjoyed a reputation as a sedative and opium substitute, but scientists declare that there is no experimental evidence to support these claims. Although not to everyone's taste, the young tender leaves of this lettuce relative are sometimes added to salads or cooked as a vegetable.

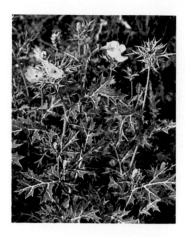

Prickly Poppy

Argemone mexicana L.

Mexican Poppy, Mexican Prickly Poppy, Thorn
Poppy, Yellow Prickly Poppy, Yellow Thistle

POPPY FAMILY

Papaveraceae

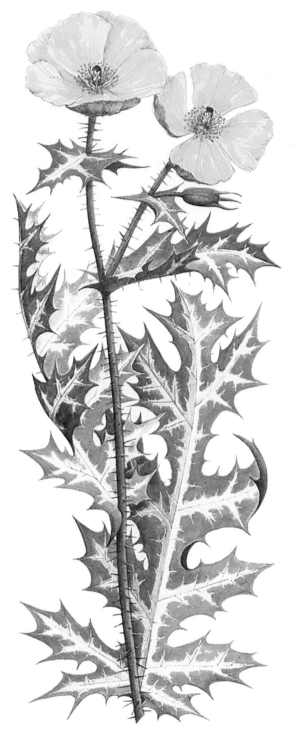

Anyone so foolhardy as to pick prickly poppy
soon learns that its name is well earned: the
leaves and seedpods are armored with needle-
sharp spines. Although this arsenal does not
contribute to the plant's popularity, it does
protect both humans and animals from the ill
effects of the toxic substances it contains. If an
animal, such as a goat, should persist in grazing on this punishing fare, not only will the
beast suffer but so will those who drink its
milk, because the poisons are passed along in
the milk. In humans prickly poppy can cause
dropsy, or edema (an abnormal retention of
fluid in the body).

Despite its bad effects when taken internally, the plant once had external applications.
The Comanche Indians employed an extract of
the seeds to treat sore eyes, and other folk
healers later prescribed the juice as a remedy
for warts and lesions.

The genus name *Argemone*, mentioned in
the first-century A.D. writings of the Roman
naturalist Pliny, is derived from the Greek
word *argemon*, meaning loosely "cataract of the
eye"—a reference to a poppylike flower that
was used to clear vision in Pliny's day.

X Prickly poppy and its seeds are poisonous if
taken internally and may cause edema (an abnormal retention of water in the body) and glaucoma.
Habitat: Dry roadsides, waste places, old fields,
meadows, and orchards.
Range: A native of tropical America, prickly poppy
can now be found as far north as New England,
and has escaped cultivation in some places.
Identification: An erect annual herb reaching 3
feet and sometimes higher. The spiny-toothed,
thistlelike leaves are stalkless and often blotched
with white. Yellow or orange flowers (June–September, or year-round in southern climates), about
2–2½ inches across, are followed by inch-long
prickly seedpods.
Uses: Prickly poppy is no longer recommended by
modern practitioners of folk medicine.

Privet

Ligustrum vulgare L.

Common Privet, Prim
OLIVE FAMILY
Oleaceae

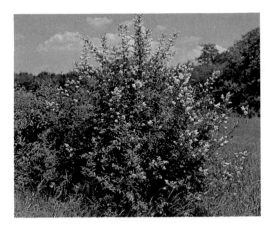

In colonial times privet was transported to North America for cultivation as a hedge plant, and it has been highly esteemed here ever since. Its abundant leaves form a thick screen, and if the plant is allowed to grow, it can reach 15 feet. In warm areas the foliage often remains on the plant year-round, and it is seemingly impervious to air pollution. Privet responds well to clipping, swiftly sending out new growth to replace what is lost. Skilled gardeners may clip it into animal shapes and other fanciful designs—an art called topiary.

In view of such virtues many gardeners may be surprised to learn that privet has also had a solid reputation as a medicinal plant. A century ago, physicians used its berries as a strong laxative. The flowers were placed on the forehead as a headache remedy, and the leaves found use as an astringent in the form of mouthwashes and gargles. Both leaves and flowers have been relied on for assuaging such female problems as irregular menstruation and vaginal irritations. Privet's assets do not end there, however. The bark produces a yellow dye, and the berries yield green and black dyes. The young branches are sometimes used for basketry.

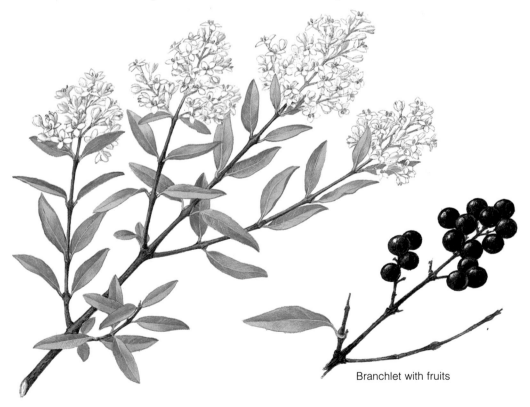

Branchlet with fruits

X Do not take internally. The fruits and leaves can cause gastrointestinal irritation, liver damage, and reduction in blood pressure.

Habitat: Thickets, roadsides, open woods.

Range: Introduced from Europe, privet has escaped cultivation in North America and grows from Ontario south to Pennsylvania and North Carolina.

Identification: A shrub normally growing 3–9 feet tall. Its lance-shaped to elliptical leaves, 1–2½ inches long, are smooth and dark green and grow in opposite pairs. Numerous small white flowers (June–July) appear in loose terminal clusters and are followed by oval black berries.

Uses: Privet leaves have long been held to have astringent properties, and pharmacologists state that this belief is valid. A few herbals still recommend them for this use—suggesting that they be boiled and the extract used as a douche for vaginal irritations or as a gargle for sore throat.

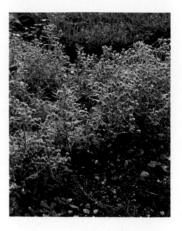

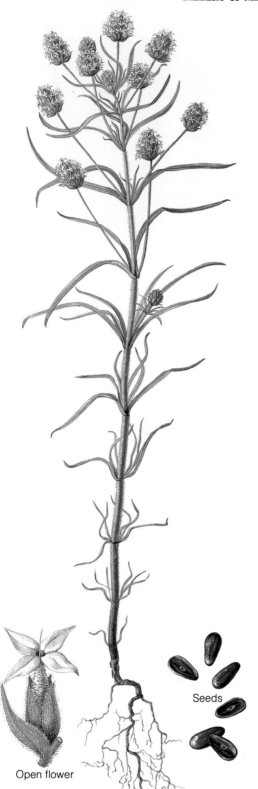

Seeds

Open flower

Psyllium

Plantago psyllium L.

Fleaseed, Fleawort, Plantain
PLANTAIN FAMILY
Plantaginaceae

An annual herb, psyllium occupies an important place among medicinal plants. Its seeds—whose smallness leads to the plant's name *psyllium,* from *psylla,* the Greek word for flea—contain a mucilage that, when combined with water, swells tremendously. A gram of seed will expand 8 to 14 times its volume in water. The enlarged mass is highly gelatinous, and since ancient times psyllium seed has been used with great effectiveness as a laxative. Its special asset is that, being a vegetable substance, it has a purely mechanical action, lubricating and cleansing the intestines simultaneously. Thus, there are no harmful side effects, either physiological or chemical. *P. psyllium* is cultivated largely in France and Spain. A related species native to India, *P. ovata,* bears seeds that are richer in mucilage and is currently used in over-the-counter preparations for a wide range of maladies, including irritable bowel syndrome.

Psyllium is also said to relieve an ailment known as autointoxication, in which the body poisons itself by producing and absorbing an excess of intestinal waste products. Psyllium, some herbalists maintain, removes the offending substances.

X Psyllium powder, if inhaled, may cause asthma, and eating unsoaked seeds may cause gastrointestinal problems. See a doctor before using psyllium if you have an intestinal disorder.
Habitat: Poor soils and waste places in full sun.
Range: A native of southern Europe, North Africa, and western Asia, psyllium is cultivated in North America and has escaped from gardens in the eastern United States.
Identification: An annual herb growing up to 15 inches tall. Very narrow lance-shaped leaves grow in opposite pairs or in whorls of three to six. Small whitish flowers (June–July), borne in dense round spikes, produce capsules containing tiny brown glossy seeds.
Uses: Psyllium has been long used as an intestinal lubricant and laxative. Because of its gentle lubricating action, it is especially useful to hemorrhoid sufferers. Both *P. psyllium* and *P. ovata* were listed in the 1980 edition of the *U.S. Pharmacopeia.*

Pumpkin

Cucurbita pepo L.

Field Pumpkin
GOURD FAMILY
Cucurbitaceae

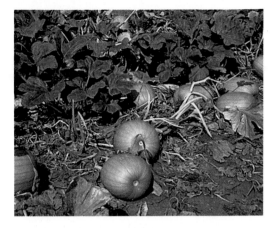

In autumn, across a large part of North America, cultivated pumpkins are seen in fields, on farm stands, and in store-window and other displays heralding the start of fall and its holidays. The shells make decorative lanterns at Halloween time, and the pulp becomes the traditional Thanksgiving pumpkin pie. In addition to pie pumpkins, this particular species of the gourd family includes such squashes as crookneck, straightneck, zucchini, acorn, and marrow. The species name comes from the Greek word *pepon*, meaning "sun ripened."

When the first explorers arrived in America, they noticed the pumpkin plant in the cultivated maize fields of the Indians. The red men, they discovered, utilized the plant for medicine as well as for food. An emulsion made from a mixture of pumpkin and watermelon seeds served to heal wounds for members of the Yuma tribe. The Catawbas ate the fresh or dried seeds as a kidney medicine, while the Menominees drank a mixture of water and powdered squash and pumpkin seeds to ease the passage of urine. In settler folk medicine the ground stems of pumpkin were brewed into a tea to treat "female ills," and the ripe seeds were made into a palatable preparation to dispel worms. Modern folk healers advocate pumpkin seeds to rid the body of intestinal worms, and they point out that the seed oil is helpful for healing burns and wounds.

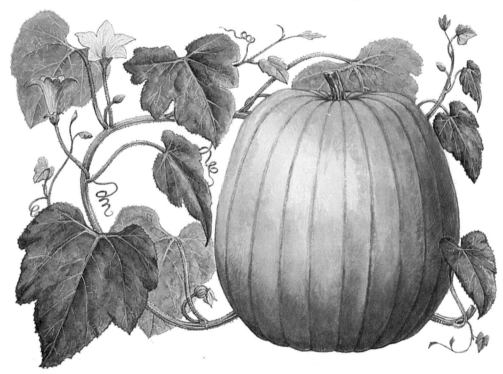

Habitat: Waste places, open fields.
Range: Native to tropical America, pumpkin has been cultivated almost everywhere in the world, including North America. It sometimes escapes from gardens.
Identification: An annual vine with tendrils and a creeping prickly stem reaching 30 feet in length. Large, rough, dull green leaves, ½–1 foot wide, are triangular with three to five lobes. Bright yellow funnel-shaped flowers (June–August) are followed by the familiar orange fruit, which is furrowed when mature in late summer or early autumn and contains numerous flat white seeds.
Uses: The seeds of pumpkin have traditionally been recognized as an anthelmintic, or agent that kills intestinal worms or expels them from the body. Modern proponents of herbal medicine still recommend the seeds for this purpose, and scientists assert that this use is valid.

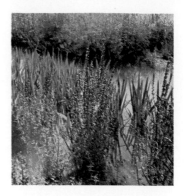

Purple Loosestrife

Lythrum salicaria L.

Rainbowweed, Spiked Loosestrife

LOOSESTRIFE FAMILY

Lythraceae

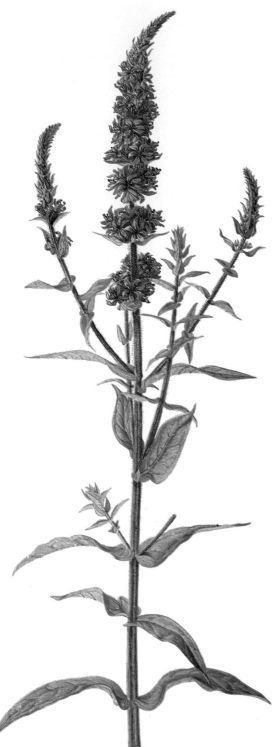

Here is a wildflower that motorists can enjoy from their cars. During the summer, vast vivid patches of purple loosestrife, with its long, showy spiked blossoms ranging in color from rose to red to deep purple (whence the common name rainbowweed), are seen from roads and highways near riverbanks, in wet meadows, and in other marshy areas in the Atlantic Coast states and as far west as Minnesota.

Purple loosestrife is one of the most interesting wild plants, as Charles Darwin and other naturalists and botanists discovered. It has three different forms of flower, but only one type of bloom appears on any one plant.

Mankind has taken notice of loosestrife since antiquity. The Greeks thought that garlands of the herb hung around the necks of oxen would encourage a team to plow a field in harmony. More practically, they used the plant in a hair dye and also burned it to drive away insect pests. Because purple loosestrife is rich in tannin, herbalists later employed it for its astringent values as an eyewash and as a remedy for diarrhea. They also used the herb to halt bleeding, a use that may explain its botanical name, *Lythrum*, from the Greek word for gore.

Habitat: Along the banks of rivers and streams, in wet meadows, wet roadsides, and swampy areas.
Range: Native to Europe, purple loosestrife is naturalized from Newfoundland as far south as Virginia and as far west as Minnesota.
Identification: A perennial herb growing to 5 feet tall. The stem is squarish; the leaves are narrow and lance-shaped, and occur in pairs or in whorls of three. Rose to deep purple flowers (June–September) with four to six petals bloom in long spikes. The plant usually grows in dense patches.
Uses: Purple loosestrife has long been established as an astringent because of its tannin content. Modern-day herbalists value this quality and recommend the herb for diarrhea. They also suggest an infusion of the plant's green parts and flowers as a gargle for sore throats, as a douche, and to clean wounds.

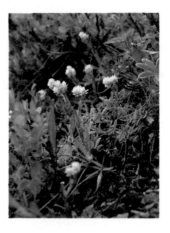

Pussytoes

Antennaria neglecta Greene

Field Cat's-foot, Field Pussytoes
COMPOSITE FAMILY
Compositae

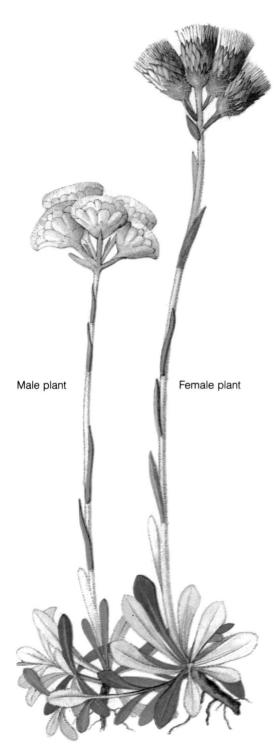

Male plant   Female plant

The soft white flowerheads, resembling tufts of white plush, bring to mind a kitten's soft, delicate paws, for which the plant pussytoes was named. Botanists saw in the tall, fine stamens of the flowers a resemblance to the antennae of insects, and so named the plant's genus *Antennaria*.

In spite of its delicate appearance, pussytoes is a strong and persistent plant. It spreads itself by a network of runners that appear to discourage other plants from growing near it. Long ago, people living in rural areas noticed this characteristic and decided that the plant was probably good for warding off insects. They added pussytoes to hair shampoo to discourage head lice, and they packed the plant in with woolen clothing to repel moths.

Pussytoes seems to have had no specific use in folk medicine, but it is reported that North American Indians, and later herbalists, extracted a gum from the plant stalks and used it for a chewing gum. A European relative of pussytoes, *A. dioica*, may be found growing in the wild in Alaska. This species has been employed in herbal medicine as an astringent, to soothe coughing, and to reduce fever, but it is seldom recommended today.

Habitat: Pastures, prairies, open woods.
Range: A native of North America, pussytoes is found from Nova Scotia and southern Ontario south to Virginia, Kansas, and Arizona.
Identification: A perennial herb growing 4–12 inches high, pussytoes spreads by runners and often forms thick mats. The lance-shaped basal leaves, about 2 inches long, usually have one main vein, and are green on the upper side and whitish below, as are the alternate upper leaves, which are stalkless and smaller. Tiny tubular flowers (April–July) form dense white terminal flowerheads surrounded by white bracts on the male plant and pink to purple bracts on the female plant.
Uses: Pussytoes was once employed as a moth repellent and for discouraging head lice. A related species, *A. dioica*, served as an astringent and cough remedy and to break fevers. No scientific studies have been made that would prove or disprove the validity of these uses.

277

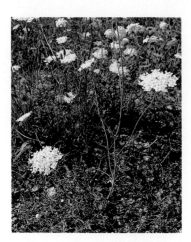

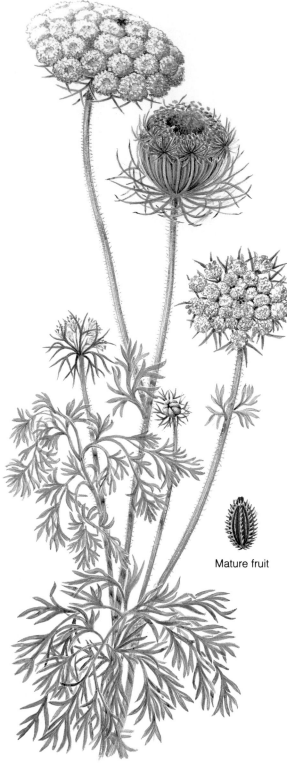

Queen Anne's Lace

Daucus carota L.

Bee's Nest, Bird's Nest,
Devil's Plague, Wild Carrot

CARROT FAMILY

Umbelliferae

By midsummer, fields and roadsides across most of temperate North America are crowded with the intricately patterned flat flower clusters of Queen Anne's lace. Each main cluster is composed of perhaps 500 flowers and has at its center a single, tiny deep red or purple flower. According to one folk belief, these red flowers, when eaten, prevent epileptic seizures. The deep red flower also figures in a story of how the plant received its name. According to this legend the red flower symbolized a drop of the blood of Queen Anne (1665–1714), who pricked her finger making lace.

Over the years extracts from boiled wild carrots were used medicinally as a diuretic and to dissolve kidney stones. The seeds were eaten to eliminate intestinal worms and gas.

The first colonists arriving in America brought carrot seeds with them, since carrots were a popular vegetable in England. The plant soon escaped from gardens in America (as it had done in England) and reverted to the wild state that we know as Queen Anne's lace.

Mature fruit

X Do not confuse Queen Anne's lace with the poisonous water hemlock (*Cicuta maculata*), poison hemlock (*Conium maculatum*), or fool's parsley (*Aethusa cynapium*). The red or purple flower in the center distinguishes *Daucus carota*.
Habitat: Fields, roadsides, other open places.
Range: Temperate North America.
Identification: A biennial growing to 3 feet tall. White, flat flower clusters (May–October) top tall branching stems. After pollination, the clusters become cup-shaped when they dry and bear seeds (actually fruits). The leaves are finely divided and arranged alternately along the stem. The root is vertical, slender, white, fleshy.
Uses: Scientific experiments have verified the effectiveness of the seeds in dispelling flatulence (intestinal gas). The wild root, like the cultivated one, is rich in vitamin A, which is good for night vision, but the vitamin is harmful when taken in excessive amounts.

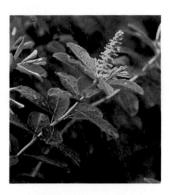

Queen's-delight

Stillingia sylvatica L.

Queen's-root, Silverleaf, Yawroot
SPURGE FAMILY
Euphorbiaceae

Native to a large part of the southern United States, queen's-delight was once a popular home medicine with settlers in the region. They claimed that its root had many virtues: as a laxative, an emetic (to induce vomiting), an expectorant (to bring up phlegm), a so-called blood purifier, and a treatment for syphilis. In 1828 a certain Dr. T. Y. Symons brought queen's-delight to the attention of the medical profession by publishing in the *American Medical Record* his findings on it as a valuable drug in treating syphilis, for which mercury (a dangerous drug) was used. Queen's-delight soon met with physicians' approval and was listed in the *U.S. Pharmacopeia*.

Unfortunately, doctors found that queen's-delight had to be fresh to be effective. And doctors and herbalists later decided that the plant was more reliable for the laxative or emetic properties that many other plants also afforded than as a remedy for syphilis, for which no cure existed. Some modern herbals recommend the plant for "purifying" the blood system and restoring it to normal, but another herbal reference mentions queen's-delight as an "empiric"—that is, a drug of doubtful value.

Habitat: Pine barrens and other sandy soils.
Range: Native to the United States queen's-delight grows from Virginia south to Florida and Texas, and west to southeastern Colorado.
Identification: A perennial herb growing to 4 feet tall. Leathery, elliptical alternate leaves, about 1–3 inches long, are finely toothed and nearly stalkless. Yellow flowers (March–August or all year in warm climates) are petalless and occur in dense terminal spikes, with the male blossoms along the upper part of the spike and the female blossoms along the lower part.
Uses: The root was once a widely prescribed home remedy in the U.S. South. In folk medicine it was promoted mainly as a blood purifier (restoring health by cleansing the blood of so-called impurities that were thought to cause certain sicknesses) and as a syphilis cure; however, it no longer enjoys wide acceptance among herbalists. There is no scientific evidence regarding any of its medicinal uses.

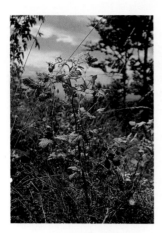

Raspberry

Rubus idaeus L.

Red Raspberry
ROSE FAMILY
Rosaceae

The plump, red fruits of the raspberry shrub are known to everyone who has ever spent a summer in the eastern part of the country, for these delectable berries grow wild along roadsides and in thickets. Less familiar are the wild raspberry's medicinal virtues. American Indians used the shrub as an astringent, making an infusion, or tea, of the root bark, which they applied to sore eyes. Europeans in the 17th century regarded the raspberry as an antispasmodic, and they made a syrup of the juice, which they employed to prevent vomiting. Herbals of the time recommended the fresh fruit for dissolving tartar on the teeth. In the 18th century physicians and herbalists deemed the berries useful as a remedy for heart disease.

Modern herbals prescribe the plant chiefly for the medical problems of women. The shrub contains a substance that is both a relaxant and a stimulant of the uterine muscle. Herbalists value an infusion of the leaves for parturition (the process of giving birth) in order to help relax and stimulate the uterus and make the process less painful. In addition, herbalists use raspberry leaf tea as a treatment for diarrhea, sore throat, colds, and fevers.

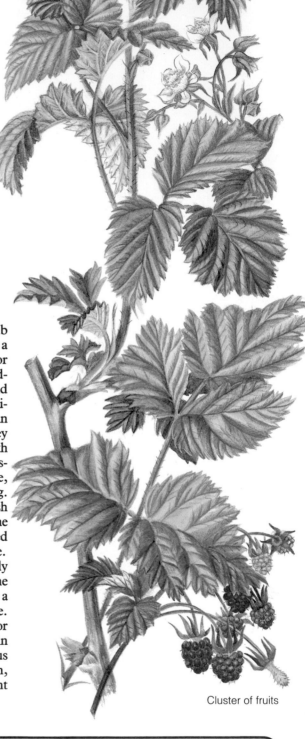

Cluster of fruits

Habitat: Thickets and roadsides near towns and villages.

Range: A native of Europe, the raspberry is naturalized in North America from Newfoundland to Ontario, south to New England, New York, Michigan, and South Dakota.

Identification: A biennial or perennial shrub, growing 3–6 feet tall. The upright canes that arise from underground suckers and stolons (runners) are usually prickly. Pinnately divided leaves have three to seven toothed leaflets, which are velvety gray underneath. Small white flowers (May–July) are followed by red fruits (June–October).

Uses: Scientific studies support the traditional use of the raspberry as an astringent in the treatment of diarrhea. On the basis of animal experiments, pharmacologists have validated the use of the leaves as an antispasmodic for dysmenorrhea (painful menstruation) and have found some evidence to validate its uses as an aid in childbirth.

Red Clover

Trifolium pratense L.

Beebread, Cow Clover, Meadow Clover,
Purple Clover, Trefoil
PEA FAMILY
Leguminosae

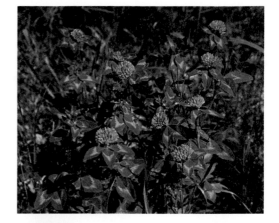

Among the largest of the various clover species, red clover is also the most celebrated for its magical powers. Since pagan times, people have credited it with the ability to protect against witchcraft and evil spirits. Those venturing forth into territory where spirits were said to lurk routinely carried a sprig of clover as traveler's insurance. Four-leaf clover, an occasional variety resulting from mutation, was and still is considered a sign of luck.

As for red clover's medicinal virtues, it long had a reputation for helping coughs (including whooping cough), colds, sore throats, and skin eruptions. American Indians employed the plant for sore eyes and as a salve for burns. In springtime they ate the leaves of the plant, which is a relative of the pea, as a vegetable. One 19th-century American newspaper article reported the usefulness of red clover extract in curing a case of cancer.

Modern herbalists, more cautious in their praises, sometimes recommend the plant as an alterative, or drug used to alter the course of an ailment and restore healthy body functions. They also mention red clover as a sedative and as an antispasmodic.

Red clover is used in agriculture as a soil-improving cover crop, a source of nectar for honeybees, and as grazing and fodder for cattle. It is Vermont's state flower.

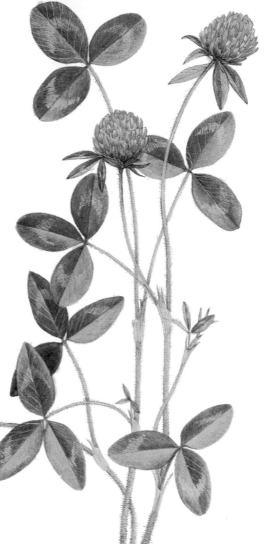

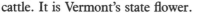

Habitat: Clearings, pastures, meadows and fields, along roadsides.

Range: Introduced from Europe, red clover has become naturalized throughout almost all of temperate North America.

Identification: A biennial or short-lived perennial reaching heights of nearly 3 feet, red clover grows in clumps that are made up of several smooth or hairy stems. Green leaves are stalked and consist of three oval leaflets, each one usually carrying a distinctive whitish V-shaped marking. Rose to pink flowerheads (May–October) are round and about 1 inch across.

Uses: Red clover tea is still used today in folk medicine as a remedy for sore throats, colds, and coughs. Pharmacologists state that no scientific data have been reported to validate these medicinal uses for the plant.

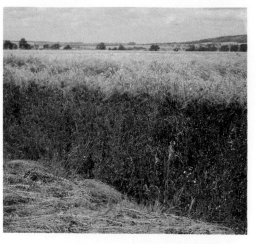

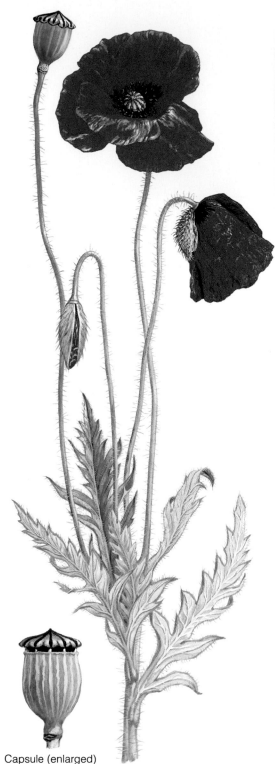

Capsule (enlarged)

Red Poppy

Papaver rhoeas L.

Corn Poppy, Corn Rose,
Field Poppy, Flanders Poppy

POPPY FAMILY

Papaveraceae

Even though it is not a native plant, the red poppy has become a symbol of America's remembrance of its war dead. This is the flower that flourished in the fields surrounding the cemeteries of the Flanders region of France and Belgium, where thousands of Allied casualties of World War I are buried—a fact immortalized by John McCrae's poem, "In Flanders Fields." The paper version of this poppy worn on Memorial Day is more familiar to most Americans than the real flower because, although the red poppy has escaped cultivation, it is seen mainly in gardens.

Medicinally, the red poppy has served mankind both as a sedative and as an analgesic. The plant contains a mild and nonpoisonous sedative alkaloid called rhoeadine. (Unlike its cousin the opium poppy, it is not a source of narcotics.) In bygone days mothers added red poppy juice to babies' food to put infants to sleep. The blossoms were also compounded into a cough syrup for children. Today the poppy is mainly in demand for its seeds, which are used in baking.

Habitat: Fields, meadows, roadsides.
Range: Native to Europe and Asia, the red poppy is widely cultivated in North America and often escapes from gardens.
Identification: An annual herb, the red poppy averages 2–2½ feet in height. It has an erect, hairy stem that bears bristly, pinnately divided leaves. Scarlet flowers (late May–October), 2 inches across, have blue-black stamens and four large petals, each with a purplish-black dot at the base. The fruit of the red poppy is a capsule containing many black seeds.
Uses: The red poppy has been employed medicinally over the ages as a mild sedative to induce sleep in babies. The flowers contain traces of alkaloids that would act as a sedative, but no scientific studies have been carried out to prove this effect. Herbalists use the blossoms and seeds in a pediatric cough syrup. The flowers are used to color teas, wine, ink, and medicines.

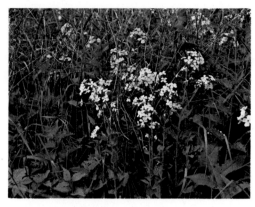

Rocket

Hesperis matronalis L.

Damask Violet, Dame's-rocket, Dame's-violet,
Mother-of-the-evening, Sweet Rocket

MUSTARD FAMILY

Cruciferae

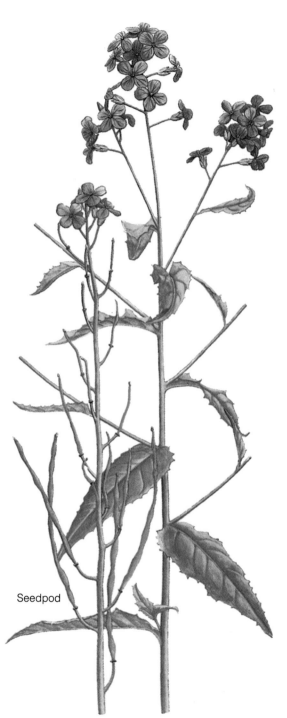

Seedpod

Although it has little odor in daytime, at night rocket fills the air with a sweet violetlike fragrance. Its genus name, *Hesperis*, is a Greek word meaning "evening"—a reference to the plant's lovely evening perfume. As its species name, *matronalis*, and the list of common names imply, rocket was once a great favorite of women. Perhaps its most famous admirer was the doomed French queen Marie Antoinette (1755–1793), who, according to legend, had bouquets of rocket, pinks, and tuberoses smuggled to her while she was imprisoned during the French Revolution. Rocket was especially popular in Europe and was brought to North America as a garden flower.

In modern herbals rocket is occasionally mentioned as a diuretic and an expectorant and for inducing sweating. As early as the 16th century the herbalist John Gerard noted that "the distilled water of the flowers is counted to be a most effectual thing to procure sweat," which would break a fever. In the next century Nicholas Culpeper emphasized that the plant was good for treating wounds and excellent for obstructions of the internal organs. In Maud Grieve's herbal, published in England in the 1930's, rocket was listed chiefly for scurvy.

Habitat: Roadsides, thickets, wet ditches, open woods, fields.

Range: A native of Europe, rocket has escaped cultivation in North America and is found growing wild from Newfoundland to Ontario, south to Georgia, Kentucky, and Kansas.

Identification: A biennial or perennial herb growing to a height of 3 feet. The upper leaves are lance-shaped and stalkless; the lower leaves are larger, about 4 inches long, and attached to the stem by very short stalks. Dainty four-petaled flowers (May–August), about 1 inch across, range in color from purple to pink to white and have a faint scent in daytime, a stronger aroma during the night. The seedpods, called siliques, are cylindrical and up to 5 inches long.

Uses: Rocket is not widely used in herbal medicine. Its principal modern application has been as a diuretic, but there is no scientific evidence that this use is valid.

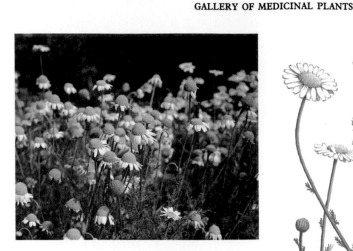

Roman Chamomile

Anthemis nobilis L.

Common Chamomile, English Chamomile,
True Chamomile

COMPOSITE FAMILY

Compositae

As readers of *The Tale of Peter Rabbit* remember, it was chamomile tea that Peter's mother administered to him after he had overindulged in Mr. McGregor's vegetable garden. Generations of humans, too, have relied upon chamomile tea to help comfort an upset stomach, and it is still used for this purpose. English chamomile, as the plant is sometimes called, has also been named explicitly in modern herbals as an antispasmodic, useful for menstrual cramps; as an appetite stimulant; as a mild sedative; and as an agent that reduces pain and swelling resulting from injury. Its use as a medicinal herb can be traced to ancient Egypt, where certain priests employed the flowers to help patients who were suffering from fever. It was the Greeks of antiquity who named the plant *khamaimelon* (loosely "ground apple"), since it creeps along the ground and the flowers have an applelike aroma. The Romans advocated chamomile as an antidote for poisonous serpent bites.

Roman chamomile is frequently confused with German chamomile, botanically known as *Matricaria chamomilla*. The two plants are members of the same family, and do resemble each other. Both have pale green, feathery-looking leaves, both produce daisylike flowers, and both have an applelike fragrance.

Habitat: Waste places, near gardens.
Range: Native to western and southern Europe, Roman chamomile is a garden escape and has spread locally in North America.
Identification: A much branched perennial herb growing up to 12 inches long, with almost prostrate downy stems. Pale green leaves are finely divided and feathery. Daisylike flowerheads (June–September), about 1 inch across, with yellow centers and white petallike ray flowers, grow singly at the ends of branches and have an applelike odor.
Uses: Generations have used Roman chamomile tea as a remedy for simple cases of indigestion. Herbalists also use it as an appetite stimulant and as an anti-inflammatory, or agent that reduces the pain or swelling resulting from an injury. Research seems to validate these uses as well as chamomile tea's efficacy in treating upset stomach and menstrual cramps.

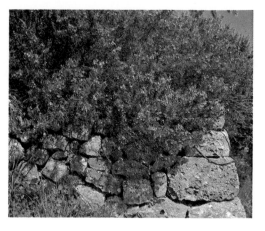

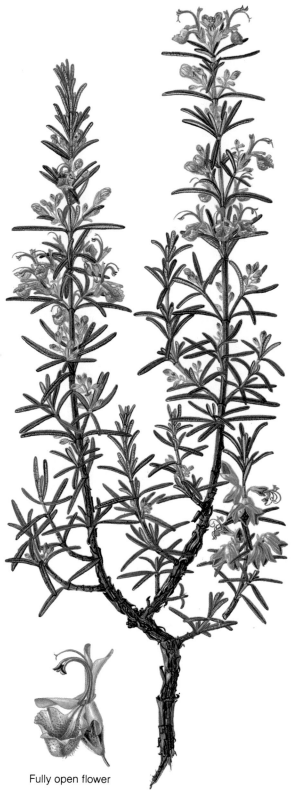

Fully open flower

Rosemary

Rosmarinus officinalis L.

Old Man

MINT FAMILY

Labiatae

History records that in ancient Greece, where rosemary was said to strengthen the memory, students of the time wore sprigs of the herb in their hair while they studied. As a result of this reputation, rosemary became a symbol of remembrance. Brides wore it to show that they would always remember their families, and the dead were buried with it to signify that they would not be forgotten.

Over the centuries people found a host of benefits in the plant. According to one belief rosemary could incapacitate a robber: wash the thief's feet with a lotion made from the root and he will be deprived of the strength to steal. When the populace desperately sought protection against rampant diseases, they burned the aromatic branches as a disinfectant. Apothecaries of the 16th and 17th centuries prescribed rosemary for the relief of intestinal gas and as a tonic and digestive aid. They suggested different preparations of the plant for toothache, headache, gout, coughs, and even baldness. Rosemary has also been used as an antispasmodic. Long ago, cooks discovered rosemary's culinary properties; the leaves are a basic item in the modern herb rack and herb garden.

X The undiluted oil should never be taken internally.
Habitat: Mild, sunny regions.
Range: Native to the Mediterranean area, rosemary is cultivated outdoors in mild regions of North America and grown indoors in harsher climates.
Identification: A perennial shrubby herb, averaging 2–4 feet in height. Its leathery leaves are dark green above and silver below. They are ½–1½ inches long, needlelike, and narrow, and have a spicy, resinous smell. The flowers (May–July) are usually pale blue but sometimes pink or white.
Uses: Many toiletry preparations are scented with rosemary, and cooks flavor meat dishes, soups, and stews with it. Pharmacologists find that oil of rosemary's use in diluted form as a carminative (a substance that rids the intestines of gas) is valid. There is some evidence for the plant's effectiveness as an antispasmodic.

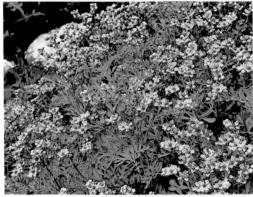

Rue

Ruta graveolens L.

Common Rue, Countryman's-treacle,
Garden Rue, German Rue, Herb-of-grace
RUE FAMILY
Rutaceae

Highly regarded since ancient times, rue was recognized as medicinally helpful for more than 80 complaints by the time of the early Roman Empire. The first-century A.D. scholar Pliny reported that it preserved eyesight and noted that painters and engravers ate a good deal of rue. In the 16th and 17th centuries, herbals advocated it as an antidote for all sorts of poisons, from toadstools to serpent bites. Because of rue's strong, rather musty odor, it enjoyed particular prominence for warding off pestilences. In the Middle Ages the well-off carried nosegays of rue out of doors to drive away the lice of beggars, and even into the 18th century, bouquets were placed in law courts to counteract prisoners' vermin and germs. At one time in Catholic churches, brushes made of rue were used to sprinkle holy water before Mass—a practice that may explain another of the plant's common names, herb-of-grace.

After settlers introduced rue into America, it became a popular folk remedy, and doctors and apothecaries specified it for many uses—as an antispasmodic, an emmenagogue (an agent that brings on menstruation), and an anthelmintic (an agent to destroy intestinal worms), to name a few.

X Rue may cause mild poisoning. Even handling the fresh leaves may cause the skin to blister. Pregnant women especially should not take it internally.
Habitat: Pastures, roadsides, abandoned lots.
Range: Introduced from Europe, rue is now naturalized in North America from Vermont south to Virginia and west to Missouri.
Identification: A perennial herb growing to 3 feet tall. The erect branching stems bear aromatic blue-green alternate and pinnately divided leaves. Bright yellow flowers (June–July), about ½ inch across, with green centers, occur in loose clusters.
Uses: Scientific studies validate the effectiveness of rue as an antispasmodic. There is little or no evidence, however, to support the plant's efficacy in bringing on menstruation or in suppressing coughs—two of its common uses in modern herbal medicine.

Running Clubmoss

Lycopodium clavatum L.

Clubfoot Moss, Clubmoss, Foxtail, Ground Pine,
Staghorn, Staghorn Moss, Vegetable Sulfur
CLUBMOSS FAMILY

Lycopodiaceae

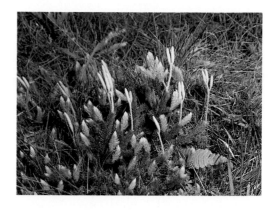

Forests of giant clubmosses that reached 100 feet in height encircled our planet many millions of years ago. Today these ancient relatives of the running clubmoss constitute, in their petrified form, an important source of coal. Eventually the primeval giant clubmoss evolved into its present form: a smallish plant with a ground-hugging stem that grows up to 4 feet long. The botanical name of the plant means "club-shaped wolf's claw," a reference both to the plant's club-shaped spore cases and to a fancied resemblance between the plant's root and a wolf's claw.

The fine yellow powder formed by the spores of running clubmoss is extremely rich in oil and flammable—hence its old name vegetable sulfur. Stage designers once employed the powder to create stage lightning for plays, and in the pioneering days of photography the spores served as a flash powder. The yellow powder was once used as an absorbent dusting powder in surgery and as a baby powder. Both the spores and the whole plant figured in medications once prescribed for various ailments such as kidney stones and urinary tract infections.

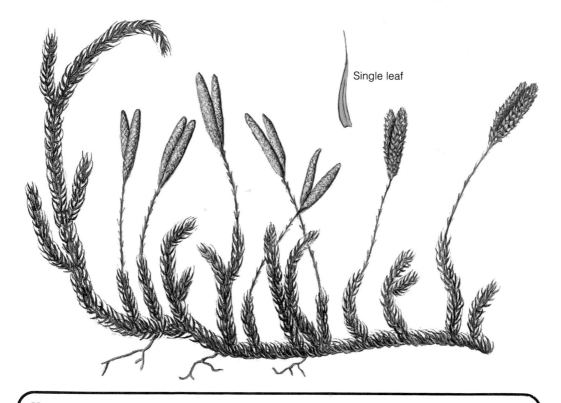

Single leaf

X The spores irritate mucous membranes.

Habitat: Barren hills and mountainsides, forests and heaths with poor soil.

Range: Running clubmoss is native to temperate regions worldwide.

Identification: A perennial herbaceous evergreen, running clubmoss is a flowerless plant, reproducing by spores. Its creeping stem, up to 4 feet long, branches freely and is densely covered with tiny green leaves that are slender, soft, and arranged spirally along the stem. Spore-bearing cones (June–September) are borne in pairs at the ends of erect branches.

Uses: The spores of running clubmoss make a fine yellow powder that served as an absorbent powder for rashes, wounds, and surgical incisions, but since the spores are known to be an irritant to mucous membranes, the powder cannot be recommended for these medicinal uses.

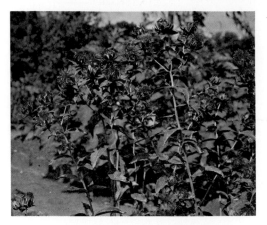

Safflower

Carthamus tinctorius L.

American Saffron, Azafran, Bastard Saffron,
Dyer's-saffron, False Saffron

COMPOSITE FAMILY

Compositae

When scientists found that the presence in man's diet of polyunsaturated fats tends to lower the levels of blood cholesterol—now recognized as contributing to heart disease—attention was focused on a variety of vegetable oils as substitutes for the animal fats that tend to raise cholesterol levels. Safflower oil, it turned out, had one of the highest percentages of polyunsaturates, with the result that the plant is nowadays grown mainly for its oil.

That was not always so. Safflower was originally valued for the yellow and red dyes that its flowers yield. The red dyestuff was employed for centuries as a rouge ingredient and to color silks. Safflower's textile-dyeing use may be very old indeed—ancient mummy wrappings apparently dyed with the flowers have come to light. In the 1700's the Portuguese, it was said, added safflower to foods, probably as a saffron substitute. But safflower does not have the true saffron flavor—hence the names bastard saffron and false saffron.

Aside from its effectiveness in lowering cholesterol levels, safflower's medicinal value is limited. It has been used in the treatment of fevers and as a laxative.

Habitat: Light, dry soil in sunny places.
Range: Native to the Middle East, safflower is widely cultivated in Europe and North America.
Identification: An annual growing to 3 feet tall with a single smooth upright stem, safflower has shiny, oval, spiny-edged alternate leaves, each ending in a sharp spiny point. The plant flowers profusely (June–July), with 1- to 1½-inch solitary heads that turn from deep yellow to deep red. The seeds (August) are hidden in a mass of thistly down.

Uses: A tea brewed from chopped or granulated flowers is given to induce perspiration and thus reduce fever; pharmacologists investigating the plant's medicinal uses indicate that this one is probably valid. However, scientists question that safflower has any effect as a laxative. The flowers still serve as a dyestuff in some parts of the world, but the oil-producing seeds, which are used in paints and varnishes as well as cooking and salad oil, are the reason for safflower's cultivation.

Sage

Salvia officinalis L.

Common Sage, Garden Sage, Meadow Sage,
Scarlet Sage, True Sage
MINT FAMILY
Labiatae

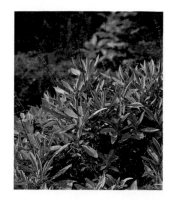

"Why should a person die, when sage grows in his garden?" This is not really a question, but a saying that originated in the Middle Ages at the famous medical school of Salerno, Italy. Sage has enjoyed a high reputation as a health giver ever since antiquity, to judge by its Latin name *salvia*, which comes from a word meaning "healthy." Greco-Roman medicine viewed sage as a diuretic with specific usefulness for certain women's complaints. A boiled-down brew of sage reputedly checked heavy menstrual bleeding, whereas a similar extract mixed with wine was held to bring on delayed periods. The ancients also wrote that sage mixed with white wine or wormwood tea relieved dysentery and, when applied externally, healed certain wounds. Later herbalism, up until the 20th century, carried on the tradition, and sage also figured in prescriptions for colic and fevers, to expel worms, and to prevent epileptic seizures.

The learned 17th-century diarist John Evelyn wrote: "'Tis a plant indeed with so many and wonderful properties, as that the assiduous use of it is said to render men immortal." Science casts grave doubt, however, on all but the humblest of sage's reported medicinal powers—its ability to ease gas pains.

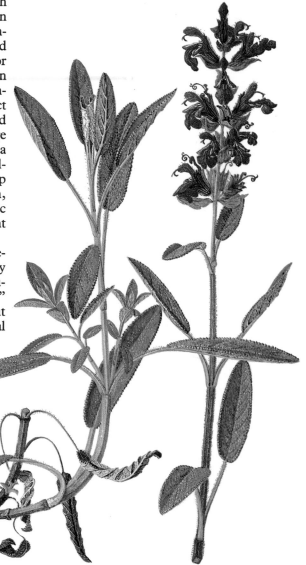

Habitat: Well-drained soil in sunny areas.
Range: Native to southern Europe, sage is now cultivated throughout temperate North America and occasionally escapes from gardens.
Identification: An aromatic evergreen perennial, sage grows up to 2 feet high, with oblong, woolly, gray-green leaves that grow in opposite pairs on square stems. Violet-blue flowers (June–September) are arranged in whorls at the ends of the stems and branches.

Uses: Present-day herbalists sometimes recommend sage tea for excessive sweating, for nervous disorders, to reduce a nursing mother's milk flow when she is weaning her baby, and as a carminative (a substance that relieves gas pains). They also specify its external use as a gargle and lotion for wounds. Research confirms only sage's effectiveness as a carminative and, possibly, for lowering a fever. Today the main use of the plant is as a culinary herb.

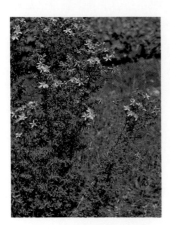

St. John's Wort

Hypericum perforatum L.

Amber Touch-and-heal, Goatweed,
Klamath Weed, Rosin Rose
ST. JOHN'S WORT FAMILY
Hypericaceae

Here is a plant to conjure with, a plant with supernatural powers. The ancient Greeks believed that the fragrance of St. John's wort would cause evil spirits to fly away. The early Christians converted the herb into a symbol of St. John the Baptist because it flowers about June 24, the day the church designated as St. John's Day. But Christian priests in the Middle Ages continued to follow their pagan forebears' example by using the plant in exorcisms, and European peasants employed a sprig of St. John's wort as a charm against witchcraft. The plant's use in the treatment of melancholia and madness seems to have been based on these ancient beliefs.

St. John's wort was long thought to have soothing properties that made it of special value in the treatment of wounds. Although a tea from the flowers is still used in herbal medicine, some researchers who study herbal teas warn against taking it because the plant contains hypericin, a photosensitizing substance that reacts with light to cause skin burns in light-skinned persons.

X Drinking the flower tea can cause skin burns.
Habitat: Meadows, dry pastures, roadsides.
Range: Native to Europe, St. John's wort is naturalized in Quebec and Ontario and in the eastern half of the United States, the Pacific Northwest south to northern California, and central Nevada.
Identification: An erect perennial herb that grows up to 32 inches tall and has a somewhat woody base. Oblong-oval leaves grow in opposite pairs. The flowers (June–September) have five yellow petals, which often have black dots at the margins.
Uses: Herbalists have long employed an ointment made from St. John's wort as an astringent for bruises, skin irritations, insect bites, and other wounds. American Indians used a tea brewed from the plant for tuberculosis and other respiratory ailments. Plant extracts have exhibited anti-inflammatory activity in laboratory animals, and in test tube experiments extracts have been active against the bacterium that causes tuberculosis.

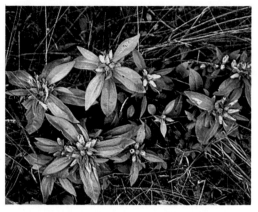

Sampson's Snakeroot

Gentiana villosa L.

Marsh Gentian, Pale Gentian,
Straw-colored Gentian, Striped Gentian
GENTIAN FAMILY
Gentianaceae

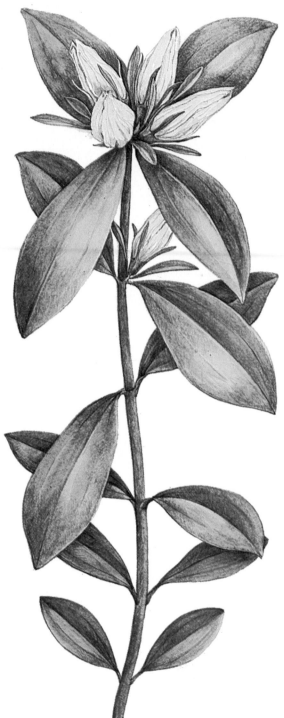

The genus is named for Gentius, a king of Illyria, on the Adriatic Sea, during the second century B.C. According to the first-century A.D. Greek physician Dioscorides and his Roman contemporary the naturalist Pliny, Gentius discovered the power of these plants. But in actual fact the use of gentians in medicine is recorded on a papyrus found in an Egyptian tomb at Thebes and dating from about a thousand years before Gentius' time.

One of many so-called snakeroots, Sampson's snakeroot is esteemed in herbal medicine not only as an antidote for snakebite and the "bites of mad dogs." It has also been specified for the treatment of gout and rheumatism. But the plant's foremost use, generally in the form of a tea, has been to stimulate the appetite and help digestion. Sampson's snakeroot is a popular home remedy in Appalachia, where the people sometimes carry a piece of the root to increase physical strength.

Among the various gentian species, the European *Gentiana lutea* has the most potent and versatile medicinal applications.

Habitat: Semishaded sites, dry coastal plains, pinelands, meadows, and open woods.
Range: A native of North America, Sampson's snakeroot is distributed from New Jersey, Pennsylvania, and southern Ohio and Indiana south to Florida and Louisiana.
Identification: A perennial herb with smooth stems growing to a height of about 18 inches. The leaves are lance-shaped to oval and reach up to 3 inches long. The small funnellike greenish-white to purplish-green flowers (August–October) have purple stripes inside and are borne in dense terminal clusters.
Uses: Researchers have found that the use of Sampson's snakeroot as an appetite stimulant is valid. The plant contains bitter chemical substances that would have this effect.

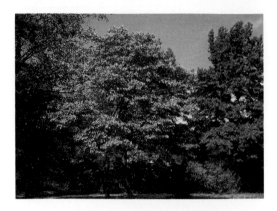

Sassafras

Sassafras albidum (Nutt.) Nees

Ague Tree, Cinnamonwood, Smelling-stick
LAUREL FAMILY
Lauraceae

When the Spanish arrived in Florida in the early 16th century, they mistook the fragrant sassafras for a cinnamon tree, an error still perpetuated in one of the tree's common names. The local Indians used the bark of its roots to treat fevers and rheumatism, and as a general tonic and "blood purifier"—a medicine that by causing urination and sweating cleanses the blood of "impurities" once thought to cause a range of ailments from skin diseases to malaria. Word of sassafras's amazing curative powers reached Europe, and for a time it became a major colonial export, second only to tobacco. The Europeans also discovered sassafras tea, and it soon became a fashionable beverage. A growing (but unjustified) reputation as a cure for syphilis cost sassafras its respectability, however, and as a result, its economic importance.

An oil extracted from the tree remained in use as an antiseptic for dentistry and as a flavoring for toothpastes, root beer, and chewing gum until the early 1960's. At that time the U.S. Food and Drug Administration declared that the chemical compound safrole, found in the oil of the root bark, was a potential carcinogen.

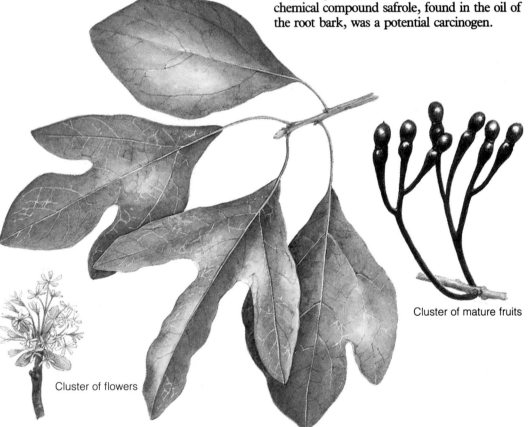

Cluster of mature fruits

Cluster of flowers

X The U.S. Food and Drug Administration lists sassafras oil as "unsafe" because of determinations that the safrole in the oil is a potential carcinogen.
Habitat: Woods, roadsides, fields.
Range: A native of eastern North America, sassafras is found from Ontario south to Florida and Texas and as far west as Missouri.
Identification: An aromatic deciduous tree, averaging 10–40 feet tall, with a rough gray bark. Bright green alternate leaves are oval, with one to three lobes. Greenish-yellow flowers (April–June) appear before the leaves and are followed by pea-sized fruits.
Uses: Sassafras root bark was long considered a virtual cure-all, but only its effectiveness in relieving intestinal gas and as a diuretic have been substantiated. Because of the designation as "unsafe," the bark is no longer sold or used commercially, nor should it be used by anyone.

Scotch Pine

Pinus sylvestris L.

Scotch Fir, Scots Pine

PINE FAMILY

Pinaceae

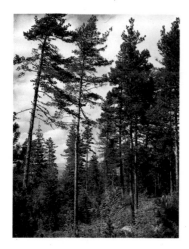

Americans know Scotch pine best as an ornamental tree, either in the garden or in the house at Christmas. But the tree is also used in reforestation projects because it matures rapidly and will endure extremes of temperature, rainfall, and soil conditions.

Scotch pine has an impressive history as a useful medicinal plant too. In 19th-century North America it was employed as a diuretic and to induce perspiration and thus help break a fever. It was also specified for constipation and chronic bronchitis. Externally, the tar was incorporated into an ointment, or tar water, employed as a remedy for such chronic skin diseases as psoriasis and eczema and for open sores. Scotch pine pitch, the result of distilling the tar, also yielded medicinal preparations for eczema and similar skin problems, and it was recommended internally for skin diseases and hemorrhoids as well.

In Europe, where Scotch pine is native, it serves as a light and durable building material. At one time in North America, the needles of Scotch pine were made into a mattress stuffing known as pine wool, which was said to ward off lice and fleas.

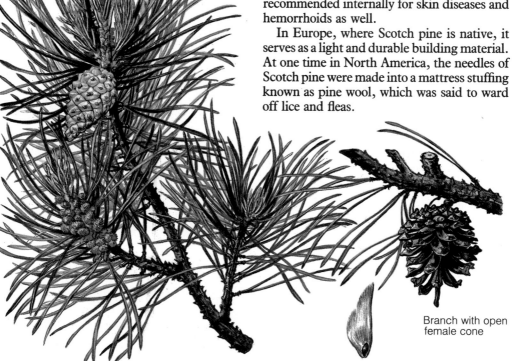

Branch with open female cone

Winged seed

Habitat: Temperate and northern climates.
Range: A native of Eurasia, Scotch pine was introduced into North America and is now naturalized from Ontario south to New Jersey and west to Ohio and Iowa.
Identification: An aromatic evergreen tree growing to heights of 65–115 feet. The bark on the lower trunk is grayish brown, and on the upper trunk and branches it is orange-red, deeply fissured, and flaky. Bluish-green needles occur in pairs and are about 1½–3 inches long. Yellowish-brown male cones form dense clusters. The female cones are brown when young and usually solitary; they turn green and grow to 1–2½ inches long, then turn brown again when mature.
Uses: Scotch pine tar and pitch once served as home remedies for chronic skin diseases such as eczema. Pine oil is used today as a disinfectant in commercial products. Scientists report that when used externally it acts as an antiseptic.

293

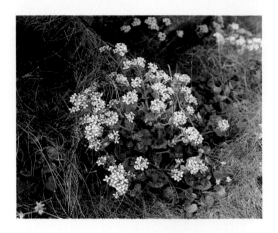

Scurvy Grass

Cochlearia officinalis L.

Scurvy Weed, Spoonwort
MUSTARD FAMILY
Cruciferae

A plant of the seashore and salt marsh, scurvy grass proved a good friend to seafarers. In the old days, scurvy—a devastating disease caused by a prolonged deficiency of vitamin C—was a scourge of sailors, who might pass months at sea without fresh fruits or vegetables. But if a captain stowed a supply of scurvy grass, as the 18th-century English explorer Capt. James Cook did, the sailors were safe, for the herb is rich in that vital nutrient.

Perhaps because it flourishes in salty soils, some herbalists thought scurvy grass would dissolve the "salts" of gout and rheumatism. Because it contains tannin, scurvy grass is astringent and can be used to stanch a nosebleed or other bleeding wound. The plant has also been classified as a diuretic, recommended for use in the treatment of kidney stones and dropsy (edema, or accumulation of fluids in the body). Herbalists claim, too, that the juice and leaves clear up skin blemishes.

Wild-food enthusiasts use the young leaves and stems as salad greens and a potherb, comparing the taste to that of the plant's relatives watercress and horseradish.

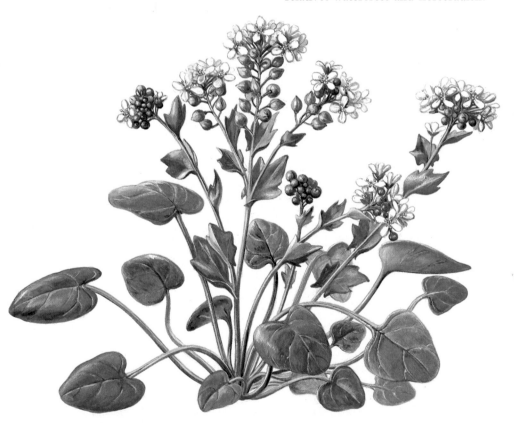

Habitat: Salty soils near coasts, salt marshes, springs, rivers, and moist mountain areas.
Range: A native of subarctic regions, scurvy grass is distributed in North America from Newfoundland to Alaska and south along the Pacific coast to Washington and Oregon.
Identification: A biennial herb growing 4–12 inches high. Its curving or upright stems bear fleshy, dark green, long-stalked leaves that are oval to heart-shaped. Small white flowers (June–August) with four petals that form a cross are borne in terminal clusters.
Uses: An excellent source of vitamin C, scurvy grass has served both physicians and herbalists as an antiscorbutic, or remedy for scurvy. Those who enjoy wild foods use the raw leaves as a potherb and add the tender young leaves and stems, which have a pungent flavor, to salads and sandwiches.

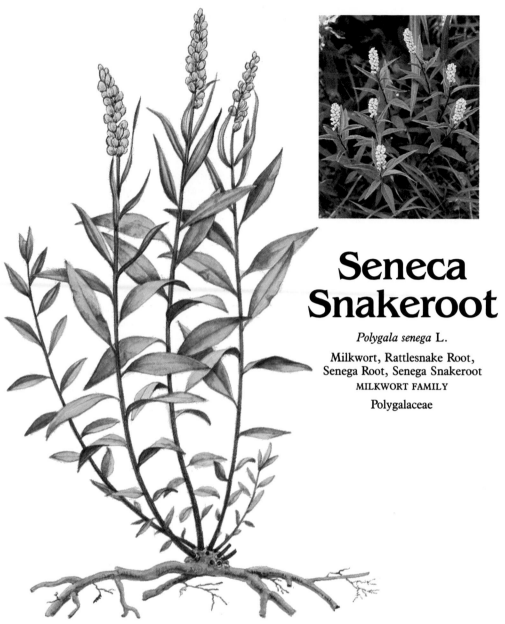

Seneca Snakeroot

Polygala senega L.

Milkwort, Rattlesnake Root,
Senega Root, Senega Snakeroot
MILKWORT FAMILY
Polygalaceae

The Greek-derived genus name *Polygala* means "much milk" and originally designated seneca snakeroot as an herb believed to increase the flow of milk in cattle. *Senega*, which is the species name of this native American plant, is Latin for "seneca" and reflects early reports that the Seneca Indians used the plant medicinally. It was dubbed rattlesnake root because the Senecas and other tribes considered the root an antidote for rattlesnake bites. They chewed the woody roots and then applied the pulpy mass to the bite, but there is no evidence that the treatment worked. Indians also brewed teas from the roots to control fevers and to ease heart trouble and asthma.

Starting in 1736, seneca snakeroot was promoted as a cure for pleurisy by Dr. John Tennent, a Scottish physician who had done research among the Indians, and the plant was taken up as a wonder drug for a host of other respiratory ills. Today it is used only occasionally, for coughs and colds.

Habitat: Dry, rocky woods, prairies, and hillsides at higher elevations.
Range: Native to North America, seneca snakeroot is found in Canada from Newfoundland to Alberta, and in the United States from New England to Georgia and Arkansas, and west to the Dakotas.
Identification: A perennial herb with greenish-purple erect stems growing up to 1 foot tall. The leaves are lance-shaped and almost stalkless. Small whitish-green to pinkish pealike flowers (May–July) are borne in dense terminal clusters.
Uses: Although seneca snakeroot was dropped from the pharmaceutical reference book the *National Formulary* in 1960, herbalists still recommend preparations made from the roots to bring up phlegm in cases of asthma and bronchitis. Scientific data indicate that this use is probably valid. In Europe the root is an ingredient in commercial cough drops and syrups and herbal teas.

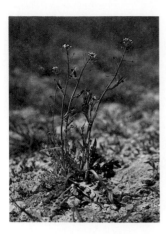

Shepherd's-purse

Capsella bursa-pastoris (L.) Medic.

Caseweed, Mother's-heart,
Shovelweed
MUSTARD FAMILY

Cruciferae

A native of the Old World that now thrives around the globe, shepherd's-purse is well suited for survival: a single plant can produce up to 40,000 seeds. The name shovelweed comes from the plant's heart-shaped seedpods, which resemble pointed shovels. But the pods were most commonly compared to the leather pouches in which shepherds carried their food—hence the name shepherd's-purse.

According to the Greek physician Dioscorides (first century A.D.) and the Roman naturalist Pliny (A.D. 23–79), the seeds were effective as a laxative. But in the 1500's the Italian physician Pietro Mattioli cited shepherd's-purse as helpful in stopping excessive bleeding, and this use remained. During World War I, when certain German drugs that controlled bleeding were not available, British doctors used extracts of shepherd's-purse. The herb is also reported to halt bleeding from internal organs and from hemorrhoids. The 17th-century English herbalist Nicholas Culpeper wrote of its virtues: "The juice dropped into the ears, heals the pains, noise, and matterings thereof. A good ointment may be made of it for all wounds."

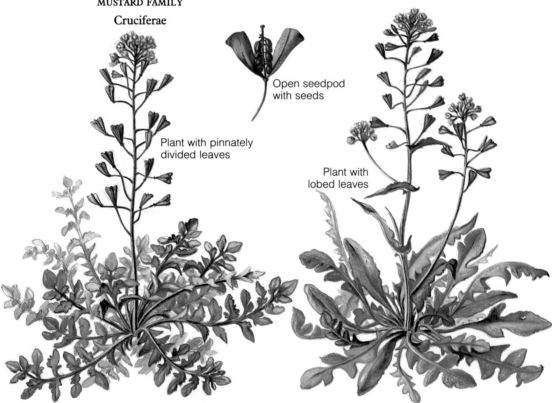

Open seedpod
with seeds

Plant with pinnately
divided leaves

Plant with
lobed leaves

Habitat: Sandy or loamy soil in sunny, open waste places, pastures, lawns, gardens.
Range: Temperate areas throughout the world.
Identification: A hardy self-pollinating annual growing to 18 inches high. The stem rises from a basal rosette of lobed or divided leaves; smaller, alternate, clasping leaves grow along the stem. Small white flowers that bloom throughout the year have four petals and produce small, distinctive, heart-shaped seedpods.

Uses: The chief use of shepherd's-purse in medicine has been to stop bleeding from internal organs and to control profuse menstruation. Human and test tube studies show that the plant has hemostatic properties—that is, the ability to stop bleeding. The peppery young leaves can be eaten like spinach or used to season stews, and the seeds can be substituted for mustard.

Silverweed

Potentilla anserina L.

Argentine, Crampweed, Goosewort,
Moon Grass, Wild Tansy
ROSE FAMILY
Rosaceae

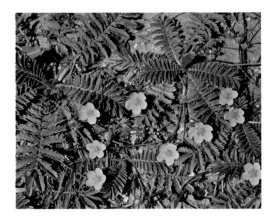

Roasted, boiled, or raw, silverweed's starchy rootstock has served as food for North American Indians, Eskimos, and northern Europeans for many years. At times silverweed rootstock—which is said to taste like parsnips, sweet potatoes, or chestnuts—has kept regional populations alive when nothing else was available to eat. Silverweed is also food for many wildlife species. The leaves are evidently a favorite of geese, because the common name goosewort means "goose plant," and the species name *anserina* is Latin for "of or pertaining to geese." The plant reproduces by sending out runners, which develop roots that penetrate the soil and produce leaves. When the main plant dies, the newer portions that have developed along the runners become separate plants. This mode of propagation helps the plant stand up to grazing by animals.

The genus name *Potentilla*, derived from the Latin *potens*, or "powerful," refers to the plant's reputed power to cure various ailments. Tea made from silverweed was formerly much used to treat menstrual cramps and indigestion. Boiling the plants produced a decoction used as a mouthwash for sore gums and toothache. An infusion of silverweed and honey has also been taken to relieve sore throat.

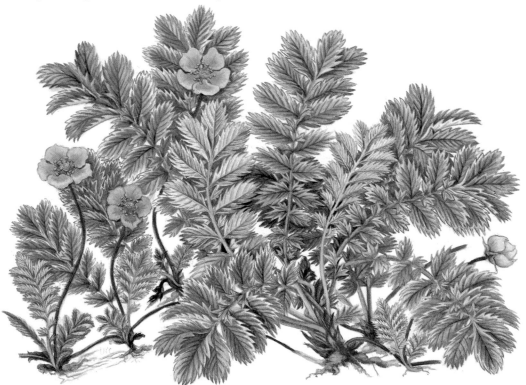

Habitat: Damp ground, streamsides.
Range: Native to Eurasia, silverweed is found in North America from Nova Scotia to Alaska, south to New York, Iowa, New Mexico, and California.
Identification: A ground-hugging perennial growing 8–16 inches tall. Runners, 3–6 feet long, link new plants bearing tufts of leaves that are pinnately divided into toothed leaflets with silvery undersides. Each tuft bears a single five-petaled, bright golden yellow flower (June–August) atop a 2- to 12-inch-long leafless stalk. The flowers close at night and on cloudy days.
Uses: Silverweed contains much tannin, which is an astringent and may account for its use as a gargle and mouthwash. No scientific data have been made available to validate the plant's use for cramps, indigestion, toothache, and sore throat.

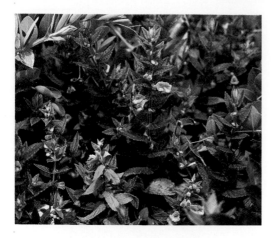

Skullcap

Scutellaria lateriflora L.

Blue Pimpernel, Blue Skullcap, Helmetflower,
Hoodwort, Mad-dog Skullcap,
Mad-dog Weed, Madweed

MINT FAMILY

Labiatae

Publicized as a cure for rabies, skullcap caused a stir in medical circles when, about 1773, Dr. Lawrence Van Derveer announced that he had successfully treated hundreds of cases with it. His claims for skullcap were discredited—but not before earning the plant no less than three common names referring to its association with rabies. Today some scientists conclude that Dr. Van Derveer's claims may not have been completely without basis. Skullcap has achieved a reputation as a sedative and antispasmodic—properties that may account for its sometimes being effective in alleviating the symptoms of rabies.

Equally extravagant have been the claims for skullcap's effectiveness as a "nervine," or tranquilizer. For years herbalists have acclaimed the plant as "one of the finest nervines ever discovered" and have prescribed it for a gamut of so-called nervous disorders, from mild anxiety to epilepsy. But there has been less controversy over the calming effect of the tea made from the whole plant.

Skullcap is a native American plant, which some Indian tribes used as a sedative and to promote menstruation. The name refers to the shape of the flower, which resembles a helmet with the visor raised. "Skullcap" was the word for a type of military helmet that was familiar to early colonists.

X Large doses may cause giddiness, confusion, twitching, and stupor.

Habitat: Moist woods and swampy areas.

Range: Native to North America, skullcap is found in temperate regions of the continent.

Identification: A perennial with an erect, smooth, branching stem growing to 3 feet. Broadly lance-shaped, toothed leaves grow in opposite pairs. Small tubular blue, pinkish, violet, or white flowers (July–August) have two lips, the upper one hooded.

Uses: Skullcap contains scutellarin, a flavonoid with sedative and antispasmodic properties. This substance was probably the active ingredient in the skullcap extract used in 19th-century medicine for nervous disorders ranging from insomnia to epilepsy. It is still used in modern herbal medicine for the prevention of epileptic seizures. More cautious pharmacological opinion concedes as "possible" the validity of skullcap's use as a sedative, but only on the basis of animal tests.

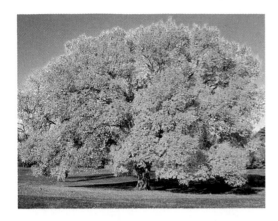

Slippery Elm

Ulmus rubra Muhl.

Indian Elm, Moose Elm,
Red Elm, Sweet Elm

ELM FAMILY

Ulmaceae

North American Indians were the first to discover the healing powers of the native slippery elm. They found that when the tree's inner bark comes in contact with water, the gummy substance, or mucilage, surrounding its fibers swells and produces a soothing and softening ointment. They used the salve externally to treat skin problems ranging from chapped lips to burns and wounds. Surgeons in the American Revolution treated many gunshot wounds with poultices of slippery elm. From Indian medicine men settlers also learned of the effectiveness of brews made from the tree's bark in treating diarrhea, constipation, kidney disorders, and numerous other internal complaints. Midwives once used slippery elm sap as a lubricant to ease labor.

Since the early days, herbalists not only have used slippery elm for skin and internal problems but also have found that the tea has nutritional value and is good for babies and invalids. The plant was once listed in the *U.S. Pharmacopeia,* and its use as a soothing medication continues today in many rural areas.

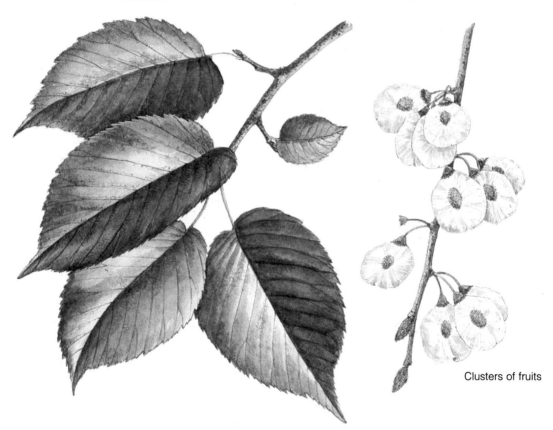

Clusters of fruits

Habitat: Poor soil in open and elevated areas; also found in woods and by streams.
Range: Native to North America, slippery elm is found mainly in southern Canada and south to Florida and west to Texas and the Dakotas. It is a rare or threatened species in some states.
Identification: A deciduous tree, 50–80 feet tall. The trunk is dark brown to reddish brown; the bark is rough and thick. Alternate dark green toothed leaves, 6–8 inches long, are oval and asymmetrical. They are rough above and hairy below. Dark brown flower buds with orange tips open into small flowers (March–May) in inconspicuous clusters at the tips of the branches.
Uses: Slippery elm is used as a soothing medication in many rural parts of the United States. Research has established that it does have the demulcent (soothing to the mucous membranes) and emollient (skin-softening) properties that have been ascribed to it in folk medicine.

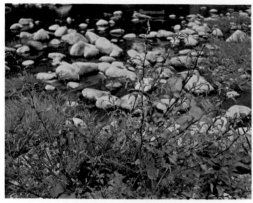

Smartweed

Polygonum hydropiper L.

Biting Knotweed,
Red Knees, Water Pepper
BUCKWHEAT FAMILY

Polygonaceae

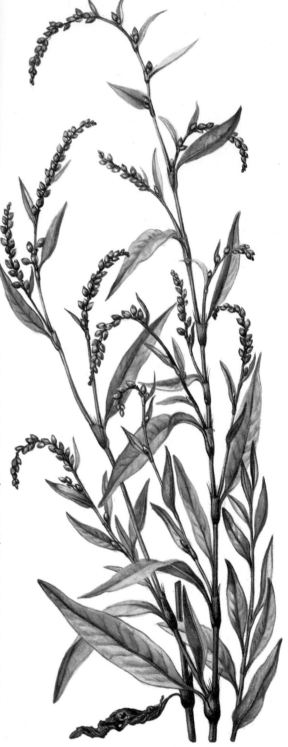

Just one taste of smartweed is enough to explain its name. Its acrid burning flavor does indeed cause a smarting sensation—so much so that livestock avoid the plant. Its fondness for streamsides and other damp places inspired another of its common names, water pepper, while its jointed stems account for such names as red knees and biting knotweed.

According to the herbalist Maud Grieve, man has ascribed a strange assortment of powers to the plant: a bit of smartweed tucked beneath the saddle was said to keep a horse from feeling hunger or thirst; strewing the plant on the floor was supposed to rid a room of fleas; and just a few drops of the juice reportedly destroyed the insidious worms that were believed to cause earaches. Cholera victims were sometimes wrapped in sheets that had been soaked in a brew made of boiled smartweed. The plant was also added to baths to help ease the pain of rheumatism. Smartweed has been called effective as a cure for everything from toothaches and epilepsy to gangrene and gout. Today smartweed is used in folk medicine as an external astringent, a remedy for diarrhea, and a contraceptive.

Habitat: Damp soils, streambanks, ditches.
Range: Native to Eurasia and America, smartweed is common throughout North America except in southern Georgia and in Florida.
Identification: An annual herb with reddish jointed stems, 1–2 feet long, and narrow lance-shaped leaves. Tiny greenish-white, often red-tipped flowers (June–November) are borne on long, slender, drooping spikes. The leaves and stems have a pronounced peppery taste.

Uses: Because of its hot, biting flavor, common smartweed is believed to have been used as early as prehistoric times as a seasoning for food. The plant also yields a golden yellow dye. Experiments indicate that extracts of smartweed have hemostatic properties (help stop bleeding) and lower the blood pressure. Animal studies suggest the plant has contraceptive effects. There is little evidence that it remedies diarrhea.

Solomon's Seal

Polygonatum biflorum (Walt.) Ell.

True Solomon's Seal
LILY FAMILY
Liliaceae

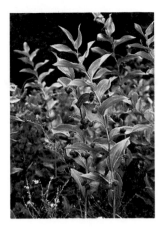

So strongly did medieval herbalists trust in the power of Solomon's seal to heal wounds that they fancied that the deep scars along its rhizome, or rootstock, had been set there by that wise king and legendary magician Solomon as a testimony to its medicinal virtues.

Each year the rhizome produces a new stem that withers in the summer, leaving a scar resembling the wax seals once used to close letters. The plant's age is estimated by counting the scars. These seallike knobs also inspired its botanical name, *Polygonatum*, meaning "many-jointed," and gave rise to the belief that it was effective in curing water on the knee. A European species, *P. officinale*, unmistakably resembles the American species; they and other *Polygonatum* species not only look alike but have had similar medicinal uses.

The 16th-century herbalist John Gerard claimed Solomon's seal rhizome was a panacea for cuts, wounds, and bruises of all kinds, including those "gotten by falls or women's willfulness in stumbling on their hasty husbands' fists." Solomon's seal roots contain a substance called allantoin, which when derived from other plant sources is used in modern medications for the external treatment of wounds and skin ulcers.

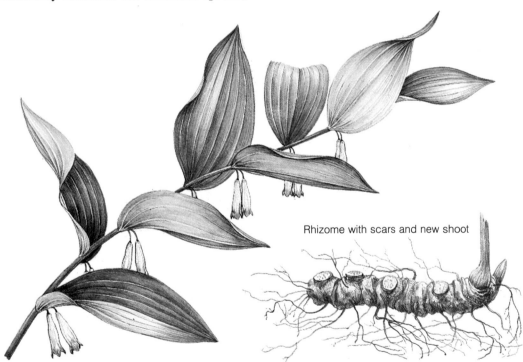

Rhizome with scars and new shoot

Habitat: Moist woods, thickets, roadsides.
Range: Native to North America, *P. biflorum* is distributed from Ontario south to Florida and west to Texas and Nebraska.
Identification: A perennial herb with a fleshy rhizome and an erect, angular stem growing 1–3 feet high, curved like a bow at the top. Large elliptical outward-pointing leaves are arranged alternately along the stem. White to greenish-yellow cylindrical flowers (May–June) with six green-spotted lobes at the tips hang in pairs from the sides of the leaf axils. The berries are blue-black.
Uses: Pharmacologists doubt that Solomon's seal is effective as a hemostatic (an agent that stops bleeding), the most common traditional use of the plant. Nor do they find evidence to support its reported efficacy as an antiemetic—an agent that stops vomiting.

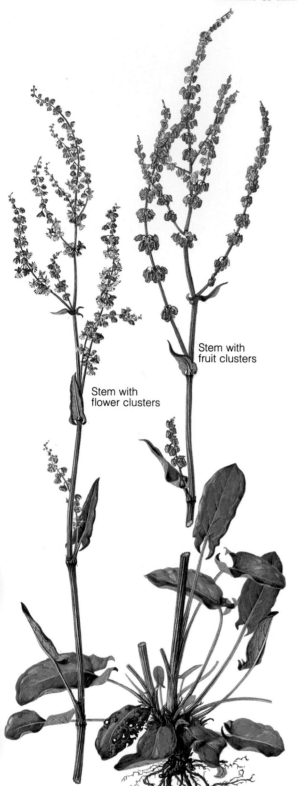

Stem with
fruit clusters

Stem with
flower clusters

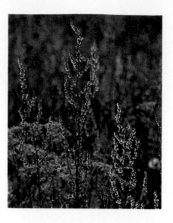

Sorrel

Rumex acetosa L.

Garden Sorrel, Greensauce, Soursuds
BUCKWHEAT FAMILY
Polygonaceae

A common summertime sight in the North American wild, sorrel came to the New World as a salad green. Its jade-green, arrow-shaped leaves were a regular feature of European vegetable gardens from the Middle Ages until the 1700's. Mashed sorrel leaves mixed with vinegar and sugar were popular as a green sauce with cold meat—hence one of the plant's names, greensauce. The herb's sharp taste is due to its oxalic acid and vitamin C content; the latter led to its use in folk medicine to prevent scurvy. But because even small amounts of oxalic acid are toxic to some extent, sorrel should not be served indiscriminately. In particular, persons with gout, rheumatism, or kidney ailments should avoid sorrel. In large amounts oxalic acid is extremely poisonous. The oxalic acid content of sorrel can be reduced by parboiling before cooking.

A tea made from sorrel root was long recommended by herbalists as a diuretic, but its use is inadvisable because of the plant's potential toxicity. A leaf tea has also figured in herbal medicine as an appetite stimulant, a scurvy preventive, and an antiseptic; it is also somewhat laxative. A tea of leaves also appears in herbal literature as a coolant for fever.

X Sorrel contains oxalic acid and can be dangerous to small children, old people, or persons in delicate health. It should be parboiled before cooking. The medicinal tea may be poisonous in large doses.
Habitat: Meadows, old fields, roadsides.
Range: Introduced from Europe, sorrel is widely naturalized in North America.
Identification: A perennial 2–2½ feet tall, sorrel has an erect stem branching at the top into several stalks bearing clusters of small reddish-green to brown flowers (June–September). Smooth, bright green leaves shaped like arrowheads, each on its own slender stalk, form a basal rosette when the plant is young and grow alternately along the stem as the plant matures. The leaves on the upper stem embrace it.
Uses: Research has determined that sorrel and other *Rumex* species contain chemical compounds that have a mild antiseptic effect and also act as a laxative.

Sourtop Blueberry

Vaccinium myrtilloides Michx.

Velvet-leaf Blueberry

HEATH FAMILY

Ericaceae

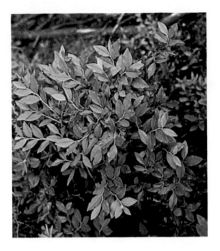

Handfuls of tangy purple berries eaten on the spot make for memories of climbing favorite mountains, of seeing autumn slopes washed with deep blue or purple where sourtop blueberry, huckleberry, or blueberry bushes cover the ridges. Closely related and near look-alikes, these plants are best known for their delicious edible fruits, but their medicinal properties have long been valued too. They are members of the heath family and occur in many varieties, which frequently hybridize. Locations vary, too, ranging from mountains to bogs, but the requirements are the same everywhere—acid soil that is sandy or peaty.

Herbalists have traditionally recommended a tea brewed from the leaves or berries to prevent the formation of kidney or bladder stones, and people have long gargled with such brews to ease mouth sores. They have also drunk the tea as a diabetes remedy and to relieve the miseries of diarrhea and bladder irritation. The leaf tea has also served as an antiseptic skin lotion. Whatever their medicinal properties, the fresh tender springtime leaves make an excellent tea.

The Chippewas used the flowers of blueberry, *V. angustifolium*, as a medicine for "craziness."

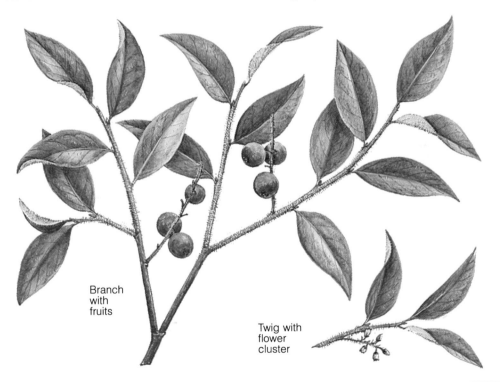

Branch
with
fruits

Twig with
flower
cluster

Habitat: Moist woods and clearings, swamps.
Range: Native to North America, sourtop blueberry grows wild from Newfoundland to British Columbia, in the mountains of the eastern United States, and in parts of the Midwest.
Identification: A low-growing shrub, usually about 3 feet tall, that grows in dense colonies because of its intertwining roots. Alternate oval leaves are 1–2 inches long, entire (not toothed), and hairy or velvety and whitened on their lower surfaces. They grow on very short stalks, which turn wine-red in autumn. Tiny light green or pink flowers (May–June) are shaped like drooping vases. The berries (July–September) are a white-powdered dusky blue.
Uses: Pharmacologists have studied sourtop blueberry's use as a diuretic and astringent for disorders of the genitourinary tract and find it of questionable value. Research indicates, however, that the leaf tea may help rid the body of worm infestations.

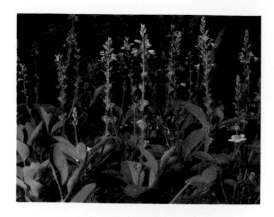

Although the flowers are easily ignored when larger and showier plants are nearby, the small pale blue, lavender, and white blooms of speedwell are a common summer sight in woods. Herbalists once employed speedwell in the treatment of a wide variety of ills. In modern herbal medicine, speedwell tea, brewed from the dried flowering plant, sometimes serves as a cough remedy or as a lotion for irritated or infected skin. The somewhat bitter and astringent taste and tealike smell of speedwell led to its use as a tea substitute in 19th-century France, where it was called *thé d'Europe*, or "Europe tea." The French still use this term as a name for speedwell.

Speedwell

Veronica officinalis L.

Gypsyweed, Low Speedwell, Veronica
SNAPDRAGON FAMILY

Scrophulariaceae

The name speedwell comes from an old meaning of the word *speed*, "thrive." The scientific term *Veronica* goes back some 500 years and is apparently connected with the name of the legendary Veronica, who is said to have wiped the face of Jesus as He went to Calvary. It is possible that the genus *Veronica* was named after her because the flowers supposedly resemble the markings left on the cloth with which she wiped Jesus' face.

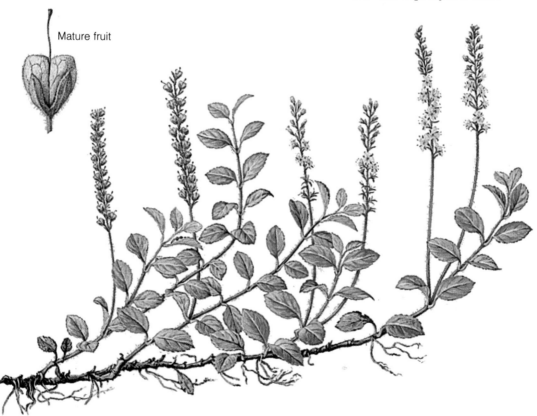

Mature fruit

Habitat: Stony or gravelly acidic soils, in meadows, fields, open woods, and clearings.

Range: Native to temperate regions of the Northern Hemisphere, speedwell is found from Newfoundland to Ontario, south to North Carolina and Tennessee, and west to Wisconsin.

Identification: A low-growing perennial, it has hairy creeping stems with grayish-green, opposite, oval leaves. Flowering stalks shoot straight up as much as 16 inches above the recumbent portion of the plant,

bearing small blue, lavender, or white flowers (May–July) in racemes (elongated flower clusters). The plant reproduces by seed and by runners.

Uses: A tea prepared from the dried flowering plant serves as a diuretic and expectorant (to bring up phlegm), but pharmacologists question the effectiveness of both these uses. They also doubt that the tea has value as a lotion for skin infections and irritations.

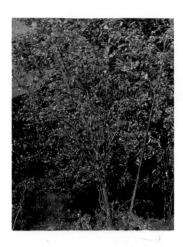

Spicebush

Lindera benzoin (L.) Blume

Benjamin Bush, Feverbush, Spiceberry,
Spicewood, Wild Allspice
LAUREL FAMILY

Lauraceae

Twice the native shrub spicebush has come to the aid of Americans at war. During the Revolution spicebush berries were used by American housewives to replace allspice, which had previously been imported from England. Later, during the Civil War, spicebush leaves and twigs furnished the blockaded South with a substitute for foreign teas.

Colonial surveyors believed that where spicebush grew, the soil would prove to be fertile farmland. The men and women who settled these lands also valued the spicy-smelling bush for its medicinal properties. They made an extract of the leaves or bark to induce perspiration and thus break a fever. In the past, folk doctors also placed great faith in spicebush's powers as a tonic and as a cure for intestinal worms, dysentery, colds, and coughs. Some herbalists distilled from the oil in the berries a liniment for rheumatism, bruises, and neuralgia. The Indians made a tea from the twigs, which their women drank to promote menstruation or to ease its pain.

Sometimes called the "forsythia of the wilds," spicebush produces countless yellow flowers that appear while the twigs are still barren of leaves.

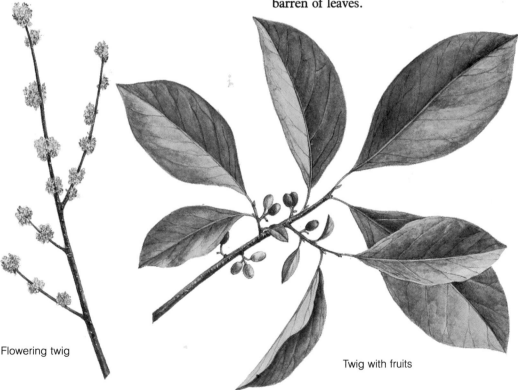

Flowering twig

Twig with fruits

Habitat: Moist woods, streambanks.
Range: A native of North America, spicebush is found from southern Ontario and Maine south to Florida, and west to Kansas and Texas. It is an endangered species in some states.
Identification: A deciduous shrub growing 3–15 feet tall. Clusters of tiny yellow flowers (March–April) appear before the smooth, pointed, alternate leaves, which give off a spicy fragrance when crushed. Small, shiny, bright red fruits (July–September) emit a spicy scent when squeezed.
Uses: The prime medicinal use of spicebush has been as a febrifuge, or agent that reduces fever. Folk healers still use the shrub for this purpose and they also recommend it for colds and as a tonic. There is very little scientific data available to validate these claims. Since colonial times, the berries have served cooks as a substitute for allspice. The leaves make a refreshing tea, and in spring the blossoms can be added for extra sweetness.

Spikenard

Aralia racemosa L.

American Sarsaparilla, American Spikenard,
Indian Root

GINSENG FAMILY

Araliaceae

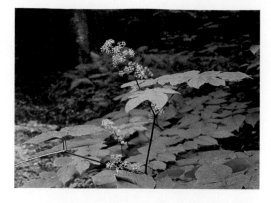

A large, handsome perennial plant, spikenard was a popular herb among American Indians, who gathered its pleasantly scented roots for a variety of medicinal uses. Herbalists record that the Cherokees drank spikenard tea for backache and that the Shawnees used it to treat gas pains, coughs, asthma, and chest pains. Other tribes gave the tea to women in labor to make childbirth swifter and less painful. The Micmacs reportedly applied a salve of spikenard to cuts and wounds, while the Ojibwas used the root in a poultice for healing broken bones.

Early settlers added spikenard to their own herbal medicine shelf and found even more uses for it. Juice from the dark purple berries and oil from the seeds were poured into ears to cure earache and deafness. Medical practitioners in the 19th century prescribed the root to treat gout, rheumatism, syphilis, and other diseases in which it was deemed necessary to "purify the blood."

Closely related to spikenard is wild sarsaparilla, *Aralia nudicaulis*, whose root is similarly aromatic and was likewise used for medicinal purposes—as a tonic, stimulant, and perspiration inducer. Wild sarsaparilla was also brewed into a root beer.

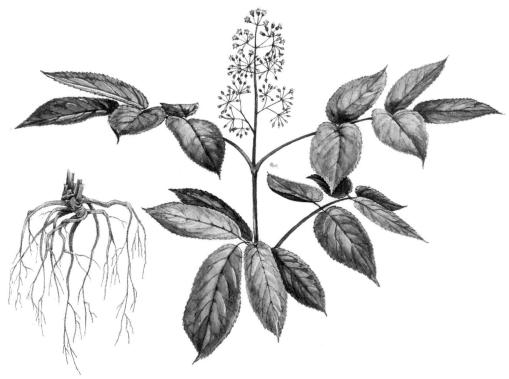

Rootstock with stems and roots

Habitat: Rich woods and thickets.
Range: Quebec to Manitoba, south to Georgia and Mexico, west to South Dakota.
Identification: A perennial growing to 10 feet in height, spikenard produces tiny green flowers (June–August) in clusters on branched stalks. The flowers later develop into dark purple berries. The leaves are divided into many oval leaflets. Wild sarsaparilla is smaller, growing to about 1 foot; its leaves are divided into five toothed, oval leaflets.

Uses: Spikenard is not widely used today as a medicinal ingredient. Herbalists may use a tincture of the root in cough syrups, alone or with such other ingredients as wild black cherry bark, elecampane, and coltsfoot. There is some evidence that the root may be effective against rheumatism. Whether or not spikenard root helps, it is pleasant-tasting and harmless.

Spindletree

Euonymus europaeus L.

European Spindletree
STAFF-TREE FAMILY
Celastraceae

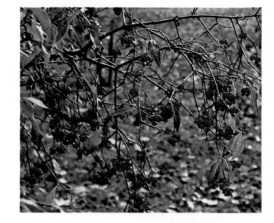

With its pretty red autumn leaves and showy red berries, this is a most ornamental shrub or tree, but its festive appearance belies its poisonous nature. The fruit, leaves, and particularly the bark of the spindletree contain a substance that supplies a valuable laxative for pharmaceutical manufacturers. Early herbalists used these parts as a purgative, or strong laxative, but laymen should never take any part of the tree internally, for colon pain and drastic purging can result. The U.S. Food and Drug Administration has declared the tree "unsafe" and dangerous for this reason.

The Swedish botanist Carolus Linnaeus labeled the tree *Euonymus* ("of auspicious name"). This name, which the 3rd-century B.C. Greek naturalist Theophrastus first recorded in his works, was euphemistically bestowed in recognition of the plant's toxicity.

At one time sculptors favored the wood of the spindletree, and artists used its charcoal for sketching. In the past, some tanners preferred the bark to that of all other trees for tanning and dyeing leathers, which they sold for the manufacture of fine leather gloves.

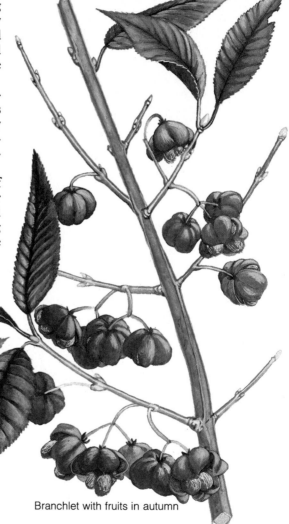

Branchlet with fruits in autumn

Branchlet with open flowers

X The U.S. Food and Drug Administration lists the spindletree as "unsafe" because of its violent laxative properties.
Habitat: Roadsides and other waste places.
Range: A native of Europe, spindletree has escaped cultivation in parts of Canada and in parts of the United States from Massachusetts to Wisconsin and southward.
Identification: A bushy shrub or small tree growing to 20 feet tall. Small, dark green, finely toothed oval to lance-shaped leaves, 1¼–3 inches long, grow in opposite pairs. White to greenish-yellow flowers (May–June) are borne in loose clusters near the axils of the leafstalks. Red fruits, when ripe, reveal orange seeds.
Uses: Experimental evidence appears to validate spindletree's harsh laxative effect, and pharmacologists warn against using any part of the plant.

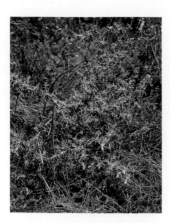

Star Thistle

Centaurea calcitrapa L.

Caltrops
COMPOSITE FAMILY
Compositae

On European battlefields long ago soldiers planted caltrops (metal traps with four spikes) to damage the feet of the enemy and the hooves of their horses. Quite possibly it was these soldiers, returned from the wars, who gave the name caltrops to star thistles, the bristly plants that resembled the battle traps and that impeded a farmer's march through his fields or a walker's stroll along the roadside.

Despite its prickly nature, star thistle has a number of virtues. The young scales of the flowerhead are edible like an artichoke, and in parts of North Africa the young, tender stems and leaves complement the salads. Camels, too, are fed this herb. Star thistle has also had medicinal use, most notably for reducing fevers. In the 19th century, one botanist noted that Americans were employing the plant for kidney complaints such as nephritis and gravel (small kidney stones). A modern European herb book lists the seeds as a diuretic and suggests a palatable prescription made by crushing them in white wine. It also recommends an infusion (tea) of the leaves and flowers for fevers and general debility. For a more potent remedy, the herbal mentions brewing the leaves with angelica, wormwood, or white willow bark.

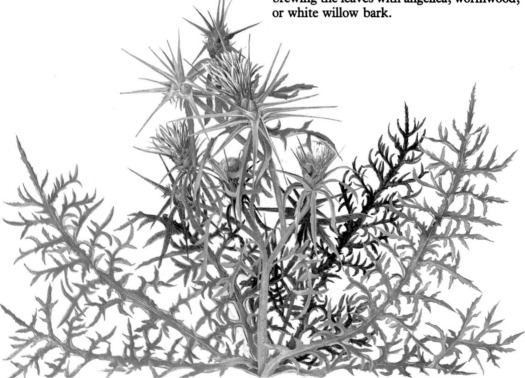

Habitat: Fields, waste places, roadsides.
Range: A native of Europe, star thistle is naturalized in eastern North America from eastern Canada, New England and New York south to Virginia, and in western North America from British Columbia to California.
Identification: An annual or biennal herb, 8–20 inches tall, rising from a basal rosette of twice-divided spiny leaves, 4–7 inches long. The pinkish-purple flowerheads (June–October) are surrounded by straw-colored prickly bracts.
Uses: Star thistle has been specified as an antipyretic (an agent that helps reduce a fever), a diuretic, and a tonic. There is some experimental evidence that the leaves and flowers have an antidiabetic effect, but this needs confirmation. Other claims for the plant have not been studied scientifically.

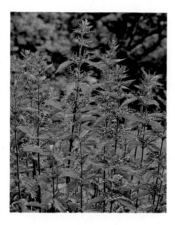

Stinging Nettle

Urtica dioica L.
Common Nettle
NETTLE FAMILY
Urticaceae

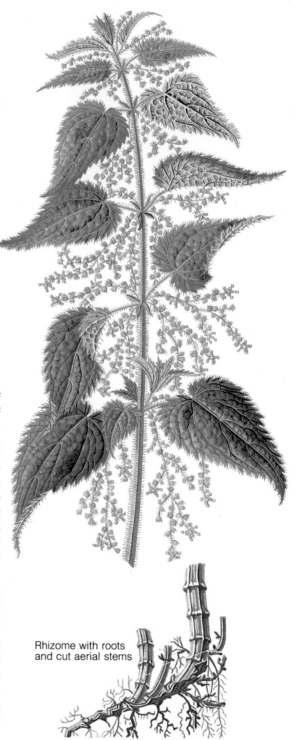

Rhizome with roots
and cut aerial stems

Although it is best known today for the burning rash it produces upon contact with the skin, stinging nettle deserves greater appreciation. Once widely consumed as a spring tonic, the plant's tender young stalks (boiling removes the irritating material) are rich in protein, iron, and vitamins A and C and make a healthful tea, soup, or green. Stinging nettle was formerly cultivated in Scotland for the fibers in the stalks, which served to make a durable linenlike cloth. This use goes back to the Bronze Age; the very name nettle is said to derive from words meaning "textile plant."

Herbalists also made good use of the nettle, which they considered a cure for everything from baldness to tuberculosis. But the nettle seems to have been most popular as a counterirritant—an agent that, by irritating the skin of an inflamed area, causes increased blood flow to the area and thereby reduces the inflammation. Victims of gout and rheumatism allowed themselves to be scourged with nettles in the dubious belief that this would alleviate their sufferings.

Habitat: Waste places, roadsides.
Range: Native to Eurasia, stinging nettle now grows as a weed throughout southern Canada and in most of the United States.
Identification: A perennial herb with erect stems up to 4 feet tall, nettle has opposite, heart-shaped, coarsely toothed leaves covered with stiff, stinging bristles (the bristles also cover the stems). Tiny light green flowers (June–September) are borne in long slender spikes at the axils of the leaves.

Uses: A tea made from the seeds is used in modern herbal medicine as a hair tonic and growth stimulant and antidandruff shampoo; a poultice of the leaves reportedly alleviates pain due to inflammation; and the dried powdered leaf is said to stop nosebleed. Pharmacologists doubt that the plant is effective in any of these uses. Nettle is a commercial source of chlorophyll and yields a green dye. The young shoots are edible after boiling.

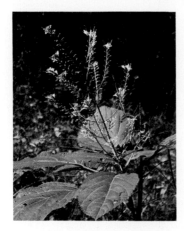

Stoneroot
Collinsonia canadensis L.

Horse Balm, Horseweed, Ox Balm, Richweed
MINT FAMILY
Labiatae

A strong lemon fragrance, which has earned stoneroot the common name richweed, is the most conspicuous feature of this native American member of the mint family. Its leaves and rhizome (underground stem) were brewed to make medicinal teas and washes, or lotions, for cuts and wounds by generations of American Indians and pioneering white settlers in the mountains of Virginia, the Carolinas, Kentucky, and Tennessee. As with many plants, the different names provide important background. The name stoneroot refers either to the plant's knobby, stone-hard rhizome or to the mountaineers' use of a tea brewed from the rhizome as a diuretic in the treatment of an affliction known as the stone—possibly kidney or bladder stone. The names with "horse" and "ox" refer to the species' large size.

American Indians and white settlers treated wounds with stoneroot preparations, which they applied externally as a poultice or wash. The tea brewed from the rhizome served not only as a diuretic—as in the treatment of the "stone"—but also as a general tonic, a headache remedy, and a laxative. The plant enjoyed some further use among 19th-century physicians in the United States.

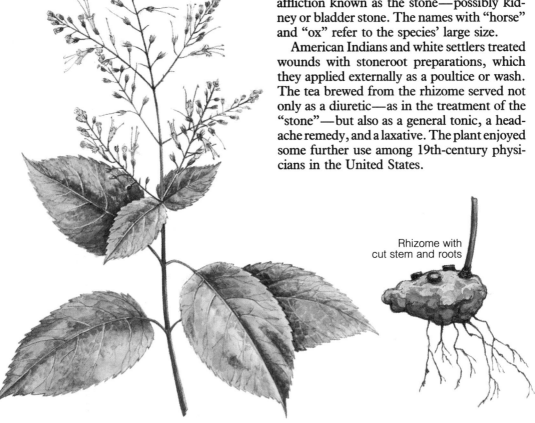

Rhizome with
cut stem and roots

Habitat: Moist woodlands or in shade on rich soil.
Range: Native to North America, stoneroot is found growing wild from Massachusetts and Vermont south to Florida and west to Ontario, Wisconsin, and Arkansas.
Identification: A perennial herb growing up to 4 feet tall, with a single, erect, square stem. Oval, toothed leaves grow in opposite pairs along the stem, which culminates in a cone-shaped, branched cluster of small, tubular, light yellow flowers (July–September). The flowers have a strong lemony smell.
Uses: A tea brewed from the rhizome of stoneroot once served as a tonic and diuretic and as a household remedy for headaches and constipation. It was also applied in poultices on wounds, cuts, and bruises. Scientific evidence does not support any of these uses.

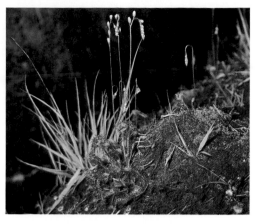

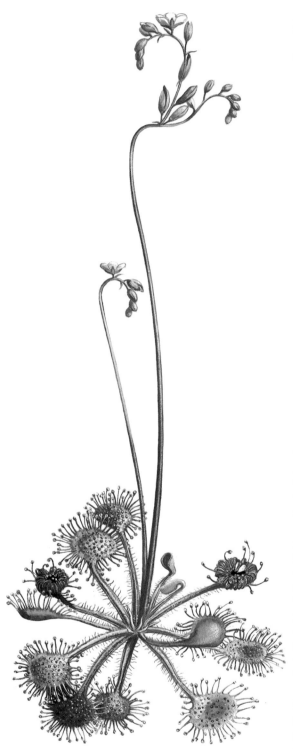

Sundew

Drosera rotundifolia L.

Common Sundew, Red Rot,
Round-leaved Sundew

SUNDEW FAMILY

Droseraceae

The moment a small unsuspecting insect alights upon a leaf of sundew, it is hopelessly trapped. At the base of the plant's long flowering stems are dish-shaped leaves covered with hairs that exude a substance at their tips. In sunshine this sap sparkles and attracts insects. Upon an insect's touch, the hairs bend in and down upon the creature, and additional amounts of sap, which contains digestive enzymes, convert the insect's protein into food for the plant.

As early as the 13th century, alchemists noted positive results from the use of sundew's sap in the treatment of consumption, or tuberculosis. In 16th-century England John Gerard observed in his *Herball* that "physicians have thought this herb to be a rare and singular remedy for all those that be in a consumption of the lungs." Today herbalists recommend sundew sap for soothing coughs due to irritation and ascribe to it antispasmodic properties that would also help stop coughing.

The genus name *Drosera* comes from a Greek word meaning "dew." The plant's dew-like sap is usually discharged by the leaves about noon—the same time that the flowers open briefly when there is sun.

Habitat: Wet peaty soils, bogs, swamps.
Range: Native to North America and Eurasia, sundew grows from Newfoundland to Alaska, south to Florida, Illinois, Montana, and California.
Identification: A perennial herb growing up to 8 inches tall. Round, dish-shaped, long-stalked leaves grow in a rosette and are covered with glandular hairs that secrete a sticky sap that attracts and snares small insects. The sap contains a powerful digestive juice that changes the protein in the insect into a substance absorbable by the plant through the surface of the leaves. Pinkish-white flowers (June–August) are borne in elongated clusters at the ends of leafless stems.
Uses: For centuries sundew sap was used to treat tubercular coughs. Herbals today prescribe it to soothe coughs due to irritation of the mucous membranes, and for spastic coughing, as in the case of whooping cough. Scientists confirm only its use as a soothing agent for coughs.

311

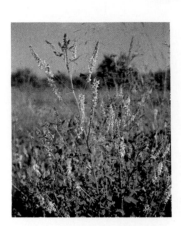

Sweet Clover

Melilotus officinalis (L.) Lamk.

King's-clover, Sweet Lucerne,
Yellow Melilot, Yellow Sweet Clover

PEA FAMILY

Leguminosae

The nectar of sweet clover seems to have an intoxicating effect on bees, drawing them to the blossoms in swirling clouds. Equally attractive to horses and cattle, the plant is one of their favorite fodders. In the 1920's, farmers began to store sweet clover for fodder. When cattle feeding on the hay began hemorrhaging, it was discovered that the clover they had eaten had been stored before it was completely dry, and so had fermented. Further investigation showed that coumarin, a substance in the plant that gives it its vanilla taste, becomes an anticoagulant, dicoumarol, when fermented.

Medicinally, sweet clover's popularity goes back many centuries. The ancient Egyptians made a tea from the plant to treat intestinal worms and earache. The Greek physician Galen prescribed using a similar infusion in a poultice for inflammations and swollen joints. In Anglo-Saxon England, sweet clover earned a reputation for preserving eyesight. The plant was also made into a salve for wounds and sores, a purpose it still serves in England, where some pharmacists sell "melilot plasters." A pleasant vanilla-flavored tea made from the blossoms and leaves can be drunk for its own sake or to relieve chronic flatulence.

X Rotted sweet clover is an anticoagulant that causes hemorrhaging in animals. Unrotted sweet clover is entirely safe.

Habitat: Fields, roadsides, waste places.

Range: A native of Europe, sweet clover is now naturalized across North America and widely planted for fodder.

Identification: A biennial herb, growing to 5 feet, with many branches. Each leaf consists of three leaflets with toothed margins. Light yellow flowers grow in towering spikes (June–September) and are about ¼ inch across. The whole plant has a sweet vanilla smell that is more intense when the plant is dried.

Uses: Because sweet clover is a mild astringent, its chief use through the ages has been as a poultice for inflammations and wounds of tender parts of the body, such as the eyes. Commercially, the plant is now used mainly as fodder.

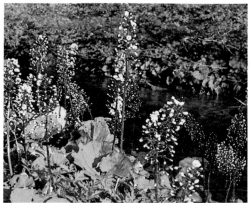

Cluster of
fruiting heads

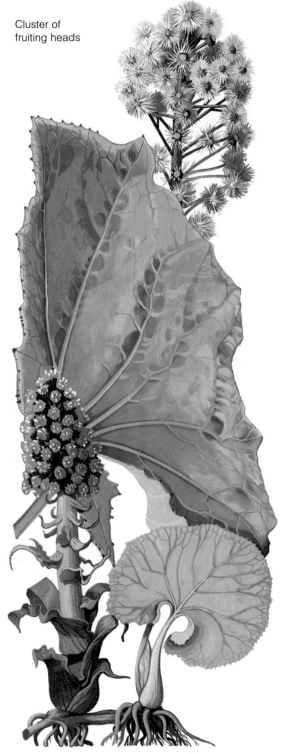

Sweet Coltsfoot

Petasites hybridus (L.) Gaertn., Mey., and Scherb.

Butterbur

COMPOSITE FAMILY

Compositae

Because the leaves are big enough to protect a person's head from sun or rain, the Greeks styled sweet coltsfoot "hat plant." The name of the broad-brimmed hat, somewhat like a sombrero, worn by travelers in Greco-Roman times was *petasos*, and the plant name derived from it survives in botanical usage. According to the Elizabethan John Gerard's *Herball* (1597), the dried powdered root of sweet coltsfoot mixed with wine was a superior medicine against the plague and other pestilential diseases. The powdered root worked as a remedy for intestinal worms, as a diuretic, and to stimulate menstruation, Gerard wrote, and was effective if dusted on ulcerating sores. In subsequent herbal tradition sweet coltsfoot acquired a reputation as a remedy for gravel (small kidney stones), as an antispasmodic, and as a colic medicine. Some herbalists cited a poultice of the fresh leaves or of the leaves and flowers for external application on wounds. The dried leaves have served as a tobacco substitute—a particularly rank and unpleasant substitute, according to some people who have tried smoking them in a pipe.

X Do not take sweet coltsfoot internally. Laboratory tests on rodents indicate that it may cause cancer if taken in large doses or repeated small doses.
Habitat: Riverbanks, near woods, waste places.
Range: Introduced from Europe, sweet coltsfoot now grows wild in North America from Massachusetts to Pennsylvania.
Identification: A stout perennial herb arising from a coarse rhizome (underground stem) and having a hollow, thick, reddish-brown leafless aerial stem (called a scape) covered with lance-shaped scales and terminating in a dense club-shaped cluster of flowerheads. Large leaves, up to 2 feet wide, are spiky around the edges. Lilac-pink flowers (April–May) are small and tubular.
Uses: Although some modern herbalists recommend the rootstock of sweet coltsfoot to break a fever and as a diuretic, antispasmodic, and pain reliever, scientific evidence indicates that the plant is unsafe.

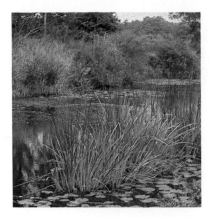

Sweet Flag

Acorus calamus L.

Calamus, Flagroot, Sweet Cane,
Sweet Grass, Sweetroot, Sweet Rush
ARUM FAMILY

Araceae

A denizen of the water's edge and wetlands, the yellow-flowered sweet flag is native to Asia and North America. Settlers—who knew the plant in Europe, where it was widely grown by the 17th century—scattered the lemony-smelling leaves on the floors of their homes to mask the stench of poor sanitation and ventilation.

When not in bloom sweet flag looks like blue flag—a dangerous resemblance because the rhizome of blue flag is poisonous and sweet flag rhizomes were once eaten as a candy. Once people smoked or chewed the powdered rhizome of sweet flag because it was supposed to destroy the taste for tobacco and thus help break the smoking habit. In 1968 the U.S. Food and Drug Administration reported that an Asian variety of the species produced cancerous tumors in experiments with rats. It therefore declared the species "unsafe."

American Indians had so many medicinal uses for the rhizomes and roots that sweet flag became a valuable commodity, and some tribes used it as a medium of exchange. Most medicinal uses pertained to stomach disorders, but Indian healers also used the root for toothache, fever, and menstrual problems.

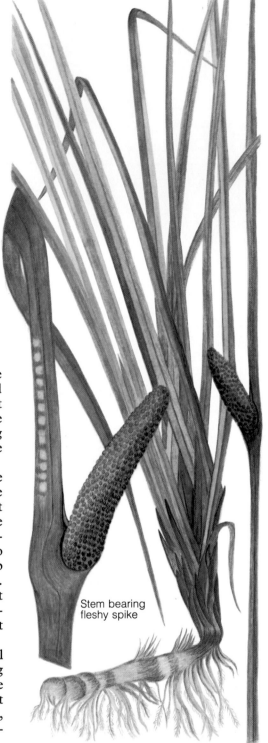

Stem bearing
fleshy spike

X The U.S. Food and Drug Administration has classified sweet flag as "unsafe."
Habitat: Streambanks, swamps, wet meadows.
Range: Native to North America and Asia, sweet flag is found from Nova Scotia south to Florida and Texas, and west to Oregon. The species is rare or threatened in some states.
Identification: A perennial herb, sending up from its underground stem flat, leaflike stems with swordlike leaves at the base. The stems may reach 5 feet and over. Halfway to the top each bears a 2- to 4-inch-long fleshy cylindrical structure, in which tiny yellowish-brown flowers (May–August) are embedded.
Uses: Sweet flag was listed in the *U.S. Pharmacopeia* (1820–1916) and the *National Formulary* (1936–1950). During those years, physicians used it for stomach cramps and gas and as a tonic and stimulant. Experimental evidence suggests that extracts of sweet flag rhizome and roots may alleviate stomach cramps.

Sweet Gum

Liquidambar styraciflua L.

Bilsted, Gum Tree,
Red Gum, Star-leaved Gum
WITCH HAZEL FAMILY

Hamamelidaceae

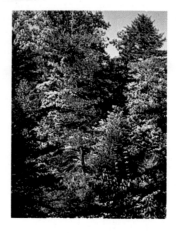

When the Spanish explorer Hernando Cortez dined with the Aztec emperor Montezuma, cigarettes of tobacco flavored with sweet gum were brought on after the meal. The amber-colored "gum," or balsam, gives the sweet gum tree its name. Indians of the southern United States reportedly made a preparation of the balsam to treat fevers and wounds. In some areas the pioneers made an extract of the bark and leaves to cure diarrhea, but in the South they chewed the leaves for this purpose. In the Appalachians, people dipped the twigs in whiskey and nibbled them to clean their teeth. Mixed with tallow or lard, the balsam served as an ointment for hemorrhoids and for ringworm of the scalp and other skin infections. The balsam alone was believed to be a cure for herpes and skin inflammations.

Dried balsam, called storax, is currently listed in the *U.S. Pharmacopeia.* Guatemala and Honduras are the main sources of storax, which, besides its medicinal applications, is used to flavor soft drinks, tobacco, candy, and chewing gum and to scent perfumes.

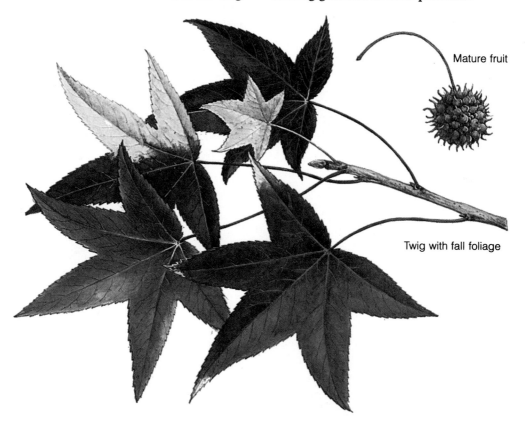

Mature fruit

Twig with fall foliage

Habitat: Moist woodlands, on rich, well-drained soils; bottomlands; swamps.

Range: Native to North America, sweet gum grows from Connecticut west to southeast Missouri and eastern Texas, and southward into Mexico and Central America.

Identification: Growing up to 140 feet tall, but more commonly to 60–80 feet in temperate regions, the sweet gum tree has a gray bark, with deeply furrowed, corky ridges on its twigs. The leaves are star-shaped with five to seven finely toothed, pointed lobes. Tiny yellowish-green flowers (April–May) cluster in separate spherical male and female flowerheads.

Uses: Several parts of sweet gum have had medicinal uses, the most important part being the balsam, called storax, whose chief applications are as an expectorant and an antiseptic. The food industry uses the balsam as a flavoring. Gardeners plant the tree for its brilliant fall foliage.

315

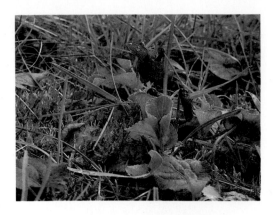

Sweet Violet

Viola odorata L.

Blue Violet, English Violet,
Sweet-scented Violet
VIOLET FAMILY
Violaceae

Nature lovers know that springtime has arrived when they see the first delicate but fragrant bluish-purple blossoms of sweet violets nodding gently at the woodland's edge or in the meadows. Sweet violets have been much admired for more than 2,000 years. Ancient Athenians held the plant in high regard for its power both to moderate anger and to cure insomnia. The Roman naturalist Pliny said its roots, if steeped in vinegar, would cure gout, and added that a garland of violets worn about the head would banish headaches and dizziness. Later the Celts mixed the flowers with goat's milk to make a cosmetic. In the 16th century the English made a syrup of the flowers and used it as a mild laxative for children. They also employed the syrup to treat a number of adult ailments, including epilepsy, pleurisy, and jaundice.

In modern times violet blossoms have been used principally as a coloring agent, as the fragrance in perfumes, and in cough syrups.

At different times and places, folk healers have touted the plant as a cure for growths. Since about 500 B.C., the fresh leaves have been used in poultice form to treat skin cancer, and this belief in violets' efficacy as a cancer cure unfortunately continues to this day—with virtually no scientific proof to back it up.

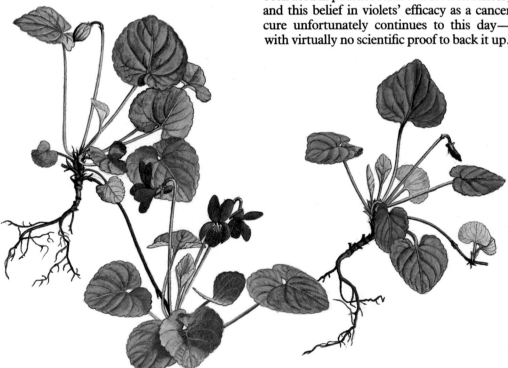

X Large doses of the root cause nausea and vomiting.
Habitat: Poor soils in partially shaded sloping meadows and woods.
Range: Native to Europe, Asia, and North Africa, sweet violet is now naturalized in North America.
Identification: A creeping perennial, sweet violet reproduces by long-stalked rooting runners called stolons. The leaves, produced in rosettes near the ground, are heart-shaped and slightly downy.

Sweetly scented solitary flowers (April–June) appear on long stalks and are generally deep violet but may range to rose and white.
Uses: Claims that the leaves of the sweet violet offer a cure for skin cancer have not been substantiated by medical research. Today the plant's chief medicinal use is as an expectorant, although this use has not been scientifically validated. The plant has also been used as a diuretic, and this effect has recently been confirmed in animal studies.

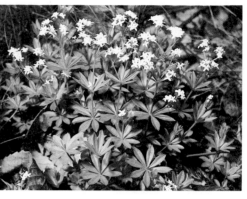

Sweet Woodruff

Asperula odorata L.

Waldmeister

MADDER FAMILY

Rubiaceae

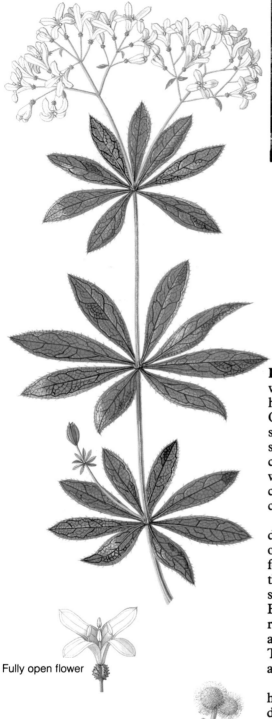

Fully open flower

Mature fruit

In Germany, spring would not be complete without sweet woodruff, since sprigs of this herb are essential for making May wine, which Germans drink both as a spring tonic and to salute the new season. Mixed with fodder, sweet woodruff gives the milk of cows a delicious aroma. But when it becomes wet, sweet woodruff, like sweet clover, may rot and become moldy, producing an anticoagulant that can cause hemorrhaging in the cattle.

Unlike the fragrance of most herbs, which dissipates soon after drying, the haylike odor of dried sweet woodruff intensifies and persists for years—a fact explained by the presence of the chemical substance coumarin, which is sometimes used as a fixative for perfumes. Because of its pleasant fragrance, sweet woodruff was once used as a scenting herb for homes and churches and as a stuffing for mattresses. The dried leaves give linen closets a sweet aroma and reportedly keep moths away.

Sweet woodruff has also been a medicinal herb of some importance: the fresh leaves for dressing wounds and cuts, a decoction of the leaves as a stomach digestive and cordial, and a leaf tea for liver disorders and as a diuretic.

X The tea in large doses may cause dizziness and symptoms of poisoning, such as vomiting.
Habitat: Gardens, roadsides, woods.
Range: Native to Europe and Asia, sweet woodruff has become naturalized in parts of southern Canada and of the northern United States.
Identification: A perennial spreading into clumps 8–15 inches tall. The square stems are slender and smooth, the rough-edged leaves borne in whorls of six to eight. Small white funnel-shaped flowers (May–June) bloom in loose clusters. The sweet hay scent of the flower increases as it dries.
Uses: Sweet woodruff has a historic reputation as a tonic for liver disorders. World-famous as an aromatic ingredient in May wine, sweet woodruff is also used today in punches and other drinks. Modern herbalists recommend the herb as a laxative and as an antiarthritic. Research indicates that it may be effective in these roles. The plant is mainly grown today as a ground cover.

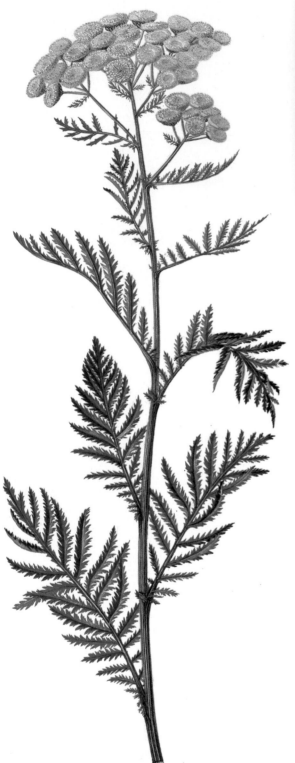

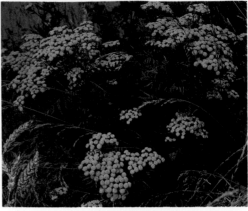

Tansy

Tanacetum vulgare L.

Scented Fern, Stinking Willie
COMPOSITE FAMILY
Compositae

A strong-smelling garden favorite, tansy resists frost and cold, and its attractive yellow flowerheads are extremely long lasting, both when they are in bloom and after they have been picked and dried. Patches of tansy can survive for decades in the same location. The very name tansy, herbalists declare, is a corruption of the Greek word for immortality—*athanasia.*

Because of its strong smell, tansy is a natural insect repellent. In the Middle Ages dried tansy was one of the "strewing herbs" scattered across floors to keep pests away. Housewives also hung it from rafters, packed it between bedsheets and mattresses, and rubbed it on meat to discourage lice, flies, and other vermin. In more recent times, they have used it to repel moths and get rid of fleas.

Tansy also has a long history as a seasoning and medicinal plant. In England, the leaves were once used to flavor small tansy cakes eaten during Lent—their bitter taste symbolized Christ's suffering. A tea from the leaves was once commonly taken for colds, stomachaches, and intestinal worms. Folk healers also made a poultice from the leaves to place on cuts and bruises.

Habitat: Roadsides, abandoned land.
Range: Introduced from Europe, tansy has escaped from gardens from Newfoundland to British Columbia and in much of the United States.
Identification: An extremely hardy aromatic perennial with stiff, erect stems up to 3 feet high. Feathery, dark green, narrow, lance-shaped leaves with deeply toothed leaflets grow alternately along the stem, at the top of which bloom many dense clusters of small, buttonlike yellow flowerheads (July–October). Tansy grows in clumps.
Uses: The dried leaves are an effective insect repellent. In folk medicine today, tansy still serves as a vermifuge (to expel worms), an emmenagogue (to bring on menstruation), and an antispasmodic. Pharmacologists studying the plant for its medicinal value find some evidence for its use as an antispasmodic but little or no evidence for its use as a vermifuge or an emmenagogue.

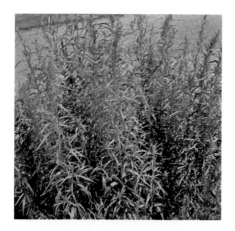

Tarragon

Artemisia dracunculus L.

Dragon's-mugwort, French Tarragon
COMPOSITE FAMILY
Compositae

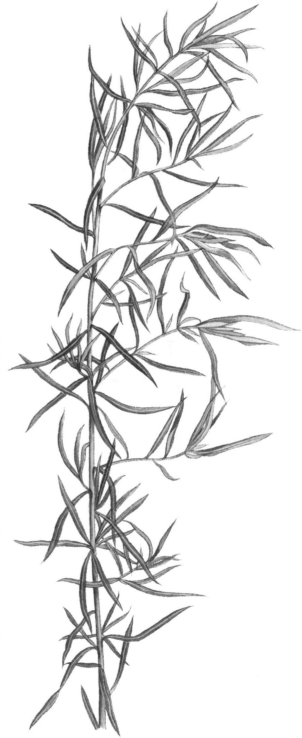

Charlemagne, king of the Franks (768–814) and Holy Roman emperor (800–814), liked tarragon so much that he ordered it planted on all his estates. Even today no French cook would be caught without it. The herb's delicate licorice taste makes it a complementary seasoning in meat, fish, and chicken dishes, salads, dressings, and sauce béarnaise.

No one knows when tarragon became medicinally classified as a "dragon herb," the name herbalists gave to plants they used as antidotes against the bites of venomous animals. Tarragon arrived in England from southern Europe in the 1500's. There, as the diarist John Evelyn later disclosed, it was recognized as a "friend to the head, heart, and liver." Records show that by 1650 tarragon had been transported to the Dutch settlements in the New World. It was one of 33 common plants listed there by the settlers.

In modern folk medicine herbalists advocate the use of tarragon for alleviating rheumatism and arthritis. They also prescribe it to stimulate appetite, to promote menstruation, and as a diuretic. Do not confuse French tarragon with the tasteless variety called Russian tarragon, which looks similar but has paler leaves.

X There is evidence from experimental animals that tarragon's essential oil can cause cancer if taken in large doses and over a long period of time.

Habitat: Plains, prairies, dry slopes.

Range: Native to the Northern Hemisphere, tarragon grows wild from British Columbia south throughout the western United States.

Identification: A perennial herb growing up to 5 feet tall. The leaves are simple, alternate, narrow, and either oblong or lance-shaped. They grow ¾– 3½ inches long. Tiny, gray-green, globular flowerheads (July–October) are ⅛ inch across. The fresh leaves have an aniselike odor when crushed.

Uses: Tarragon is best known as a culinary herb. Current herbals list the plant as a diuretic, an appetite stimulant, and an emmenagogue (for bringing on menstruation). Pharmacologists who have investigated tarragon's use as an emmenagogue find some evidence but no positive proof of the validity of this use.

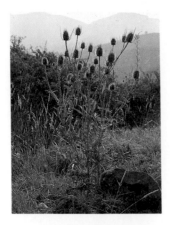

Teasel

Dipsacus sylvestris Huds.
Venus' Basin, Water Thistle, Wild Teasel
TEASEL FAMILY
Dipsacaceae

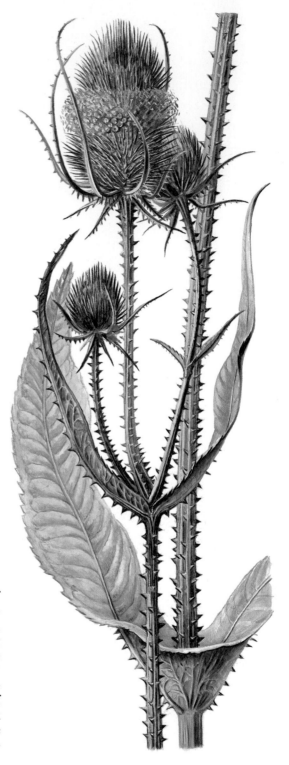

The upper leaves of the teasel plant join to form a basin in which rainwater collects, and this structure inspired the plant's other common names, Venus' basin and water thistle. The water was once believed to be cooling to inflamed eyes and was recommended "as a cosmetic to render the face fair." The Greek physician Dioscorides maintained that the root had a cleansing property and advocated boiling the root in wine and applying the decoction to fistulas and warts. Other early herbalists favored a root tea as an appetite stimulant, a remedy for jaundice, and a diuretic.

Wild teasel is a close relative of the cultivated species, *D. fullonum.* The main difference between the two plants is that the bracts of wild teasel's flowerheads are straight while those of the cultivated species have hooked tips, which will, however, revert to growing straight if the plant is returned to the wild. The Romans used these hooked tips for "teasing" and raising the nap of woolen cloth. At one time in the United States the cultivation of teasel was a sizable industry in New York State. Modern machinery has replaced the domestic teasel, but cannot match the luxurious finish it imparts.

Habitat: Ditches, old fields, and other wastelands.
Range: A native of Europe, wild teasel is naturalized in North America from Quebec to Ontario, from New England south to North Carolina and west to Utah, and in the Pacific Northwest states, especially in areas where it was once cultivated.
Identification: A prickly biennial herb with a bristly stem growing 3–6 feet tall. The prickly lance-shaped to oblong leaves occur in pairs with their bases fused. The small bluish-lavender flowers (July–October) are tubular and are borne in a flowerhead surrounded by sharp spiny bracts.
Uses: Teasel is seldom recommended in herbal medicine today. Those sources that do mention the plant include the following uses: as a diuretic, in treating skin inflammations and fistulas, to promote sweating, and as an aid to digestion. No scientific data are available to confirm any of these effects. In winter many people use the seed heads in floral decorations and bouquets.

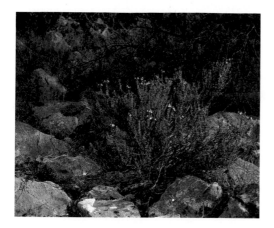

Thyme

Thymus vulgaris L.

Common Thyme, Garden Thyme
MINT FAMILY
Labiatae

No cook worth her or his salt needs to be told what to do with thyme. Fresh or dried, alone or combined with parsley and bay leaves to make a bouquet garni, the herb adds a distinctive aromatic flavoring to sauces, stews, stuffings, meats, poultry—indeed, to almost anything from soup to salad.

In medieval times the plant symbolized courage, and to keep up their spirits, knights departing for the Crusades received scarves embroidered with a sprig of thyme from their ladies. There was a popular belief, too, that a leaf tea prevented nightmares, while another held that a tea made of thyme and other herbs enabled one to see nymphs and fairies.

Herbalists of the Middle Ages regarded thyme as a stimulant and antispasmodic and recommended sleeping on thyme and inhaling it as a remedy for melancholy and epilepsy. In 1725 a German apothecary discovered that the plant's essential oil contains a powerful disinfectant, called thymol, that is effective against bacteria and fungi. Thymol also acts as an expectorant, loosening phlegm in the respiratory tract so that it can be coughed up. Later herbals listed thyme for these uses and as a remedy for numerous other complaints, including diarrhea and fever. They prescribed the oil externally as an antiseptic for fungal infections such as athlete's foot.

X Excessive use of oil of thyme may cause gastrointestinal disorders.

Habitat: Warm and sunny fields.

Range: Native to southern Europe, thyme is widely cultivated in North America, where it has escaped from cultivation in some places.

Identification: A perennial herb growing up to 15 inches tall. The stems are woody and stiff; the twigs are velvety white. Narrow gray-green leaves about ¼ inch long are borne in opposite pairs. Lavender-pink to whitish flowers (April–July) occur in small clusters. The leaves are highly aromatic.

Uses: Traditionally thyme has been used to relieve spasms and coughing. Scientific tests have validated the plant's continued use in modern folk medicine as an antispasmodic and antitussive, or remedy that relieves coughing. The oil is used in cosmetic and pharmaceutical preparations.

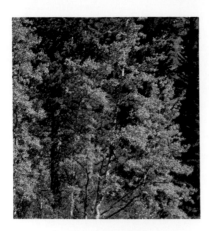

Trembling Aspen

Populus tremuloides Michx.

American Aspen, Mountain Aspen,
Quaking Aspen, Quiverleaf, White Poplar
WILLOW FAMILY

Salicaceae

So lavish with its gifts is the trembling aspen that it feeds no less than 500 species of animals, fungi, and other life-forms. The beaver prefers its bark to all others and builds his dams of its poles; its winter buds are fare for grouse; the moose browses on its foliage all year round.

Man, too, once relied on this tree as a source of foods and medicines. Various North American Indian peoples ate the inner bark or drank the syrup derived from it as a spring tonic or energy source. The Crees boiled the bark for a cough medicine. The Delawares boiled the root to obtain a tonic for debility, and they made a cold remedy from the bark. The Mohawks used the bark tea to expel worms. The Fox people boiled trembling aspen buds in fat as a salve for a cold sufferer's sore nostrils. The Chippewas brewed a drink from the roots to prevent premature childbirth, prepared a heart medicine from various parts of the tree, and applied the chewed-up bark to cuts. In the 19th century, herbalists, picking up where the Indians left off, experimented with tinctures of the bark as a remedy for fever, rheumatism, arthritis, and the common cold, as well as for worms.

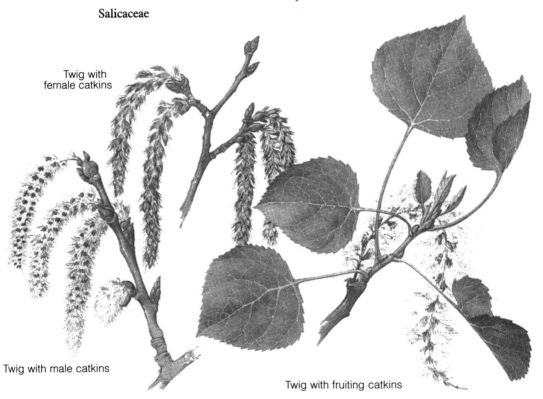

Twig with female catkins

Twig with male catkins

Twig with fruiting catkins

Habitat: All terrains except swamps.
Range: Native to North America, trembling aspen is found from Newfoundland west to Alaska, south to Virginia, Kentucky, and Iowa, and in mountain areas as far south as western Mexico.
Identification: A small, short-lived tree growing up to 40 feet tall, trembling aspen has a smooth, nearly white bark that roughens and darkens with age. Roundish-oval leaves, which flutter in a slight breeze, are borne on slender flattened leafstalks.

Male and female flowers (April–May) appear in long clusters called catkins on separate trees about one month before the leaves.
Uses: Pharmacologists state that trembling aspen has chemical qualities similar to those of aspirin, and would therefore be expected to be useful for fevers, mild pain, and inflammations. The tree is economically valuable for reforestation, and its wood is made into magazine pulp and has been used for matches and cheap crates.

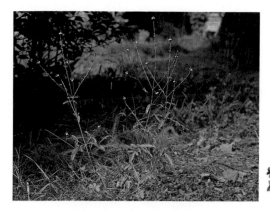

Vervain

Verbena officinalis L.

Herb-of-the-cross, Pigeon's-grass
VERVAIN FAMILY
Verbenaceae

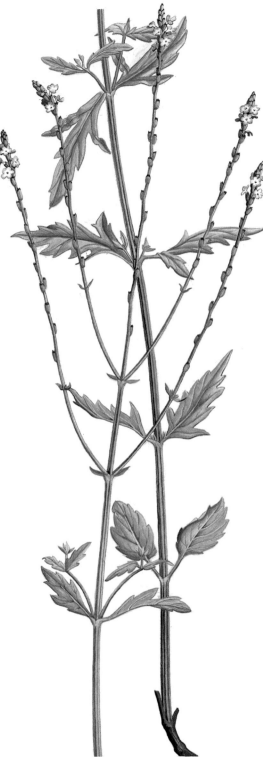

Even though it is undistinguished in appearance and not at all rare, vervain was long regarded with awe throughout its natural range. The Romans consecrated it for the purification of their temples and private homes, and also used it medicinally. Various preparations of the plant served as remedies for snakebite and diarrhea, while chewing the plant and its root was supposed to strengthen gums and teeth. It was both an ingredient of medieval witches' love potions and a charm against their evil spells. Vervain even made its way into Christian lore as the plant that had served to stanch Christ's wounds on Calvary— hence the name herb-of-the-cross.

Vervain achieved a reputation as a virtual panacea. Colds, fevers, so-called nervous complaints, skin infections, and gout were among the disorders it was supposed to cure. Herbalists still recommend vervain tea occasionally as a tonic, astringent, diuretic, diaphoretic (for reducing fever by inducing sweating), sedative, antispasmodic, and aphrodisiac.

Brought to North America by the Puritans, *Verbena officinalis* is now nearly as common on the continent as the native American *Verbena* species. One of them, *V. hastata*, is also credited with medicinal properties.

Habitat: Roadsides, pastures, waste places.
Range: Native to the Mediterranean region, but early spread throughout Eurasia, vervain is now widely naturalized in temperate North America.
Identification: A perennial herb 1–2 feet tall with thin, erect, stiff stems. The leaves are opposite; the lower ones are oblong and coarsely toothed, the upper ones slender, lance-shaped, and deeply lobed. Small lilac-hued flowers (June–October) with five petals are borne on a slender spike.

Uses: Many of vervain's medicinal uses have been subject to scientific scrutiny. Pharmacologists find no evidence to support the plant's use as an antispasmodic or as a contraceptive. Nor can they substantiate its efficacy in treating fevers, skin infections, and dysentery. They do, however, find evidence that the plant is effective as a diuretic, gout remedy, and anorexic (appetite supressant).

Virginia Snakeroot

Aristolochia serpentaria L.

Birthwort, Pelican Flower,
Sangrel, Snakeweed
BIRTHWORT FAMILY

Aristolochiaceae

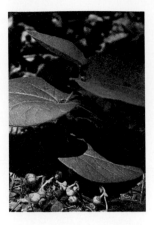

The most exotic feature of the Virginia snakeroot is its brownish-purple flower, a long curved tube resembling a meerschaum pipe, the kind old-time Germans used to smoke. Often completely hidden in the leaf litter of its forest habitat, the low-growing flower is pollinated by carrion flies attracted by its strong, fetid odor. Upon entering the flower in search of food, the flies are trapped by the hairs lining the tube. In their struggle to escape, the insects cover themselves with pollen, which they then carry on to the next flower they visit.

Snakeroot, as its name indicates, was used as a cure for snakebite. The Indians of its native North America chewed the root and applied it to the wound as well as swallowing some of it.

Its effectiveness as an antidote was never proved, but colonial and European doctors tried it as an antidote for the bites of rabid dogs and for poisons and as a treatment for malaria, typhus, and infectious fevers of all kinds.

The plant's heart-shaped leaves led Kentucky mountaineers to favor a tea from the root as a heart tonic. Up to the early 1900's, herbalists and physicians used the plant as an appetite stimulant and a digestive aid. In country hotels the bartender often kept a bottle of snakeroot steeped in spirits, which he served to customers as digestive bitters or as a heart tonic.

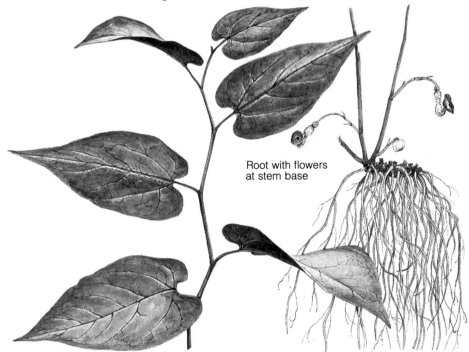

Root with flowers
at stem base

X Snakeroot contains an acid that is toxic to the kidneys and liver and causes potentially cancerous genetic mutations.
Habitat: Rich and dry woodlands.
Range: Connecticut south to Florida and Texas and west to Kansas. The species is endangered or threatened in some states.
Identification: An erect perennial herb growing up to 2 feet tall. The leaves are sparse, 1½−4½ inches long, and heart-shaped with pointed tips.

Small purplish- to reddish-brown flowers (May−July) are almost buried in the ground. They arise from the stem base and emit a foul smell.
Uses: In folk medicine snakeroot has been chiefly used to treat fever. Modern herbalists prescribe snakeroot as an aphrodisiac, to prevent convulsions, and to promote menstruation. None of these uses has been scientifically validated. Snakeroot contains an acid that may cause genetic mutations. Some countries forbid the plant's sale.

Virgin's-bower

Clematis virginiana L.

Clematis, Devil's-darning-needle,
Old-man's-beard, Traveler's-joy
BUTTERCUP FAMILY
Ranunculaceae

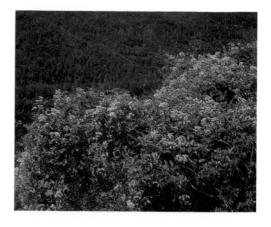

This lovely trailing vine climbs as high as 15 feet on top of other plants, creating a shaded shelter, or bower. The vine is also known as old-man's-beard because of the long feathery beardlike tail on its fruit. There are some 250 known species of *Clematis* in the world, many of which have been hybridized and have become favorite plants of home gardeners.

C. virginiana is native to North America and has had a place in the pharmacopeia of the continent. According to one source, Indians made a decoction (extract) of the plant, which they applied to cuts and sores. The European botanist Constantine Rafinesque, who studied American plants and wrote *Medical Flora*

(1828–1830), made the following comment on virgin's-bower: "Bark and blossoms acrid, raising blisters on the skin; a corrosive poison internally, loses the virulence by cooking." He wrote that an oily liniment made from the plant would cure the itch and that the plant, in minute doses, was good for chronic rheumatism, palsy, and ulcers. Modern herbal studies cite virgin's-bower as an external remedy for skin diseases, but report that experience and scientific studies have confirmed Rafinesque's observations on the plant's toxicity.

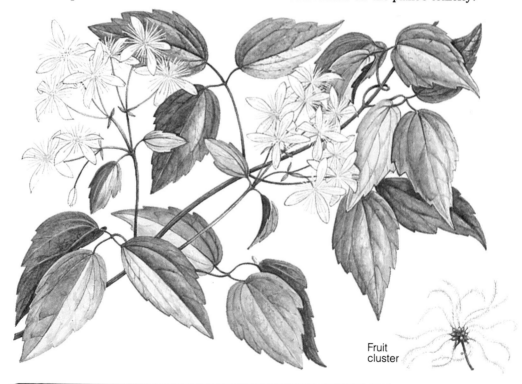

Fruit
cluster

X Virgin's-bower causes blistering of the skin and mucous membranes. If the plant is taken internally symptoms include salivation, bloody vomiting and diarrhea, and, in extreme cases, convulsions.
Habitat: Streambanks, thickets, woods, roadsides.
Range: A native of North America, virgin's-bower grows from Quebec to Manitoba, south to Alabama and Louisiana, and west to Kansas.
Identification: A perennial herbaceous vine that climbs over other plants, up to a length of 15 feet.

The leaves are divided into three toothed oval leaflets, each on a long stalk; the stalks act as tendrils. Numerous creamy white flowers (July–September) bloom in large clusters and are followed by fruit heads with long plumy tails.
Uses: Virgin's-bower was popular in pioneer medicine as a treatment for the itch, skin diseases, and venereal eruptions. Modern herbalists cite these uses but warn that the juice is a powerful irritant, and scientific studies bear out this effect.

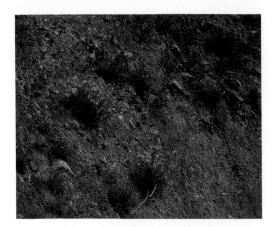

Wallflower

Cheiranthus cheiri L.

English Wallflower, Handflower
MUSTARD FAMILY
Cruciferae

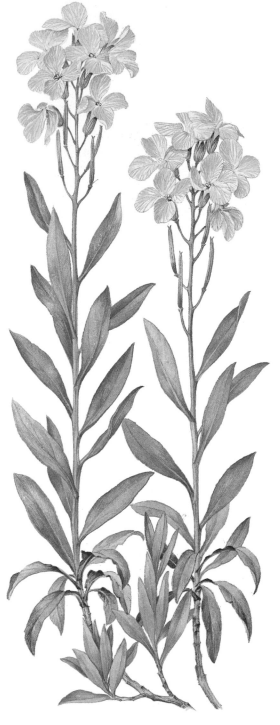

Young women relegated to the sidelines at social functions are often called wallflowers, perhaps because they, like the plant, have the habit of clinging to walls. Long ago, however, this sweet-smelling plant had more romantic associations. In 14th-century Scotland, the story goes, Elizabeth, daughter of the earl of March, dropped a wallflower from her castle window as a signal to her beloved, the son of an enemy clan, that she was ready to elope. As she made her escape, she fell to her death. Her unhappy lover placed a wallflower in his cap and left Scotland forever. The plant thereafter became a symbol of adversity in love.

Ever since the time of the Greek physician Galen (about A.D. 130–200), doctors have acknowledged wallflower's medicinal attributes. It was used to promote menstruation, relieve pain in childbirth, clear up cataracts, and cleanse the kidneys and liver. The 17th-century English herbalist Nicholas Culpeper also mentioned the plant as a treatment for palsy and apoplexy. Early in the 20th century, pharmacologists discovered that wallflower's seeds, leaves, and flowers contain a substance, similar to digitalis, that acts on the heart. The plant is therefore not recommended for domestic use.

X Do not use except under a physician's direction.
Habitat: Old walls and rocky places.
Range: A native of Europe, wallflower is a popular garden plant in temperate North America.
Identification: A short-lived perennial with erect stems growing up to 2½ feet tall. Narrow oblong to lance-shaped leaves 3 inches long are arranged alternately along the stems. Fragrant flowers (May–June), 1 inch across and with four rounded petals, range in color from yellow to orange to yellowish brown. Like other mustards, wallflower produces long narrow siliques, or many-seeded capsules, after flowering. They grow in elongated clusters at the ends of the stems.
Uses: Wallflower was traditionally used over the centuries as a diuretic. After the discovery that the plant contains glycosides that have properties like the digitalis in foxglove, herbalists stopped recommending the plant because of the danger that an overdose will cause heart failure.

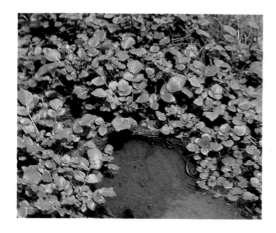

Watercress

Nasturtium officinale L.

Nasturtium

MUSTARD FAMILY

Cruciferae

As the Latin words *nasus tortus*, or "twisted nose," imply, watercress gives off a pungent odor that makes the nose wrinkle. The leaves and edible seedpods have a sharp, peppery taste, which accounts for watercress's longtime popularity as a salad green.

Watercress has long been known for its medicinal properties. The Greeks and Romans thought it improved the brain, and later, in medieval Europe, it became an ingredient in a salve for sword wounds. Early settlers brought the plant to America chiefly because of its effectiveness in preventing scurvy, for the plant is rich in vitamin C. The Indians adopted watercress as a food and also used it to treat liver and kidney problems.

Rich in mineral salts as well as vitamins C, A, B_2, D, and E, watercress was used not only as a scurvy preventive and remedy but as a springtime tonic and appetite stimulant. In various parts of the world it found use in an assortment of ways—as an aphrodisiac, contraceptive, laxative, cough medicine, and asthma remedy, and to clear up the complexion.

Watercress often grows near deadly water hemlocks. Hemlocks are easy to distinguish, however; they are much taller, with leaves divided into narrower, paler green leaflets, and they have umbel-shaped flower clusters.

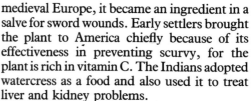

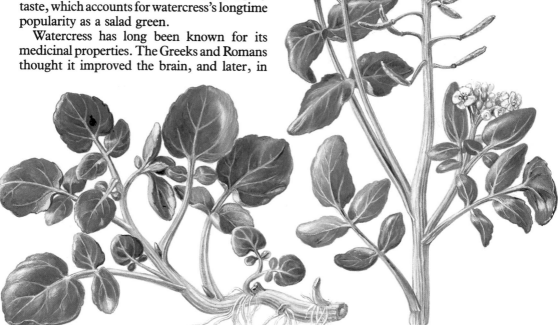

X Wash watercress thoroughly before eating it; the water it grows in may be polluted.

Habitat: Cold, fresh water in springs, brooks, and streams and on nearby banks.

Range: Introduced from Europe, watercress is widely naturalized in southern Canada and most of the United States.

Identification: A perennial aquatic plant with leaves divided into three to nine dark green, glossy, ovate to elongated leaflets. Spikes of white flowers (March–November) ¼ inch across develop into sickle-shaped seedpods called siliques.

Uses: For centuries watercress was eaten as an antiscorbutic because of its high vitamin C content. Today its appeal is both nutritional and culinary. Cooks make salads, soups, and sandwiches of watercress and use it as a garnish. Herbalists recommend the plant for nervousness and rheumatism, but there is no scientific evidence that watercress is effective in these roles.

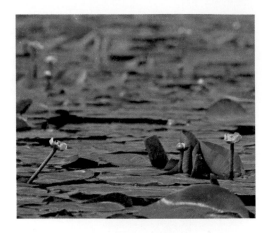

Water Lilies

Nymphaea alba L.

White Water Lily

Nuphar lutea (L.) Sibth. and Smith

Yellow Pond Lily

WATER LILY FAMILY

Nymphaeaceae

When the English botanist Richard Anthony Salisbury (1761–1829) gave the water lily family its scientific name, he chose the term *Nymphaeaceae*. The name is an allusion to the nymphs—minor divinities of Greek mythology who inhabited natural places, including streams, rivers, and lakes. Like some nymphs, the flowers of this family are not only beautiful but live in water. Often a small pool is covered with water lilies, and occasionally an entire pond is filled with their bobbing heads.

One of the best-known family members is the common white water lily, which has been prescribed as an anaphrodisiac, or agent that inhibits sexual drive. (It may be that the chaste-looking blossom emerging from a murky pond suggested the plant's application for cooling ardor.) *Nymphaea alba* shares many medicinal properties with the yellow pond lily, a close relative belonging to the genus *Nuphar*. Both plants contain tannin and mucilage and have been employed as astringents to halt diarrhea and as demulcents to help soothe irritated, sore throats. The rootstock of the yellow pond lily, bruised and steeped in milk, is said to kill beetles and cockroaches, and the smoke of the rootstock will drive away crickets.

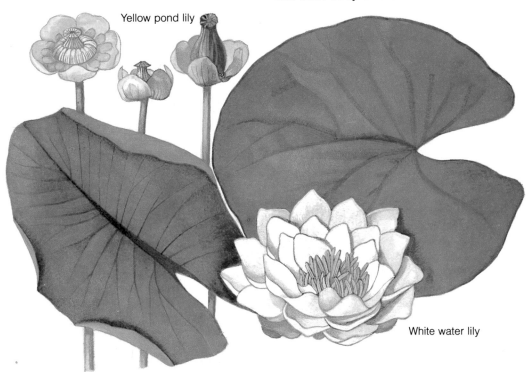

Yellow pond lily

White water lily

Habitat: The white water lily prefers marshy streams, lakes, rivers; the yellow pond lily favors still freshwater, slow streams, tidal waters.

Range: A native of Eurasia, the white water lily has been introduced and naturalized locally in North America. The yellow pond lily, native to Eurasia and North America, is found from Ontario to Florida, west to Wisconsin, Missouri, and Texas.

Identification: Water lilies are aquatic perennials growing from an underwater stem, which is buried in the mud and sends down rootlets for anchorage. The white water lily has round, leathery leaves, deeply notched at the base, and a multipetaled white blossom (June–September). The yellow pond lily has heart-shaped leaves and produces a cup-shaped yellow blossom (May–October).

Uses: No scientific evidence supports the white water lily's use for suppressing sexual desire. No scientific studies have been made of either plant's effectiveness as a demulcent or an astringent.

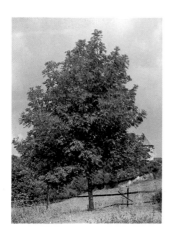

White Ash

Fraxinus americana L.

American Ash, Biltmore Ash,
Cane Ash, Smallseed White Ash
OLIVE FAMILY
Oleaceae

Sometimes called American ash, the regal white ash could well be called the all-American tree. Not only does it provide the wood for baseball bats but it is also one of the most common shade trees in the eastern half of the United States, where it is native. The timber is tough and pliant, supplying wood for everything from church pews to bowling alleys.

The American Indians showed the early settlers a medicinal use for almost every part of the tree. The Connecticut Indians used the sap to treat external cancerous growths—one Mrs. Loomis attested to the cure. In Maine the Penobscot tribe valued a decoction (extract) of white ash leaves as an antiseptic for internally cleansing women after childbirth. Other tribes specified a tea made from the bark as a treatment for an itching scalp and sores, and a leaf tea as a vermifuge, or agent that expels worms from the body. Even the seeds were used: as an aphrodisiac, a diuretic, an appetite stimulant, and a remedy for fevers. In the 19th century American physicians prescribed white ash preparations as a styptic, to stop minor bleeding; as an emetic, to promote vomiting; and for a variety of other purposes.

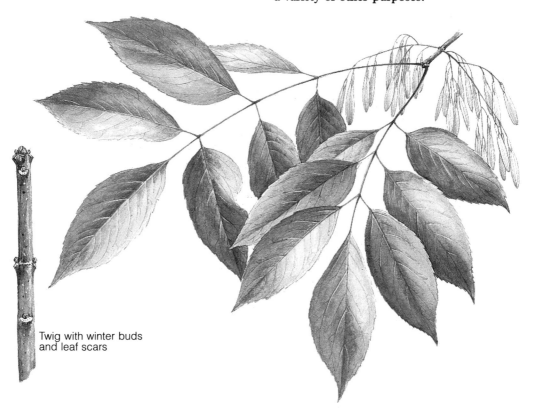

Twig with winter buds
and leaf scars

Habitat: Streambanks, hills, mountain slopes.
Range: Native to North America, white ash is found from Nova Scotia to southern Ontario, south to northern Florida, and west to eastern Kansas.
Identification: A deciduous tree, commonly growing to 80 feet but sometimes reaching over 100 feet. The scaly bark is dark brown to gray. The branches and twigs are stout. The leaves are pinnately compound, with five to nine pointed oval leaflets. Clusters of purplish male and female flowers (April–May) appear on separate trees; the male blooms every year, the female flowers heavily only every two or three years. The winged fruits are 1–2½ inches long.
Uses: Experimental evidence does not support white ash's use in herbal medicine as either an emmenagogue or a diuretic. White ash lumber is used in many consumer goods, including furniture and athletic equipment.

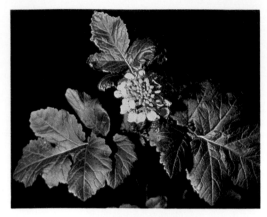

White Mustard

Sinapis alba L.

Kedlock, Yellow Mustard

MUSTARD FAMILY

Cruciferae

Jesus, in talking to His disciples, remarked: "If you have faith as a grain of mustard seed, you will say to this mountain, 'Move from here to there,' and it will move." Some biblical scholars believe that this reference is to the tiny seeds of the white mustard plant.

In the Mediterranean world, mustard has been recognized as a good medicine and good food since time immemorial. A 4,000-year-old Sumerian tablet mentions it; the very name *Sinapis* is ultimately of Egyptian origin. Mustard's power prompted the first-century A.D. physician Dioscorides to write: "It is good in general for any pain of long continuance when we would draw out anything from the deep within to the outside of the body . . . ." The name mustard comes from the practice of blending the crushed seeds with fermenting grape juice, or must, to make the sauce known as mustard—a practice dating back at least to Roman times. Since ancient times it has been known that the oil of mustard could be applied externally to soothe bodily aches. Mustard plaster—consisting of a paste of mustard seeds, flour, and water—served as an external application for pulmonary ailments. Powdered mustard as a condiment and mustard greens as a highly nutritious food have entered the culinary traditions of many nations.

X Mustard plasters require careful application; if the plaster is too strong or is left on too long, severe blistering can result.

Habitat: Roadsides, vacant lots, waste areas.

Range: Native to Eurasia, white mustard was introduced into North America long ago and now grows wild throughout the continent.

Identification: A coarse, hairy annual with an erect stem and a few ascending branches bearing pinnately divided bristly leaves, white mustard grows about 2 feet in height, with yellow flowers (June–August) that produce four to six round white to yellowish seeds in bristly pods tipped with a long flat beak and standing out from the stem.

Uses: Small amounts of the ground seeds mixed with water act as a laxative and can relieve acid indigestion. Homemade plasters from the seed are applied to sore muscles, and oil of mustard is an ingredient in ointments for external relief of minor aches and pains. Scientists state that these uses are valid.

White Oak

Quercus alba L.

Stave Oak, Stone Oak, Tanner's-oak
BEECH FAMILY
Fagaceae

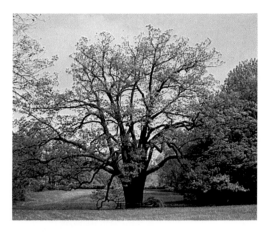

One of the largest and most valuable forest trees, the mighty white oak gives its wood to the finest furniture and flooring, its acorns as a food source, and its bark as a medicinal remedy. Although the tree tends to be slow growing, some of the old giants found in virgin forests have a ring count attesting to a life of 300 to 500 years. The wood is close-grained, hard, and tough, and that is why it came to be preferred for timber, furniture, and flooring. For centuries, too, white oak was essential in ship construction—from the gun deck of the famous frigate *Constitution* to the keels of World War II minesweepers and patrol boats. North American colonists also used this native species for barrel making because the wood held liquids, including the all-important rum.

The oak's fruits, the acorns, were a food staple for some Indian tribes, who boiled them or crushed them in water and ate them raw. The bark has a high tannin content and is therefore astringent. In Indian medicine it was brewed into a tea for treating diarrhea and bleeding hemorrhoids. Modern herbals still specify white oak as an astringent, recommending its external use for wounds, open sores, and hemorrhoids and for poison oak and insect bites.

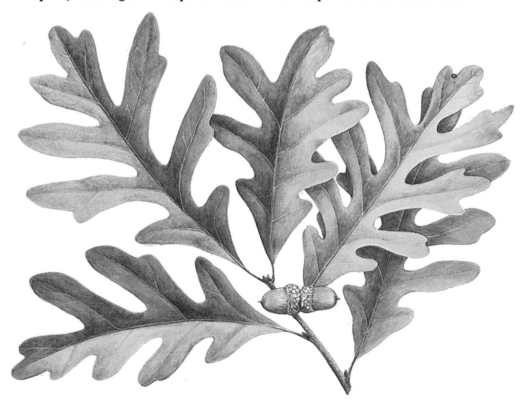

Habitat: Moist valleys and riverbanks to dry hillsides and sandy plains.
Range: Native to North America, the white oak grows in the wild from southern Canada to northern Florida and west to Minnesota and Texas.
Identification: A medium-sized to tall deciduous tree, rarely reaching a height of more than 115 feet. The light gray bark is thick and sometimes has a reddish-brown shade. Alternate leaves, divided into 7–10 rounded lobes, are bright green on the upper side, paler below. The brownish-green male and female flowers (May–June) are borne in separate clusters called catkins. The fruits (acorns) are light brown when mature.
Uses: Scientists state that white oak bark's use is valid as an external astringent, causing the capillaries and skin to constrict and thereby stopping minor bleeding. Its usefulness as an external hemostatic, or agent that arrests more serious bleeding, may be valid but has not been proved.

331

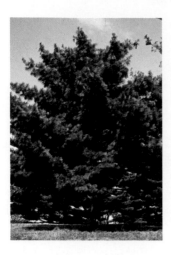

White Pine

Pinus strobus L.

New England Pine, Northern Pine,
Pumpkin Pine, Soft Pine
PINE FAMILY
Pinaceae

So vast were the native white pine forests in northeastern America that pioneers claimed a squirrel could travel all its life without coming down from the trees. The strong, light wood was unrivaled as a building material, and the colonists exported huge quantities to Europe. After the British crown declared that the largest trees had to be reserved for mast wood for its navy, the colonists poached the pine at night for their own use. When the American Revolution erupted, the tree was the emblem on the first flag of the Revolutionary forces.

To the Indians, the tree was a source of medicine. They drank a boiled extract of the inner bark, which contains some tannin, as an astringent for diarrhea, but mainly they soaked the bark and applied it to wounds as a soothing plaster. They also used the inner bark in cough remedies. It contains considerable mucilage, which soothes the mucous membranes lining the repiratory tract and may help loosen phlegm so that it can be coughed up. A boiled extract of the gum was also given as a pain reliever for rheumatism, and a syrup made from the resin for colds. Settlers adopted the Indians' medicinal uses of white pine.

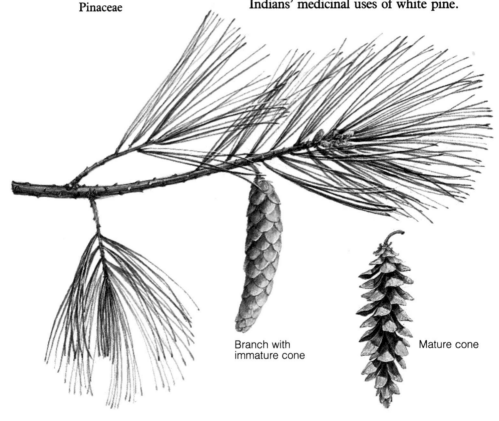

Branch with
immature cone

Mature cone

Habitat: Many different types of soil but prefers well-drained soils in a cool climate.
Range: Native to eastern North America, white pine is found from Newfoundland to Manitoba, south to northern Georgia and Illinois.
Identification: An evergreen tree reaching up to 230 feet. The bark is gray or dark brown. The leaves are bluish-green needles, 3–5 inches long, borne in bundles of five. Yellowish-green male and light red to pinkish-green female flowers (May–

June) are produced in cones. The female cone is 4–8 inches long, the male much smaller.
Uses: The inner bark of white pine is an ingredient in some cough medicines. Research by pharmacologists indicates that it may be an expectorant and that it does soothe irritated mucous membranes of the throat and so is of some benefit in cough preparations. Since white pine is no longer commonly used as an astringent, there is no modern research on the validity of this use.

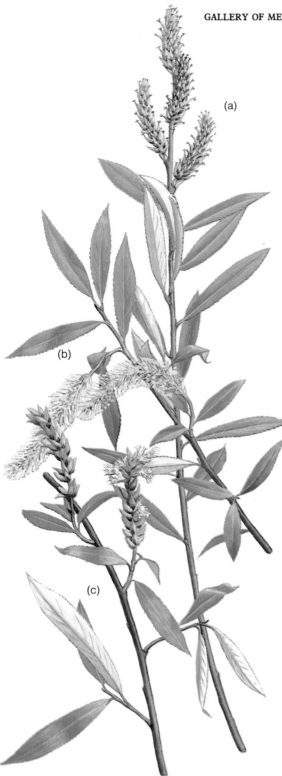

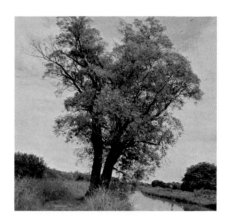

White Willow

Salix alba L.

Common Willow, European Willow
WILLOW FAMILY
Salicaceae

More than 300 species of willow range across the northern temperate and frigid zones, from the weeping willow with its trailing boughs to the tiny ground-creeping willow of the Far North. The Greek physician Dioscorides, writing in the first century A.D., was probably the first to describe the use of willow to reduce fever and pain—the tree's bark and leaves are rich in salicin, a glucoside closely related to acetylsalicylic acid, the active ingredient in aspirin. Over the centuries the list of willow's medicinal uses expanded to include remedies for insomnia, colds, rheumatism, and dysentery. It owed its effectiveness in these uses to salicin's fever-reducing, anti-inflammatory, antiseptic, and painkilling properties.

In the 1830's, researchers isolated salicin and its derivative salicylic acid from white willow and various other plants. But they found that its side effects—stomach pains and nausea—greatly limited its value. In the 1850's a derivative, acetylsalicylic acid, was synthesized from salicylic acid. This was the prototypical aspirin, but it took researchers close to 50 years to recognize that the new drug had all of salicylic acid's therapeutic properties without the side effects. Aspirin contains no willow derivatives but is entirely synthetic.

(a) Twig with female catkins
(b) Twig with male catkins
(c) Twig with maturing fruit

Habitat: Damp, low places, especially along rivers and streambanks.
Range: Native to Europe and central Asia, white willow is now naturalized in North America, especially from Nova Scotia down the Appalachian chain to Georgia.
Identification: A deciduous tree growing up to 70 feet tall or taller, white willow has finely toothed, lance-shaped, short-stalked, silky leaves, several times longer than they are broad, and a gray bark that is heavily ridged in older trees. The flowers (April–May) are borne in catkins (long clusters).
Uses: White willow preparations, such as teas brewed from the leaves or inner bark, serve as home remedies for fevers and chills, rheumatic pains, and digestive problems. Externally they work as a disinfectant and astringent on cuts and sores. Young, pliable shoots are good for weaving baskets and wicker furniture. Willow charcoal has been used for charcoal artists' pencils.

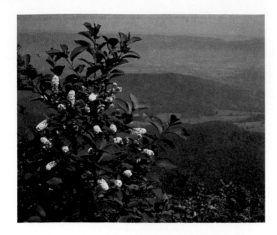

Wild Cherry

Prunus virginiana L.

Chokecherry, Common Chokecherry
ROSE FAMILY
Rosaceae

Among the plants most endowed with nature's gifts are the many species of *Prunus*—including the cherry and plum trees whose delicate blossoms have for centuries inspired the Japanese art of flower arranging. Not only has the cherry been a source of food and drink since time immemorial, but its wood has been used in furniture making. And few have gone through life without tasting wild cherry cough drops made from the bark of *P. virginiana* or a commercially prepared wild cherry syrup.

Early colonists probably first learned of the plant's medicinal benefits from the Indians, who used a bark tea for diarrhea and lung ailments. The colonists included the bark in cough medicines, and from about 1800 until 1975 it was listed in the standard pharmacopeias. Wild cherry—also called chokecherry because the raw fruit is sour—was thought to help cause sweating and so to bring down a fever. The bark was also used in folk medicine as an ingredient in tonics and as a decoction, or extract, to expel worms, and extracts of it were applied externally to ulcers and abscesses.

The sloe, *P. spinosa*, is a European species used medicinally and to make sloe gin.

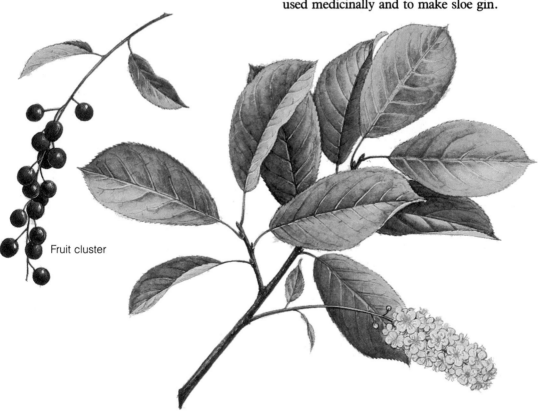

Fruit cluster

✗ Do not eat the leaves and fruit pits; they contain poisonous hydrocyanic acid, which causes difficult breathing, loss of balance, and convulsions.
Habitat: Moist woodlands, thickets, riverbanks.
Range: Native to North America, wild cherry is found from Newfoundland to Saskatchewan, south to North Carolina and Tennessee.
Identification: A large shrub or small tree growing up to 20 feet tall. The bark is smooth and usually reddish brown. It has lustrous, dark green, saw-tooth-edged, alternate leaves that are pointed at the tip and oval. Showy white flowers (April–July) produce one-seeded purplish-red fruits.
Uses: The bark of the wild cherry is best known as an ingredient in cough remedies, but pharmacologists state that this use of the plant is only slightly effective. The fruit is popular in jellies and jams, and it is sometimes used to make wines.

Wild Ginger

Asarum canadense L.

Canada Snakeroot, Colicroot, False Coltsfoot,
Indian Ginger, Vermont Snakeroot

BIRTHWORT FAMILY

Aristolochiaceae

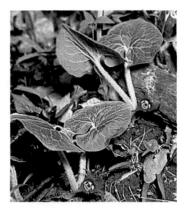

Don't try to find wild ginger by looking for its flowers. The plant's large heart-shaped leaves tend to obscure its tiny reddish-brown blossoms, which are even more difficult to see because they either droop with their heads down beneath the leaves or are half-buried on the forest floor. You are more likely to detect the flowers by their foul odor, like that of rotting meat; but this stench attracts the flies that are necessary for pollinating the plant.

There are about 70 plants in the wild ginger genus, but they are not related to the "true," or commercial, ginger, although some wild-food enthusiasts report that they have pulverized the rootstock into a powder or candied it as a substitute for the commercial product.

North American Indians often used wild ginger to disguise spoiled meat and to flavor food. In Canada a preparation of the plant served as a remedy for heart palpitations for some tribes. In 1837 this heart medicine was offered to Dr. Stephen Williams of Deerfield, Massachusetts, who said he offended the visiting red men when he refused it. Indian women liked wild ginger for another reason—they favored it to induce a normal menstrual cycle. The pioneers used the plant to ease intestinal and stomach gas, to promote sweating to break a fever, and as a tonic and appetite stimulant.

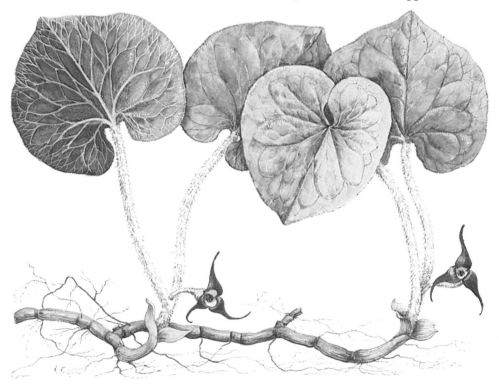

X Studies indicate that wild ginger has the potential for causing cancer.

Habitat: Shady moist woods with rich soils.

Range: A native of North America, wild ginger is found from Quebec to Ontario, south to Florida, and west to Minnesota and Illinois.

Identification: A prostrate and matted perennial herb arising from a rhizome (underground stem). Hairy stalks support the plant's heart-shaped, veined, and hairy leaves, 5–6 inches wide. Tiny dark reddish-brown flowers (March–June), ½–1½ inches across, are found at the fork between two leafstalks and are hidden by the leaves. They are followed by leathery round capsules.

Uses: Wild ginger has been prescribed in folk medicine as a tonic; as an agent that relieves gas; as an agent that increases perspiration and thus helps break a fever; and as an appetite stimulant. Studies show that use of the plant for stimulating the appetite and relieving gas pains may be valid.

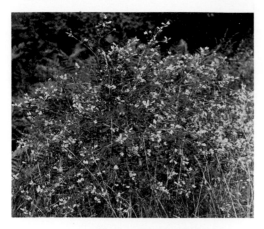

Wild Indigo

Baptisia tinctoria (L.) R.Br.

Baptisia, Clover Broom, Horsefly Weed, Indigo
Broom, Rattlebush, Shoofly, Yellow Indigo
PEA FAMILY
Leguminosae

The word "indigo" in a plant's name invites
the assumption that a rich blue dye must be
forthcoming. Unhappily, wild indigo is a poor
substitute for the indigo dye that has furnished
the world with a distinctive deep blue color for
4,000 years. The wild indigo native to North
America is a bushy plant with blue-green
leaves and yellow flowers similar to those
found on pea plants, and it has some history as
a North American Indian medicinal plant. The
Mohegans of southern New England steeped
the root to obtain a medicine with which they
bathed cuts and wounds, and the pioneers
followed them in this practice. The plant had a
reputation as an effective antiseptic, especially
when fever accompanied the wound.

For a decade during the early 19th century
the *U.S. Pharmacopeia* carried wild indigo, as
doctors made trials of extracts derived from the
plant to treat typhoid fever. Experimental
doses and overdoses of the root tincture and
powder resulted in symptoms similar to those
of the onset of typhoid, and this led practitioners of homeopathy (a medical system based
on the doctrine that "like cures like") to hope
for cures in actual cases of the disease.

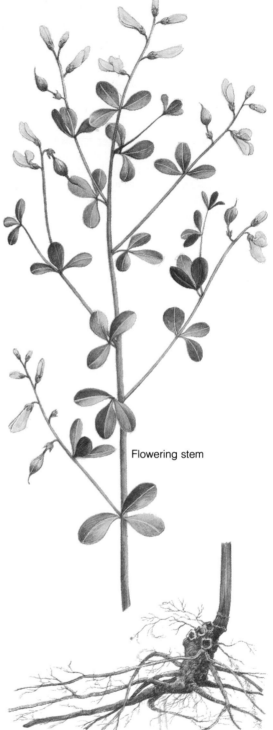

Flowering stem

Rootstock

Habitat: Dry soil in open woodlands and fields,
especially near sandy coastlines.
Range: A native North American plant, wild indigo
is distributed from Maine to Minnesota and south
to Florida and Louisiana.
Identification: An erect annual growing up to 3
feet tall, with smooth, round, branching stems.
Blue-green leaves, divided clover-fashion into
three ¾-inch-long leaflets, turn blue-black when
dried. Canary-yellow flowers (May–September),

½ inch long, are borne atop the tallest branches.
The seed capsule is an oblong pod.
Uses: Wild indigo roots have served as an antiseptic for cuts and wounds since Indian days.
Herbalists still recommend preparations of the
plant as a gargle and external antiseptic. There is
no scientific evidence, however, to support the
effectiveness of the plant in these uses.

Wild Licorice

Glycyrrhiza lepidota (Nutt.) Pursh

American Licorice

PEA FAMILY

Leguminosae

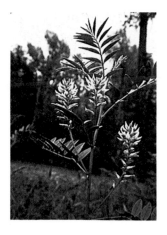

Among the Sioux Indians wild licorice was valued as a pain reliever. They put the root in the mouth to ease toothache, and they steeped the leaves to make drops for treating earache. Other peoples used the extract of the root to cure fever, to induce menstrual flow, and to expel the placenta after childbirth. Preparations of the plant were also taken internally for stomach ulcers, arthritis, and rheumatism.

The native wild licorice is little used today, and not at all in official medicine. Its close European relative, *G. glabra,* is imported and used commercially by the U.S. pharmaceutical, confectionery, and tobacco industries. This species has been valued medicinally for about 3,000 years—it is mentioned on Assyrian tablets and Egyptian papyri. The alleged benefits of licorice root preparations are end-less, but there is evidence that its high mucilage content may make it effective as a soothing cough remedy and that it contains cortisone-like substances, which may justify its use in the treatment of inflammations. *G. glabra* has also been prescribed as a mild laxative. The root of the plant yields a substance (glycyrrhizin) that is about 50 times sweeter than sugar but, unlike most sweets, quenches rather than increases thirst. It is reportedly a safe sugar substitute for diabetics.

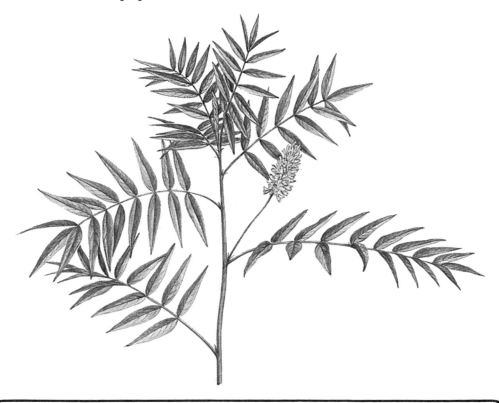

X Excessive amounts of the root, herbal teas, or candy derived from *G. glabra* may be harmful. Licorice increases salt retention and depletes the potassium in the body, causing lack of energy, weakness, and even death. People with high blood pressure or heart problems should avoid licorice.
Habitat: Meadows, prairies, waste places.
Range: Native to North America, wild licorice is found from Ontario west to Washington and south to Missouri, Texas, and Mexico.

Identification: An erect perennial herb reaching up to 3 feet tall. The leaves are pinnately divided into lance-shaped leaflets, which are dotted with minute brown scales (*lepidota* means "scaly"). White to pale yellow flowers (May–August) appear in dense spikes at the ends of branches. The seedpod is brown and prickly.
Uses: Pharmacologists state that the mucilage content of wild licorice probably makes it effective as a soothing cough remedy.

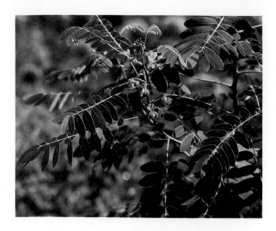

Wild Senna

Cassia marilandica L.

American Senna, Locust Plant, Maryland Cassia
PEA FAMILY
Leguminosae

There is hardly a better illustration of the folly of trusting blindly in "health foods" than the true story told of a woman who bought a packet of senna, made a tea from it, and proceeded to drink several cups. After a day of intestinal agony, she realized what herbalists have known for thousands of years—that a large dose of senna tea is a potent cathartic. Modern herbals recommend one cup of leaf tea for laxative purposes, and some suggest mixing an aromatic herb with the leaves to dilute the tea and lessen the intestinal cramps that are possible side effects.

Arab herbalists introduced two species of senna to Europeans in the 9th or 10th century. American pioneers discovered that the Indians had a native senna, *C. marilandica*, or wild senna, which is a laxative like the Old World species, but a milder one. The Indians had other uses for senna. They applied poultices of the crushed roots to sores and drank an extract of the boiled roots for fevers. Modern herbals list wild senna tea as a treatment for worms and excessive production of bile by the liver, as a breath sweetener, and as a diuretic. But wild senna's chief fame in herbal circles rests on its effectiveness as a laxative.

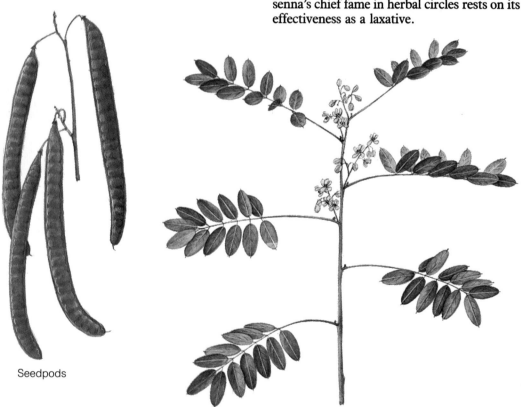

Seedpods

Habitat: Thickets, roadsides; near streams in extremely dry areas.

Range: Native to the United States, wild senna is found from Pennsylvania south to Florida and Texas, west to Iowa, Kansas, and Oklahoma.

Identification: A perennial herb growing to about 4 feet tall. Pinnately compound leaves consist of four to eight pairs of leaflets, each about 1–2½ inches long. Bright yellow flowers with brown centers (July–August) appear in short clusters in leaf axils at the ends of the twigs. They produce thick, curved seedpods, 2–3 inches long, that resemble locust insects and give the species another of its common names, locust plant.

Uses: A tea made from wild senna leaves has been taken as a laxative for centuries. Scientific studies show that this remedy is valid. The leaves are used in many pharmaceutical laxative preparations found on market shelves today.

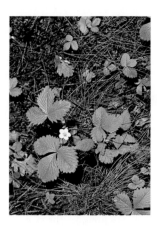

Wild Strawberry

Fragaria vesca L.

Wood Strawberry, Woodland Strawberry

ROSE FAMILY

Rosaceae

During the carefree days of summer, hikers frequently pause on slopes to taste wild strawberries. The tiny berries give off a delicate aroma that is subtly reminiscent of roses. Apothecaries and herbalists had a high regard for the wild strawberry's medicinal properties and recommended the plant for many complaints. One 17th-century herbalist noted: "The berries cool the liver, blood, and spleen, or a hot choleric stomach. They refresh and comfort fainting spirits and quench the thirst. They are good for inflammations, but it is best to refrain from them in a fever, lest they putrefy in the stomach and increase the fits." The 18th-century botanist Carolus Linnaeus, who was also a physician, ate large quantities of the berries to keep himself free of gout—a pleasant prescription, but its effectiveness has not been proved. In 20th-century folk medicine strawberry tea has served as a tonic. The tea has a slightly astringent taste, owing to the presence of tannin, which also accounts for the use of the tea as a remedy for diarrhea and as a gargle for sore throat. Herbalists also prescribe the fresh fruit as a laxative.

New plant
from runner

Cluster of fruits

Habitat: Meadows, woods, along roadsides.
Range: Wild strawberry is found from Newfoundland to Alberta, south to Virginia and New Mexico. The species is rare and endangered in Indiana.
Identification: A perennial herb, spreading by means of runners, from which stems with clusters of leaves grow. Each leaf is borne on a long slender stalk and consists of three toothed leaflets. Shortly after pollination, the white petals of the flowers (May–August) fall off and the flower receptacle enlarges to form a compound fruit on whose surface tiny one-seeded fruitlets are embedded.
Uses: Modern herbalists hold that the leaf tea stimulates the appetite. Scientific investigations have not proved this claim, but suggest it may be valid. Research does not support the plant's use in herbal medicine as an hematinic (an agent that stimulates blood cell formation or increases hemoglobin in the blood) and an antidyspeptic (a substance that helps to remedy indigestion).

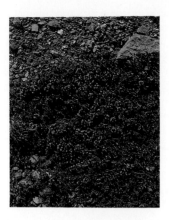

Wild Thyme

Thymus serpyllum L.

Creeping Thyme, Lemon Thyme,
Mother-of-thyme

MINT FAMILY

Labiatae

"**I know a bank** whereon the wild thyme blows," confides Oberon, referring to the sleeping place of his fairy queen, in Shakespeare's *A Midsummer-Night's Dream*. In 17th-century England theatergoers may well have perked up their ears at this statement, because wild thyme to them was a valuable medicinal plant, and they knew it as "a certain remedy for that troublesome complaint, the nightmare." A family herbal of the times also mentioned the plant "for headache due to inebriation" and "for nervous disorders." An herbalist coming to America with the early settlers saw to it that wild thyme was brought to the New World. The colonists used the herb for women's problems, especially to promote monthly menstruation.

Like its close relative thyme, the plant contains thymol, familiar to most druggists as a strong disinfectant and an active ingredient in antiseptics, mouthwashes, and gargles. Pharmacists are acquainted, too, with wild thyme's lemony scent in toiletry goods—a discovery made by ancient Athenian men, who made themselves elegant by rubbing their chests with a thyme-scented lotion after bathing.

Though less pronounced in flavor than the cultivated thyme (*T. vulgaris*), wild thyme can be substituted for it as a condiment in stews, soups, stuffings, sauces, and poultry and meat dishes. The meat of sheep that graze upon wild thyme is said to be extra flavorful. Its scientific name, *serpyllum*, reflects the plant's serpent-like, creeping habit of growth.

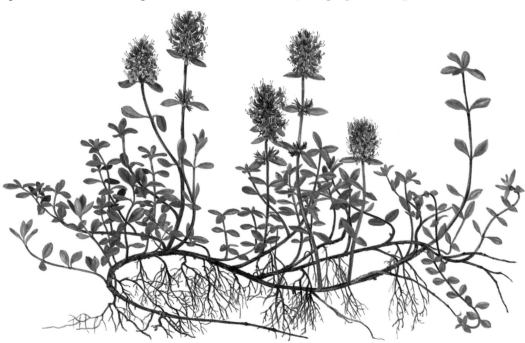

Habitat: Fields, roadsides, woods.

Range: Native to Europe, wild thyme is naturalized and found from Quebec to Ontario, south to North Carolina, west to Indiana, and sporadically west of the Cascade Range.

Identification: A perennial herb with creeping woody stems growing up to 1 foot long. The leaves are opposite, narrow, oblong or oval, and seldom more than ½ inch long. Rosy pink to purplish flowers (June–September) bloom on erect branches in small heads. The leaves exude a lemony odor.

Uses: Folk healers cite wild thyme as a sedative, antiseptic, diuretic, expectorant, antispasmodic, and carminative, or substance that alleviates intestinal gas. Wild thyme's uses as an antiseptic, an expectorant, an antispasmodic, and a carminative have all been validated by pharmacologists.

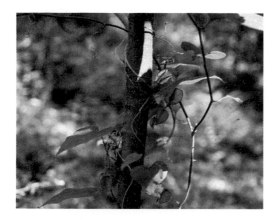

Wild Yam

Dioscorea villosa L.

Colicroot, Devil's-bones

YAM FAMILY

Dioscoreaceae

Not at all closely related to the yams that figure in the traditional Thanksgiving dinner, wild yam root (actually a rhizome) has a disagreeable taste. Growing mainly in the central and southern parts of North America, wild yam once played a prominent role in folk medicine in the United States. Preparations from the boiled root were taken by Indian women to relieve the pains of childbirth and were recommended as a diuretic, emetic, expectorant, and remedy for colic and muscle spasms. Southern black people esteemed it especially as a treatment for rheumatism.

In the 1930's scientists began searching for plant sources for such steroids as cortisone and the sex hormones because the cost of isolating these substances from animal sources was prohibitively expensive. Eventually researchers discovered steroidlike substances in *Dioscorea villosa* and related species. Today quantities of *Dioscorea* species are collected in the wild or cultivated in Mexico to supply diosgenin, the basic substance from which birth control pills and several other steroid drugs are made.

Just how this plant came to be called devil's-bones is unknown, but the name is apt. The long, thin, twisted roots that creep along below the surface of the soil have a skeletal look.

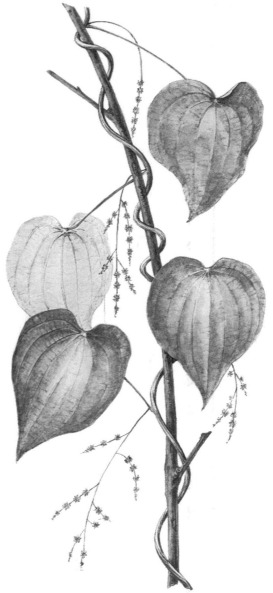

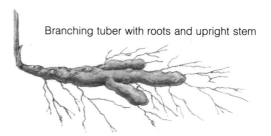

Branching tuber with roots and upright stem

Habitat: Damp woodlands and thickets.
Range: New England west to Minnesota, south to Georgia and Texas. The species is threatened in Rhode Island.
Identification: A perennial vine climbing to 20 feet. Heart-shaped alternate leaves, hairy on the under surface, are borne singly along the slender stem. Flowers (June–July) are greenish white, tiny, and borne in loose clusters. Seeds form in yellowish-green winged triangular capsules.

Uses: Although there seems to be no scientific basis for most of the folk remedies for which wild yam was used, various *Dioscorea* species are an important source of diosgenin used by the pharmaceutical industry in the manufacture of birth control pills and certain other steroid drugs. The steroidlike properties of wild yam may account for its effectiveness in treating rheumatism and similar inflammatory diseases.

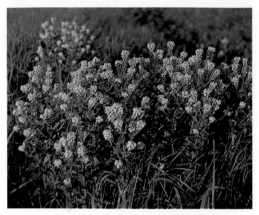

Winter Cress

Barbarea vulgaris R.Br.

Herb of St. Barbara, Upland Cress,
Yellow Rocket
MUSTARD FAMILY
Cruciferae

The herb of St. Barbara, as winter cress has been called, became associated with that legendary saint because its seed was traditionally sown on December 4, which was her feast day. As the name winter cress implies, this wild relative of broccoli stays green all winter, sprouting afresh each time the snow melts. In the days before rapid transportation made possible the shipment of southern produce to northern markets, winter cress was one of the few fresh greens available in the North during winter. About 1900, winter cress seed still appeared in the catalogs of mail-order nurseries, but its strong flavor has made it unpalatable to modern tastes, and scientists have discovered that the plant may be harmful.

Another link to its namesake, the martyr St. Barbara, is found in the plant's soothing powers. St. Barbara, who refused to renounce her belief in God, was traditionally invoked against lightning and fire, and thus she became the patron saint of military architects, artillerymen, and miners, who run risks from the gunpowder and flames with which they work. Traditionally, they have relied on winter cress as a dressing for wounds.

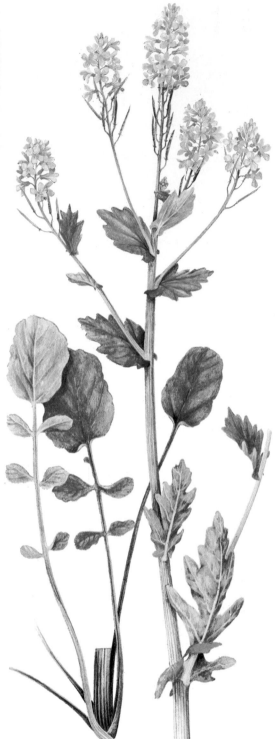

Long-stalked basal leaves

X Do not use plant for any purpose internally; recent tests indicate winter cress may produce kidney malfunction.
Habitat: Waste places, wet meadows, streamsides, moist woods.
Range: Introduced from Europe, winter cress now grows wild from Newfoundland to Ontario and south to Arkansas, in some north central states, and in Washington and Oregon.
Identification: A short-lived perennial growing 1 – 4 feet tall. Long-stalked lower leaves are pinnately cut into one to four pairs of lateral lobes and one large, oval, terminal lobe. The upper leaves are stalkless and deeply toothed. The lemon-yellow flowers (April–August), ½ inch across, appear in clusters and produce needlelike seedpods ½ – 1½ inches long.
Uses: Winter cress is no longer used medicinally. Although some seed catalogs list it, scientists warn against its use because of its potential danger.

Wintergreen

Gaultheria procumbens L.

Boxberry, Checkerberry, Mountain Tea,
Partridgeberry, Teaberry

HEATH FAMILY

Ericaceae

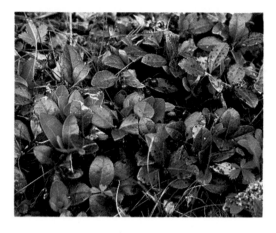

Rheumatism seems to have been a common complaint among North American Indians, to judge from the number of remedies they had for it. One of these was a tea brewed from wintergreen leaves. When American patriots boycotted British tea before the American Revolution, wintergreen tea was one of their substitutes, and they too began to use it as a remedy for headache, muscle aches, and colds. In the 1800's pharmacologists discovered that the oil from wintergreen leaves has aspirinlike properties, which explain its effectiveness as a pain reliever. Today herbals largely recommend wintergreen oil applied externally to reduce painful swelling from injury and to treat inflammation of the joints and muscles.

Wintergreen once supplied flavoring for candies, cough drops, and toothpastes—and the names of such products with a wintergreen flavor suggest it still does. But wintergreen has been replaced by synthetics, and the genuine article—an evergreen—is now enjoyed mainly by deer, partridge, and other animals as a winter food.

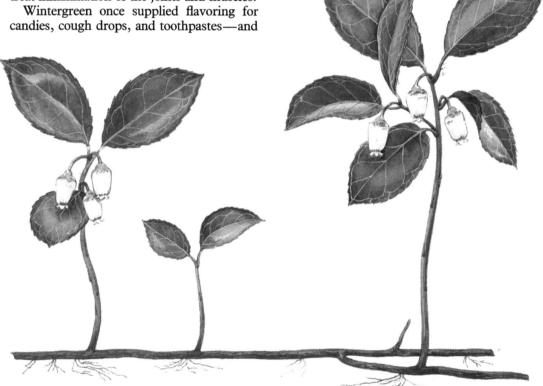

X Oil of wintergreen is poisonous except in small amounts, as for flavoring. Children have died after drinking the oil.

Habitat: Acidic soils, woods, mountains.

Range: A native of North America, wintergreen is found from Newfoundland to Manitoba, south to Georgia, and west to Minnesota.

Identification: A shrubby evergreen perennial growing up to 6 inches tall. Finely toothed oval leaves are pale or yellowish green when young; mature leaves are leathery and glossy, dark green above, paler below. Bell-shaped white flowers (July–August) are followed by red fruits.

Uses: Wintergreen leaf tea has traditionally been employed as a pain reliever. Present-day folk healers prescribe wintergreen oil in external preparations to reduce joint and muscle inflammation and pain, especially that caused by rheumatoid arthritis and rheumatism. Scientific data indicate that the oil is probably effective in these uses.

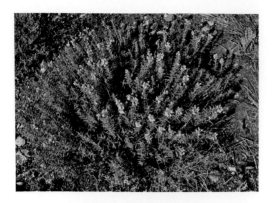

Winter Savory

Satureja montana L.

Mountain Savory
MINT FAMILY
Labiatae

Perfuming dry hillsides throughout its Mediterranean home territory, winter savory is a plant of the sun and a hardy perennial, unlike its smaller, softer garden relative, summer savory (*S. hortensis*), which lives only a year or so. The two plants have similar properties: they contain some active substances that, according to some herbalists, render them antiseptic, expectorant, and tonic. For a very long time both winter and summer, or garden, savory were thought to be psychological and physical stimulants, and they enjoyed a special reputation as aphrodisiacs. Because the word *satureia* was a synonym for the aphrodisiac made from savory, people speculated on a possible connection between the genus name and the lecherous satyrs of mythology, but the link is strictly an imaginary one.

Although some authorities say winter savory has no medicinal uses, others list the plant as a remedy for gas pains, as an appetite stimulant, and as an antiseptic gargle. Winter savory leaf serves as a fragrant culinary herb, to be hung up to dry in bunches and then crumbled and sprinkled onto the food at the moment of preparation. The leaf is also a traditional ingredient in salami.

Habitat: Light, well-drained soil; dry, rocky hillsides.

Range: A native of the Mediterranean region, winter savory has been introduced and is cultivated in North America.

Identification: A perennial shrub with stiff upright stalks growing up to 20 inches high, winter savory has smooth, shiny, leathery leaves that are narrow, pointed, and bordered with fine hairs. The leaves have an aromatic smell and a hot, bitter taste. Pink to white flowers (June–September) are borne on leafy terminal spikes.

Uses: Researchers confirm that winter savory's uses as a carminative (an agent that relieves gas pains) and as an antiseptic gargle are valid. The crumbled dried leaves are a fragrant seasoning, making some foods more digestible. The oil derived from the plant serves as a flavoring in some liqueurs.

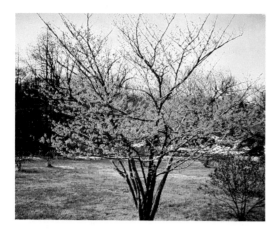

Witch Hazel

Hamamelis virginiana L.

Snapping Hazel, Winterbloom
WITCH HAZEL FAMILY
Hamamelidaceae

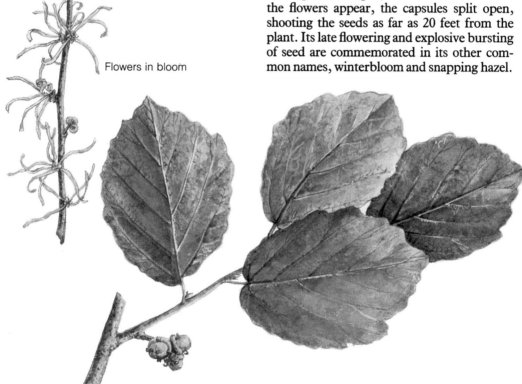

Flowers in bloom

Witch hazel is one of the commonest home remedies in the United States today. Consisting of a distillation of witch hazel bark, twigs, and leaves mixed with alcohol and water, it is used mainly as an astringent. It is also sometimes applied with a steam towel to bruises and strains or in a cold compress to a fevered brow.

Indians taught the early settlers how to make decoctions of witch hazel bark, twigs, and leaves in various strengths for use as a liniment and eyewash and in the treatment of hemorrhoids, internal hemorrhages, and excessive menstrual flow. (These decoctions probably contained astringent tannins.)

The name witch hazel was given to the North American shrub *Hamamelis virginiana* by the English settlers, who attached some of their own lore to the American species. Back home, the forked twigs of various European trees had been used as divining rods to locate water and minerals. The "witch" in the name witch hazel does not refer to magic or broomsticks but comes from an Anglo-Saxon word meaning "to bend."

Witch hazel blooms in the fall, after its seeds have ripened in capsules. At the same time that the flowers appear, the capsules split open, shooting the seeds as far as 20 feet from the plant. Its late flowering and explosive bursting of seed are commemorated in its other common names, winterbloom and snapping hazel.

Habitat: Woods.
Range: Nova Scotia south to Georgia and west as far as Minnesota and Missouri. The species is endangered in Minnesota.
Identification: A twisted shrub or small tree with gray-brown bark, witch hazel grows 5–15 feet high. The buds occur in clusters at the bases of the leaves. The flowers (September–November) have petals resembling twisted yellow straps and open after the leaves have fallen from the branches. The leaves are lopsided at the base, with shallow-toothed edges. The shiny black seeds are contained in hard brown capsules.
Uses: A distillation of the extract of witch hazel bark, twigs, and leaves mixed with alcohol and water is today a widely available household remedy for external use, mainly as an astringent. Some after-shave lotions also contain an astringent extract of witch hazel.

Wood Sorrel

Oxalis acetosella L.

Shamrock, Sour Trefoil,
True Wood Sorrel, White Wood Sorrel

WOOD SORREL FAMILY

Oxalidaceae

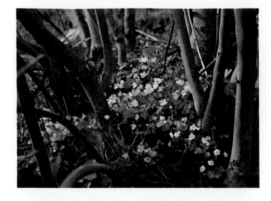

As any true Irishman knows, the shamrock's tripartite leaf was the means by which the great St. Patrick is said to have explained the doctrine of the Trinity to the heathen Celts, and now this plant serves as the symbol of the Emerald Isle. Opinions vary about which plant is the true shamrock, but a strong case can be made for wood sorrel, which is native to the British Isles. In England wood sorrel was called cuckoo bread because it sprouted from the ground when that bird began his springtime serenade.

Wood sorrel has a pleasantly sour flavor. In Elizabethan England it was a popular culinary herb, used as a salad ingredient, a potherb, and a sauce herb. After garden sorrel (which is not botanically related to wood sorrel) was introduced, it replaced wood sorrel in the kitchen.

The herbalist Nicholas Culpeper, writing in England in the 1600's, reported wood sorrel's medicinal virtues. He recommended the plant "to quench thirst, to strengthen a weak stomach, to stay vomiting," and he noted that it was "excellent in any contagious sickness or pestilential fever." By the 1800's this species of sorrel had been introduced into North America. One herbalist noted that a decoction, or extract, of wood sorrel was being used to treat inflammatory disorders, fevers, and diseases of the kidneys and bladder.

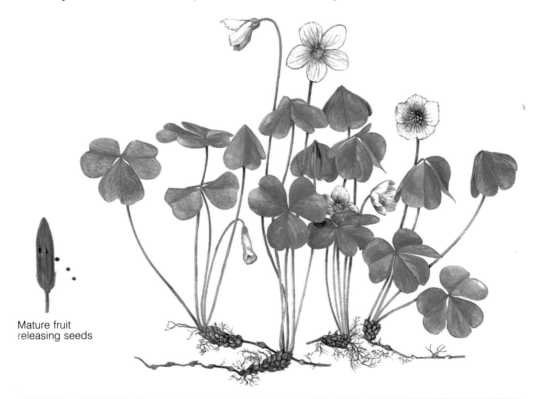

Mature fruit
releasing seeds

X Leaves contain oxalic acid, which may cause diarrhea, kidney stones, kidney failure, or hemorrhaging if taken internally in very large amounts.
Habitat: Moist shady soils in woods; near rocks and on mossy banks.
Range: Native to Eurasia, wood sorrel is grown and sometimes escapes from gardens in North America from Newfoundland to Saskatchewan, south to Wisconsin, Tennessee, and North Carolina.
Identification: A perennial herb growing up to 6 inches tall from a creeping rootstock. Bright green basal leaves, three to eight together, are borne on long slender leafstalks; each leaf is divided into three leaflets. Solitary white flowers (April–July) on long slender stalks have pinkish or purple veins.
Uses: Traditionally, wood sorrel was prescribed as a diuretic for kidney and bladder problems. Today herbalists name it as an external wash, or lotion, in treating skin infections. There is no scientific basis for these claims.

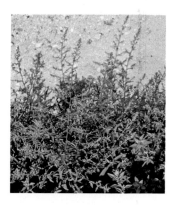

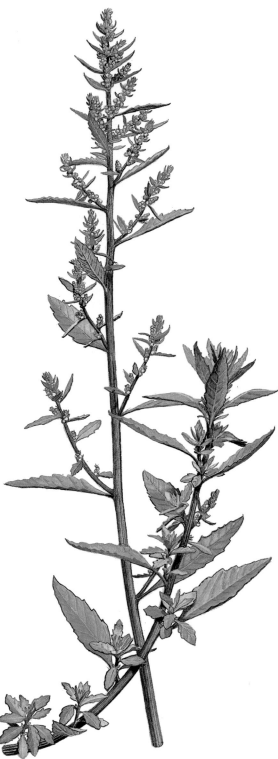

Wormseed

Chenopodium ambrosioides L.

American Wormseed, Jerusalem Oak,
Jesuit Tea, Mexican Tea, Stinking Weed

GOOSEFOOT FAMILY

Chenopodiaceae

The homely, strong-smelling wormseed had its day in the 19th century, when official medicine in North America recognized it as a most effective cure for roundworm and hookworm. Official recognition had been tardy, however. For centuries American Indians had known about this remedy, which paralyzes the offending intestinal worms. A strong laxative administered after the wormseed has had its effect drives the parasites from the body.

This worm remedy probably came north into the United States and Canada from Mexico and South America, where the species is indigenous, and pioneers and settlers learned of its use from Native Americans. In the 19th century wormseed was cultivated in vast amounts in Maryland to supply the commercial demand of the pharmaceutical industry. Chenopodium oil, the effective substance, is found in the whole plant but is most concentrated in the seeds. Wormseed was official in the *U.S. Pharmacopeia* for more than a century, from 1820 to 1947.

For some years physicians have ceased to recommend wormseed because it can cause harmful side effects ranging from nausea and dizziness to paralysis and death.

X Both the plant and the seeds may be fatal. Symptoms include nausea, dizziness, convulsions, and paralysis.
Habitat: Open fields, waste places, cultivated land.
Range: A native of tropical America, wormseed has become naturalized from southern Ontario and New England south throughout the United States.
Identification: A strong-smelling annual or perennial, growing up to 5 feet tall, with an erect stem that is somewhat woody at the base. Alternate, coarsely toothed leaves are oblong to lance-shaped. Dense spikes of tiny greenish flowers (August–November) are borne in the leaf axils.
Uses: Tests by scientists confirm that wormseed oil is a valid anthelmintic, or agent that rids the body of worms. The chenopodium oil derived from wormseed is especially effective against roundworms and hookworms, causing them to lose their grip on the intestines.

347

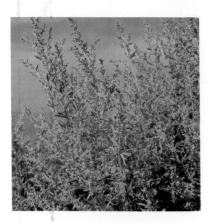

Wormwood

Artemisia absinthium L.

Absinthe, Absinthium, Green Ginger,
Madderwort

COMPOSITE FAMILY

Compositae

Gray-green and almost shrublike, wormwood grows mainly in temperate regions of eastern North America. The plant is an immigrant from Europe, where it was used for centuries for a host of diseases and disorders: to promote menstruation; as an antidote for drunkenness and all sorts of poisons; as a bitter tonic, for stimulating the appetite; as a remedy for intestinal worms; as a treatment for gout, kidney stones, and jaundice; as a compress to ease the pain of swellings and bruises; as an external antiseptic; and as a strewing herb to mask bad odors and drive away vermin.

Wormwood was also used in the infamous liqueur called absinthe, which was much in vogue in 19th-century Europe. Because so many cases of narcotic poisoning (causing damage to the nervous system and mental deterioration) were reported, in the early 1900's absinthe was banned in the United States and other countries. The U.S. Food and Drug Administration lists wormwood as an unsafe and dangerous herb.

Today, wormwood is used sparingly to flavor vermouth. Some horticulturists plant the decorative gray-green herb in gardens to provide a contrast with more colorful blossoms.

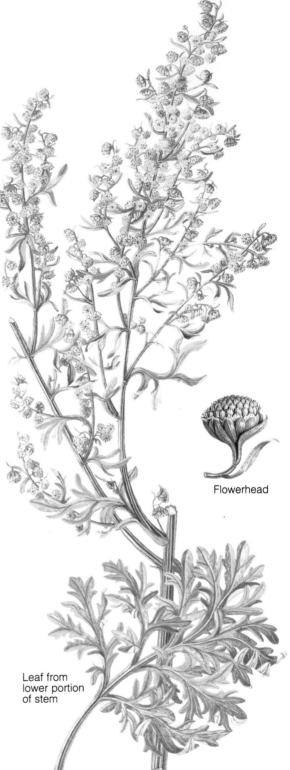

Flowerhead

Leaf from
lower portion
of stem

X Wormwood has been declared "unsafe" by the U.S. Food and Drug Administration.

Habitat: Roadsides and other waste land.

Range: Native to Europe, wormwood is cultivated and grows wild in North America from Newfoundland to Manitoba, south to Pennsylvania.

Identification: A shrubby perennial herb with a gray, finely hairy, erect stem growing up to 4 feet tall. Silky gray-green leaves are much divided and featherlike. Tiny yellow flowerheads (July–September) are borne in loose clusters on the upper ends of branches.

Uses: Scientists have not been able to validate wormwood's longtime use as an anthelmintic (an agent that destroys intestinal worms) nor have they been able to confirm the plant's value as an emmenagogue (an agent that induces normal menstruation). Scientists state that wormwood may have a narcotic effect and that it is most likely an effective external antiseptic.

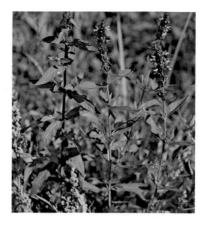

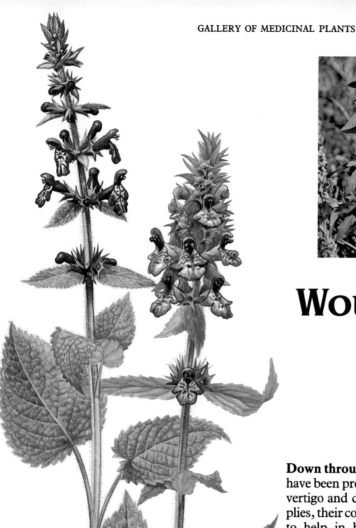

Stachys sylvatica   *Stachys palustris*

Woundworts

Stachys palustris L.

Marsh Woundwort

Stachys sylvatica L.

Hedge Woundwort

MINT FAMILY

Labiatae

Down through the centuries the woundworts have been prescribed for ailments as diverse as vertigo and dysentery. But as their name implies, their commonest traditional use has been to help in healing surface sores and open wounds. The leaves are applied as a poultice or simply bruised and placed on a wound to stop the flow of blood.

Look for *S. palustris*, often called marsh woundwort, in wet meadows, beside streams, and in damp roadside ditches. Its less common relative *S. sylvatica*, or hedge woundwort, prefers drier sites such as hedgerows and open woodlands. But despite one old-time herbalist's claim that toads are fond of such places, don't expect to find one beneath every hedge woundwort you happen upon.

Because of their hairy stems and leaves, the woundworts are sometimes known as hedge nettles. Unlike true nettles, however, they have no stinging hairs and so are entirely safe to touch. The marsh woundwort, in fact, is sought out by some as a food plant. Its abundant underground tubers can be dug up in the fall for eating raw, boiled or baked, or pickled.

Habitat: Marsh woundwort grows in wet meadows and other damp places. Hedge woundwort is found in drier locations such as hedgerows, woods, and waste places.

Range: Marsh woundwort ranges from Newfoundland to Alaska south through most of the United States. Hedge woundwort is found in scattered locations from New England to Virginia. Both species are native to Europe.

Identification: Both plants are rank-smelling herbaceous perennials 2–3 feet tall, with square hairy stems and toothed opposite leaves. Their mottled pink-red to rose-purple flowers (June–September) are tubular with lobed lower lips and grow in clusters at the ends of the stems. The leaves of marsh woundwort are lance-shaped and usually lack leafstalks.

Uses: Both plants have been used to stop bleeding from open wounds and promote their healing, but no scientific evidence exists to support these uses.

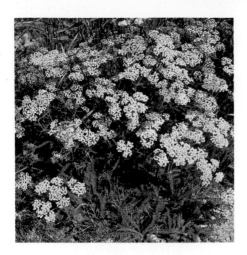

Yarrow

Achillea millefolium L.

Bloodwort, Milfoil, Sanguinary,
Stanchgrass, Thousand-leaf

COMPOSITE FAMILY

Compositae

Since at least the time of the ancient Greeks, yarrow has been used to treat cuts, wounds, burns, and bruises. Its genus name, *Achillea*, refers to the hero Achilles, in Homer's *Iliad*, who is said to have given yarrow to his soldiers to stanch the blood from their wounds. The species name *millefolium*—"of a thousand leaves"—describes the fine, feathery leaves of the plant.

In ancient times and on through the Middle Ages, yarrow kept its place as a medicinal plant—and even a magical potion. Yarrow is one of a handful of plants called allheal in the English herbal tradition; on the other side of the world it is the "life medicine" and general panacea of the Navajos. People used yarrow as an astringent, made a salve of it to heal sores, and chewed the leaves to lessen the pain of toothaches. American Indians poured an infusion of the plant tops into the ears of those with earaches, and pioneers drank it for everything from urinary problems to head colds.

Yarrow makes a fine decorative plant for gardens, and its lingering spicy odor enhances dried flower arrangements.

Flowerheads with disc flowers
and five petallike ray flowers

Habitat: Fields, roadsides, and other open places.
Range: Native to Europe, yarrow is now naturalized in temperate regions of North America, except southern Texas and the southwestern states.
Identification: A perennial herb growing from 8 inches to 3 feet tall, with stems branching near the top to support heads of cream-colored flowers (May–November). These heads, about ¼ inch across, consist of yellow disc and five petallike ray flowers. Feathery, delicate leaves resembling tiny fern fronds grow alternately along the stem.
Uses: An infusion of the leaves and flower tops is drunk to reduce fever and as a mild tonic to stimulate the appetite. A poultice made from the whole plant or a powder of ground-up dried yarrow tops is applied to cuts and wounds. Modern researchers find good experimental evidence for yarrow's use as an anti-inflammatory agent and possibly as an astringent.

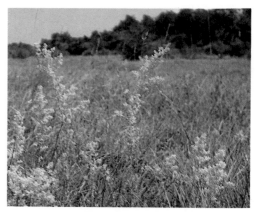

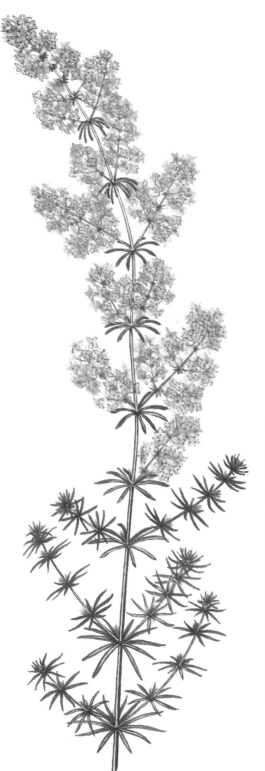

Yellow Bedstraw

Galium verum L.

Cheese Rennet, Maid's-hair,
Our-Lady's-bedstraw

MADDER FAMILY

Rubiaceae

The Virgin Mary prepared the manger in Bethlehem with yellow bedstraw according to legend, and perhaps she did, because this herb's honey-scented flowers and hay-scented dried foliage were traditionally used as mattress stuffing. The plant's chief employment, going back to early Greece, was in cheese making. A strong decoction, or extract, of the leaves and stem acts as a curdling agent. Some herbals still suggest making cheese by this method, but bedstraw is no longer employed in the commercial product. The plant also furnished two dyes: a red one from the roots and a yellow one from the flowers. During the reign of Henry VII (1485–1509) in England the ladies of the court used the yellow dye to tint their hair blond—hence the common name maid's-hair. Dairymen in Cheshire, England, used the yellow dye to color cheese.

The red root extract suggested to herbalists of long ago that the plant might be useful for halting bleeding. In Elizabethan England herbal healers also recommended a decoction of the plant as a soothing foot bath.

Habitat: Dry fields and meadows, sunny slopes, open woods, roadsides.

Range: Introduced from Europe, yellow bedstraw has become naturalized in North America from Newfoundland to Ontario, south to Virginia, and west to Ohio, Missouri, Kansas, and North Dakota.

Identification: A perennial herb growing up to 3 feet tall. Rough-surfaced, narrowly lance-shaped leaves, about 1 inch long, are borne in whorls of four to eight around the stem nodes and are covered with soft hairs on the underside. Numerous tiny bright yellow flowers (June–August) occur in dense elongated clusters.

Uses: Yellow bedstraw has long been used in folk medicine as a styptic (a substance that stops minor bleeding) and for making foot baths. Herbals still list it for these purposes, and they also specify a tea made from the plant as a diuretic and for the treatment of epilepsy. There is no scientific evidence to support any of these uses.

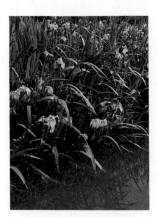

Yellow Flag

Iris pseudacorus L.

Yellow Iris, Yellow Water Flag
IRIS FAMILY
Iridaceae

Legend tells that Clovis, king of the Franks
(A.D. 481–511), prayed to the Christian God
during a decisive battle and, upon emerging
victorious, converted to Christianity. He took
the yellow iris, a symbol of the Virgin Mary, as
his emblem—the fleur-de-lis that was the
royal emblem of France until recent modern
times. Actually, the fleur-de-lis was usually
identified with the white iris, but the legend is
much loved.

Yellow flag received the species name *pseudacorus* because when not in flower it resembles *Acorus calamus*, or sweet flag, another
medicinal plant. Yellow flag was once credited
with healing properties it did not actually
have—it was used as a diuretic, purgative, and
emetic. It has also been recommended for
making a cooling astringent lotion for external
application, and is reputedly effective when
applied to wounds. A tea prepared from the
rhizome (underground stem) was once used as
a remedy for certain gynecological complaints,
but is no longer recommended. Yellow flag
flowers yield a yellow dye; the roots yield both
brown and black dyes, as well as black ink. A
French chemist of the early 19th century
discovered that the ripe seeds, when well
roasted, make a good coffee substitute.

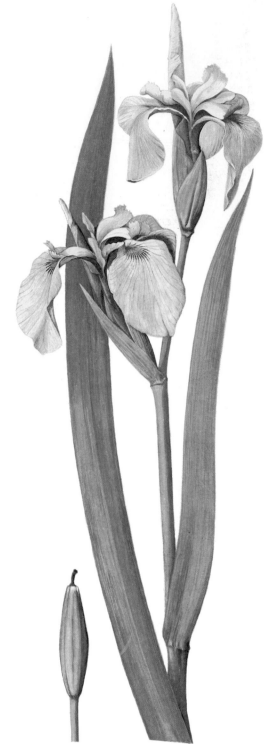

Mature fruit

X The rhizome and root, if taken in large amounts,
may cause stomach and intestinal pain, nausea,
and vomiting.
Habitat: Marshland and other wet, open places.
Range: Introduced from Europe to North America,
yellow flag has escaped cultivation to grow wild
from Newfoundland to Minnesota and throughout
the southeastern United States.
Identification: A perennial growing up to 3 feet
tall, yellow flag has an underground stem (rhizome) and slender grasslike leaves. Yellow flowers (April–August) grow out of papery envelopes
known as a spathes. The petals are erect and
spoon-shaped; the sepals curve outward and
down and are marked with dark lines and flecks.
Uses: A lotion made from the juice of the fresh
rhizome is sometimes recommended by herbalists
for wounds. Pharmacologists report that there is
some evidence that yellow flag shows anti-inflammatory activity.

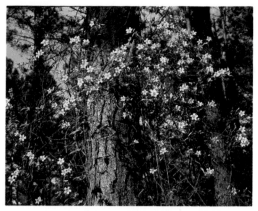

Yellow Jessamine

Gelsemium sempervirens (L.) Ait.f.

Carolina Jasmine, Carolina Jessamine,
Evening Trumpet Flower, Woodbine
LOGANIA FAMILY
Loganiaceae

The allure of the sweetly perfumed, brilliantly colored flowers of yellow jessamine masks the fact that it contains a deadly poison whose fatal effects have been compared to the hemlock's. A person or animal that eats any part of it can pass from paralysis to death without intervening loss of consciousness. Even bees that pollinate the plant are occasionally poisoned by it.

Despite its deadly properties, yellow jessamine once served as a medicine. During the 19th century, various preparations made from the roots were used as sedatives, painkillers, antispasmodics, and fever-reducing agents. The plant was popular in the treatment of whooping cough and asthma. A tea made from the flowers was once recommended for coughs, shortness of breath, pleurisy, and upset stomachs. Fortunately, by the early 20th century, medicinal use of yellow jessamine had declined with the increasing recognition that all parts of the plant are dangerously toxic.

A beautiful evergreen climbing vine, yellow jessamine is the state flower of South Carolina.

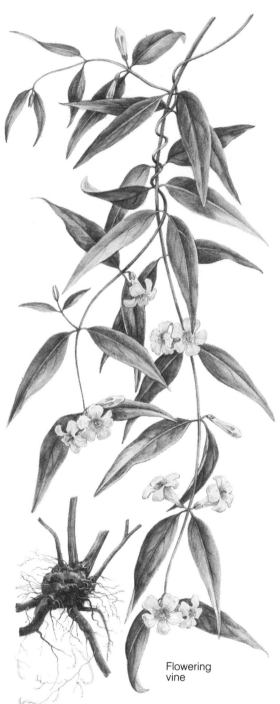

Flowering vine

Rootstock

X All parts of yellow jessamine contain toxic alkaloids that can cause paralysis and death, and none must be taken internally.
Habitat: Rich, moist soils on streambanks, in thickets, at forest edges; a climber, on fences or trees.
Range: Native to North America, yellow jessamine grows wild from southeast Virginia south to Florida and west to Tennessee, Arkansas, and Texas.
Identification: A woody perennial evergreen vine that forms tangled carpets or grows up to 40 feet high, depending on its support system. Shiny lance-shaped leaves grow in opposite pairs. Fragrant, bright yellow, trumpetlike flowers (January–May), 1 inch long, bloom singly or in clusters of two or more.
Uses: Yellow jessamine contains substances that depress the central nervous system, making it effective as a sedative, painkiller, and antispasmodic. It was once listed in the *U.S. Pharmacopeia,* but because even a small dose can have dire consequences, it is no longer used medicinally.

Yellowroot

Xanthorhiza simplicissima Marsh.

Shrub Yellowroot

BUTTERCUP FAMILY

Ranunculaceae

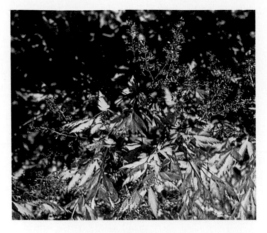

A pure, bitter taste, due mainly to the presence in the roots of a yellow crystalline alkaloid known as berberine, made yellowroot a standby in the 19th century as tonic bitters to be taken before meals to stimulate the appetite. Native to eastern North America, the shrub has been in continuous use in Appalachia ever since Daniel Boone's day as a remedy for stomach upsets. American Indians chewed the root for the same purpose and boiled the roots to prepare a concoction that they used for treating colds. According to one source, they sometimes used a medicine brewed from the roots as an aid in childbirth.

Yellowroot survives to this day as a folk remedy in parts of the U.S. South, where the root is chewed to freshen the mouth and sharpen the taste buds. Tea brewed from the roots serves as a mouthwash and as a medicine for throat and stomach disorders. According to a 19th-century authority, the best seasons of the year for collecting yellowroot are late fall and early spring. The bitter alkaloid constituting the medicinal ingredient is concentrated in the gray-brown outer layer of the root.

Xanthorhiza means "yellowroot"; *simplicissima* translates literally as "simplest," but in a specialized sense it means "mostly single-stemmed, having few branches."

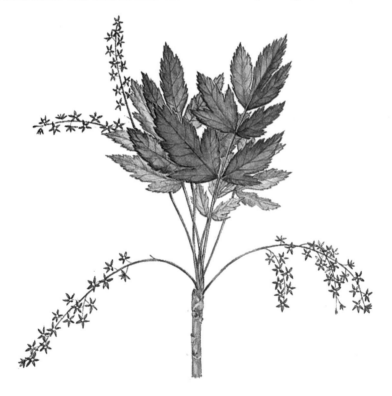

X Excessive doses of yellowroot may be harmful.
Habitat: Damp woods and along streambeds.
Range: Native to eastern North America, yellowroot grows wild, mostly in mountainous areas, from southwestern New York to northwestern Florida.
Identification: Growing up to 2 feet tall from a twisted rhizome (underground stem), yellowroot sends up one or more gray-brown aerial stems, each of which bears a cluster of bright green leaves at the end. At the base of the leaf clusters, small brownish-purple flowers (April–May) are borne in loose drooping clusters.
Uses: The clean, bitter taste of yellowroot accounts for its former popularity as a tonic. Various strengths of tea brewed from the roots have served in folk medicine as a wash for an ulcerated mouth, as a sore throat remedy, and as a tea for stomach upset, but current pharmacological opinion is that the plant has little medicinal value.

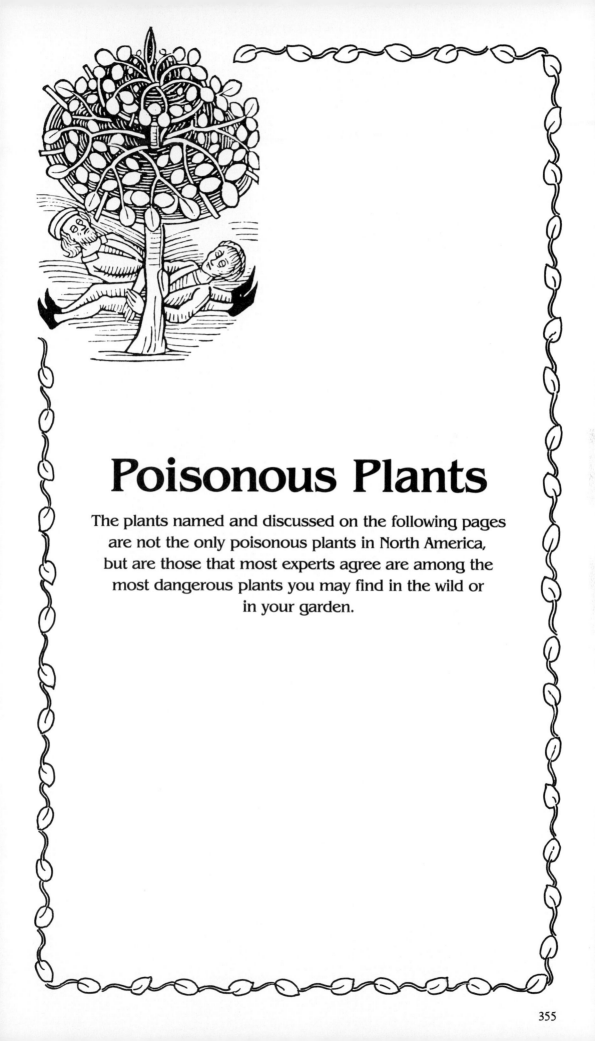

Poisonous Plants

The plants named and discussed on the following pages are not the only poisonous plants in North America, but are those that most experts agree are among the most dangerous plants you may find in the wild or in your garden.

The dangerously poisonous plants listed below are described and illustrated either in the "Gallery of Medicinal Plants" (pages 74–354), where each is distinguished by a red **X**, or in "Exotic Plants" (pages 359–391). All contain toxic chemicals that can cause serious illness or death. Twelve other common poisonous plants are described on these pages.

American mistletoe (*Phoradendron flavescens*)
Arnica (*Arnica montana*)
Autumn crocus (*Colchicum autumnale*)
Belladonna (*Atropa belladonna*)
Bird's-foot trefoil (*Lotus corniculatus*)
Bittersweet nightshade (*Solanum dulcamara*)
Black locust (*Robinia pseudoacacia*)
Bloodroot (*Sanguinaria canadensis*)
Blue flag (*Iris versicolor*)
Broom (*Cytisus scoparius*)
Castor oil plant (*Ricinus communis*)
Celandine (*Chelidonium majus*)
Chinese lantern (*Physalis alkekengi*)
Cotton (*Gossypium hirsutum*)
Daffodil (*Narcissus pseudonarcissus*)
Ergot (*Claviceps purpurea*)
Figwort (*Scrophularia nodosa*)
Foxglove (*Digitalis purpurea*)
Goldenseal (*Hydrastis canadansis*)
Hedge mustard (*Sisymbrium officinale*)

Hemp dogbane (*Apocynum cannabinum*)
Henbane (*Hyoscyamus niger*)
Horse chestnut (*Aesculus hippocastanum*)
Indian pink (*Spigelia marilandica*)
Indian tobacco (*Lobelia inflata*)
Jimsonweed (*Datura stramonium*)
Larkspur (*Delphinium ajacis*)
Lily of the valley (*Convallaria majalis*)
Marsh marigold (*Caltha palustris*)
Mayapple (*Podophyllum peltatum*)
Moonseed (*Menispermum canadense*)
Virgin's-bower (*Clematis virginiana*)
Wallflower (*Cheiranthus cheiri*)
White false hellebore (*Veratrum album*)
Wild cherry (*Prunus virginiana*)
Wild licorice (*Glycyrrhiza lepidota*)
Winter cress (*Barbarea vulgaris*)
Wormseed (*Chenopodium ambrosioides*)
Wormwood (*Artemesia absinthium*)
Yellow jessamine (*Gelsemium sempervirens*)

American Yew

Taxus canadensis Marsh.   All parts of all yews except the cuplike red aril (seed cover) are poisonous. You can tell a yew from other needled evergreens by its lack of cones and its berrylike red fruits. The flat single needles are dark green on top and pale green to yellow below, and they seem to be on opposite sides of the stem, although close examination shows that they grow all around it. *T. canadensis* is a low shrub that grows in most northern states and in Canada. Other yew species, both shrubs and trees, are found all across the continent.

Black Nightshade

Solanum americanum Mill.   All parts are poisonous. Although the ripe black berries of *S. americanum* have been used for pies and jams, children have died from eating the unripe fruit; it is best to avoid the plant altogether. A sun-loving, upright plant 1 to 3 feet tall with oval to lance-shaped leaves, the black nightshade bears white flowers with five backswept petals, shaped like the purple blossoms of the bittersweet nightshade (*S. dulcamara*).

Death Camas

Zigadenus elegans Pursh.   All parts are poisonous. Several *Zigadenus* species grow in the same western plains, woods, and mountain meadows as the edible camases (*Camassia*), and their onionlike bulbs are easily confused. *Z. elegans* (also called elegant camas and alkali grass) bears a wandlike cluster of star-shaped greenish-white flowers atop its erect stem. The flowers of other death camases are white to yellow. True camases have blue flowers.

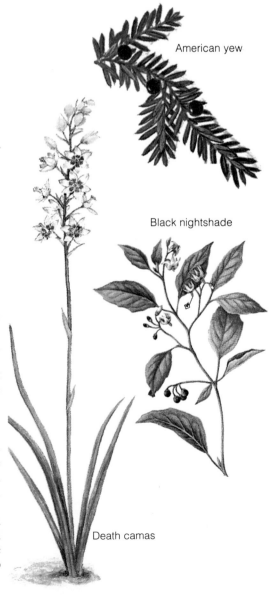

American yew

Black nightshade

Death camas

Desert Plume

Stanleya pinnata (Pursh) Britt. Leaves and stems may be poisonous if eaten raw. Stanleyas, also known as prince's-plumes, accumulate the poisonous element selenium, often found in the arid western soils where they grow. Vigorous cooking can eliminate the poison. The bright yellow flowers of *S. pinnata* are borne in long, showy spires atop stems up to 5 feet high. The flowers of the 2-foot-tall *S. elata* are lemon-yellow to white.

Green False Hellebore

Veratrum viride Ait. All parts are poisonous. Like *V. album*, described on page 391, *V. viride* has large leaves that clasp its stem. It may grow 7 feet tall, and is topped in spring by a branching cluster of greenish flowers.

Monkshood

Aconitum uncinatum L. All parts of all monkshoods are poisonous. At least one *Aconitum* species (more than 100 exist) is found in nearly every part of North America except the deserts. They are recognizable by their palmately lobed or cleft leaves and their more or less upright stems of hooded, blue or purple (occasionally white) flowers.

Mountain Laurel

Kalmia latifolia L. Leaves and flowers are poisonous. A shade-tolerant evergreen shrub with showy clusters of starlike pinkish-white flowers, the mountain laurel graces open forests throughout eastern North America. The smaller, less showy sheep laurel (*K. angustifo-*

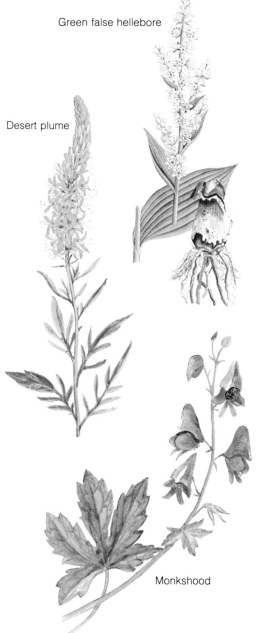

Green false hellebore

Desert plume

Monkshood

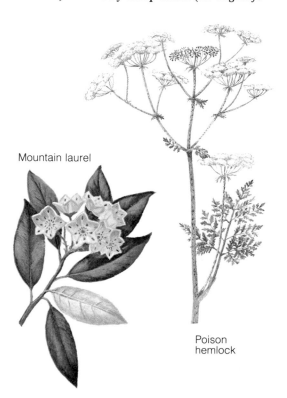

Mountain laurel

Poison hemlock

lia), with deep pink flowers, grows in sunny fields and waste places. The toxin in the nectar of both species can poison honey.

Poison Hemlock

Conium maculatum L. All parts are poisonous, especially the seeds and roots. Like Queen Anne's lace and several edible members of the carrot family (Umbelliferae), *C. maculatum* has lacy leaves and small white flowers arranged in umbels—clusters whose branches radiate from a central point like the ribs of an umbrella. It grows in open places throughout North America. Its root is white, and its crushed leaves emit a sour, mousy odor. Another deadly umbellifer, the water hemlock (*Cicuta maculata*), grows in wet or swampy ground. Its umbel is flat, and its leaves resemble those of angelica; a yellow sap with a parsniplike odor flows from its cut stem.

357

Pokeweed

Phytolacca americana L.   Leaves, roots, and berries are poisonous. A malodorous upright perennial weed up to 12 feet high, the sun-loving pokeweed grows in damp fields, open woods, and waste places in eastern North America, California, and Hawaii. Its branching stem is reddish; its large pointed leaves taper at both ends. Upright spikes of greenish-white flowers develop into hanging clusters of purple to black berries.

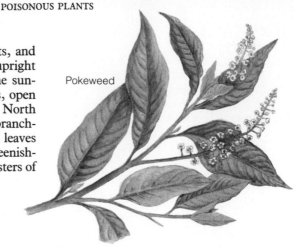

Pokeweed

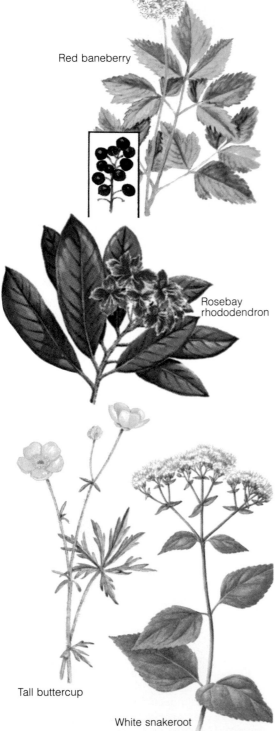

Red baneberry

Rosebay rhododendron

Tall buttercup

White snakeroot

Red Baneberry

Actaea rubra (Ait.) Willd.   Berries and roots are poisonous, as are those of the white baneberry, or doll's-eyes (*A. pachypoda*). The leaves of both species are divided into several sharply toothed leaflets and form knee- to waist-high canopies in shady woods. Both species bear dense, rounded clusters of small creamy white flowers above the leaves in late spring. The clustered berries of *A. rubra*, which grows throughout North America, are red on slender stalks; those of the eastern *A. pachypoda*, on thick red stalks, are white with black dots.

Rosebay Rhododendron

Rhododendron maximum L.   The leaves and flowers of all rhododendrons and azaleas are poisonous, as is honey made from their nectar. *R. maximum* is one of 23 North American species; several hundred other species exist, many of which are cultivated and may escape to the wild. Most have oblong to oval, alternate leaves, often clustered at the ends of branches, and most bear showy terminal clusters of bell-shaped or tubular flowers.

Tall Buttercup

Ranunculus acris L.   The sap of all buttercups is poisonous. That of *R. acris* and a few others can also cause blisters or ulcerous sores if it touches the skin. Most of the 300-odd species are sun lovers that grow in moist fields, ditches, or swamplands, and most are recognizable by their splayed leaves and bright yellow flowers. There are exceptions, however; be sure of identification before eating any wild plant.

White Snakeroot

Eupatorium rugosum Houtt.   All parts are poisonous. You can tell this white-flowered species from its white-flowered medicinal relative boneset (*E. perfoliatum*) by its stalked, oval to heart-shaped leaves; boneset's lance-shaped leaves seem to surround the stem. Joe-pye weed (*E. purpureum*), another medicinal cousin, has pink to purple flowers. Cattle rarely eat the plant. Those that do are afflicted with "the trembles" and may give poisonous milk.

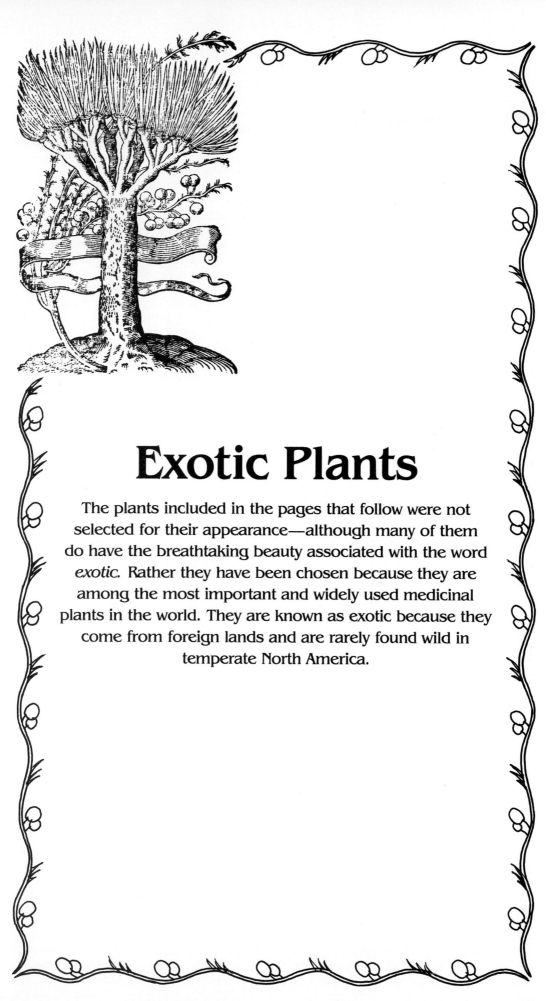

Exotic Plants

The plants included in the pages that follow were not selected for their appearance—although many of them do have the breathtaking beauty associated with the word *exotic*. Rather they have been chosen because they are among the most important and widely used medicinal plants in the world. They are known as exotic because they come from foreign lands and are rarely found wild in temperate North America.

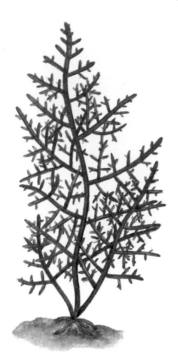

Agar

Gelidium cartilagineum (L.) Gaill.
AGAR FAMILY
Gelidiaceae

At first glance the comparatively plain red seaweed *G. cartilagineum* does not appear to be an important plant. However, it has abiding medicinal value, and it makes a vast contribution to the bacteriological sciences.

Agar, as *G. cartilagineum* is more familiarly called, is a red seaweed, a member of a large group that includes some of the world's most beautiful seaweeds. The colors of the red seaweeds, ranging from a soft rosy pink to a striking purplish red, are due to pigments that camouflage their green chlorophyll. These pigments serve to soak up light when it is scarce, and so those seaweeds that inhabit deep, dark waters are more colorful than those that dwell near the light in shallow tidal areas.

Small, reddish brown, and cylindrical in appearance, *G. cartilagineum* reaches only about 6 inches in height, but its diminutive size belies the toughness of its bushy stems and branches. The cells of this and other red seaweeds contain an odorless, tasteless, colorless, and transparent substance commonly called agar. To produce agar, the manufacturers first boil the seaweed in plain water or in water to which sulfuric acid has been added; then they dry and clean the gelatinous result.

One of the most interesting properties of agar is that it is indigestible by practically all bacteria. Hence, it is an excellent base on which to control the growth of laboratory bacterial cultures—the bacteria consume the medium in which they are grown but not the agar itself. This significant fact was discovered

in the 1880's by the pioneering German bacteriologist Robert Koch. Because agar is also indigestible by humans, it is a common ingredient of packaged diet foods; it fills the stomach without adding calories. In the Far East, agar has been a popular food additive for centuries. The Japanese are particularly partial to it and put it into sauces, soups, jellies, and desserts. It is sometimes used in the West as a gelling and stabilizing agent by meat and fish canneries and by manufacturers of baked goods, dairy products, and candies.

Agar's extremely useful medicinal asset is that it is hydrophilic; that is, it absorbs water. Hence, it is effective as a bulk laxative: the agar soaks up the water in the intestines and increases the bulk of waste material; the increased bulk, in turn, stimulates peristalsis (the rhythmic motions of the intestinal wall), which prompts evacuation of the wastes. Because of its water-absorbent capacity, agar has also been employed commercially in the impression materials used by dentists and in the manufacture of some emulsions, lubricants, suppositories, and cosmetic gels.

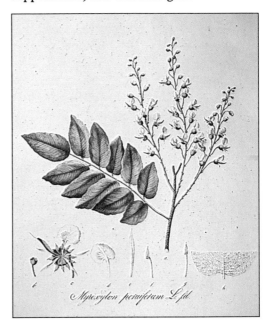

Myroxylon pereiferam L. fil

Balsam of Peru

Myroxylon balsamum var. *pereirae* (Royle) Harms
PEA FAMILY
Leguminosae

Although it thrives chiefly in El Salvador, in the region bordering the Pacific Ocean known as the Balsam Coast, this imposing tree is popularly called balsam of Peru. It received its geographically confusing name in the 16th century, because the Spanish shipped its thick resin, or balsam, to Europe from ports in Peru. Today the tree grows wild throughout much of Central America, in southern Mexico, and in parts of northern South America.

Easily grown from seeds or cuttings, the balsam of Peru is sometimes cultivated in the tropics as a shade tree and is often planted for shade on coffee plantations. It averages 50 to 65 feet high, but has been known to grow much taller. Its evergreen leaves are divided into glossy, oblong or oval, 2- to 3½-inch-long leaflets, each besprinkled with transparent dots. Clusters of fragrant white flowers are borne at the ends of the branches.

But it is not its leaves, nor its flowers, nor its graceful form that gives the balsam of Peru its commercial value. Rather it is the balsam itself—the thick, delightfully fragrant resin (it smells like cinnamon when fresh, like vanilla when aged) found in the trunk—that people have sought for centuries. The Indians in Central and South America, including the mighty Incas who ruled Peru, knew that the balsam was effective in stopping bleeding and in promoting healing. They also used the leaves as a diuretic and to expel parasitic worms. The Indians introduced the tree's medicinal virtues to the Spaniards, who quickly recognized it as a potentially lucrative item of trade and began sending it home.

Today the trade in balsam is vigorous. The resin finds its way into antiseptic and fungicidal ointments used for such varied skin diseases or disorders as scabies (an itch caused by parasitic mites) and ringworm (a fungus infection). In the United States, the resin is also an ingredient in dental cements and in suppositories marketed to relieve the itching of hemorrhoids. It is employed, too, to flavor cough drops and to perfume toiletry goods.

Benzoin Tree

Styrax benzoin Dryand.
STORAX FAMILY

Styracaceae

On his voyage in 1497–1498 around the Cape of Good Hope to India, the Portuguese navigator Vasco da Gama was presented with a gift of benzoin, a substance highly valued by the Indians. Because of its appealing vanillalike aroma, they chose benzoin for an incense in their temples. Medicinally, they used it to relieve shingles, ringworm, and a number of other skin disorders. In other parts of southern Asia, benzoin was employed to mend sores on the feet and was traditionally applied to heal the wound made by circumcision.

A member of the storax family, *S. benzoin*, like many of its relatives, is a fast-growing tree that ranges in height from about 15 feet to an imposing 115 feet. Its fragrant clusters of silky white blossoms are followed by round, 2-inch fruits that hold one or two round seeds. The bark of the tree, covered with a silky whitish down, contains the valuable aromatic resin.

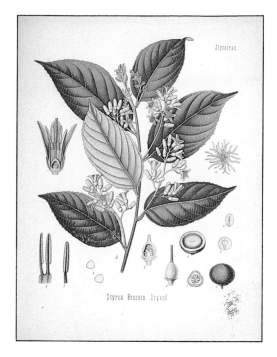

Styrax Benzoin Dryand

Commercial growers in warm, tropical areas of the Far East find that benzoin trees are fairly easily cultivated. In some regions, seedlings are put in before a crop of upland rice so that the advancing grain can shade the young trees. When a tree reaches six or seven years of age, workers slash it with a hatchet or cut deep triangular holes in the bark with a knife, and the resin—a yellowish-white to reddish-brown fluid—begins to flow and to harden into tears, or lumps. The flow is greatest during the first three years of tapping, and can continue for another three. A tree usually dies before it reaches the age of 17 years.

Benzoin is quite bitter, and so it is seldom administered internally. Because it has expectorant properties, helping to loosen phlegm in the mucous membranes of the respiratory passages, it has been prescribed for acute obstructive laryngitis—better known by parents of young children as croup. The child inhales vapors from a small amount of boiled water to which a teaspoon of a benzoin tincture has been added. Benzoin is also an antiseptic and an astringent for healing small cuts. The resin is a common ingredient in skin-protective products, where it aids the healing of chapped or blistered skin. Benzoin's preservative qualities make it much in demand by the cosmetic industry for use as a fixative in soaps, perfumes, and creams. Small amounts of benzoin are added to many foods, from beverages to baked goods, as a flavoring.

Benzoin is obtained from *S. benzoin*, generally known as Sumatra benzoin, and from its close relative *S. tonkinensis*, often called Siam benzoin. In the United States, Sumatra benzoin is employed chiefly in pharmaceutical preparations, while Siam benzoin is used as a food flavoring and in fragrances.

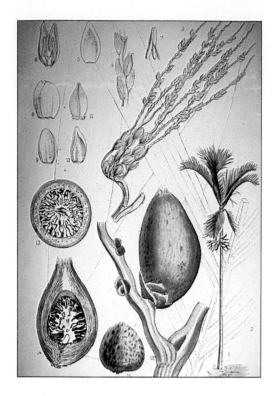

Betel Palm

Areca catechu L.
PALM FAMILY
Palmae

Slender and handsome, the betel palm is a common and delightful sight in tropical Asia, where it thrives in areas with heavy rainfall. The graceful palm, which can attain heights of 100 feet but usually averages 30 to 50 feet, has a narrow trunk—never wider than 6 inches in diameter—and a relatively small crown. Its erect and feathery divided leaves (fronds) are 3–6 feet long and are sometimes variegated in color. The fragrant whitish male flowers are borne on the upper part of the flowering branches, the large female ones at the base. The egg-shaped, orange-red fruits contain small seeds, about 2 inches long, that are commonly called betel nuts.

The betel nut was made famous in James Michener's *Tales of the South Pacific.* Anyone who has read the book, or seen the stage or movie musicals that were based on it, probably remembers the native woman Bloody Mary. Michener depicted her thus: "She had few teeth . . . and had thin ravines running out from the corners of her mouth . . . usually filled with betel juice which made her look as if her mouth had been gashed by a rusty razor." The description shows that the author knew something about the centuries-old Southeast Asian habit of chewing betel nuts. (The Chinese discovered the practice when they conquered the Malay Archipelago in 150 B.C.)

The Asians wrap a leaf of the local spicy betel pepper vine (*Piper betle*) around a small piece of freshly roasted betel nut, add a pinch of powdered lime, and chew the mixture as a stimulant that imparts a feeling of general well-being, aids digestion, sweetens the breath, and strengthens the gums. The betel nut contains tannins, which give it an astringent effect, and several powerful alkaloids—especially one called arecoline—which promote the secretion of saliva and intestinal juices. The nut also turns saliva red, which accounts both for Bloody Mary's appearance and for her name.

It was not until about 1863 that the betel nut's active alkaloid substances were identified by Western scientists. Arecoline was found to be an effective taeniacide, or agent that destroys tapeworms. It has also been employed to treat problems of the urinary tract. Western physicians have generally abandoned the use of the drug in favor of purer synthetic substitutes because it has been found that large doses can have severe toxic side effects in humans, but it is still in use in veterinary medicine.

The beautiful betel palm is extensively cultivated in India and Sri Lanka, and betel chewing is still widely practiced throughout most of southeastern Asia.

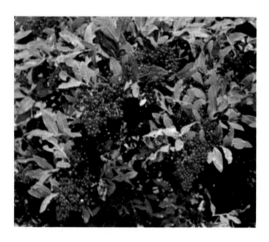

Black Pepper

Piper nigrum L.
PEPPER FAMILY
Piperaceae

No plant since the apple of Eden has had a larger, more telling effect on human history than the black pepper vine. Beginning in 327 B.C., when Alexander the Great invaded India and discovered the pleasures of well-seasoned food, wars have been fought, kingdoms overthrown, unknown oceans braved, and continents discovered—all for the sake of the shriveled, beadlike fruits known as peppercorns. Attila the Hun, holding all of Rome hostage, demanded 3,000 pounds of them as tribute. Throughout medieval Europe, pepper was commonly traded, ounce for ounce, for gold. In 1488, in search of a water route to the spice markets of India, Bartholomeu Dias first sailed the raging waters around Africa's Cape of Good Hope. Four years later, looking for an easier route to the same markets, Columbus landed in the New World. In the centuries that followed, European nations vied viciously with each other in colonizing tropical lands and trying to corner the spice market.

The fruits that inspired these deeds are produced by a woody, broad-leaved evergreen vine that is cultivated today in many tropical lands, from India, Indonesia, and Malaysia to South America and the West Indies. The stout vine, which is allowed to climb poles or small trees in cultivation, bears many slender, densely packed flower spikes. The fruits that develop upon these spikes are generally harvested while still green; the signal is the reddening of the lowest fruits on a spike. The green fruits are dried until the flesh around the single hard seed is wrinkled and grayish black, then ground into black pepper or packaged and sold as whole peppercorns. The milder white pepper is made from the same plant; but the fruits are allowed to ripen, and the flesh is removed before the seeds are ground.

Black pepper's aromatic, slightly musty odor comes from the volatile oils found largely in the flesh and skin; its pungent bite comes from the alkaloids—piperine and piperidine—and resins found mostly in the seeds. The oils go into perfumes and flavorings. The searing substances have served many purposes: they have gone into liniments and gargles; they have been used as carminatives, reducing stomach and intestinal gas; and they have been found to stimulate the activity of the heart and kidneys. Piperine is also an effective insectide against houseflies, and gardeners use pepper sprays against several kinds of pests.

Cubeb berries, the fruits of the closely related cubeb pepper, *P. cubeba*, contain substances that have been used as antiseptics, carminatives, and diuretics. Ground into powder and added to cigarettes, they are smoked, in the tropical areas where they grow, for the relief of throat inflammations. Oil of cubeb is a constituent of some throat lozenges.

Calabar Bean

Physostigma venenosum Balf.
PEA FAMILY
Leguminosae

The line between a deadly poison and a beneficial drug is often very fine. Exactly how fine is illustrated with terrible clarity by the fruit of a twining woody vine native to the area of Africa once known as Calabar. Here the River Niger, nearing the end of its 2,600-mile journey to the sea, spawns scores of streams that run like blue veins across the Niger Delta.

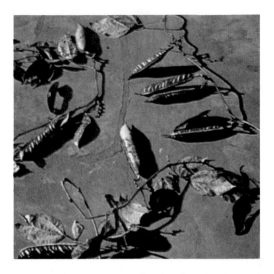

The Calabar vine roots in the riverbanks and sends its stem climbing 50 to 60 feet high among the trees. Long clusters of its big purple flowers hang in spring like bloated wisteria blossoms. After the flowers have fallen, 6-inch-long, brownish-yellow seedpods develop, and when they ripen they split, revealing two or three fat maroon seeds called Calabar beans.

Until the past century or so, the Calabar bean served the people of the region as a sort of botanical judge, jury, and executioner. Someone accused of a serious crime was given a drink made from the powdered beans. If he regurgitated the concoction, he was presumed innocent; if it killed him, he was guilty. It was a simple and direct system of justice, but when the British colonized the area, they disapproved. Hoping to end the practice of trial by ordeal, they banned the cultivation of Calabar beans. The vines grew wild, however, and so the measure had little effect. In the mid-19th century they outlawed the practice altogether.

The potency of the beans remained a mystery. What poison was in them? And more important, could it be used to help rather than to kill people? In time, scientific research answered both questions. The beans contain several alkaloids, the key one being physostigmine, a powerful stimulant of muscular contractions. It kills by contracting the heart, diaphragm, and pulmonary muscles to the point of rigid paralysis. Because of this property, the drug has proved useful in reversing the action of such poisonous substances as atropine and curare, which kill by relaxing the same muscles. Doctors have also used physostigmine and its synthetic counterpart, neostigmine, to stimulate intestinal muscles after the shock of surgery and to counteract the symptoms of the serious muscle-weakening disease myasthenia gravis. Today, the drug's major applications are in the field of ophthalmology: it is a miotic, causing the pupil of the eye to contract; and it helps to reverse the buildup of pressure inside the eye that can lead to blindness in the disease glaucoma.

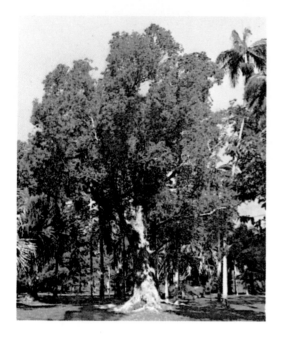

Camphor Tree

Cinnamomum camphora (L.) J.S.Presl
LAUREL FAMILY
Lauraceae

The fragrant wood of the camphor tree has traveled the world over in the form of finely wrought sailors' chests. Strong and durable, resistant to the ravages of salt air, repellent to moths, and immune to the attacks of most insects, the wood has protected the clothes of many a seaman. Its most important constituent in this regard is a chemical known as 2-bornanone. Better known as camphor, this chemical is a potent moth repellent.

The camphor tree is native to eastern Asia. Standing as tall as 100 feet, spreading its crown equally wide, and filling the air with sweet fragrance during the flowering season, it graces terrain between 4,000 and 7,000 feet above sea level. In cultivation, the trees are not nearly so impressive. Grown for the sake of their leathery leaves rather than their durable wood, they are kept pruned to 5 or 6 feet high. The aromatic leaves are harvested three or four times a year, and the oil is extracted and distilled into colorless camphor crystals, which are shipped all over the world.

Camphor extraction has been going on in the Orient for well over 1,000 years, but only in the past century have the leaves been the main source. Previously the trunks, roots, and branches of 70- to 80-year-old trees were chopped and steam-distilled. But world demand surged in the 19th century, when camphor came to be regarded as an all-around nostrum in Europe and the United States, and the supply of trees became depleted. Hence, more efficient methods were developed.

It was once a common practice to wear a little bag of camphor crystals around the neck to cure a cold or related illness. Camphor oil was freely applied to ease the pains of bruises, sprains, inflammations, gout, and rheumatic joints, and it was taken internally to treat hysteria, epilepsy, and heart problems. In addition, the fumes were used in the treatment of asthma, bronchitis, emphysema, and a host of other respiratory maladies.

But science has found that prolonged exposure to the fumes—and to an even greater extent, ingestion of the substance itself—can cause poisoning, and so camphor's medicinal use in the United States is limited to lotions that relieve superficial pain and itching. White camphor oil, from which the poisonous substance has been removed, goes into some cough drops, candies, and soft drinks.

Among the nonmedicinal products in which camphor is used are deodorants, disinfectants, explosives, insecticides, paint solvents, perfumes, and soaps. You can still get camphor wood, too, if you wish to make a mothproof chest, but it is extremely expensive. The aromatic oil of cinnamon, a common constituent of such products as soap, mouthwash, incense, and scented candles, comes from a close relative of the camphor tree, *C. cassia*. Cinnamon, the popular spice, comes from *C. zeylanicum*.

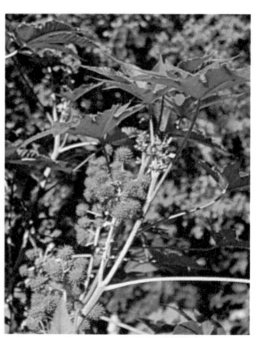

Castor Oil Plant

Ricinus communis L.
SPURGE FAMILY
Euphorbiaceae

When archeologists first went into 4,000-year-old Egyptian tombs, their eyes were drawn to sparkling gems, precious metals, finely carved statuary, and the stone sarcophagi in which ancient mummies rested. Only later did they and other researchers pay much attention to the tiny oval objects found in the tombs. Glossy and mottled, seldom more than ½ inch long, these objects looked like nothing more than polished bits of marble. But further study showed the "stones" to be millennia-old castor beans, the seeds of an African tree that now grows in warm areas throughout the world and is cultivated by American and European gardeners as a foliage plant.

In its native habitat, the castor oil plant is a tree 30 to 40 feet high, bearing broad, deeply lobed leaves on long stalks. The leaves are purple-bronze when young, gray-green or dark maroon when mature. The petalless female flowers, borne in clusters above the male flowers, develop into burlike capsules containing three seeds each. When the capsules mature and dry out, they explode, scattering their beans. Shrubby dwarf strains no more than 5 feet high have been developed in cultivation, bearing nonexplosive capsules.

The Egyptians used castor oil, derived from the beans, as lamp oil and as an unguent; they also purged their systems three times a month by drinking the oil mixed with beer. The Greeks and Romans—taking note, no doubt, that the beans are poisonous—used the oil only externally. It was not until the late 18th century that the foul-tasting substance regained its ancient role as a laxative.

The bean's poisonous substance, ricin, is one of the deadliest toxins known; eating a single castor bean can kill a child. Fortunately, extracting the oil without the ricin is a fairly simple process. The key is temperature. Heat is used to extract oil from most seeds, but when castor beans are heated, the ricin from the bean is distributed throughout the oil. When the beans are hulled and crushed at temperatures below 100°F, however, they yield a clear or yellowish poison-free oil rich in another substance, ricinolein, which irritates the intestines, causing them to expel their contents.

Castor oil has several commercial application as well. Because it is insoluble in benzine and has a very low freezing point, it is well suited for the lubrication of airplane engines. It is also used in hydraulic brake fluids and in biodegradable laundry detergents, as well as in paints and varnishes. Oil meant for these purposes is extracted by heat and is poisonous.

Chat

Catha edulis (Vahl) Forsk. ex Endl.
STAFF-TREE FAMILY

Celastraceae

From the air, the upland hills of Ethiopia's Harar Province look like an immense, carpeted staircase to the sky. Closer inspection reveals the textured carpet that covers the vast

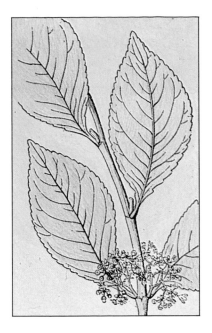

steps to be made up of undulating rows of small, leafy trees. In bloom, the trees' little white flowers seem to dust the landscape like a light snowfall. But this is not the reason that the African evergreen has sometimes been called the flower of paradise. It has earned the idyllic name by virtue of the effect its leaves have on people.

The trees are generally called chat (also spelled khat, kat, or qat), and although they may grow 20 to 50 feet high in the wild, they are kept in a shrublike state, no higher than 10 feet, in cultivation so that the upper leaves can be easily reached and harvested.

For hundreds of years, perhaps for much longer, the farmers of the region have taken bunches of the leaves to chew as they worked. They would chew these quids for about 10 minutes, swallowing the juice as it accumulated and finally swallowing the leaves themselves. The effects are much the same as those of the coca leaves chewed by South American Indians: increased alertness, relief from hunger and fatigue, mild euphoria.

The substance that has this effect—a boon to farmers who must labor under difficult conditions from dawn till dark—is a stimulant to the central nervous system known by the jaw-breaking name D-norpseudoephedrine. Although Western scientists report that insufficient research has been performed to determine the substance's medicinal value, if any, its use is on the increase in Africa.

In Ethiopia, the major exporter of chat, the upper branches of the tree are harvested and wrapped in protective banana leaves, then shipped by air to nearby countries. Time is of the essence; the active ingredient loses much of its potency within three days. While some of the leaves are chewed, most are brewed with water and honey to make Arabia tea, an important beverage among Arab peoples.

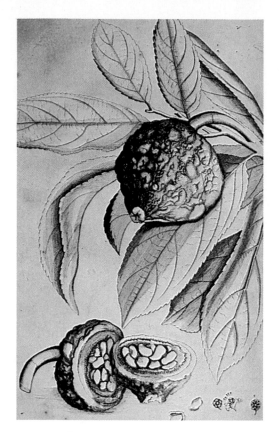

Chaulmoogra

Hydnocarpus wightiana Blume
FLACOURTIA FAMILY
Flacourtiaceae

Leprosy. The word has struck terror in human hearts since the beginnings of recorded history. As carriers of an incurable disease, thought to be highly communicable, lepers have been outcasts. Small wonder, for the ravages of leprosy were horrifying—in advanced cases, faces would be eaten away, bodies covered with rotting sores, fingers and toes falling off. At various periods of European history victims were killed, or required to wear bells so people could avoid them, or isolated in nightmarish leper colonies.

And yet a cure has existed for thousands of years. Ancient Hindu and Chinese documents described an oil that was effective against the disease, and reports of the cure occasionally reached Western ears. Only about the middle of the last century, however, was the miraculous chaulmoogra oil taken seriously by Western physicians; it was investigated and tested, and soon it was being imported from China. The supply was severely limited, however, and its source remained a mystery.

In 1920, an adventurous botanist named Joseph Rock arrived in Singapore to begin his search for the tree that was said to be the source of the oil. He knew the chaulmoogra tree existed, but he did not know what it looked like, where it grew, or how it yielded the valuable oil. To find out, he wandered Far Eastern hinterlands, climbing mountains and exploring jungle lowlands. Finally he found seeds for sale in native markets in India. They came, he found, from a tall, leathery-leaved tree with large white flowers (in fact, three species supplied the seeds, the most important of which was later called *H. wightiana*). Rock collected a large supply of seeds and sent them to Hawaii, where a plantation was established to supply the world with chaulmoogra oil.

Rock himself, having become enthralled by the Orient, returned to the Far East and spent nearly 30 years in the mountainous region near the Chinese-Tibetan border. He sent thousands of unknown plants and birds to Western museums and botanical gardens, and eventually he translated more than 8,000 books from the obscure Na-Khi language of the region into English. Driven out by the Chinese Communist revolution, he went to Hawaii, where he died in 1962, at the age of 79.

The chaulmoogra tree can reach a height of 50 to 60 feet. Only after eight years of growth does it bear the round, hairy fruits that house the valuable seeds. These contain strongly antibacterial chemicals, two of which, hydnocarpic and chaulmoogric acids, are responsible for destroying the bacterium, *Mycobacterium leprae*, that causes leprosy. In Indian medicine, the oil has also been used to treat intestinal worms and skin diseases. In many places today, the ingredients of chaulmoogra oil, modified by chemists, are still used to cure early cases of leprosy—advanced cases do not yield to the treatment—but they have generally been replaced by synthesized sulfones.

Chili Pepper

Capsicum frutescens L.
NIGHTSHADE FAMILY
Solanaceae

It should be no surprise to anyone who has bitten into a hot pepper that the fleshy scarlet fruit contains a rubefacient; that is, a substance that causes human skin to glow fiery red. The substance is called capsaicin, and it reddens the skin because it triggers increased blood circulation to the area that it touches.

If that skin area overlies sore muscles, the excess blood can reduce pain and promote healing. For this reason, capsaicin is a key ingredient in many liniments and, together with other chemical compounds found in chili peppers, is prescribed in the treatment of rheumatism, bursitis, and other such ailments. It is also used to treat stomachaches that involve poorly functioning stomach muscles. And because the red-hot chili pepper is an inhospitable place for bacteria, its extracts have been used as antibacterial agents.

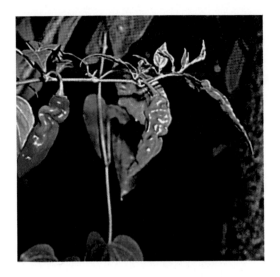

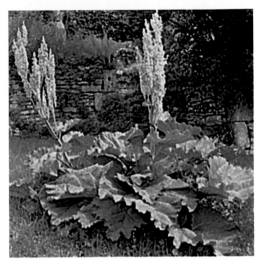

Capsaicin was not isolated until 1876, but the fruit of the shrubby plant that produces it had served mankind for centuries. Long before 1494, when the plant was described by Diego Álvarez Chanca—a physician who accompanied Columbus on his second voyage to the West Indies—the Indians of the American tropics had cultivated chili peppers and had used them in cooking. Surely the early Indians noticed the way in which food containing peppers was slower to spoil and easier to digest than food without them. They probably also noticed that the juice of the peppers brought a warming flush to the skin and eased soreness.

The Spanish and Portuguese carried chili peppers to many ports of call, and before long the plants became established in Africa and India. Today, they are grown in warm climates throughout the world, and their annual relatives, including the familiar bell pepper, are common in gardens everywhere. Much of the world's supply of capsaicin today comes from plants grown in India and Japan.

Chinese Rhubarb

Rheum palmatum L.
BUCKWHEAT FAMILY

Polygonaceae

A Chinese herbal more than 2,000 years old included a plant called *tahuang* ("great yellow"), so named because of the mild but effective purgative contained in its yellow rhizomes (underground stems). Chinese rhubarb (*R. palmatum*) and its close relative *R. officinale*, both native to the cool mountains and high plateaus of western China and Tibet, have been medicinally important in the Orient from that time to this. The bright yellow powder derived from the rhizomes of these Far Eastern plants has also played an important role in European medicine and commerce.

As early as 114 B.C., caravans carried the dried rhizomes eastward over the high mountains to Bokhara in central Asia, whence they found their way to Europe by way of the Black Sea. Dioscorides and Pliny wrote of the plant in the first century A.D. In later centuries, Arabs conducted a busy trade in rhubarb by way of Persia and other parts of the Mideast. In the 1650's, two major routes had been established for importing the drug from China: one through India, the other through Moscow via the Gobi desert and Siberia. By 1687, the Russians had established a monopoly on the trade, in part because they rejected inferior imports and built a reputation for high quality. The monopoly was not broken until about 1860, when the port of Canton was opened to direct trade between China and Europe.

Meanwhile, 18th-century Europeans had begun cultivating the edible garden rhubarb, *R. rhabarbarum*, for medicinal purposes. Although its rhizomes served folk medicine as a mild laxative, they do not have the medicinal properties that give Chinese rhubarb its powers. In fact, they contain a poisonous substance—as do the leaves—so they probably did more harm than good.

Chinese rhubarb's medicinal components fall into two categories: anthraglycosides and tannins. The first cause the laxative effects; the second are astringents, which have the opposite effect. Hence, depending on the size of the dose and the way in which it is given, the rhizome is effective in treating both constipation and diarrhea. The rhizome is no longer used medicinally in the United States, but its extracts serve as laxatives.

The stalks of *R. palmatum* can grow up to 6 feet high and are topped by large, deeply lobed leaves that resemble the human palm in shape (hence the species name). For the sake of these leaves, as well as the spikes of tiny red flowers, Chinese rhubarb is sometimes grown as an ornamental. It is difficult to start from seed, so the plant is almost always propagated from cuttings or by root division.

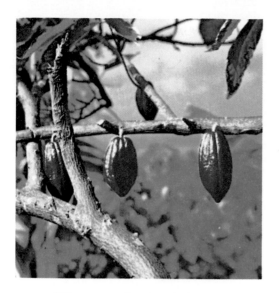

Chocolate Tree

Theobroma cacao L.
STERCULIA FAMILY
Sterculiaceae

"Food of the gods"—that is the literal and apt translation of the name *Theobroma*. It was given to the chocolate tree and its genus by the great botanist Carolus Linnaeus, creator of the modern system of scientific nomenclature. The name reflects not only the flavor of chocolate, but its history as well.

In 1519, the Spanish explorer Hernando Cortez and his soldiers witnessed a strange ceremony at the court of the Aztec emperor Montezuma. Seated high on a golden throne, observed by his subjects with reverent awe, the "living god" repeatedly drank from a golden goblet containing a beverage called *chocolatl*. When the Indians honored the Spanish by offering them the bitter, dark brown drink, they explained that the beans from which it was made had come from paradise, and so each sip would bring wisdom and knowledge. So valuable were the beans to the Aztecs that they served as a form of currency: 4 beans could buy a wild turkey; 100 could purchase a live slave.

Cortez praised chocolate effusively in a letter to the Spanish ruler, Charles V, and brought a supply of the beans home with him. Enthusiasm for the new drink, made more palatable by the addition of sugar and vanilla (an improvement said to have been made about 1550 by the nuns of a Mexican cloister), spread to the French court. There it was considered an aphrodisiac and happily imbibed by those who could afford it. The English added milk to the formula and established chocolate houses, as did the Dutch, where aristocrats sipped the heavenly drink in privacy.

Native to the tropics of Central and South America, the chocolate tree is a widely branching evergreen that may reach 40 feet in height, but is pruned to about 20 feet on plantations. Small fragrant clusters of pink or creamy flowers, borne directly on the trunk or main branches, develop into woody, football-shaped fruits up to 1 foot long. These range in color from yellow to reddish purple to brown. Within each fruit, embedded in a gelatinous pinkish pulp, are about 50 bitter seeds, or cocoa beans.

Harvesters scrape the beans and pulp together into fermenting troughs, where the sweet pulp liquefies and the beans lose their astringency. Then the beans are dried, roasted, shelled, and processed into their constituent parts. Fat—more than 50 percent of a cocoa bean—is rendered into yellowish cocoa butter. Unlike most fats, it is not greasy. It also has a pleasant odor and does not easily become rancid, and so it is prized for use in soaps and other toiletry products, as well as in suppositories and soothing ointments.

The fat-free powdered residue is cocoa; mixed with sugar and hot milk or water, it is the warming, energizing drink that northerly peoples still regard as the food of the gods. Various grades of chocolate candy, from smooth milk chocolate to the hard, bitter blocks used by bakers, are made by combining the cocoa with assorted mixtures of cocoa butter, milk, vanilla, and sweeteners. Because it is rich in the stimulants caffeine and theobromine, chocolate combats fatigue and gives a burst of quick energy. This is why soldiers have carried chocolate into battle from the period of the Civil War to modern times. In addition, recent research has found that chocolate has a soothing effect on troubled minds.

Clove Tree

Syzygium aromaticum (L.) Merr. and Perry
MYRTLE FAMILY
Myrtaceae

According to the writings of Chinese physicians, during the Han dynasty (207 B.C. to A.D. 220) court visitors were required to hold cloves in their mouths when addressing the emperor—presumably so that he would not be offended by their bad breath. By the 4th century A.D. Europeans had heard about the pungent and aromatic flower buds, and trade had begun with Arabs who acquired the dried buds from the east. In later centuries, cloves were among the precious spices for which European nations competed.

The competition for cloves heated into a fierce trade war between the Portuguese and the Dutch in the 17th and 18th centuries. The clove tree was native to many of the Moluccas, or Spice Islands. But the Dutch established a monopoly by destroying all of the trees except those that grew on one island, Ambon, which they owned. Eventually the French managed

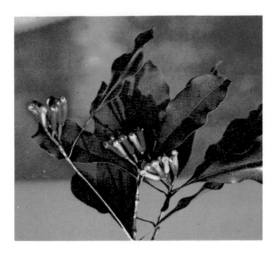

Coca Shrub

Erythroxylum coca Lamk.
COCA FAMILY
Erythroxylaceae

Long before the coming of the Spanish Conquistadores, the coca leaf was regarded as a divine gift by the Inca rulers of Peru. Its use was reserved for priests and royalty, for the wealthy and talented, and for others of rank and privilege.

There were exceptions. The common Indians who carried bales of the sacred leaves across the Andes mountains from what is now Bolivia were probably allowed to chew bits of their burden as they trudged along, for under the influence of the drug contained in the leaf, they hardly felt the sharp mountain chill and could travel for days with little food or water. And surely the natives of the steep valleys along the eastern face of the Andes, where the coca shrub grew, chewed the leaves regularly—as their descendants do today—to still the hunger pangs and numb the fatigue that are constant facts of life in such a poor, harsh land.

But by the time the Spaniard Pizarro arrived

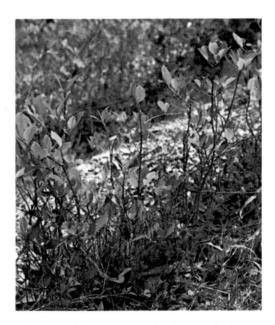

to cultivate the tree on their islands, and by the start of the 19th century, cloves were being grown on plantations in many tropical lands. Zanzibar (now part of modern Tanzania) has long been a major grower. Other clove-producing countries include Jamaica, Sri Lanka, Malaysia, and Indonesia (which includes the Moluccas). Indonesians consume half of the world's clove supply; they mix the spice with tobacco to make a special kind of cigarette.

The handsome clove tree is a pyramidal broad-leaved evergreen that may reach a height of 30 to 40 feet. Its smooth, shiny leaves are dotted with glands that emit the tree's characteristically aromatic fragrance. Even more fragrant are the tiny yellow flowers that appear in loose clusters at the ends of branches, but these flowers are seldom allowed to bloom. When the pink buds turn fiery red at the base, they are plucked and sun-dried to a deep reddish brown. These dried buds are the delicious-smelling cloves known to pharmacists and gourmet chefs around the world.

Although kitchens are among the primary consumers of cloves, a large percentage of the small, hard buds go to processing plants, where clove oil is extracted by distillation. This essential oil, which holds such chemicals as eugenol and eugenyl acetate, accounts for most of clove's culinary and medicinal properties. Oil of clove is widely used by dentists in fillings and cements and in post-extraction treatment. The warm pungent smell of clove also lends itself to soaps, lotions, and toothpastes.

Possessed of both antiseptic and anodyne, or pain-relieving, qualities, cloves have long been popular in folk medicine. Generations of folk healers, pharmacists, and dentists have prescribed cloves or clove oil to relieve toothache. The herbal literature of many lands recommends clove tea, made by steeping the buds in boiling water, to cure nausea and to rid the stomach and intestines of gas. The Chinese use oil of clove to treat diarrhea and hernia. Tinctures of clove oil are also effective against such disease-causing fungi as those that cause athlete's foot.

with some 200 men, the rigid control of coca leaves had been relaxed. Nearly everyone chewed them, and they were a coin of exchange in the marketplace. The Spanish, having disposed of the Inca nobility, used Indians to till their newly conquered land and to work their mines. Because they found it cheaper to provide the slave laborers with coca than with food and water, they continued to import the divine leaves from across the mountains. And so the drug of the wealthy and powerful became—not for the last time in its history—a device to enslave the common people.

Although the Spanish brought news of the

magical coca leaf to Europe, it was more than 300 years before anyone found a use for it. Then its exploitation burgeoned.

In 1860 a German researcher isolated the chemical responsible for the plant's power. He called it cocaine. In 1884 Dr. Carl Koler, a colleague of Sigmund Freud's, discovered that the drug could act as a local anesthetic in eye surgery. As the years passed, other scientists learned that cocaine paralyzed nerve endings responsible for transmitting sensations of pain, and so it became a valuable local anesthetic, revolutionizing many surgical and dental procedures. However, because it also stimulated heart and respiratory rates, besides elevating arterial blood pressure, it sometimes did more harm than good to surgical patients.

Meanwhile a French merchant became wealthy by selling a tonic made from coca leaves. A few years later an American druggist was to become much wealthier by combining coca leaves with the juice of the cola nut in a sweet syrup that he called Coca-Cola. (The use of cocaine in soft drinks was prohibited in the United States in 1904.) Freud and a few other pioneers in the study of the human mind became interested in cocaine's ability to intensify concentration, negate fatigue, and induce a feeling of well-being. Poets, novelists, and painters began to use it, and Sir Arthur Conan Doyle gave the practice the legitimacy of literature when he had his detective, Sherlock Holmes, take cocaine to keep his wits occupied when he had no case to work on.

Today the medicinal uses of cocaine are performed by such synthetics as lignocaine, benzocaine, and procaine (sold under the trade name Novocain), which have cocaine's anesthetic properties but lack its stimulatory side effects. But the widespread nonmedical use of cocaine, both as a drug of the rich and powerful and as an means of exploiting the poor, is among the serious problems of our age.

Coffee

Coffea arabica L.
MADDER FAMILY
Rubiaceae

Imagine a sunny day in the distant past—perhaps a thousand years ago, perhaps much longer. A band of African warriors enters a damp highland forest, dense with the glossy undergrowth of 12- to 15-foot-high broad-leaved evergreens. Clustered at the leaf axils of these shrublike trees are rounded, deep red berries, no larger than the first joint of a man's little finger. The men know that something in the berries helps them to perform great feats of strength and bravery, and so they pluck a large supply of the berries to chew in preparation for the battle that lies ahead.

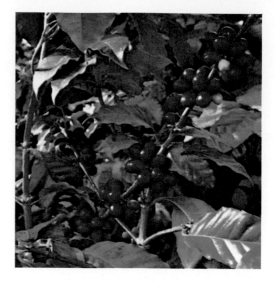

That "something" is caffeine, the same substance that a modern American seeks from a steaming breakfast brew. It stimulates the central nervous system: the flow of blood is increased, especially through the coronary arteries that feed the heart; the heart itself beats a bit faster; muscles respond to the urgent pulse; the kidneys work a little harder; breathing is stimulated; so is cerebral activity. One is more alert and ready to face the day.

After five or six cups of coffee, however, the mild stimulation is transformed into restlessness, irritability, feelings of nausea, even muscle tremors and mental instability. One has overdosed on the world's most popular drug.

Caffeine, derived from the two grayish seeds that dwell within each fruit of several *Coffea* species, was identified in 1821, by a scientist who mistakenly thought that the seeds might contain quinine. Today it is possible to enjoy the flavor of coffee without the effects of caffeine. Decaffeinated coffee is made by removing the caffeine while leaving the oil, called caffeol, which is responsible for the beverage's distinctive aroma and flavor. The extracted caffeine is not lost, however. It is sold to the pharmaceutical industry for incorporation into pain remedies, where its stimulating effect helps to rush such substances as aspirin and phenacetin into the system. It is also a cardiac and respiratory stimulant, of particular value in fighting overdoses of such central nervous system depressants as alcohol, barbiturates, and morphine.

C. arabica, which originated in Ethiopia, was introduced into Persia, Egypt, and Arab lands at some unknown date in antiquity. For a long time, the roasting, grinding, brewing, and consumption of the beans were the province of priests and medicine men. But by the 15th century, Mecca boasted several public coffeehouses. Similar establishments were later to spring up in Constantinople, in Venice, and (despite efforts by the church to ban the "infidel drink") in Rome. By the mid-17th century, coffee drinking had become highly fashionable in London, Paris, and Berlin.

The Arabs held a monopoly on coffee, most of which moved through the port of Mocha—hence one popular name for coffee. Arabs were forbidden to export the plants or unroasted seeds, but in 1690 the Dutch smuggled out some seedlings. They set up coffee plantations in Java—hence another popular name. In the early 18th century, coffee trees were taken to Martinique and Jamaica, where they flourished. They soon went to other islands, to Central America, and to Brazil, which eventually became the world's leading coffee producer (a distinction that is today claimed by Colombia). In recent decades several African and Asian countries have taken large shares of the market, deriving their product from such species as *C. canephora* and *C. liberica*.

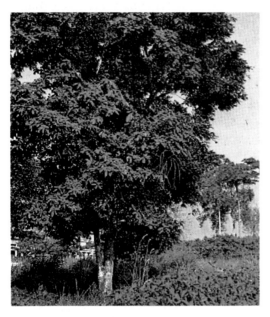

Cola Tree

Cola nitida (Vent.) Schott and Endl.
STERCULIA FAMILY
Sterculiaceae

According to the claim in an early Coca-Cola ad, the explorer Henry Morton Stanley might never have found Dr. David Livingstone in deepest Africa had it not been for the cola nuts that his native bearers chewed on the long jungle trip. For centuries many Africans have chewed cola nuts for the same reasons that the inhabitants of southeastern Asia enjoy betel nuts—they are stimulants (about three times richer in caffeine than coffee) and breath sweeteners. Widely sold in African marketplaces, cola nuts are also used to depress the appetite during religious fasts and are believed to have aphrodisiacal powers.

There are some 125 *Cola* species in the world, all indigenous to the rain forests of

tropical West Africa. *C. nitida* is one of only two species (the other is *C. acuminata*) that are used commercially. Both are extensively cultivated in the West Indies, Brazil, India, and Sudan. The stately evergreen usually grows 40 to 60 feet high, and bears leathery leaves that are about 10 inches long. The small, petalless, yellow flowers produce long chocolate-colored pods, within which are 4 to 15 reddish-brown seeds, or cola nuts. The seeds give off a heady aroma of roses, but their taste is extremely bitter on the first bite. The flavor deepens with chewing, however, and the aftertaste is sweet.

In the United States, the cola nut is best known as an ingredient of cola beverages. Unlike the beans of chocolate and coffee, the nuts require no intricate preparation. They are simply boiled in water to extract the basis of the soda pop. In its early days the original cola beverage, Coca-Cola, contained coca leaf extract (the source of the drug cocaine) and generous amounts of cola nut extract. Today, although the formula is jealously guarded, the drink is known to contain decocainized coca leaf extract, and the cola content is so minute that it does not register in laboratory tests.

Caffeine, extracted from cola nuts as well as from coffee beans and other sources, is a cardiac and respiratory stimulant and is included in many nonprescription pain remedies, soft drinks, and energizers. Because the effects of the caffeine in cola beverages are heightened by carbonation, such beverages are commonly used to ease headaches and hangovers and to settle queasy stomachs.

Corkwood

Duboisia myoporoides R.Br.
NIGHTSHADE FAMILY
Solanaceae

Crowded below the decks of the many troopships that rode the rolling waves of the North Atlantic during World War II, thousands of American GI's battled an unarmed but formidable enemy—seasickness. To combat the debilitating malady, military doctors prescribed scopolamine.

One of the drug's major sources is the corkwood, an Australian tree found in the thickets and open woodlands of the coast of Queensland, as well as in the interior of north and central New South Wales. The tree sometimes reaches a height of 40 feet in the wild, but in cultivation it is generally kept shrubsized. It has gray, fissured bark and pretty, bell-shaped, white to pale lavender flowers. But it is the broad, lance-shaped leaves that yield the drug for which the tree is cultivated. Since the mid-20th century, Australian corkwood plantations have been an important source of scopolamine.

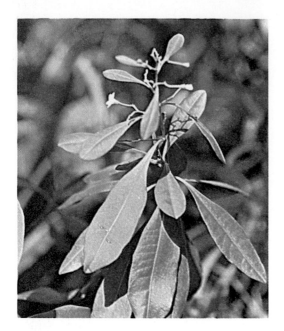

The aborigines of Australia have long been aware of the corkwood's powers. They would submerge branches of the tree in eel-populated waters because they knew that something in the tree caused the eels to become lethargic, and consequently easy prey. About 1861, European settlers in Australia first learned of the aboriginal eeling practices, but it was some time before they found out exactly which plant was being used. Eventually scientists discovered that corkwood leaves are rich in the narcotic scopolamine, as well as in atropine and several other alkaloids found in many members of the nightshade family, including belladonna and bittersweet nightshade. One expert has estimated that scopolamine and atropine are prescribed for at least 50 maladies in present-day medicine.

Scopolamine's sedative properties were dramatically demonstrated in the early part of the 20th century, when the German doctor Carl J. Gauss used the drug to produce his famed "twilight sleep," which made the experience of childbirth relatively painless. Today scopolamine is also administered as a tranquilizer in the treatment of drug or alcohol withdrawal and of various psychotic problems. In combination with morphine, scopolamine is often given as a truth serum and is used as an anesthetic in surgery. Because scopolamine has a blocking action on the nerves that control a variety of organs, physicians have also recommended it for controlling the kind of violent muscular spasms of the respiratory system that can be life-threatening to an asthma sufferer. And just as it was an excellent medication for seasickness in World War II, it is considered one of the best remedies for combating both airsickness and car sickness.

Atropine, the other important narcotic derived from the leaves of the corkwood tree, is especially efficacious in drying up such moist areas of the body as the upper throat or the nasal passages. For this reason it has proved invaluable in treating hay fever and the common cold. Atropine is valuable, too, in diagnostic and postoperative procedures involving the eye because it has the ability to relax certain eye muscles, dilating the pupil.

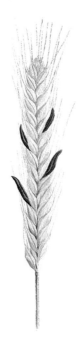

Ergot

Claviceps purpurea (Fries) Tul.
SAC FUNGI FAMILY
Clavicipitaceae

In many countries of the world, vast fields of rye grain are routinely and deliberately infected with a devasting fungus disease. The process starts in early July, when healthy rye flowerheads have begun to wave in the wind. Then sprayers arrive to dust the fields with spores of the fungus that causes the disease called ergot. This process is repeated several times to make certain that all the plants have been properly infected.

In about two weeks, signs of the fungus are clearly visible. Tiny dark purple to black "horns" protrude from what once were the ovaries of the rye flowers, giving off an unpleasant, fishy odor. There will be no grain from these fields again this year, yet the farmers are elated. Their crop—the fungus that replaces the kernels of grain—is in great demand by pharmaceutical companies, who extract valuable drugs from it.

Throughout medieval times, and as recently as the mid-20th century, grain that had been contaminated by ergot caused widespread epidemics of a dreaded affliction known as St. Anthony's fire, or holy fire. Entire communities were sometimes devastated: pregnant women spontaneously aborted their fetuses, people lost fingers and toes to gangrene, others went mad, some went into convulsions and died. It is likely that the witchcraft trials of 1692 in Salem, Massachusetts, were inspired by cases of ergot poisoning.

Scientists studying such accidental poisonings of the past found that the fungus causes strong uterine contractions—accounting for the abortions. They also found that it narrows blood vessels, preventing blood from reaching the body's extremities (this caused the gangrene) and the brain (hence the madness, convulsions, and death).

The alkaloids that were responsible for these afflictions are also the substances that give ergot its medicinal worth. The drug ergonovine, identified in 1920, is now used—as it was for many centuries by Chinese and European midwives who did not know its name—to stimulate the smooth muscles of the uterus and bring about strong rhythmic contractions during childbirth. The drug also constricts blood vessels, thereby preventing excessive bleeding. This asset is expecially useful during the third stage of childbirth, when the placenta is expelled and the threat of hemorrhage is great.

Ergotamine, another drug obtained from ergot, was isolated in 1935 and is reported to be particularly effective in contracting blood vessels in the head. This property has made it a helpful agent in the treatment of migraine headaches, which many scientists believe to be triggered, at least in part, by the dilation of these cranial blood vessels.

Today, farmers in the United States do not deliberately infect grain with ergot. As a result, pharmaceutical companies import the fungus or buy it from growers whose crops have been accidentally contaminated. Although many kinds of grain can be infected with forms of ergot, only the ergot that grows on rye is acceptable for pharmaceutical purposes.

Ginger

Zingiber officinale Roscoe
GINGER FAMILY
Zingiberaceae

Encased in a delicate, silvery-brown skin, the gnarled and knobby rhizome, or underground stem, of the ginger plant, known as gingerroot, has been prized since ancient times both for its flavor and for its medicinal properties. In ancient India it was known by the Sanskrit name *shringara*, and the Greeks of the first century A.D. wrote of it as *zingiberis*. At that time, and for several centuries thereafter, Europeans obtained gingerroot in trade from the Arabs—as they did many other spices. By the early 16th century it was being grown in Spain. Today it is cultivated wherever the climate is humid and frost-free, the best ginger

reputedly coming from the island of Jamaica.

The plant's long slender leaves grow along 2- to 4-foot-tall stalks, which arise like cornstalks from the creeping rhizome, as do the separate flower stalks. The rhizome produces the volatile oil that contains such aromatic substances as camphene, phellandrene, zingiberene, and zingerone. These, along with several other chemicals, have made ginger one of the world's oldest and most popular medicinal spices, used in folk medicine almost everywhere. The tangy taste is due to the oily liquid gingerol, also contained in the rhizome.

In China, the warm, pungent tang of ginger tea—made by boiling pieces of fresh gingerroot in water—has long been prescribed for colds, coughs, flu, and hangovers. The Chinese say that the tea has the power to strengthen lungs and kidneys. Tibetans use ginger to

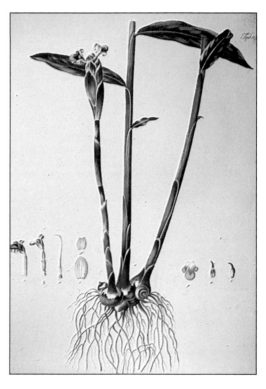

stimulate the vital energies of one who is debilitated, lethargic, or convalescing from an illness. In Japan, a ginger-oil massage is a traditional treatment for spinal and joint problems. Other herbalists have recommended hot ginger compresses and baths to relieve gout, arthritis, headaches, and spinal pain. Ginger compresses are also used in many parts of the world to relieve sinus congestion, kidney problems, menstrual cramps, and various other aches and pains. A warm ginger footbath is said to envigorate the whole body, and a piece of cotton soaked in ginger oil is a common treatment for an earache. Candied gingerroot, a favorite treat of children the world over, has recently regained some of its old-time popularity in this country, largely because it is very nearly as healthful as it is pleasurable to eat.

Modern medicine recognizes many of the spice's time-honored virtues. It is known to be a rubefacient, reddening the skin by stimulating the flow of blood to a given area, and this property alone accounts for much of its ability to ease soreness. It is also a carminative (ridding the stomach and intestines of gas) and an aid in the digestion of fatty foods. Recent research has even shown that ginger can be as helpful as scopolamine in preventing motion sickness and vertigo.

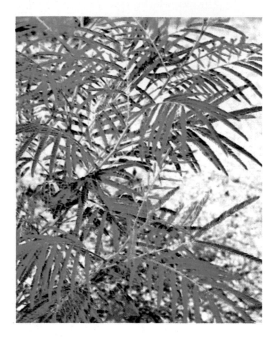

Gum Arabic

Acacia senegal (L.) Willd.
PEA FAMILY
Leguminosae

The sand dunes of northwest Africa may seem unlikely havens for ornamental trees. Yet it is in this largely barren landscape, as well as in other parched areas of Africa, India, and the Mideast, that the gum arabic tree thrives, often forming dense thickets. It is a scraggly specimen much of the time, seldom more than 15 feet high. Its branches, sparsely covered with fernlike leaves, are lined with the same kind of talonlike thorns for which its close American relative, *A. greggii*, came to be named the catclaw. But after the seasonal rains, fat red buds swell, and the tree comes alive with color. The buds open to become fluffy wands of ivory-white flowers, soon to be joined by a new crop of foliage.

Lovely as it is, this seasonal show is the least of the tree's virtues. In time of drought the deeply fissured gray bark splits, and resinous sap wells slowly out, hardening into beadlike tears an inch or two across. As the Egyptians discovered more than 3,700 years ago, this sap is of great value. They used it for centuries as a

glue to hold together gems and shards of colored glass and as a base for long-lasting paints, so that today we can see, among other things, their depictions of heaps of *kami* (as the Egyptians called gum arabic) and of the tree from which it came. Perhaps they also used it as a medicine; we cannot be sure. But we *do* know that medieval Arab physicians treated a wide range of ailments with gum arabic—hence its name.

In the old days, the sap was harvested largely by nomadic bedouins. These wanderers first followed a long, circular route across the desert, slashing the bark of wild trees as they went, and then they retraced their steps to gather the precious tears. Today, although some gum arabic is still taken in the old way, most comes from cultivated plantings. The vast majority of these plantings are in Sudan's Kordofan Province. Here, long strips of bark are cut away after the seasonal rains have ended—usually in February and March or in August and early September. After three or four weeks, when the translucent pinkish or yellowish tears have hardened, reapers sweep them off using long-handled nets to avoid the needle-sharp thorns. Brittle, virtually odorless and tasteless, the tears are cleaned, sorted, and sun-bleached, then packed in 100-pound sacks and taken to market.

Because it soothes irritated mucous membranes, gum arabic is a key ingredient in many products for the treatment of sore throats, coughs, and diarrhea; it is also the glue that holds some pills and tablets together. However, most of the more than 11,000 tons that is imported into the United States each year goes to the food industry—bakers use it to give body and texture to some of their products, candy makers to coat some of theirs with a hard sheen. It is also used in wax polishes, in watercolors and other paints, and on the flaps of envelopes and the backs of postage stamps.

Ipecac Shrub

Cephaelis ipecacuanha (Brot.) A. Richard
MADDER FAMILY
Rubiaceae

The year was 1682. The Grand Dauphin, son of France's Sun King, Louis XIV, seemed to be dying of a severe and prolonged case of dysentery. The king was frantic with worry and anxious to try any remedy, but there was little that doctors were able to do. Then word reached Jean Baptiste Colbert, the king's chief minister, that a man called Jean Adrien Helvetius was curing similar cases in Paris with a secret remedy. Helvetius was sent for, the mysterious concoction was administered, and in due time the symptoms of the dread disease vanished. Louis's gratitude was effusive. Hel-

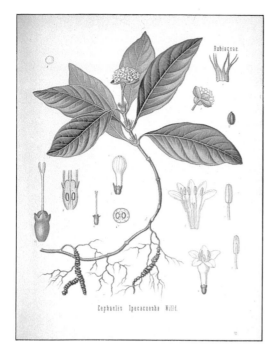

vetius was honored by the court, received a small fortune for the formula, and was appointed inspector general of French hospitals. Later he became personal physican to the duke of Orleans. His son was to become physician to the queen of France and his grandson, Claude Adrien Helvetius, one of the outstanding poet-philosophers of his time.

The secret remedy that saved the dauphin and wrought such a change in the fortunes of the Helvetius family was ipecac (pronounced *IP-uh-kak*), made from the dried rootstock of an 18-inch-tall shrub that grows rampant in the steamy forests of Amazonian Brazil and Bolivia—places where annual rainfall often exceeds 80 inches. The Indians of those regions had used it for many years, perhaps for many centuries, to treat amebic dysentery, and it is still used for that purpose throughout the world. It is also wielded in India and Pakistan against other serious parasitic diseases, including bilharziasis, caused by a flatworm. The component that acts against these invaders of the human body is an alkaloid called emetine. Given by mouth in small doses as part of a syrup, it also acts as an expectorant in the treatment of persistent coughs.

Ipecac is a strong emetic as well. A standard item in family first aid kits for many years, ipecac syrup has been used to induce vomiting, especially in people who have swallowed certain poisons. Although it is still widely used, it has become the subject of controversy. Research has shown that cephaeline, the emetic agent in ipecac, is itself a powerful irritant that can cause poisoning, and so ipecac syrup should be administered only in measured doses by trained medical personnel.

Ipecac is grown commercially in several tropical regions of the world, but in South America it is still gathered from the wild. Local Indians arrive with digging tools and pointed sticks in November and set up camp. Gently they pry up each plant's musty-smelling rootstock and cut away much of it, leaving just enough to allow the shrub to survive and produce a new crop. They may still be at work in January and February, when globelike clusters of tiny, white, funnel-shaped flowers bloom among the dark green leaves. But by May, when the small, oval, deep purple fruits ripen, the harvesters are gone.

Irish Moss

Chondrus crispus (L.) Stackh.
CARRAGEEN FAMILY
Gigartinaceae

During the potato famine of the mid-19th century, thousands of beleaguered Irish saved themselves from starvation by eating the bushy seaweed known as Irish moss. They were following the example of many generations of hungry poor folk in their own land and in other lands that border the North Atlantic Ocean. It is an example that has been followed by many since, when hard times have pressed. In more bounteous times, the same humble seaweed has served as an effective laxative and as a home remedy for sore throats and chapped skin. It is also commonly employed as a filler and stretcher of other foods.

Also known as carrageen, from a village in

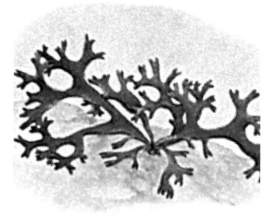

southeastern Ireland where the seaweed is plentiful, Irish moss is found clinging to submerged rocks along the shorelines of Canada, New England, the British Isles, and Europe as far south as Portugal. Irish immigrants who found Irish moss growing on the rugged shores of Canada and New England were the first to gather and use it in America.

Irish moss is harvested throughout the summer months by men in boats, who use rakes to gather the 2-foot-long stems from among the submerged rocks where they grow. (Hand-gathered Irish moss, while rare in commerce, is preferred because it is unmixed with other seaweeds.) Then workers rinse the curly red, purple, or yellow-green plants and let them dry in the sun for as long as two weeks, in the course of which the colors bleach to a grayish or yellowish white. The dried seaweed is soaked in cold freshwater until it swells back to its original bulk. Then it is boiled until it dissolves. The resultant liquid turns to a jelly as it cools, and it is this jelly that serves both medicinal and culinary purposes.

It may be eaten as is, or it may be used as a thickener for soups and stews. Boiled with milk and sugar, it makes a tasty white pudding with a high mucilage content—a soothing food for people with sore throats. Irish moss is also used commercially as a stabilizing agent and thickener in chocolate milk, ice creams, baked goods, and other foods. Irish moss is also a soothing emollient, or skin softener, and is incorporated as an emulsifier into cosmetics and skin lotions.

Jaborandi Tree

Pilocarpus jaborandi Holmes
RUE FAMILY
Rutaceae

If you hold a leaf of the jaborandi tree up to the light, you will see that its surface is sprinkled with translucent dots, as though it were under attack by tiny insect pests. Each dot is a gland that secretes an alkaloid-rich oil, and it is for the sake of this oil that jaborandi leaves are regularly harvested in the wild. From them are extracted several substances, the most important of which is the alkaloid pilocarpine, a weapon in the medical battle against the blinding disease glaucoma.

The shrublike jaborandi tree, native to northern Brazil, is only 5 to 10 feet high and grows in dense stands. Its starlike white or pinkish flowers, borne on spikes at the ends of the branches, are mildly scented and, like the leaves, are covered with tiny oil-producing glands. When crushed, the petals fill the air with the aromatic scent of the oil they contain. Only the oil contained in the grayish-green leaves, however, is extracted for medicinal use.

A tea made from the leaves has long been important in Brazilian folk medicine. When drunk, it acts as a diuretic and sweat-inducer. Applied to the scalp, it is said to prevent baldness, although no scientific study yet supports this belief. Elsewhere, an infusion of the powdered dried leaves has been used as a stimulant and expectorant, and has been incorporated into the treatment of a number of diseases, including rheumatism and pleurisy. In the United States, doctors once used extracts of the leaves to stimulate the flow of urine in patients whose normal bladder functions had been shocked into inactivity by

surgery, but this job is now done in other ways.

All these effects hint at the way pilocarpine works in the human body. It behaves much like a substance in the body that helps transmit impulses from the ends of autonomous nerves—the ones that trigger the body's auto-

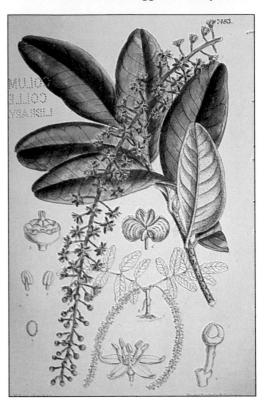

matic functions, such as the beating of the heart and the focusing of the eye—to the muscles that do the work. As such, it stimulates the heartbeat, peristaltic contractions in the intestine, and contractions of the uterus.

When applied to the eye of someone suffering from the early stages of glaucoma, it stimulates the muscles that contract the pupil, and in the process relieves the pressure within the eye. Since the disease blinds by building up pressure until the mechanisms of the eye can no longer function, this relief—while no cure for the disease—can save the eyesight of its victim. An application of pilocarpine takes effect in less than 15 minutes and continues to protect the eye for about 24 hours.

Jamaica Quassia

Picrasma excelsa (Swartz) Planch.
QUASSIA FAMILY
Simaroubaceae

No insect pests ever attack the tall, graceful Jamaica quassia tree. The whole plant—and especially the whitish wood—is permeated by an extremely bitter resin whose major chemical constituent, a bitter compound called quassin, is an effective natural insecticide. It serves mankind in other ways, too, both medicinally and nonmedicinally.

The ashlike tree itself, native to Jamaica and several other West Indian islands, grows to a height of 45 to 60 feet. It has pinnately compound leaves with many pointed leaflets, and it bears attractive clusters of small rose-colored flowers. The wood was long used by West Indians to make quassia cups, which they filled with water and allowed to stand undisturbed for a time. Then, when the resin-tinged water was needed as a tonic to settle an upset stomach, to sharpen an appetite, or to combat a fever, they drank it. Stronger mixtures, made by chipping the wood fine and soaking it in water, were used in enemas to destroy parasitic threadworms and in lotions to get rid of body lice.

The extracted quassin, about 50 times as bitter as quinine, has been used in medicinal preparations for many of the same purposes. It

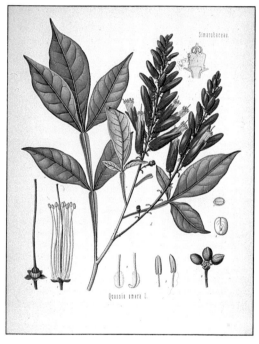

stimulates production of stomach secretions, as well as those of the liver, kidneys, gallbladder, and intestines, and so it is both a laxative and an aid to a flagging appetite. Another extract of the resin, quassimarin, has been reported by researchers to be of possible value in the fight against leukemia.

Quassin is also popular as a bitter constituent of tonic wines, aperitifs, and liqueurs; of marmalades, candies, and baked goods; and of frozen dairy desserts and gelatin puddings. The wood chips, roasted and ground to a powder, have served as a substitute for hops in brewing beer and ale.

As a pesticide, quassin is regarded as one of the safest for home gardens because it kills many pests while sparing such beneficial insects as ladybird beetles and bees. In fact, even though the tree itself repels most insects, its

flowers attract honeybees—much to the consternation of beekeepers, for honey made from the bitter quassia nectar is inedible.

Organic gardeners generally buy bags of quassia wood chips, then extract the quassin as West Indians do, by soaking the chips in water. The mixture is then sprayed on plants to rid them of aphids, mealybugs, sawflies, thrips, leafhoppers, caterpillars, and even slugs. It is also sprayed on fruit trees to discourage hungry birds.

Karaya Tree

Sterculia urens Roxb.
STERCULIA FAMILY
Sterculiaceae

Every spring Indian harvesters enter forests on the tablelands of the subtropical Himalayas in search of the soft-wooded trees called karaya, which stand up to 30 feet high. It is April, and the monsoon rains will come in June. In the interim, the workers selectively wound some of the larger trees of the forest, cutting away two sheets of the smooth, glossy, grayish-white bark, each about 1 foot square, from opposite sides of the trunk. Avoiding the large leaves, which resemble the leaves of grapevines except that their stalks are armed with stinging hairs, the harvesters make the cuts at a slant, so that rainwater will not collect in the wounds. The pieces peel off as easily as birch bark, and a gummy, brownish, vinegary-smelling sap begins to flow. It solidifies into ropy strips or into huge tears, some of which may weigh as much as 10 pounds. The wounds bleed heavily for a day or so, then less heavily for several days more, and the workers return periodically to collect the hardened residue.

In October, after the monsoons have come and gone, the workers will return for another harvest, but they will choose different trees. A karaya tree needs three to five years to recover from its wounds, and no tree should be so wounded more than five times during its life.

Variously called karaya gum, sterculia gum, kadaya, and *mucara*, the hardened sap of the karaya tree is a polysaccharide—a complex form of carbohydrate—whose individual molecules have been reported to outweigh those of water by more than 500,000 times. When in contact with water, the absorbent granules of the dried gum swell up like sponges to as much as 100 times their original size. To a physician, this property spells "bulk laxative," for in the intestine such swelling triggers peristalsis, the rhythmic, rippling action that pushes food through the digestive system. Dentists use powdered karaya gum as a denture adhesive that is resistant both to bacteria and to the enzymes of the mouth.

In the food industry, karaya gum serves as a

stabilizer for salad dressings, a binder for such meat products as bologna, a gummy base for candies, and a thickener of meringue, ice cream sticks, sherbet, whipped cream, and cheese spreads. Beauticians take advantage of the gum's water-retentive and thickening properties when they use hair-setting lotions and skin-softening creams into which it has been incorporated. It is also used by the paper industry as a binder of the fibers of tissue paper, and in the construction industry to bind the particles of some composition boards.

Kava

Piper methysticum G.Forst.
PEPPER FAMILY
Piperaceae

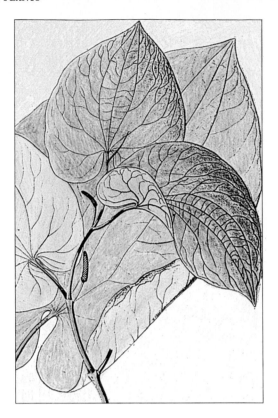

As though giving a clue to one of its dangerous effects on the human body, the kava shrub that grows wild on many South Pacific islands sports broad, heart-shaped leaves webbed with a network of prominent veins. In large enough doses, the narcotic drugs that the plant contains can increase the force of heart action while decreasing the pulse rate, induce a hypnotic state, and paralyze large skeletal muscles such as those of the legs.

The storehouse of drugs lies in the erect, 8- to 20-foot-tall shrub's roots and large, woody rhizomes (underground stems). Islanders have long used these rootstocks to make a potent beverage called *kava-kava*, which has played a role in virtually all their ceremonies of life: it has been drunk to celebrate marriages, births, and other rites of passage, to mourn deaths, to placate the gods, to cure illnesses, to remove curses, to herald the beginnings of work projects, and to bid such projects farewell. Its effect is not intoxicating, in that it does not dull mental processes, but narcotic. It induces a euphoric state of tranquil well-being that eventually leads to a deep, dreamless sleep.

The time-honored method of activating the drugs is still the most effective, although outsiders may find it repellent. To the accompaniment of song and ceremony, pieces of the dried rootstock are chewed—generally by young girls with strong teeth—until they are reduced to a soft, pulpy mass. This is spit into a wooden bowl, mixed with water or coconut milk, and kneaded by hand. After a few hours of fermentation, the solids are strained out and the liquid is drunk—in the old days, only by men.

The rootstocks are seldom chewed nowadays. They are simply pulverized, mixed with water or coconut milk, and filtered out. The result is a popular beverage, drunk by men and women alike, that has a stimulating, tonic effect but lacks the narcotic power of the chewed product. Research has shown that it is not the chewers' saliva that sets the drug's narcotic constituents free, as had been speculated, but the vigorous emulsification caused by the chewing. To approximate the chewing process, modern pharmacy can emulsify the crude drug in a suitable oil.

Several constituents of the rootstock, including methysticin, yangonin, and kawain, have been isolated and harnessed for use in sedatives, tranquilizers, and appetite stimulants. Early in the 20th century, some extracts of the rootstocks were found to have antiseptic properties, which led to their use in treating various infections, especially those of the genitourinary tract; but these have been superseded by more effective drugs.

Khella

Ammi visnaga (L.) Lamk.
CARROT FAMILY
Umbelliferae

The Arabs discovered centuries ago that the small, grayish, egg-shaped, aromatic fruits of khella could ease a multitude of ailments, including the stabbing pain of angina pectoris, caused by a reduction in the flow of blood to the heart. Khellin, the substance in the fruits that accomplishes this feat, is described by scientists today as a selective coronary vasodilator: that is, it expands only the arteries that feed the heart, giving quick relief when angina is caused by constricted or partly blocked coronary arteries.

Khellin is also a bronchodilator, expanding

the bronchi, or breathing tubes that funnel air from the throat to the lungs. Hence, as the ancient Arabs knew, it can save the life of someone who is suffocating from the terrifying bronchial spasms of asthma or severe allergies.

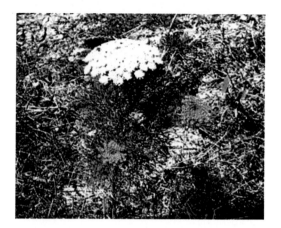

Extracts of the fruits act as a diuretic as well, increasing the flow of urine and hence getting rid of excess body fluids. The same extracts have also been used to ease the pain of kidney stones as they scrape through the ureter—the small tube that leads from the kidney to the urinary bladder.

Unfortunately, khellin is not without its side effects. Researchers have found that it has a cumulative toxicity. Its active principles build up in the body when the drug is taken over a period of time, and this build-up can cause nausea and vomiting. For this reason the drug is no longer used in the United States. However, it is still employed by doctors in the regions around the Mediterranean Sea where it originated and where it grows in profusion.

Like its relative Queen Anne's lace, the 2-foot-tall khella plant has finely cut, ferny leaves. Each of its straight flower stalks is topped by a rounded cluster of countless tiny white flowers. These clusters—called umbels, because their stalks radiate from a central point like the ribs of an umbrella—are themselves made up of smaller umbels. After the flowers have dried and the seeds have matured, the small stalks of the major umbels stiffen and grow hard; this gives the plant yet one more useful function, which is expressed in a name by which it is commonly known among Arabs: the toothpick plant.

Lignum Vitae

Guaiacum officinale L.
CALTROP FAMILY
Zygophyllaceae

Early in the 16th century, an explorer in the Caribbean heard about the *guaiac,* a tree that, according to local inhabitants, contained a drug that could cure most ailments. As it turned out, the tree, known today as lignum vitae ("wood of life"), is remarkable on several counts, all having to do with the hardness of the wood and its rich supply of fats and resins.

The wood, the hardest in commercial use, is so loaded with these fats and resins that objects made from it are self-lubricating and nearly impervious to water. Until the advent of high-quality plastics, lignum vitae was the material of choice for such items as pulley sheaves, machine bushings, and propeller shafts for steamships. It has also been used to make axles, bowling balls, chisel handles, mallets, and other objects that must absorb great stress.

The acrid-tasting, brownish resin contained in the heartwood has both medicinal and nonmedicinal applications. One highly dramatic nonmedicinal use is based on the fact that, combined with an alcohol solution, the resin turns blue when it comes into contact with bloodstains. Hence it serves police and other investigators in finding bloodstains that might go undetected.

The wood was originally taken to Europe as

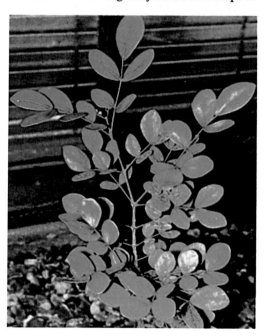

a much-needed cure for gout and syphilis. The treatment for syphilis achieved great if misplaced acclaim during the 16th century. It involved giving massive doses of the resin—gotten by boiling the wood—to patients who were wrapped in tight, head-to-toe plasters and confined to very hot rooms for a month. During this time they received little food, but in addition to the resin, they were fed large doses of mercury. Many died from this treatment; few, if any, were cured of syphilis.

In recent times, scientists have found that two of the resin's most active ingredients, guaiaretic and guaiaconic acids, are effective anti-inflammatory agents, local stimulants, and laxatives. Because of the anti-inflammatory property, the substances are used in pharmaceutical preparations for sore throats and for inflammatory diseases such as rheumatoid arthritis and gout.

The lignum vitae grows on relatively arid land in northern South America, the West Indies, and the Florida keys. An evergreen that can reach 30 feet in height (but seldom grows more than half that), it is recognizable by its furrowed greenish-brown bark. Its leaves are divided into two or three pairs of pale green leaflets 4 to 6 inches long, and its small blue flowers grow in fragrant terminal clusters.

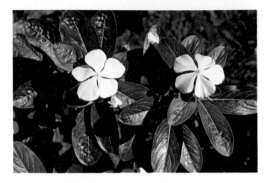

Madagascar Periwinkle

Catharanthus roseus (L.) G. Don
DOGBANE FAMILY
Apocynaceae

Few plants have generated as much recent interest among the scientific and medical communities as the Madagascar periwinkle, *C. roseus* (also known by its older name *Vinca rosea*). The interest began in the mid-1950's, when researchers, hearing of a "periwinkle tea" that was drunk in Jamaica, began to study the plant for its reported antidiabetic properties. They found much more than they had hoped for; the plant, they found, contains two anticancer alkaloids—vincristine and vinblastine—that inhibit the growth of tumors. Vincristine has proved most effective in treating childhood leukemia; vinblastine in treating testicular cancer and Hodgkin's disease (cancer of the lymphatic system). Like many drugs used in chemotherapy, both alkaloids produce such side effects as nausea and hair loss.

Along with the lesser periwinkle, rauvolfia, and other members of the dogbane family, the Madagascar periwinkle is endowed with other medicinal assets, too. In all, it contains more than 70 known alkaloid agents. Some of these decrease blood sugar levels; others reduce blood pressure.

Long before modern researchers learned of the plant's valuable and varied properties, folk healers in faraway places were using the Madagascar periwinkle for a host of medicinal purposes. In India, they treated wasp stings with the juice from the leaves. In Hawaii, they

prescribed an extract of the boiled plant to arrest bleeding. In Central America and parts of South America, they made a gargle to ease sore throats and chest ailments. In Cuba, Puerto Rico, Jamaica, and other islands, an extract of the flowers was commonly administered as an eyewash. Most of these practices are still followed.

The plant that serves so many people in so many important ways is both demure and beautiful. Although it is native to the Indian Ocean island of Madagascar, the Madagascar periwinkle is extensively cultivated, and it has become naturalized in many warm regions of the world, including the southern United States. Averaging 1 to 2 feet in height, the plant is cloaked in glossy, dark green leaves up to 2 inches long. Its flowers, borne all summer at the ends of branching stems, are fragile rosy-pink blossoms about 1½ inches across, which typically have purplish-red "eyes" in the center. There are a number of varieties available commercially, with colors ranging from hot pink to mauve and white. In seed catalogs, the Madagascar periwinkle and its varieties are often grouped with true periwinkles (*Vinca*).

Mahuang

Ephedra sinica Stapf
EPHEDRA FAMILY
Gnetaceae

An ancient Chinese prescription for asthma may have read something like this: "Take the green twigs of the mahuang shrub and boil them in water; then drink the tea." For at least 2,000 years, the Chinese have relied upon tea made from the twigs of mahuang (the name means "yellow astringent") not only to treat asthma, but also to improve blood circulation, relieve coughing fits, and break fevers. Until recent years, Western doctors and scientists scoffed at such remedies.

Today, mahuang is known to the Western world as Chinese ephedra. Like most ephedra species, including North America's Mormon tea, it is a straggly shrub, seemingly leafless to the casual eye. Its thin, pale green branches bear minute leaves that are little more than

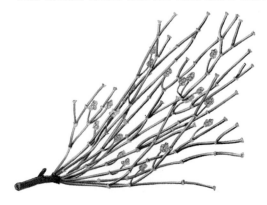

whitish scales covering the stem nodes. Tiny yellowish-green flowers are borne in clusters at the ends of spindly twigs, the male and female flowers on separate plants.

In the 19th century two Japanese scientists isolated from the twigs of the Chinese ephedra the alkaloid that accounts for the plant's time-honored medicinal powers. They called it ephedrine. In 1923, two American-educated scientists, Carl F. Schmidt and K. K. Chen, having heard a druggist in Peking discuss ephedrine's many virtues, began intensive research on it. They discovered it to be a prompt and effective decongestant with the ability to clear nasal and bronchial passages leading to the lungs. As a result of their work, ephedrine has been prescribed in the treatment of hay fever, asthma, and emphysema.

Researchers have also found that ephedrine stimulates the central nervous system. It is often administered to patients in drug- or alcohol-induced comas in order to counteract the drugs' depressant effects. And because it is a vasoconstrictor—that is, it narrows blood vessels—as well as a heart stimulant, causing blood to flow faster through the shrunken vessels, ephedrine is a remedy for hypotension, or low blood pressure. It is often used in conjuction with types of spinal anesthesia that tend to cause blood pressure to drop.

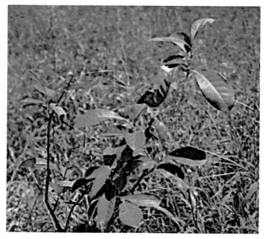

Maté

Ilex paraguariensis St.-Hil.
HOLLY FAMILY
Aquifoliaceae

Mention a holly tree to a North American or European, and you will probably conjure up visions of Christmas, with glistening green leaves and pretty red berries. But the holly tree familiar to millions of South Americans is quite different, both in appearance and in function. It is the maté, which thrives in rugged, mountainous areas of Brazil, Argentina, and Paraguay, and it furnishes the popular tealike beverage also called maté.

While the hardy English holly tree can reach

a height of 70 feet or so, its South American relative grows only about 20 feet tall. The maté's oval to oblong leaves, longer and much lighter in color than those of the English holly, also lack the glossy sheen and the prickly spines that are the northern tree's trademarks.

In Argentina and Paraguay, where maté is widely cultivated, commercial growers set the harvested leaves out to dry on special platforms over small wood fires; the leaves must dry immediately or they will quickly ferment and turn black. After 24 to 36 hours, the brittle remains are reduced to coarse powder, which is put into sacks and stored for an aging period of a year or more. Finally, the product is shipped all over South America to be made into the tealike drink that the Indians enjoyed long before Europeans reached the continent.

Like those ancient peoples, modern South Americans prize the brew as a tonic and stimulant. The maté leaves are rich in caffeine, and also contain neochlorogenic and chlorogenic acids and theobromine catechols. Together these substances give maté its tonic properties and make it a reviving and refreshing beverage with the same function that coffee or tea has in North America and Europe.

Opium Poppy

Papaver somniferum L.
POPPY FAMILY
Papaveraceae

Somewhere in Asia a vast field of flowers blooms in May, cloaking the landscape with a bright mantle of white, lavender, red, or purple. The flowers are opium poppies, and they

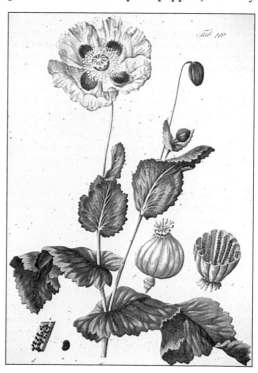

grow in many such fields in many parts of Asia and the Mideast. Beautiful though they are, the flowers are not grown for ornament but for the crop that follows.

After two or three days the tissue-thin petals fall, littering the rich soil and heralding the coming harvest. The bulbous green capsules that remain atop the 2- to 4-foot-high stalks are allowed to swell for 10 days or so. Then workers begin to walk backward among them, performing a ritual some 2,000 years old. As they shuffle along the rows, the workers make swift, precise cuts in the swollen capsules, slitting the outer flesh but never cutting through to the immature seeds inside. Almost immediately, a thick whitish fluid oozes from the incisions. The workers are careful not to disturb it as it slowly hardens and turns an earthy brown. The next morning they return to collect the gummy blobs of opium.

The powers of the opium poppy, both for good and for evil, have been known since at least 3000 B.C., when the Sumerians called it the joy plant. By 300 B.C., opium was being used by Arabs, Greeks, and Romans as a sedative and soporific. Throughout the centuries, as its use has spread into Persia, India, China, Europe, and the Americas, it has been at once a boon to humanity—the chemicals in it can bring astonishing relief to sufferers from a wide range of maladies—and a terrible curse to those who have fallen under its spell.

The most important of the opium poppy's constituents, morphine, was isolated in 1803 by a 20-year-old German pharmacist named Friedrich Wilhelm Adam Sertürner. It was the first plant alkaloid ever isolated, and its discovery set off a fire storm of research that changed medicine forever. Within half a century, dozens of alkaloids, such as atropine, caffeine, cocaine, and quinine, had been isolated from other plants and were being used in precisely measured dosages for the first time.

Morphine, reputed to be the most effective painkiller known to medicine, acts largely on the sensory nerve cells of the cerebrum, blocking messages of pain from other parts of the body. It is also a stimulant, inducing euphoria and evaporating anxieties, tensions, fears, and inhibitions—the effect sought by addicts. Unfortunately, it decreases respiration, sometimes to the point of death, and is highly addictive. Heroin, a further refinement of morphine, is so dangerous in this regard that its use is forbidden even as a medicine.

The opium poppy yields other useful alkaloids too. Codeine, an ingredient of many cough syrups because it suppresses the cough reflex, is also an analgesic that is often recommended to relieve minor pain, sometimes in combination with aspirin or an aspirin substitute. Papaverine, a muscle relaxant that blocks the nerve impulses responsible for muscular contractions, is used to treat intestinal and stomach spasms as well as the respiratory spasms triggered by asthma attacks.

All of these drugs and more come from the unripe seed capsules of the opium poppy. Yet, interestingly enough, when the capsules are allowed to ripen, they contain no trace of these drugs. They are not useless, however. Anyone who has enjoyed a hard roll sprinkled with tiny, crunchy black spheres has eaten hundreds of the seeds of the opium poppy with no ill effects.

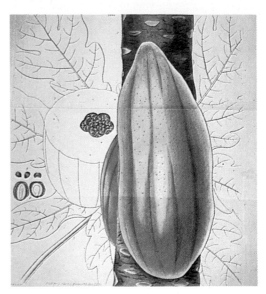

Papaya

Carica papaya L.
PAPAYA FAMILY
Caricaceae

Anyone who has vacationed in the tropics has probably enjoyed the sweet, pulpy, orange flesh of fresh papaya fruits. Many have also tasted meat that has been wrapped in papaya leaves to tenderize it. Only those who happened to visit at the right time, however, have seen groves of the treelike papaya plants in full fruit—they look a bit like giant brussels sprouts, their 20- to 30-foot-tall stems crowned by huge, long-stalked, deeply lobed leaves and festooned with as many as 40 or 50 football-sized fruits. And few tourists have ever witnessed the full-grown but unripe fruits being "milked" for papain, the substance that gives the plant its medicinal and commercial value.

Papain, contained in the plant's whitish juice, or latex, is an enzyme that breaks up protein. In its pure form, it can "digest" up to 35 times its own weight in lean meat, and so it is in great demand as a meat tenderizer. Medically, it is prescribed for people who have difficulty digesting protein and is used to break up blood clots after surgery. In addition, doctors and scientists have been studying the use of a sister enzyme, chymopapain, to shrink ruptured or slipped spinal discs.

A certain amount of papain is contained in all of the plant's juices, but the richest supply is in the leaves and in the skin of the unripe fruit. Only the latex from the unripe fruit is pure enough to make harvesting worthwhile, however, and gathering it is a labor-intensive process. Although groves of wild papaya dot the landscapes of southern Mexico and Central America, where the plant probably originated, and cultivated forests are found in nearly every tropical area of the world, only in a few places—principally in Zaire in central Africa—is the latex gathered.

There, field workers make shallow cuts in the skin of the green fruits with razor blades or with knives of bone, glass, or bamboo. This surgical technique may be performed a dozen times or more on each fruit, the latex flow being caught in devices that look like upside-down umbrellas, which are attached to the plant stems. Finally, when the crop starts to ripen or the latex supply diminishes, the harvesting season is over. Eventually, every 5 pounds of latex will yield about 1 pound of crude papain. Happily, the fruit that has been so "milked" is still edible, sweet, and juicy.

Pareira

Chondrodendron tomentosum Ruiz and Pav.
MOONSEED FAMILY
Menispermaceae

Deep in the Amazonian rain forest, an Indian stalks a young deer. The deer hesitates, sniffs the wind. The Indian raises a long blowgun to his lips and with a powerful puff of air, he sends a poison-tipped dart flying. The startled

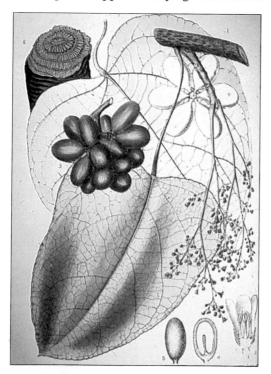

deer leaps into the underbrush, and the hunter follows. He soon finds his prey, paralyzed and dying of asphyxiation.

This primitive scene, played out in one form or another for centuries, may seem far removed from the sterile setting of a modern operating room in North America, where a surgeon performs a delicate abdominal operation. But the two are linked. The connecting thread is the drug curare, extracted from the woody stems of the high-climbing pareira vine, *C. tomentosum*.

The first European to testify to the use of curare was a Spanish soldier named Pedro de Cieza de León. About 1540 he saw several Indian tribes in what is now Peru, Ecuador, Brazil, and Colombia hunting with arrows whose tips had been dipped in the gummy substance. In 1541 the explorer Francisco de Orellana lost a companion to such an arrow. In 1595 Sir Walter Raleigh took a sample of the poison home to England.

The following centuries saw much lurid sensationalism about the mysterious poison. Speculations about its source ranged from snake venom to boiled ants to rare orchids. Expeditions found tantalizing bits of information: over 20 tribes used curare and all had different formulas; some stored it in pots, some in bamboo tubes, and some in gourds (for a time, these were regarded as the three basic types of curare); some applied it to the tips of darts, some to the detachable heads of arrows, and some to the points of wooden spears; the poison killed by asphyxiating its victims. Still, no one knew exactly what it was, how it was made, or why it worked.

The breakthrough came in 1844, when the French physiologist Claude Bernard found in experimenting with frogs that curare blocks the transmission of nerve impulses from the brain to the muscles, relaxing the muscles to the point of limpness. When chest muscles are affected, breathing stops. Not until the early 20th century, however, was it learned that—although each medicine man seemed to have his own secret formula for curare—all were based on the stems of certain climbing vines, and that among these vines *C. tomentosum* was the most lethal. When the alkaloid, tubocurarine, was finally isolated and proved to be the active muscle relaxant in the vine, modern medicine began to find applications for it. It counters such muscle-contracting poisons as strychnine and tetanus toxin. When used to relax the muscles attached to broken bones, it makes them easier and safer to set. It has been used in therapy for victims of polio and cerebral palsy, and in the treatment of epileptic seizures. Its commonest application is in abdominal surgery; injected into the muscular wall that protects the abdomen, it prevents the muscles from becoming stiff, boardlike, and all but impenetrable.

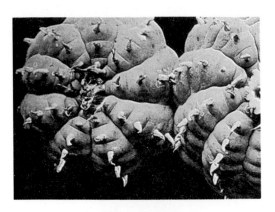

Peyote

Lophophora williamsii (Lem.) J.Coult.
CACTUS FAMILY
Cactaceae

Centuries before the Spanish explorer Hernando Cortez arrived in Mexico, the Aztec Indians were using peyote—a short, squat, button-shaped cactus that grows in the wild desert countryside. The Aztecs had discovered that the plant had certain mystical powers. During religious rites, they consumed bits of the succulent stem in order to hear and see strange sounds and images, which enhanced their spiritual experience.

The practice of chewing small slices of peyote (often called mescal buttons) continues today among many North American tribes. Although the consumption of peyote is illegal in the United States, the law allows it to be used as part of the religious ceremony of the Native American Church, whose membership is largely American Indian.

Scientists have identified some 56 individual alkaloid substances in peyote that may act as drugs within the body. The most active and best known of these alkaloids is mescaline, a powerful psychotomimetic agent—that is, a drug that can alter the mind and produce behavior similar to that exhibited by psychotic individuals. The mescaline-taker may experience various imaginary or hallucinatory effects while under the drug's influence—bold and beautiful colors and lights, the transformation of one's companions and oneself into strange beasts or abstract forms, the illusion of weightlessness, even total freedom from the body. But there is an underlying similarity in the reports of most users: it is a feeling of exaltation and a certainty that the vision is fraught with spiritual significance.

Many believe that the mescaline experience has given them valuable insights into themselves and the world around them. Others have come away with abiding anxieties, fears, even panic. While mescaline use is not habit-forming, it is possible that regular consumption of the cactus could be psychologically damaging.

For a cactus that packs such a chemical wallop, peyote is rather demure looking. It lacks the sharp spines characteristic of most other cacti, bearing only pencillike tufts of woolly white hairs along each of its 5 to 13 ribs. Only a small part of the plant—4 inches at the most—shows above the sand of the limestone deserts in Mexico and southern Texas where it grows, but the fleshy, grayish to chalky blue stem sits atop a massive, carrotlike taproot. Tiny pinkish to creamy white flowers are borne atop the stem.

As might be expected of such a chemical storehouse, peyote has been the object of much research. Because of the underlying similarity in the experiences most users, some scientists speculate that mescaline might work on a specific area of the brain; and researchers are experimenting with laboratory animals in an attempt to further define its action. And because the drug's effects so closely resemble mental illness, it is hoped that the researchers' work will lead to a more effective treatment of psychologically disturbed people.

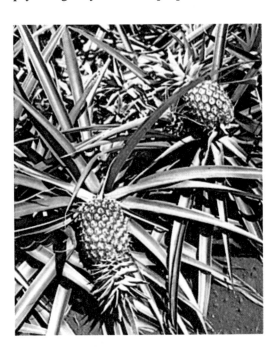

Pineapple

Ananas comosus (L.) Merr.
PINEAPPLE FAMILY
Bromeliaceae

When you think of pineapples, you think of Hawaii. So close has the association become that most people assume that the plant is native to the islands. In fact, pineapples originated in South America and probably did not reach Hawaii until early in the 19th century—the first record of their existence there is dated January 21, 1813—after having been spread by Europeans across much of the world.

Columbus came across them in 1493 on the island of Guadeloupe. The natives who cultivated them called them *ananas* and believed that they had been brought from the Amazon many generations earlier by the fierce, warlike Caribs. This bit of oral history may well be correct, for pre-Incan burial sites in Brazil have yielded pineapple-shaped jars. Columbus called the strange fruit *la piña de las Indias* ("the pine of the Indies") because, as he later told Ferdinand and Isabella, they resembled "green pine cones, very sweet and delicious." The odd name stuck, and pineapples are still called *piñas* in most Spanish-speaking countries. In fact, the word pineapple originally meant "pine cone" in England.

The new fruit was enthusiastically received in Europe and was eventually carried to India, Africa, China, and the East Indies—warm places where the tender plants could reach maturity. It takes up to 15 frost-free months for the juicy fruit to form and ripen upon the 2- to 4-foot stem that rises from a rosette of stiff, spine-edged leaves. The "fruit" is actually a complex flowerhead that forms *around* the stem; the pineapple is the only cultivated fruit whose main stem runs completely through it. Each of the familiar "eyes" on the fruit's surface is the dried base of a small purple flower. The crown of leaves on top contains a bud, and when this bud matures, the fruit is ready to be cut. Pineapples bear no viable seeds; they are grown from the crowns.

The development of greenhouses about 1700 made it possible for wealthy Europeans to grow their own pineapple plants despite the climate. Fresh pineapples became status symbols of the first rank. Ornate bedposts, desk finials, and other furniture pieces were decorated with pineapple-shaped carvings, as were doorways, gateposts, and gables of mansions in Europe and the New World.

Throughout all this history, the pineapple was valued strictly as a table delicacy. All but forgotten were the early explorers' intriguing observations that Indians had used pineapple poultices to reduce inflammation in wounds and other skin injuries. But in 1891 an enzyme called bromelain was isolated from the flesh of the pineapple and was discovered to be proteolytic—that is, it breaks down protein. Hence it is a natural meat tenderizer (the pineapple rings atop a baked ham are not there just for the flavor) and a digestive aid. It can also break down blood clots—proteins are what hold blood platelets together to form clots—and clean away the dead tissue left by burns, abscesses, ulcers, and various kinds of surgery.

How pineapples finally reached Hawaii is not known. The local name, *hala kahiki*, means "plant of Tahiti"—but in the language of the islands, all foreign lands were "Tahiti." It is known that Spanish sailors carried the fruit as the English carried limes, to avert

scurvy, and that they left the leafy crowns to take root on many Pacific islands. But the Spaniards never reached Hawaii. However the introduction occurred, the pineapple is now one of Hawaii's major crops, as well as the best-known symbol of the islands.

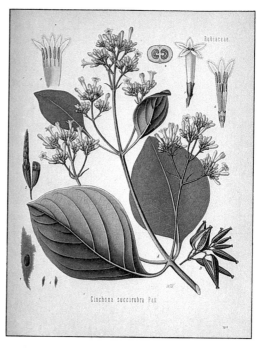

Cinchona succirubra Pav.

Quinine Tree

Cinchona pubescens Vahl
MADDER FAMILY
Rubiaceae

During World War II, as American troops fought their way from island to island across the South Pacific, they faced more than a formidable human enemy. Deadly microscopic foes also lay in wait in the tropical jungles. They were protozoans of the genus *Plasmodium* that, when injected into a human through the needle-fine proboscis of a mosquito, cause the debilitating disease malaria.

The chemical weapon of choice against malaria came from the bark of quinine trees, which were then cultivated largely on the Indonesian island of Java. But Java was in enemy hands, and so little quinine was available for U.S. troops. Only with the development of a synthetic substitute for quinine could the battle against both microscopic and human enemies be won.

Java was not the original home of these tall, broad-leaved evergreens, with their fragrant clusters of small rose-red flowers. In the early 17th century they—and the curative powers of their bitter-tasting bark—had been discovered by Spanish priests in South America's Andes mountains. It was here, in rain forests at elevations between 3,000 and 11,000 feet, that all 40 *Cinchona* species thrived.

Before too many years, all of Europe was alerted to the miracle cure contained in the bark of about a dozen species of what was then called the fever tree (for not only did the powdered bark cure malaria, it lowered fevers of all kinds). Still, most physicians refused to use the new medicine. It was being promoted by Jesuit priests, deeply hated across much of Europe at the time. For a while "Jesuits' bark," or "Jesuit powder," was all but barred in countries where malaria was exacting a terrible toll in human life. But need finally overcame prejudice, and by the end of the 17th century powdered cinchona bark was being used around the world to treat malaria. It was not a pleasant remedy—mixed in water, the powder made a bitter liquid that had to be drunk often—and the dosage was far from precise, but it worked.

In 1820 two French scientists, Pierre Joseph Pelletier and Joseph Caventou, identified the substance in the bark that cures malaria. It is an alkaloid that the scientists called quinine, after *quina*, the native Indian word for bark. Other alkaloids have since been identified in cinchona bark. Among these is quinidine, used today to treat abnormal rhythms of the heart, to relieve muscle cramps, and to aid in the treatment of headaches.

How did a natural drug factory that was native to the Americas end up in Java, out of American reach? In the 19th century, the demand for cinchona bark was so great that the trees were almost eliminated from South America. Many nations attempted to cultivate various species of quinine trees in tropical areas that they controlled. The Dutch turned out to be the most successful, and the place they chose was Java. Today, most of the world's quinine supply comes from central Africa, Indonesia, and South America—where the tree has been reestablished.

Rauvolfia

Rauvolfia serpentina (L.) Benth. ex Kurz
DOGBANE FAMILY

Apocynaceae

Holy men in India, including Mahatma Gandhi, have reportedly chewed the root of *R. serpentina* to help achieve a state of philosophic detachment while meditating. In addition, the plant—called *chandrika* (literally "moonshine plant") in Sanskrit—has long been valued in India as a sedative and hypnotic in the treatment of insanity, or "moon disease." Rauvolfia also enjoys a traditional reputation as a fever-reducing agent and as an emmenagogue (an agent that brings on menstruation), and folk healers have also employed it as an antidote for the bites of poisonous snakes. The powdered root was used to treat diarrhea and

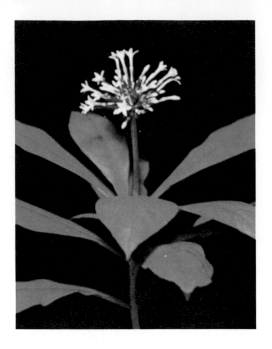

dysentery, and an extract of the root was prescribed to calm irritable babies.

Although the plant's time-honored uses are well documented, the medicinal substances that accounted for them were isolated and defined by a team of Western doctors only in 1952. The alkaloid reserpine, one of 50 isolated from the root, was to revolutionize the treatment of mental illness and high blood pressure. The researchers found that reserpine, world-famous today as "the original tranquilizer," has powerful depressant and sedative properties, and for a time it was the only such drug used in calming seriously disturbed patients. Today other tranquilizers have taken over its role in mental health therapy, but reserpine is still commonly prescribed to relieve hypertension, or high blood pressure. With all its benefits, however, reserpine has some undesirable side effects, among which are edema, nightmares, and despondency that can lead to suicidal yearnings.

There are more than 100 species of *Rauvolfia* (the genus was named for the 16th-century German physician and explorer Dr. Leonhard Rauwolf) growing in moist tropical forests of the Pacific, South America, Asia, and Africa. These milky-juiced plants range in height from a mere 6 inches to a towering 100 feet; *R. serpentina* is among the smallest, growing no higher than 1½ feet. Graceful and woody, it bears elliptical to oval leaves, dark green above and paler below, in whorls of three or four along the stem. The small pink to white flowers are borne in terminal clusters and produce tiny, oval, fleshy fruits about ¼ inch long, which turn a shiny purple-black when ripe.

Although pharmaceutical companies have tried to cultivate the plant, they have not been successful, and commercial supplies must come from the wild. Indonesia was once a major source, but its once extensive supply of the trees has been exhausted. Today's leading producers are India and Thailand.

Sea Onion

Urginea maritima (L.) Baker
LILY FAMILY
Liliaceae

Imagine a cabbage-size onion that may weigh up to 13 pounds and puts forth a flower stalk that can grow to nearly 5 feet high. The object you are envisioning is the chemically loaded bulb of the sea onion, or red squill. It grows wild in sandy coastal areas fringing the Mediterranean and in South Africa, as well as on the coast of the Canary Islands. For thousands of years it has supplied mankind with useful, and sometimes vital, medicines.

The top 1 or 2 feet of the sea onion's leafless,

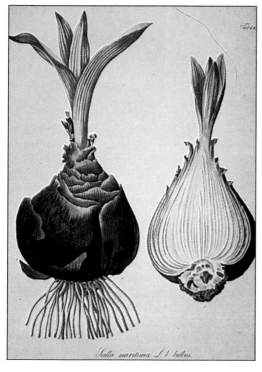

Scilla maritima L. t. bulbus

purple flower stalk bears a long cluster of whitish or rose-colored flowers. These bloom a few at a time over the course of several weeks, forming a narrow ring of blossom that starts at the bottom of the cluster and works its way to the top. This stalk appears in late summer, well after the springtime basal rosette of fleshy, lance-shaped leaves, each up to 1½ feet long, has faded. During the dormant period between the fading of the leaves and the sprouting of the flower stalk, the bulbs are harvested for the sake of the chemicals contained within them. Although sea onions are grown in cultivation, most of the world's supply of derivative chemicals comes from the wild plants.

The chemicals may differ, depending on the

color of the bulb's outer layers. Although one name for the species as a whole is red squill, two varieties exist: white and red. Both kinds contain the medicinal drugs for which the bulbs are sought, but the red variety, which is collected largely in Algeria and Cyprus, also contains a highly poisonous substance, scilliroside. Therefore, only white squill is commonly used as a medicinal source.

Ancient Egyptian, Greek, and Arab physicians knew the bulb as the source of an expectorant, diuretic, and cough remedy, and knew that large doses were a strong emetic, causing severe vomiting. The ancients may also have known of the sea onion's most important medicinal property—its ability to stimulate heart activity. The bulb was certainly treasured for this purpose in later centuries by the doctors of Europe at least, until its function was taken over by the more effective digitalis. In 1923 the hidden cardiac stimulus was finally isolated; it turned out to be a crystalline chemical called scillaren A. In combination with another less pure chemical called scillaren B, it is the basis of the modern drug.

The poison, scilliroside, is commercially important as an effective and highly selective rat poison. When ingested by most animals, including human beings, it prompts immediate vomiting before it can take effect. Because rats and other rodents are not able to vomit, they fall victim to its deadly power.

Like all bulbs, the sea onion is made up of many thin, scalelike layers. Oddly, neither the outer layers nor those near the heart of the bulb are of any value; only a few of the middle layers contain the drugs. To obtain them, the outer layers are removed and the bulb is thinly sliced, as you would slice a garden onion, and allowed to dry. Then the valuable middle layers of the dry slices are reduced to powder, from which the constituents are derived.

Senna

Cassia senna L.
PEA FAMILY
Leguminosae

Baghdad during the reign of the legendary caliph Harun al-Rashid—later to be glorified in *The 1001 Nights*—was one of the world's great cities, a hub of commerce and the center of Arab culture. Valuable spices, rare gems, and exquisite rugs were traded in the shadows of magnificent mosques. The arts flourished, but the art of medicine was barbaric at best. The standard treatment for constipation, for example, was a dose of powerful purgatives that wrenched the patient's guts so badly that most people considered the cure worse than the affliction.

And so, sometime around the turn of the 9th

century, Harun al-Rashid sent for a great and famous Christian Arab physician named Yuhanna ibn-Masawayh, known to posterity as Mesue the Elder. Among the many revolutionary medicines and treatments he brought with him from the south were senna leaves.

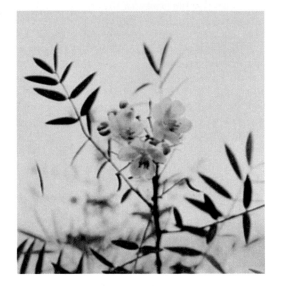

The leaves came from a yellow-flowered shrub, *C. senna*, native to the arid flatlands of northern and eastern Africa. Like its milder North American cousin the wild senna (*C. marilandica*), the plant contains a number of chemical substances that tend to stimulate peristaltic movements in the lower bowel, thus acting as a laxative. Prepared as an infusion, or tea, senna has a bitter, gluelike taste that can be improved with the addition of such spices as cloves, coriander, and ginger; the spices also help to prevent griping. It was in this form that the medicine was used in Arab lands and, later, throughout Europe for nearly 1,000 years. It has always been used with great care however; effective against many forms of constipation, it can be damaging in cases of spastic constipation or colitis, and large doses can cause severe nausea and pain.

Today, the active constituents of senna, extracted from dried leaves and green seedpods, are used in many commercial laxatives. Most of the U.S. supply comes from cultivated fields in southern India.

Smooth Strophanthus

Strophanthus gratus (Hook.) Baill.
DOGBANE FAMILY

Apocynaceae

An ambulance screeches to a halt. Paramedics leap to the pavement and rush to the side of a man lying on the sidewalk of a busy city. Quickly they determine that the man is suffer-

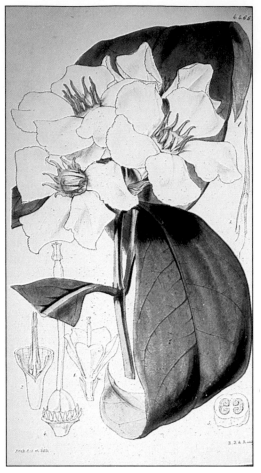

ing heart failure, and they take a number of lifesaving actions. One of these may be the injection of a substance called ouabain, obtained from the seed of a climbing African shrub. If so, within 5 to 10 minutes, the stricken heart will be beating faster and stronger; before the hour is over, the drug that stimulated it will have worked its full effect.

In an earlier time and at another place, closer to the place where the shrub grows, African hunters used long wooden spears to inject ouabain beneath the thick skins of elephants. Again within minutes, the great beasts would stagger and fall, their mighty hearts driven to the point of death.

Smooth strophanthus, the plant that yields this two-edged medicinal sword, is a woody climber native to the deciduous forests of tropical West Africa. It ascends to heights of 30 feet or more in a clambering fashion, not twining or supporting itself with tendrils as a true vine does, but using its branches almost as though they were arms to grasp the limbs of supporting trees. Its glossy evergreen leaves are thick and leathery, and it bears terminal clusters of showy, bell-shaped, purple and white flowers that resemble begonias but are fragrant at night with the scent of roses. For these reasons it is often grown as an ornamental in the tropics.

The folk healers of tropical West Africa have

found many uses for the plant. They make a rubbing compound from its leaves to reduce fevers; mash the leaves to treat skin ulcerations, wounds, and parasites; and make a decoction of the leaves as a remedy for gonorrhea. But ouabain's most common use in its native land has been as a source of arrow poison, both for hunting and for warfare, and it was this use that brought the plant to the attention of Western science.

In 1861 the famed explorer and missionary Dr. David Livingstone observed native peoples hunting with a poison that had been made from the seed of a closely related plant—a true vine called *S. kombe*—and he later reported the substance as an apparent cardiac stimulant. This led to the investigation of many similar species, of which *S. gratus* turned out to be the most valuable. (Africans who later heard that the English were using the poison from the seeds in a pure state as a medicine concluded that the English were indeed a mad race.)

Ouabain's fast action is the first quality that distinguishes it from slow-acting, digitalis-type heart stimulants. Another is that it does not constrict peripheral blood vessels as digitalis does. However, it is not without its dangers: it cannot be given orally, but must be injected in small, carefully measured doses; it cannot be given to a patient who has suffered recent heart damage; and it cannot be given within a week after a patient has taken digitalis. Within these limitations, it a valuable medicinal weapon, not only against heart disease, but against low blood pressure brought on by anesthesia during surgery.

Strychnine Tree

Strychnos nux-vomica L.
LOGANIA FAMILY
Loganiaceae

When the fabled Egyptian queen Cleopatra decided to end her life, she reportedly used her slaves as guinea pigs to test the effects of many different poisonous plants. Among the toxic sources she tried were belladonna, henbane, and the seed of the strychnine tree. No doubt the vain queen did not relish the prospect of death by strychnine, particularly as it is accompanied by violent spasms that distort the facial muscles into a hideous mask. Or perhaps it was the spectacular agony of strychnine poisoning that deterred her. Victims suffer horrific seizures without losing consciousness; in the course of them the body may be bent nearly double, so that both the head and the feet touch the ground at the same time. In any event, Cleopatra finally rejected strychnine along with all the other plant sources and selected the deadly asp as her suicidal agent.

A native of the tropics and subtropics of

southeastern Asia and Australia, the strychnine tree is a medium-sized evergreen, reaching a maximum height of about 40 feet, with a thick, frequently crooked trunk. Its deeply veined oval leaves, up to 3½ inches long, are borne in opposite pairs. Small, loose clusters of greenish flowers appear at the ends of branches and are followed by fleshy orange-red berries 1½ inches wide. These berries contain the disclike seeds that yield the poisonous substance strychnine. So bitter is this substance that it can be tasted even when diluted in a solution that is 400,000 parts water.

Strychnine is both a stimulant and a convulsant, or agent that causes uncontrolled fits or spasms, and its action can be nearly instantaneous. Long ago, primitive people discovered that the fatal seeds were effective in an arrow poison. In 15th-century Europe the seeds were imported from India to kill off the rat population. In the 19th century, physicians generally believed that strychnine was a stimulant that could affect the central nervous system, and they added small amounts of it to tonics.

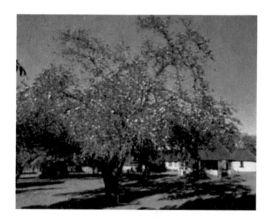

Today doctors give strychnine in controlled doses to increase muscular activity and as an antidote to poisoning caused by alcohol and other depressant drugs. It has also been administered in certain neurological treatments to stimulate specific nerve centers. Because it tends to induce intestinal movement, physicians have selectively administered the drug in the treatment of severe constipation.

Sweet Herb

Stevia rebaudiana (Bertoni) Hemsl.
COMPOSITE FAMILY
Compositae

For several weeks in the spring of 1981, an adventurous team of botanists from the University of Illinois trekked across the highlands of Paraguay, Peru, Colombia, and Mexico in search of sweet-tasting leaves. Their mission was to collect and sample the leaves of the sweet herb and related species in the hope of

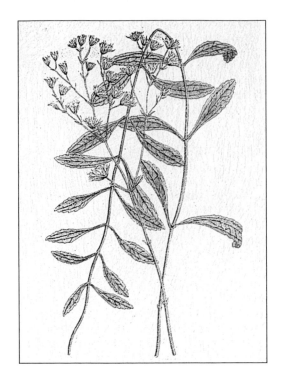

herb. The plants sampled, however, represent only about 15 percent of the genus, and so further field studies may yet produce other likely candidates for a safe sugar substitute.

In its investigations, the group discovered the alarming fact that sweet herb's natural habitat in northeastern Paraguay near the Brazilian border is being extensively exploited for timber and developed for agriculture by means of the notoriously destructive slash-and-burn method. Although concerned citizens have been trying to transplant sweet herb to plantations in other regions, they face grave problems because the plant is sensitive to environmental change and may not survive the move.

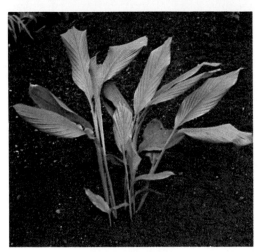

Turmeric

Curcuma longa L.
GINGER FAMILY
Zingiberaceae

discovering new sources of sweetening agents.

The Guarani Indians of Paraguay gave the sweet herb its name (*caá hê-é* in their language), and have long used it to make a sweet tea. The dried leaves and twigs of the plant are commonly sold in local markets and pharmacies; one company packages the material along with a pamphlet explaining its benefits as a sugar substitute for diabetics. Oddly enough, Paraguayans only occasionally employ sweet herb to sweeten food or maté, their tealike national drink.

Tests have shown that the plant's sweetening agent, the glycoside stevioside, is 300 times as sweet as granulated table sugar. But stevioside is potentially far more than a nonfattening sugar substitute: it actually triggers hypoglycemic activity, reducing blood sugar levels as it sweetens. Hence it can be a true lifesaver for many diabetics.

Sweet herb is one of more than 200 known species in the genus *Stevia*, all of which grow in mountainous countryside, in habitats that range from semidry grasslands and scrub forests to conifer forests and cold subalpine highlands. No taller than 3 feet, sweet herb is an erect perennial with hairy branches and stems. Its toothed, lance-shaped leaves are borne in opposite pairs along the stems, and it bears showy clusters of white flowerheads, each head made up of five tiny florets. The flowers develop into hard, one-seeded fruits (achenes).

In the course of their quest for new sweetening agents, the botanical team examined more than 30 *Stevia* species, chewing the leaves of each in the field and gathering leaves for further analysis. In addition to *S. rebaudiana*, three species in Mexico showed some trace of sweetness, but none compared with the sweet

In the marketplace of almost any town or city in southern Asia, a visitor's appetite is likely to be whetted by the tantalizing aromas of curried vegetables and meats or by the enticing smells that arise from multitudinous spice stalls. Out of sight, perhaps in a home or in the treatment room of a local physician, a doctor may be applying a yellow juice to the bruises of a young child. Elsewhere in the town, an elderly woman may be burning a heap of plant parts while directing the fumes toward a relative suffering from a head cold.

If the traveler were to observe all these events, he might not make a connection among them. Yet a simple connection exists. The odor of the curry dishes, the singular spice smell in the marketplace, the healing yellow fluid, and the aromatic smoke are all traceable to one plant—turmeric.

Turmeric flourishes in the rich, moist soils of Java, China, India, and Bangladesh and is a valuable cash crop in many other tropical areas of the Far East. The plant may grow as high as 5 feet. Its leaves are large—about 1½ feet long and 8 inches wide—and resemble those of the lily. Handsome funnel-shaped yellow flowers are borne in pairs from the leaf axils. But the rhizome, or underground stem, is the most important part of the plant. Dried and ground to a powder, it yields the substance curcumin, often sold under the name turmeric. It is this orange-yellow spice and coloring agent, one of the chief components of curry powder, that is responsible for the distinctively warm, bitter taste of curried foods. It is a common ingredient of prepared mustards as well, and is often used in making pickles. It has also long served as a fabric dye in Asia.

Curcumin has a long history as a folk remedy, and is still popular in many parts of Asia for treating a wide variety of maladies, from blood diseases to eye infections. In India, the powdered rhizome is commonly administered as an anthelmintic, or agent that rids the body of parasitic worms. Elsewhere, it is prescribed as a carminative, helping to relieve stomach and intestinal gas caused by eating certain foods, and as part of an ointment to speed the healing of smallpox and chicken pox lesions. There is evidence that the ingestion of curcumin may help stimulate the production of bile, which is produced by the liver and aids in the digestion of fats. And according to recent reports, the rhizome may also contain antibiotic properties that inhibit the growth of bacteria and fungi, but no scientific tests have yet been able to substantiate the claim.

White False Hellebore

Veratrum album L.

LILY FAMILY

Liliaceae

Like its American cousin the green false hellebore, or Indian poke (*V. viride*), the white false hellebore is a commonplace but dangerous plant. Its toxic juices, which have been used in the past to poison arrows and daggers and are still used to kill insect pests, also serve to save human life.

Native to moist meadows and open mountain woodlands in central and southern Europe as well as in central Asia, Japan, and the Aleutian Islands, the white false hellebore is considered a noxious weed by dairy farmers and shepherds, whose stock may be poisoned by it. Such poisonings are rare, however, except in badly overgrazed pastures; given a choice, few animals will eat the bitter leaves.

The white false hellebore's stout stalk, growing 3 to 4 feet high from a thick, blackish or yellowish underground stem (rhizome), is lined with large, oblong or oval, yellowish-green leaves whose bases clasp the stalk. Erect atop the stalk is a downy, branching flower spike, 1 to 2 feet long, crowded with yellowish-white flowers with greenish bases. Although

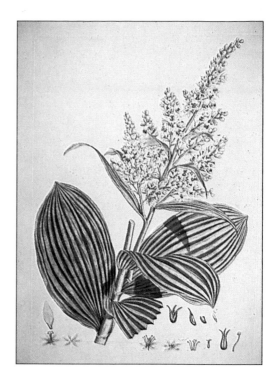

all parts of the plant are poisonous, the chemicals that give the plant its value and its virulence are concentrated in the rhizome.

To a trained botanist or herbalist, the bitter taste of the rhizome is a giveaway to the presence of potent alkaloids—a family of chemicals whose members are among the most biologically active substances known. Of the several alkaloids found in the white false hellebore, the principal ones are called protoveratrine A and B. Their value is in countering hypertension, or high blood pressure, without notably changing the patient's breathing rate or heartbeat. Protoveratrine A is the more effective in oral doses; the two are generally combined when given intravenously.

Folk healers have long made use of the plant's rhizome. Incorporated into an ointment, it has been applied to scabies, herpes, ringworm, and other skin ailments. In a shampoo, it helps to get rid of lice. Taken as a powder, it is an emetic and purgative—although a dangerous one. Carefully measured doses have been given to treat cholera and gout, and are still used in many parts of the world to treat muscular dystrophy, rheumatism, and arthritis.

The powdered rhizome, sold as an insecticide under the name hellebore, is a stomach poison against several kinds of beetles, caterpillars, grubs, cutworms, and grasshoppers. In England it is often used against the currant-worm, which can quickly defoliate a currant or gooseberry bush. American fruit growers sometimes use it to protect ripening fruits; it loses its potency quickly with exposure to air and sunlight, and a quick hosing washes away all residue. It is also used in veterinary powders to rid animals of fleas, lice, and mites.

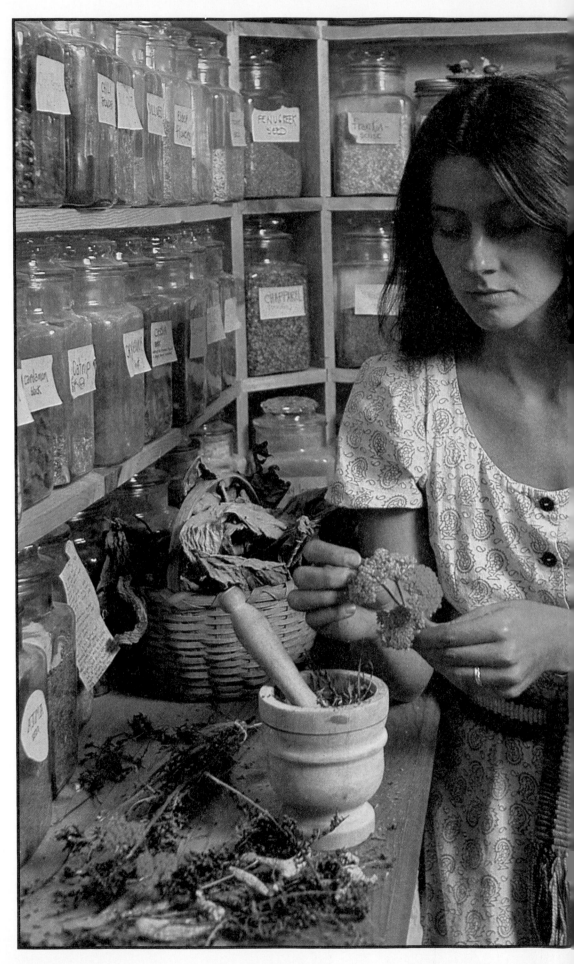

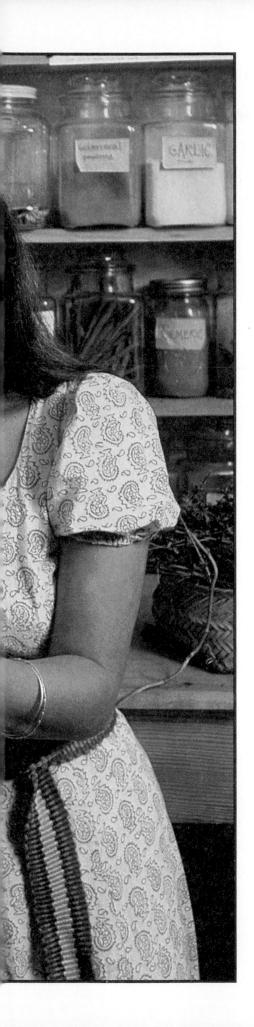

Growing and Using Herbs

The many virtues of herbs are being recognized once again—a confirmation of the wisdom and good taste of our forebears in using flowering plants, shrubs, and trees for their beauty and practical value. In this chapter, you can learn how to use many of the herbs in the "Gallery of Medicinal Plants," pages 74–354, plus some additional ones. The possibilities are numerous: you can plant your own herb garden or windowsill pots, cook with herbs in ways you might not have thought of before, brew herbal teas, create dried flower arrangements and other attractive craft items, make natural scents and beauty products, and choose from a selection of recipes for natural health aids such as lotions and tonics.

Growing Herbs

Flavorings, fragrances, refreshing teas, and soothing remedies are but a few of the ways you can use homegrown herbs—in general, plants that are used for their flavor, aroma, or medicinal properties, rather than for food or ornament. And if your plants are arranged so that you can sit near them, you will find them a delight for all the senses.

Garden size is not important. You can enjoy the bounty of herbs with just a few specimens massed in a tub or window box or tucked among your flower beds. Previous gardening experience is not needed either. Most herbs are easy to grow, resist pests, and require minimal upkeep.

The Basics

The major requirement for most herbs is sun—at least five hours of direct sunlight each day. They grow meagerly and have poor flavor without it. To gain sufficient sunlight, consider cutting back a few tree branches or growing herbs in movable tubs. If you cannot provide sun, there are a number of herbs, such as balm, borage, chervil, mint, parsley, and sweet woodruff, that tolerate partial shade.

Most herbs also need a well-drained soil. Plant them on a sloping site or make raised beds bordered with concrete blocks, bricks, stones, or old railroad ties. (Don't use ties that have been treated recently with creosote, which is poisonous.) Raised beds also help to make an herb garden neater and easier to tend.

To prepare the soil, dig deep—at least 12 inches. If your soil is heavy or has a high percentage of clay, lighten it with some peat moss and improve its draining qualities by adding some coarse sand. Also add several shovelfuls of organic matter, such as compost, well-rotted manure, or leaf mold. Herbs generally prefer a neutral or slightly alkaline soil. After conditioning with these ingredients, check the acid-alkaline balance with a kit from a gardening center. If the acidity is more than 7.5 on the pH scale, apply a light dressing of lime.

Stocking an Herb Garden

The most economical way to grow herbs is from seed, but this requires patience and often yields many more plants than you need. Such slow-growing herbs as thyme, marjoram, parsley, mint, and chives can be started indoors six to eight weeks before the last frost date; others should be planted no more than four weeks before you expect to put them outdoors.

Prepare flats or pots of sterilized potting soil mixed with perlite; plant the seeds according to package directions. Cover them with plastic and put them in a warm place with dim light. They should be kept damp until they germinate. If the soil starts to dry out, spray it with a mister or set the containers in tepid water until the top layer shows moisture. As soon as the seeds sprout, remove the plastic and move them to a bright area, but not direct sunlight. Set in full sun when the first true leaves, the second pair, develop. Make sure that there is good ventilation to prevent damping-off (rotting caused by too much dampness). Apply liquid fertilizer about 14 days after germination.

About the time of the last frost date and before the seedlings become spindly, you should harden them off—gradually acclimate them to the outdoors. You can do this by putting them outdoors in a cold frame and covering the frame on cold nights. Or put them outdoors during the day and bring them in at night. The seedlings should be transplanted into the garden preferably on a cool or cloudy day.

Parsley, dill, anise, and chamomile do not transplant well; if you sow them indoors, put them in small peat pots, which can be planted without disturbing the roots. Otherwise put the seeds in the ground where you want them to grow, after all danger of frost is past.

Prepare an outdoor seedbed of fine soil enriched with compost or add a thin layer of commercial potting soil. Scatter the seeds thinly in rows (with rows it is easier to tell the seedlings from any weeds that may emerge). Cover them with fine soil to about twice the diameter of the seeds. Keep them moist until they germinate and are well established. Thin the seedlings when they are about 1 inch high.

Certain slow-growing perennials, such as rosemary, bay, and lavender, are more easily obtained from a nursery than grown from seed. So, too, are French tarragon and true culinary (Greek) oregano; these last can be propagated only as cuttings from established plants. If possible, buy from a nursery that specializes in herbs and inquire if their plants have been hardened off. If not, you will need to follow the directions above for conditioning seedlings to the outdoors. Also examine nursery plants for pests. Brushing the foliage lightly will stir up any mature whiteflies. Examining the undersides of the leaves should reveal any insects or egg cases. Spider mites, which are difficult to see, can be detected by speckling or whitish spots on the leaves.

Propagating New Herbs From Old

Once you have a collection of thriving herbs, you can extend your garden by propagating new plants by root division, layering, or making stem cuttings. These methods are also suitable for obtaining herb specimens from, or sharing yours with, friends. See the chart on pages 396–398 for the propagating methods suitable to each herb.

Root division. In spring, any plants that grow from numerous stems can be divided this way. Simply raise the root clump out of the soil and gently break it apart with a garden fork or ease it apart with your hands.

Layering. Plants with woody, low-lying side branches can be propagated by layering. Make a slanted incision on the underside of a low, flexible branch just below a node, cutting halfway through. Anchor the branch in the soil with a stone or two heavy U-shaped wires (coat-hanger wire is suitable). Keep the soil well watered. After six to eight weeks, brush aside the earth to look for new roots. When there is a well-established root and growth is starting at the tip of the shoot, cut the newly rooted part from the branch and transplant it.

Stem cuttings. Prepare a pot or a flat (for several cuttings) with a mixture of equal parts of sand and vermiculite. Water the mixture thoroughly and tamp it down; make thin holes with a stick. Cut a healthy, flowerless shoot, 2 to 4 inches long, just below a node; strip off half of the lower leaves. Dip the cut end in rooting powder, slide the shoot gently into a prepared hole, and press the vermiculite mixture around it. To help keep the soil moist, cover the pot with a plastic bag, supported above the cuttings with sticks or a wire frame. Set the pot in the shade or a spot with indirect light. When you see new growth or a pulled-up plant reveals that the roots are 1 inch long, transplant the cuttings into regular potting soil.

Maintaining an Herb Garden

Herbs need less attention than many other types of plants, but you should keep them trimmed and remove sickly specimens and weeds from the area. In a small garden you can control the weeds by periodically cultivating around the plants. For a larger area, mulching is more practical. Around plants that prefer a rich moist, soil—for example, basil, chervil, chives, dill, mint, and savory—use a thin layer of a light organic mulch, such as dried bracken, buckwheat hulls, pine bark chips, or wood shavings. Dried lawn cuttings tend to hold in too much moisture. Small gravel is a better mulch

for herbs that prefer a drier, less rich soil: lavender, rosemary, and thyme, for example.

When you take a big harvest from the herbs for drying or freezing, work a little bonemeal, compost, or well-rotted manure into the soil to help the plants put out new growth. Avoid chemical fertilizers, if possible; they promote lush growth, but the herbs will have less flavor.

Unless the weather is very dry, water only the moisture-loving herbs, such as mint, basil, and chives, and any herbs planted in small containers. In the ground, most other herbs can withstand short droughts and generally require about one-half the water you would give to other flowering plants and vegetables.

Many culinary herbs pass their peak of flavor after they flower, and annuals begin to die off at this point. Be vigilant to pick developing buds and flower stalks of edible herbs until you are ready to let the seeds develop.

While the majority of herbs are fairly resistant to pests, a few are susceptible to aphids, whiteflies, or spider mites, and some are dearly loved by caterpillars. You can take advantage of the natural pest-repellent qualities of certain herbs to make your own nonpoisonous spray for affected plants. Pick some leaves from herbs that never seem to be bothered by pests—spearmint or rue, for example. Pour boiling water over them (three parts water to one part herb); steep for 15 minutes. When cool, strain the mixture through cheesecloth and spray it on affected plants. Make a new batch and repeat spraying every week and after rains. See also page 405 for an all-purpose spray.

Bay, rosemary, lemon verbena, and scented geraniums are perennials that tolerate only light frosts. If your winters are colder, you will have to bring these plants indoors each winter; you may want to keep them in pots rather than replant them each season.

To prepare other perennial herbs for the winter, mulch them with a thick layer of leaves, straw, or light branches as soon as the ground has frozen hard. Do not remove the covering until all danger of frost has passed. In April, check under the mulch. If new growth is turning yellow, uncover the plants on sunny days and re-cover them on frosty nights. The silver-leaved herbs, in particular, tend to rot when melting conditions and mulch combine to keep too much moisture around them.

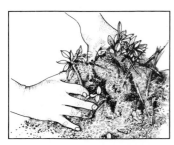

To divide plants with many stems, gently pull the roots apart.

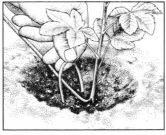

When layering, anchor the branch in the soil with U-shaped wire.

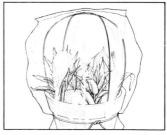

To keep stem cuttings moist, cover them with a supported plastic bag.

Cultivating Requirements and Uses

Included in the chart below is a selection of herbs that you may want to grow in your garden for use as teas, seasonings, fragrances, or dyes, or to incorporate in dried flower arrangements or beauty preparations. Most are illustrated in the "Gallery of Medicinal Plants," beginning on page 74.

Plant	How to Grow It	Common Uses
Anise	*Annual.* Sow seeds in a dry, light soil in early summer. Thin seedlings to 4 inches apart. Anise needs 120 frost-free days to produce fully ripened seed heads.	The aromatic seeds are used in cooking, in potpourris, and in some simple remedies.
Balm	*Perennial.* Grows slowly from seed. Start seeds indoors 8 weeks before the last frost. Transplant seedlings into light, sandy soil in full sun or partial shade, setting plants 18 inches apart. Balm is susceptible to disease in crowded conditions. It will self-sow.	The fragrant leaves are used in salads, soups, egg dishes, summer drinks, and in potpourris and soothing teas.
Basil	*Annual.* Grows easily from seed. Sow it indoors in early spring or outdoors after danger of frost has passed and days are warm. Set plants 12 inches apart. Basil needs medium-rich, well-drained soil and full sun. Pinch off tips to promote bushiness and flower buds to maintain growth.	The leaves are a classic complement to tomatoes; they are also used to flavor salads, sauces, and vegetables.
Bay	*Perennial (Laurus nobilis).* In areas that have more than an occasional frost, bay should be grown in a pot in a sunny location and brought into a cool, bright area in winter. Propagate by seed, cuttings, or layering in any kind of soil. Bay is a tree that can be trimmed to a desired shape.	The leaves are used for flavoring stews and sauces and for fragrance in potpourris. Bay leaves also make attractive wreaths.
Chervil	*Annual (Anthriscus cerefolium).* Resembles parsley. Sow seeds in the spring where you want it to grow; does not transplant well. Or plant seeds in the fall for a spring crop. Thin to 6 inches apart. Likes moist, well-drained soil and partial shade. Will self-sow.	The leaves, with their delicate aniselike flavor, are one of the ingredients of fines herbes. Often used in soups and salads.
Chives	*Perennial (Allium schoenoprasum).* Grows easily from seed. Provide it with moderately rich soil and full sun. Unless you are growing chives for its flowers, cut back the leaves regularly to prevent flowering and preserve its flavor. Divide clumps every third spring.	The delicate onion-flavored leaves are usually chopped and put in salads and vegetable dishes.
Dill	*Annual.* Sow dill after all danger of frost is past. It needs protection from strong winds, and a medium-rich soil. Water it frequently and pinch flowerheads unless you want seeds to develop. Dill matures quickly. For a continuous supply, sow seeds every 6 weeks. Dill will self-sow for the next year.	The leaves are used to flavor salads, sauces, fish, and vegetables. The seeds are put in pickling liquids.
Fennel	*Perennial often grown as an annual.* Grows easily from seed in alkaline soil and in full sun. Thin plants to 18 inches apart.	The leaves are used in fish dishes and soups, the seeds for flavoring baked goods. Sweet fennel stalks are eaten as a vegetable.

Plant	How to Grow It	Common Uses
Garlic	*Annual.* Plant the cloves 6 inches deep and 2 inches apart in rich soil during the fall or early spring. Pull up the heads when the leaves turn yellow, and dry them in the sun.	A basic flavoring in many recipes, garlic is also used in home remedies and to repel insects.
Horehound	*Perennial except in very cold climates.* Seeds can be sown in the early spring, but are slow to germinate; thin to 10 inches apart. Can also be propagated from cuttings or by root division. Prefers full sun and sandy soil.	Used to flavor a candy; to make a cold and cough syrup, a gargle, a tea to stimulate appetite.
Lavender	*Perennial.* Has many varieties, including dwarf. Where winters are severe, plant English lavender, the hardiest; mulch it over the winter. Propagation is easiest by root division. Likes full sun and alkaline, gravelly soil.	Grown for its fragrance in the garden and to be used in potpourris and sachets.
Marjoram	*Perennial (Majorana hortensis), grown as an annual or wintered indoors in cold regions.* Sweet, or knotted, marjoram, a creeping herb, is the most useful culinary variety. Showy marjoram, which grows to 1½ feet high, is an attractive plant. Start seeds indoors; transplant to a rich, light soil in full sun.	This herb is at its best combined with thyme as a seasoning in stuffings and meat and poultry dishes.
Mints	*Perennial.* Have many species and varieties, including orange, pineapple, and apple mint, peppermint, and spearmint; the last two are the most common. Mints grow in sun or partial shade and need an enriched soil and regular watering. They spread rapidly unless the roots are restricted by underground barriers.	Often accompany lamb and cucumber and are included in cold drinks and refreshing teas.
Oregano	*Perennial.* Prefers well-drained, slightly alkaline soil and full sun. Propagate by seed, root division, or cuttings.	The leaves are a favorite seasoning for pizza and other Italian dishes.
Oswego tea (bergamot)	*Perennial.* Likes a rich, moist soil. Will thrive in full sun or partial shade. Propagate by root division in the spring or fall.	The leaves make a refreshing tea. The flowers are used in potpourris.
Parsley	*Biennial (Petroselinum crispum) usually grown as an annual.* Curly-leaved parsley is popular as a garnish, but flat-leaved (Italian) parsley is more flavorful. Both like a rich, well-drained soil and full sun or partial shade. Parsley seeds germinate slowly. Be patient; keep the soil moist. Thin to 8 inches apart.	Used mainly as a garnish, but also is a tasty addition to salads and sauces. Parsley tea makes a healthful tonic.
Roman chamomile	*Perennial.* Can be clipped to make a fragrant drought-resistant ground cover. Sow seeds in late spring in a semirich soil; thin seedlings to 4 inches apart. Propagate by separating runners in the spring or late summer.	The dried flowers make a soothing tea.
Rosemary	*Perennial wintered indoors in cold climates.* Rosemary needs full sun, and a sandy, well-limed soil. Cut it back after flowering to prevent it from becoming leggy. Propagate by layering or cuttings.	This is an aromatic flavoring for meat and poultry dishes; also used for making wreaths.

Cultivating Requirements and Uses (continued)

Plant	How to Grow It	Common Uses
Sage	*Perennial.* Has many species and varieties, including pineapple, purple, clary, and garden, which is the hardiest and most useful for cooking. Does best in a sandy, well-limed soil in full sun. Propagate flowering varieties by seeds; others by cuttings or layering.	The leaves are favored in sauces and stuffings. They are also an ingredient in many old remedies.
Savory	Winter savory, a *perennial,* has a peppery, pungent flavor. Summer savory, an *annual,* is similar but more delicate. Plant seeds of summer savory in a rich, light, moist soil; thin to 8 inches apart. Winter savory thrives in poorer soil and with less water. It can be propagated by seed, division, or cuttings.	Savory is used to flavor sausages and other meats and is sometimes included in a bouquet garni.
Scented geraniums	*Perennials grown as annuals or wintered indoors in cold climates.* There are numerous species including rose, apple, peppermint, and lemon. All belong to the genus *Pelargonium.* They can be propagated from cuttings and like full sun and a moist, well-drained soil.	The leaves give a delicate, flowery flavor to jellies and desserts and are also included in potpourris.
Sorrel	*Perennial often grown as an annual.* Grow it from seeds in moist, rich soil and full sun or partial shade; thin to 18 inches apart.	The tangy leaves are used to flavor salads and soups.
Southernwood	*Perennial (Artemisia abrotanum).* There are three types: camphor-, lemon-, and tangerine-scented. All can be propagated in fall or spring by root division or cuttings. Set plants 4 feet apart in full sun and well-drained, average soil; cut them back in spring.	The dried leaves are an effective moth repellent.
Sweet woodruff	*Perennial.* A ground cover that spreads rapidly, sweet woodruff can be propagated in spring by root division or cuttings. Can also be started from seeds as soon as they are ripe, but seeds are slow to germinate. Prefers rich, well-drained soil and full or partial shade.	The dried leaves are used to flavor wine.
Tansy	*Perennial.* Can be started from seed or propagated by division. Will self-sow and must be controlled to prevent its becoming a weed. Plant in full or partial sun in average soil, leaving at least 4 feet between plants.	The dried flowers are lovely in flower arrangements and wreaths. The dried leaves repel moths and other insects.
Tarragon	*Perennial.* For a culinary herb, buy French tarragon from a reliable nursery. It can be propagated only by cuttings or division. (Russian tarragon, grown from seeds, has little flavor.) This delicate plant likes a well-drained, rich soil and full sun.	The leaves are used mainly as a delicate, aromatic flavoring for chicken, fish, and salads.
Thyme	*Perennial.* There are many species and varieties, including lemon, English, golden, and garden; the last is the most popular for cooking. Thyme makes an excellent ground cover on dry, sloping sites. Trim it back after flowering to keep it from getting woody. Propagate by cuttings or division.	The leaves add a slightly pungent taste to meats and vegetables; thyme sprigs are a main ingredient in bouquet garni for soups and stews.

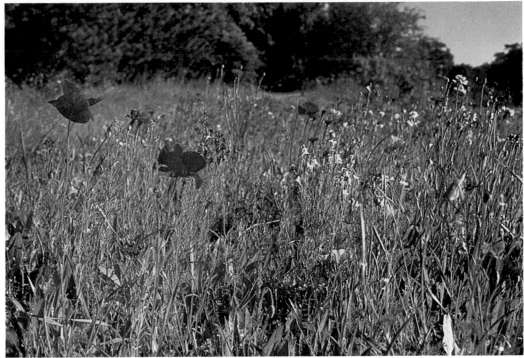

Gardeners are increasingly turning to meadow flowers for their beauty and as a laborsaving alternative to a lawn.

Creating a Wildflower Garden

"Why do you grow those weeds?" As every wildflower gardener knows, there are excellent reasons for cultivating nature's wildlings. Like a vest-pocket nature reserve, such a garden can help to keep alive rare or endangered species. Properly managed, moreover, wildflowers demand much less maintenance than traditional garden flowers or even turf. Finally, there is the unique beauty of these unimproved plants, which have not been touched by hybridizers and plant breeders.

Since these plants flourish in the wild, the novice may think they can be grown in the garden without man's assistance. In fact, however, planning and preparation are essential.

First, select plants suited to your garden. In general, each species of wildflower has evolved to fill a very specific ecological niche, and so requires a very particular kind of climate, soil, and exposure. For example, yellow bedstraw, *Galium verum*, flourishes in dry soils and full sun, knitting itself into a cover of tiny yellow blossoms. In moist soils or shade, however, it never prospers. By contrast, American ginseng, *Panax quinquefolius*, thrives only in the cool shelter of hardwood trees.

Second, limit the selection to indigenous plants. A Minnesota homeowner will be perfectly safe in planting the cup plant, *Silphium perfoliatum*, since this robust relative of the sunflower is native to the region. Likewise, a Connecticut Yankee could not go wrong in choosing liverleaf, *Hepatica americana*, as a

ground cover for the shady areas of a garden, for he will find great sheets of this handsome plant in the neighboring woods. In dry areas of the Sunbelt, cacti are an obvious choice, as alpine flowers are in northern Colorado.

Next, learn to interpret a plant's habitat. If a wildflower is described as growing on roadsides, plant it in well-drained, gritty soil exposed to the full sun, since those are the conditions from which it comes. Woodland natives usually prefer shade and moist soils rich in humus, seashore plants need sandy soils, and mountain plants grow best when their roots can hide in the cool shelter of rocks.

Site preparation and maintenance are essential too. Sprinkling seed on hard, untilled soil will serve only to feed the birds; abandoning seedlings to the summer heat without watering them amounts to a death sentence. The techniques for growing wildflowers are much the same as those for other types of gardening.

Once wildflower gardeners collected whatever they could from the wilderness. Today this practice is often illegal and never condoned by preservationists. It is also unnecessary, since many nurseries now specialize in wildflowers. But if you like, there is one way you can collect your own plants—and perform a conservationist's service to boot. With the help of a local building contractor or inspector, you can identify land slated for development, and there with the owner's permission you can dig with a clear conscience.

Planning an Herb Garden

Unless you are considering a very tight structure, such as a knot, an herb garden does not have to be put together in one season. You may start with a basic plan that appeals to you and build on it or rearrange it somewhat in succeeding years. In fact, one of the joys of herb gardening is to add new specimens encountered in one's travels or acquired from a friend.

Before undertaking an herb garden, especially an elaborate one, become familiar with as many herbs as possible. When you can picture the size, shape, and general appearance of each herb you want to include, planning will be more realistic and require fewer changes. For ideas and knowledge, consult the "Gallery of Medicinal Plants," pages 74–354, and visit herb nurseries, historical buildings that maintain traditional herb gardens, herb societies, and botanical gardens that include herb plots.

One approach to selecting the plants is to choose as a theme a particular use of herbs: a fragrance garden, a culinary garden, a garden with the makings of herbal teas or dyes, or one that attracts bees and butterflies.

To bring variety into a garden of predominantly green or silvery plants, add some types with colored or variegated leaves, such as opal basil (a deep purple), golden thyme, or golden sage. Or intersperse a few herbs that have showy flowers, such as Oswego tea and chives. You could also include a few heads of ornamental kale, the colors of which blend especially well with with the silver-leaved herbs.

Formal and Informal Plans

When you have chosen your herbs, make a sketch or cut out pieces of paper representing each plant bed and try out different arrangements. Essentially there are two basic types of garden plans: formal and informal. In the first, beds and pathways are precisely laid out, in geometric patterns, on a flat area. In the second, there are fewer divisions, and the sections or plant groupings blend naturally into one another. The informal garden is adaptable to a greater variety of terrains, such as a rocky slope, a terraced hillside, or an odd-shaped plot.

If you have the option of creating shape, a rectangular garden is an easy one to construct. A circular or oval garden is a bit more difficult to achieve, but ultimately very rewarding. One of the most challenging plans is a knot garden. Such creations, popular during the Renaissance, consist of tightly clipped herb hedges arranged in intricate patterns (see illustration, page 403).

Whatever the plan of the garden, it will benefit from a central focus, such as a pool, a sundial, an arched trellis, or a statue. Also possible is a brick or stone wall as a backdrop; not only is it attractive, but it will increase heat in the area and improve the fragrance of herbs.

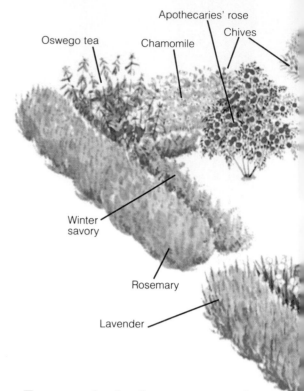

Oswego tea — Apothecaries' rose — Chamomile — Chives — Winter savory — Rosemary — Lavender

To create variety in a flat area, you can raise some of the beds to different levels. Do this by building up the sides with bricks, stones, boards, or railroad ties (not ones treated with creosote, however). Raised beds have the additional advantages of being somewhat easier to maintain and of establishing a sense of order. Just keep the beds small enough to be able to reach all the plants without straining.

Also consider using herbs as hedges or borders to establish the perimeters of your garden. Lavender, lavender cotton, rosemary, rue, and southernwood are suitable for hedges. Winter savory, thyme, and chives make attractive low borders. Curly-leaved parsley is lovely for an annual border.

Orient your herb garden toward the sun, with low, sun-loving herbs in the front and taller or shade-tolerant herbs tucked in the back. For easier maintenance you can keep perennials and annuals in separate beds, but your garden will be more attractive the year round if you space out the perennials and plant annuals between them.

If there will be pathways in your garden, decide how they will be covered: with grass or other plants, pavement, bricks, gravel, or wood chips. Well-trimmed grass not only is attractive, but is comfortable to sit or kneel on while tending the herb beds. A ground cover of creeping thyme or Roman chamomile is fragrant and drought-resistant, but needs considerable clipping and weeding to keep it neat. Paving, bricks, and gravel get hot in the sun, and although they are a less comfortable base

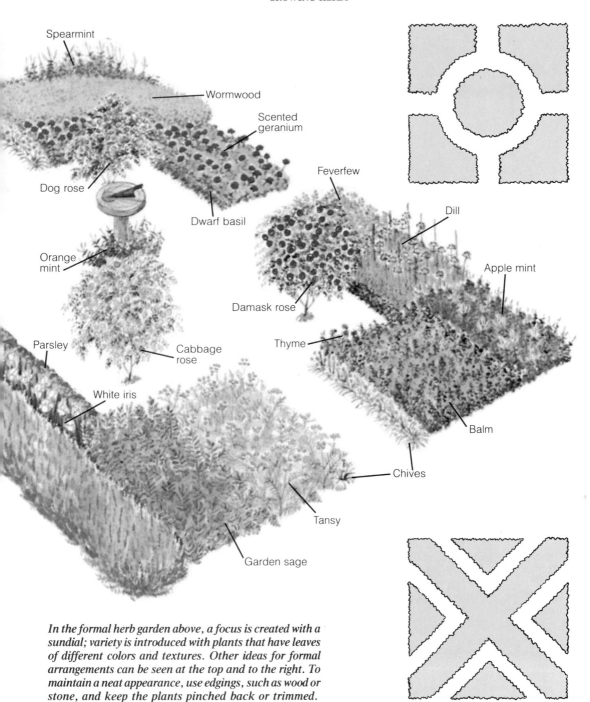

Spearmint

Wormwood

Scented
geranium

Feverfew

Dill

Dog rose

Apple mint

Orange
mint

Dwarf basil

Damask rose

Thyme

Parsley

Cabbage
rose

Balm

White iris

Chives

Tansy

Garden sage

*In the formal herb garden above, a focus is created with a
sundial; variety is introduced with plants that have leaves
of different colors and textures. Other ideas for formal
arrangements can be seen at the top and to the right. To
maintain a neat appearance, use edgings, such as wood or
stone, and keep the plants pinched back or trimmed.*

for tending beds, the extra warmth they attract
can be an advantage where summers are cool.

As part of your planning, make the most of
fragrant herbs by locating them next to paths,
where they will be brushed against or can
easily be pinched to release their fragrance. Or
put a bushy, fragrant herb in a waist-high urn,
thus bringing its fragrance closer to the nose.

Alternatives to a Planned Garden

If you do not have the space for a separate herb
garden, see page 405 for instructions on growing herbs in containers. Also consider inter-
spersing herbs with your flowers or vegetables.
The sun-loving herbs are particularly adaptable to rock gardens. Herbs with silver or pale

leaves, such as rue, lavender, and southernwood, make attractive fillers between seasonal
blooms. And the culinary herbs are natural
companions to vegetables—basil, for example,
to accompany your tomatoes, and dill and
savory to go with your homegrown lettuce.

As noted on page 395, many herbs have a
natural resistance to pests. When planted alongside more susceptible plants, they can help to
reduce problems. Some also improve the
growth and scent or flavor of particular plants
in their immediate vicinity, or help to restore
the health of an ailing plant. Although little is
understood about why companion plantings
work, many books and articles have been
written on the effectiveness of certain pairings.

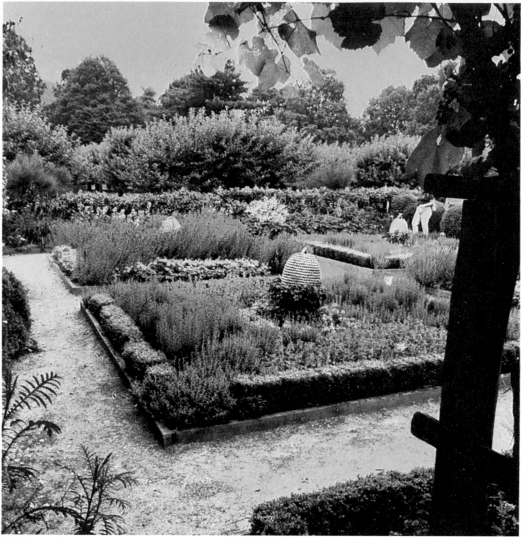

This large theme garden, part of a restored 18th-century estate, is planted with herbs that attract bees.

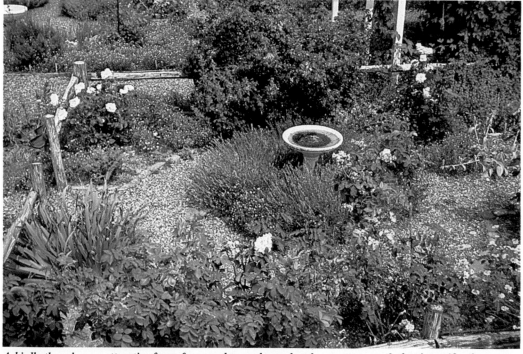

A birdbath makes an attractive focus for a garden, and gravel paths attract warmth that intensifies fragrances.

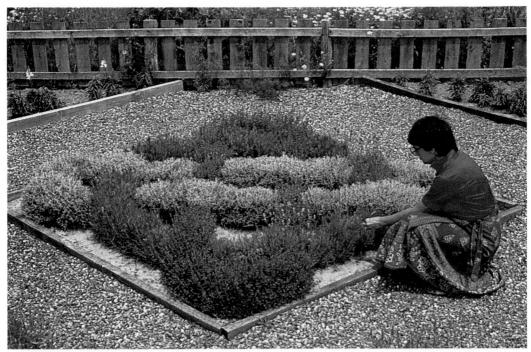

Viewed from any angle, a knot garden is a fascinating arrangement of controlled shapes and textures.

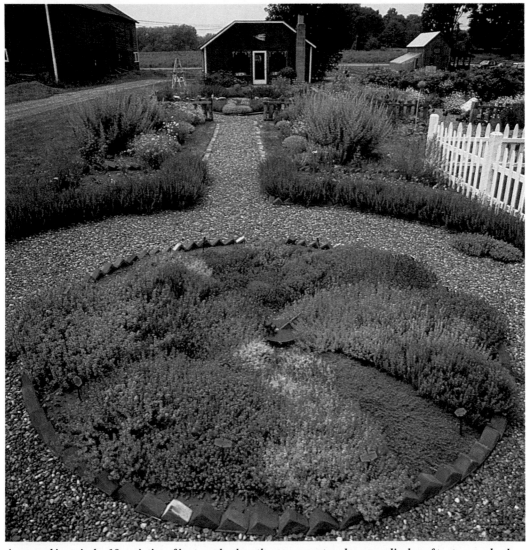

Arranged in a circle, 10 varieties of just one herb—thyme—create a decorous display of texture and color.

Making a Small Herb Garden for the Kitchen

Once you discover how delightful it is to have fresh herbs on hand, you will want to use them often. For convenience, consider planting culinary herbs as close to your kitchen as possible. You can snip a leaf or two even in the dark or in the rain. Such a garden need not be large; just 4 or 6 square feet is enough for six of the most useful herbs: basil, chives, parsley, rosemary, thyme, and mint. For a larger garden, add to this list dill, savory, oregano, bay, tarragon, and scented geraniums; the last for color as well as fragrance.

A strip of land along a wall is a good place for a culinary garden; deflected heat will intensify the flavor and scent of the sun-loving herbs. Check the planting strategies outlined on pages 400–401 for ways to group plants for pleasing effect and easy maintenance.

To create a more defined garden, and one that is also very easy to tend, consider planting herbs in the spaces between the rungs of a ladder or between the spokes of an old cartwheel, or even in an old small-paned window frame. Support a wooden frame on one or two layers of bricks; then build up each space with a soil mixture suitable for the herb it will contain—enriched and full of humus for parsley, chives, dill, mint, and savory, light and sandy for most other herbs. (See the chart on pages 396–398 for the correct soil types.)

Most culinary herbs, especially basil, dill, chives, and sage, produce more and better foliage when they are frequently trimmed back. If you cut plants back drastically, dig in some compost or add some fish emulsion to your next watering to help spur new growth.

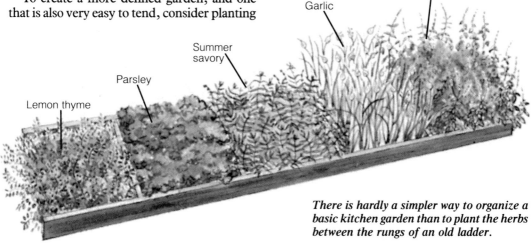

There is hardly a simpler way to organize a basic kitchen garden than to plant the herbs between the rungs of an old ladder.

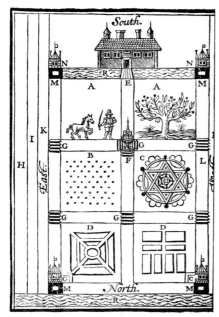

In this 17th-century plan for a country estate, not just one but two elaborate kitchen gardens are included (D).

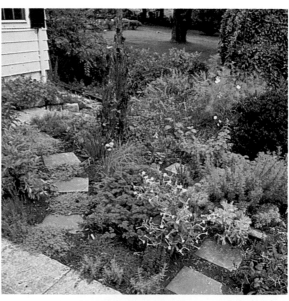

A small, informal herb garden planted near a kitchen door is a treat for the eye and the palate. To make it attractive year round, such evergreen herbs as lavender and lavender cotton have been intermingled with basic culinary herbs, including basil, sage, garden burnet, savory, and tarragon.

Growing Herbs in Containers

Most herbs can be grown in containers. If the container is a pot, the basic requirement is that it be one-third to one-half the height of the plant. Tall herbs, such as dill and lavender, are more difficult to manage, but can be grown in containers if regularly clipped back. A suitable potting mix consists of equal parts sterilized potting soil, coarse sand, and peat moss, with a little well-rotted manure added if possible.

Once herbs are established in containers, they should be watered only when dry and fed about once a month with a balanced liquid fertilizer; the leaves should be washed periodically to keep them clean and healthy.

Patio, Terrace, and Roof Gardens

During the summer, the sun-loving herbs do very well on patios, terraces, and roofs, where the heat is likely to be intense. Such plants as parsley, chives, and mint, which prefer some shade, will grow better in these locations during the spring or fall. If there is much wind, avoid such fragile herbs as dill.

It is best to start your herb seeds in pots or flats indoors, where you can keep them constantly moist; then set them outdoors in individual pots or mass them in a tub. The larger the containers, the less frequently you will have to water. If no single spot on your terrace has five hours of direct sunlight each day, set your herb containers on wheels so that you can move them to obtain maximum sun. Scented geraniums, thyme, prostrate rosemary, and marjoram can be grown in hanging baskets; they will trail attractively over the sides. Make sure that a basket is attached to a fitting firm enough to support it even in a strong wind.

If you have no patio or terrace, you can still grow herbs in window boxes. (Wooden ones should be treated with some preservative other than creosote, which is poisonous.) Make sure that they are securely attached to sound masonry or woodwork. To make the most of your limited space, discard any plant that is not thriving and replace it with a younger plant or a different species that may do better.

Growing Herbs Indoors

Given a sunny window, most herbs will grow almost as well indoors as out during the summer. The challenge and pleasure is to maintain an indoor herb garden during the winter, when fresh herbs are not generally available.

Ideal conditions are air temperature ranging between 50°F and 75°F, sunlight at least five hours a day, and humidity about 50 percent. The plants will also benefit from periodic exposure to fresh air, but not cold drafts.

A south window is the best; an east or west window should also afford adequate sunlight. However, if there is a radiator under the window or a cold draft around it, or if the temperature near the window drops at night to 40°F or less, your plants would probably be better off away from the window and under plant lights. (Exceptions are rosemary, bay, and chives, which seem to tolerate considerable coolness, but not heat.) Use incandescent plant lights according to the manufacturer's instructions. Or set the herbs under fluorescent tubes placed the same distance above the plant tops as the plants are tall. If necessary, install a timing device to ensure that the plants get at least 15 hours of light (also a minimum of 6 hours of darkness) in each 24-hour period. If the leaves turn pale, or are floppy and weak, they are probably not getting enough light. A small adjustment in the distance of the lights from the pots can make a large difference in the amount of usable light energy a plant receives.

To offset the drying effects of winter heat, set pots on pebbles in a metal or plastic tray and keep the tray filled with water to just below the bottoms of the pots. Or mist the plants at least once, or better yet twice, a day.

As a rule, it is best during the winter to water plants with tepid water. To avoid overwatering, feel the soil first to make sure it is dry. A good system is to pour the water into the saucer beneath the pot and let the plant soak it up.

Check periodically for pests; plants are much more susceptible to them indoors. If you find any, rinse the plants gently upside down in the kitchen sink (hold your hand over the soil to keep it from falling out); wash larger plants in a shower. You can also wash or spray plants with a mixture of water and dishwashing liquid (no more than 1 teaspoon per cup of water; a stronger solution can burn leaves), or spray with the following mixture: take 8 to 10 peeled, sliced garlic cloves and 1 teaspoon dried hot pepper. Pour 2 cups of boiling water over them and allow to steep for 15 minutes. Strain through a cloth and stir in 2 teaspoons dishwashing liquid. Apply every few days until the infestation clears up. The mixture can be stored in the refrigerator for up to a week. Another effective spray is one made with naturally pest-resistant herbs (see page 395). Should pests persist, discard affected plants.

If you have an outdoor herb garden, you can bring plants in for the winter. In cold climates, this is essential for certain perennials that have to be wintered indoors. In general, though, you will have more compact and attractive indoor plants if you start new ones late in the summer from seeds or cuttings, or by root division or layering (see pages 394–395).

To maintain an herb garden indoors the year round, start new plants at regular intervals. Freeze or dry the leaves of plants as they become oversized or sparse, then discard the plants.

Cooking With Herbs

For centuries herbs have been esteemed for the way they enhance the flavor and color of foods. Recently the rediscovery and the cultivation of certain herbs that were not widely known or available for many years have greatly expanded the possibilities for variety in our cooking. Below and on the following pages you can explore some of these possibilities.

Harvesting and Preservation

Throughout the summer months you will be taking fresh snippets of herbs as you need them. But to make the most of your herb garden and to keep it trim, it is a good idea also to harvest some of the leaves, flowers, and seeds to preserve for winter.

The best time to cut herbs for preserving is just as the plants begin to flower; the essence in the leaves is strongest at this point. Collect leaves about midmorning, as soon as the dew has dried but before the real heat of the day. You can prune annuals of up to one-half of their growth, perennials up to one-third; take less from slow-growing herbs such as bay and rosemary.

Cut branches with clippers or a sharp knife and arrange them in a thin layer in a basket. Take only as many leaves as you can process straightaway; never leave them in a pile.

To clean the herbs, simply swish the branches gently in a basin of cold water and spin dry or pat them between layers of clean towels. (If you mist them or apply a gentle hose spray the night before picking, there is no need to wash them.) Pick off any yellowed foliage and examine the leaves for pests; don't preserve plants with signs of infestation.

Herbs cut in early June will grow back in time for a second, possibly even a third crop. After a heavy cutting, fertilizer will encourage new growth (see page 395). Avoid cutting back perennials in the fall, as the plants need to develop mature foliage to withstand winter.

Seeds, such as caraway, coriander, cumin, dill, and fennel, should be harvested as soon as the seed heads turn brown and the stalks start to wither. Watch dill heads closely; they begin to shed almost as soon as they are ripe.

Roots can be harvested at any time, but are best in the fall, when the goodness from the year's growth is stored in them. Dig up a clump and separate out as many roots as you need. Carefully replant any extras.

Harvesting Wild Herbs

If you observe a few precautions, collecting herbs in the wild can be very enjoyable and educational. Before picking any wild plants, however, carefully research the species that interest you. Find out if there are any poisonous species that are confusingly similar and how to distinguish them from the safe plants. If you are a novice, try to find an expert on wild plants who can accompany you on a few field trips. Or take a course in the subject. Some nature preserves, botanical gardens, parks, and museums offer classes in the identification and use of wild herbs.

The best place to pick wild plants is on your own property where you know that no spray has been used. Avoid herbs growing along roadsides, where they may be contaminated by exhaust fumes or animal wastes, or in any area near a commercial farm or forest, which may have been sprayed. Be careful that watercress is not growing in polluted water.

Use common sense about quantity. Rather than pick an entire stand, always leave a good number of plants at the discovery site. It is better to leave a very small stand completely alone. (For more information on gathering plants in the wild, see pages 26—27).

Drying Foliage, Flowers, Seeds

Drying is the time-honored way of preserving herbs for the winter. It works particularly well for rosemary, thyme, oregano, marjoram, lovage, bay, balm, savory, and mint. Sage also dries well, but it sometimes gets musty. Dill, chives, parsley, chervil, fennel, and basil lose much of their flavor; it is better to freeze them.

One drying method is to tie the herbs in bunches and hang them upside down in a warm, dry place where air can circulate freely around them. An attic or shed is ideal, or you can put them outdoors in the shade and bring them in at night; drying them in sunlight destroys their flavor and color. To keep the bunches free of dust some people put them inside perforated paper bags.

Herbs can also be dried by spreading them on nonmetal screens or on frames covered with cheesecloth. These are then put in a warm, dry place, such as an attic, or a drying oven, where the temperature can be maintained between 70°F and 100°F. If you dry them in your kitchen oven, don't permit the temperature to go above 150°F or you will destroy their flavor.

A microwave oven is the fastest drying method; it takes only two to four minutes. Just follow the manufacturer's directions.

When sufficiently dry, herbs will crumble if you squeeze them. It takes up to two weeks to reach this stage, depending on the herbs, the humidity and temperature of the air, and the drying method. The next step is to strip the leaves from the stems and shake the seeds from the heads; store them in glass or china containers with airtight lids. Label each one with the name and date. During the first week of storage, check carefully for signs of condensation. If you find any, take out the herbs and dry them for another day or two.

Dried herbs keep best in a cool, dark place. While racks of herbs in glass jars look nice in a kitchen, the herbs will quickly lose their color and flavor. When properly stored, dried herbs keep for a year or longer.

Freezing Herbs

Most herbs retain fresh color and much of their flavor when frozen. They can be used in sauces, soups, stews, casseroles, and salad dressings, but are a bit too limp for garnishes.

Wash the herbs and cut off any discolored parts. Basil, thyme, and dill have better color and flavor if blanched before freezing. (To blanch, bring a pot of water to a boil. With tongs, twirl a few branches at a time in the water. After a few seconds lift them out, shake out excess water, and dry them between towels.)

Put sprigs in plastic bags; seal, label, and date them. If freezing leaves only, lay them on cookie sheets, freeze them, then put them in plastic bags. Otherwise they stick together.

Another freezing method is to mince the herbs, pack them into ice cube trays, and fill the trays with water. Or chop them in a blender or food processor with a little water. You can make up your own batches of fines herbes this way (see page 408). As soon as the cubes are frozen, put them in labeled plastic bags.

Frozen herbs will keep for up to six months. If you are using them in cooked dishes, there is no need to thaw them before use.

Preserving Herbs in Oil

Basil, tarragon, rosemary, and sorrel can be stored in oil and will keep well for up to nine months. Use vegetable or olive oil or a combination of the two. Put a layer of washed and dried leaves into a glass jar, followed by a layer of oil. Continue alternating layers, finishing with a layer of oil. Store in the refrigerator. When you use the leaves, scrape excess oil back into the jar. Use the herb-flavored oil for barbecuing, sautéing, marinades, or salad dressings.

Herb-Flavored Condiments

Another way to bring the flavor of summer to your winter table is to preserve fresh herbs in vinegar, jelly, butter, or sugar. Warm toast spread with sage butter or a salad laced with dill vinegar is not only a treat for the senses, but a pick-me-up too. Consider the following condiments not only as an adventure for yourself, but as practical and attractive gifts. Just put them in pretty crocks, jars, or bottles and affix ribbons or lovely labels that say homemade by you.

Herb vinegar. Almost any herb or combination of herbs can be used to flavor vinegar. Good choices are tarragon, sage, thyme, marjoram, basil, savory, and dill. Rosemary or any of the mints make delicious vinegars for fruit salads. Opal basil gives a lovely pink color to white vinegar.

Place several sprigs in a clean bottle, preferably one with a cork or nonmetal lid. Fill it with about a pint of any good-quality vinegar, and set in a sunny place to steep. Shake it every few days. Herb vinegar should usually steep for about three weeks. To hasten the process, bring the vinegar to a boil before pouring it into the bottle. When the vinegar tastes right to you, strain it through cheesecloth. For a nice appearance, put a fresh sprig in the bottle.

Herb jelly. Apple jelly makes an excellent base for an herb jelly. When preparing it, add ¼ cup chopped fresh rosemary, sage, or thyme leaves, or ½ cup chopped fresh spearmint, basil, or lemon verbena leaves for each 2 cups of liquid just before boiling it to the setting point. If you prefer, strain the jelly before putting it in the sterilized jars. If you do not want to prepare your own jelly, put some commercial jelly in a pan and warm it; stir in the herbs, return the jelly to the jar, and store it in the refrigerator.

For just a hint of sweet herbal fragrance, put a leaf or two of rose geranium, Oswego tea (scarlet bergamot), or balm (lemon balm) in the bottom of a jar before pouring in plain apple jelly.

Spearmint jelly is a traditional accompaniment to roast lamb. Thyme, sage, or rosemary jelly makes a delightful glaze for roast pork, chicken, or veal. Just baste the meat with it 20 minutes before the end of the roasting time.

Herb butter. To prepare herb butter, bring ¼ pound (1 stick) butter to room temperature. Cream it until fluffy, then blend in 3 tablespoons to ¼ cup of one or more minced fresh herbs (less of the more pungent ones, such as sage and rosemary). If you like, also blend in 1 tablespoon lemon juice. For garlic butter, use 1 tablespoon minced fresh garlic and 3 tablespoons minced parsley. Wrap the butter in plastic wrap; chill it for 20 minutes. Shape it into a neat roll; rewrap and refrigerate or freeze it.

Herb butters preserve the fresh flavor of herbs for up to six weeks in the refrigerator, six months in the freezer. They can be used in countless ways. Try frying an egg in marjoram butter or serving broiled steaks garnished with a knob of garlic butter. Use mint butter with carrots, rosemary butter with spinach, or dill butter with summer squash or fish.

Herb sugar. Chop some rose petals or balm, rose geranium, or mint leaves. Use 2 tablespoons of herb for each cup of sugar. Store the herb sugar in an airtight container for six weeks before use; it will keep almost indefinitely. Serve herb sugar with tea or sprinkle it on plain cookies or other simple desserts.

Basics of Herb Cookery

You might be surprised at the number of ways in which you can cook with herbs. Perhaps you have tried oregano in spaghetti sauce or served mint sauce with lamb, but have you ever put dandelions in a salad or sage in a dessert?

The recipes on the following pages, only a small sampling of ones that include herbs as a major seasoning, are intended to give you an idea of how certain herbs can be used and to inspire further experimentation. Although in most of these preparations fresh herbs are preferable to dried, the equivalent amount of dried herbs is stated when good results can be obtained by their substitution. In general, dried herbs are two to three times as potent as fresh. A reasonable substitution is 1 teaspoon of crumbled or ¼ teaspoon of powdered for each tablespoon of fresh herbs. Herbs that are frozen or preserved under oil are used in the same quantity as fresh ones.

Two terms often found in recipes that include herbs are *bouquet garni* and *fines herbes*. The first consists of herb sprigs tied together so that they can be easily removed from the dish they are flavoring. A traditional combination is four sprigs parsley, two sprigs thyme, and one small bay leaf, but you can create your own variations. An appropriate substitute for a fresh bouquet is an equivalent amount of dried herbs tied up in cheesecloth. The traditional fines herbes combination is equal parts of minced parsley, chervil, tarragon, and chives. Although these and many other herb combinations work well, it is always best to use restraint in combining herbs because too many can result in a bitter or nondescript flavor.

Heat releases herb essences. For this reason cold herbal dishes have more flavor if you bring them to room temperature before serving. To release the flavor and aroma of herbs that will go directly into such cold preparations as iced drinks, bruise the leaves lightly with a fork, pestle, meat pounder, or similar tool.

Prolonged heat can destroy or diminish the flavor of delicate herbs. It is best to put them in cooked dishes just before serving or add them as a garnish. Garnishing, in fact, is another excellent use for fresh herbs. A last-minute addition of sprigs or minced leaves adds not only a touch of color but a subtle aroma and flavor.

Appetizers

Herbed Cottage Cheese

1 pound cottage cheese
1 tablespoon minced fresh chives or 1 teaspoon dried
1 teaspoon each minced fresh marjoram, thyme, and basil or ½ teaspoon each dried
1 teaspoon each crushed caraway seeds and toasted sesame and poppy seeds

Combine all ingredients and refrigerate for 24 hours to allow flavors to blend. Serve on crackers or as a vegetable dip. Keeps up to 5 days in the refrigerator.

Eggplant Pâté With Garlic

For a more potent flavor, you can double or triple the quantity of garlic.

2 large eggplants
¼ cup olive oil
Juice of 1 medium-size lemon
1 clove garlic, crushed
Salt and pepper to taste

Preheat oven to 350°F. With a fork, puncture the eggplants in several places. Set them on a baking sheet or a piece of foil and bake for about 1 hour or until soft. When cool, cut the eggplants open, scoop out the insides, and chop them fine. Mix in the oil, lemon juice, garlic, salt, and pepper. Serve as an appetizer on crackers, toast slices, or pita bread.

Stuffed Mushroom Caps

These can be prepared a few hours ahead and baked just before serving.

1 pound large mushrooms
3 tablespoons butter
1 tablespoon chopped shallots
3 tablespoons butter or margarine
2 teaspoons each minced fresh marjoram and thyme or ½ teaspoon each dried
2 tablespoons chopped fresh parsley or 2 teaspoons dried
1 cup fresh bread crumbs or ½ cup dried
1 beaten egg
½ teaspoon salt
⅛ teaspoon pepper
Juice of 1 small lemon

Preheat the oven to 375°F. Clean the mushrooms and remove the stems. In an enamel or stainless steel pan, sauté the caps in the butter until lightly browned; remove them from the pan with a slotted spoon. Chop the mushroom stems and sauté them with the shallots in the same pan until golden.

In a bowl combine the butter, herbs, bread crumbs, egg, salt, and pepper. Stir in the stems and shallots. Fill the caps with this stuffing, sprinkle them with lemon juice, and place them, stuffed side up, on a baking sheet. Bake for 15 minutes. Makes 15 to 20 appetizers, depending on the size of the mushrooms.

Soups

Basic Beef or Chicken Stock

To accumulate enough bones or chicken parts, freeze fresh leftovers from other recipes.

5 pounds beef bones
4 quarts water
2 onions, peeled
2 carrots
2 stalks celery
2 teaspoons salt
2 cloves garlic, peeled
1 bouquet garni (see page 408)
2 sprigs rosemary (optional)
8 peppercorns

Wash the bones; brown them by baking them in a 375°F oven for about an hour. Put the bones and water in a large pot. Bring to a boil and skim off any foam. Add remaining ingredients. Simmer for about 4 hours. Remove the bulky ingredients with a slotted spoon. Strain the liquid through cheesecloth. Add more salt if necessary. If desired, chill the stock, then scrape off the fat. Makes 2 to 2½ quarts.
Chicken stock. In the above recipe substitute a 6-pound stewing hen or 6 pounds of chicken backs, necks, wings, and feet for the beef bones. Do not brown. Simmer for 2 hours.

Sorrel and Rosemary Soup

1 medium-size onion, chopped
4 tablespoons butter or margarine
1 quart chicken stock (see recipe above)
3 cups chopped sorrel leaves
2 tablespoons fresh rosemary leaves
or 2 teaspoons dried
1½ cups mashed potatoes
1 cup light cream
Parsley for garnish

Cook the onion in the butter until golden. Add the stock and bring to a boil. Add the sorrel and rosemary; simmer for 15 minutes. Stir in the potatoes; simmer for another 15 minutes. Stir in the cream and bring back to a simmer. Garnish with the parsley. Serves 6.

Tomato Soup With Tarragon

This can be eaten hot or cold. If you use a food mill to puree it, you need not skin the tomatoes.

2 tablespoons olive oil
1 medium-size onion, chopped
3 cups tomatoes (about 2 pounds), skinned and chopped, or 1 28-ounce can whole tomatoes
2 teaspoons chopped fresh tarragon or 1 teaspoon dried
1 clove garlic, minced
1½ cups chicken stock (see recipe above)
1 teaspoon salt
¼ teaspoon pepper
2 teaspoons grated orange rind

In a heavy pot, heat the oil and cook the onion in it over low heat until translucent. Stir in the tomatoes with their juice, the tarragon, and the garlic. Add the stock, salt, and pepper. Cover and simmer for 20 minutes. Puree the soup in a food mill, blender, or food processor. Add the orange rind and bring back to a simmer. Garnish with tarragon. Serves 4 to 6.

Cauliflower Soup With Chervil

With its subtle, aniselike flavor, chervil complements the cauliflower in this delicate soup.

1 medium-size cauliflower, cut into florets
1 stalk celery, diced
1 clove garlic, minced
1 tablespoon minced fresh chervil or 1 teaspoon dried
1 tablespoon minced fresh thyme or 1 teaspoon dried
1 bay leaf
¼ teaspoon pepper
2 cups chicken stock (see recipe above)
1 cup light cream or half-and-half
Chervil sprigs for garnish

In a heavy pot, combine all the ingredients except the cream. Bring to a boil; reduce heat and simmer for 30 minutes. Stir in the cream; bring back to a simmer. Add salt if necessary. Serve with the chervil sprigs. Serves 4 to 6.

Squash Bisque

If you use a food mill to puree the soup, there is no need to peel the squash, apple, or potato.

1 small butternut squash, peeled, seeded, and cut up
1 apple, peeled, cored, and chopped
1 small potato, peeled and chopped
1 leek, washed and chopped
1 onion, peeled and chopped
1 carrot, peeled and sliced
1 stalk celery, sliced
2 cloves garlic, peeled
1 tablespoon fresh oregano leaves or 1 teaspoon dried
2 teaspoons fresh rosemary leaves or ½ teaspoon dried
¼ cup chopped parsley
3 cups chicken or beef stock (see recipe above)
½ cup milk
Salt and pepper to taste

Place all ingredients except the milk, salt, and pepper in a large pot. Cover and cook over medium heat until the vegetables are tender, about 40 minutes. Puree in a food mill, blender, or food processor. Stir in the milk, adding a bit more if the bisque is too thick. Add the salt and pepper. Serves 4 to 6.

Main Dishes

Roast Lamb With Rosemary

A traditional favorite, this dish is also very easy to prepare, and it's a great guest pleaser.

Choose one of the tender cuts of lamb—the leg, the loin, or the rib—and allow ⅓ to ½ pound per serving for a boneless roast, ½ to ¾ pound per serving for one with bones included.

Preheat the oven to 450°F. With a small, sharp knife, make slits ½ inch deep into the fat side of the roast, spacing them about 2 inches apart lengthwise and crosswise. Insert a sliver of peeled fresh garlic and two fresh or dried rosemary leaves in each slit. Coat the meat lightly with more rosemary leaves. Place it fat side up on a rack in a roasting pan; insert a meat thermometer in the thickest part (unless you use an instant-read thermometer). Roast for 15 minutes at 450°F. Reduce heat to 350°F; continue roasting to desired doneness.

Opinions vary as to when lamb is properly done. The trend today is to cook it to medium rare (140°F to 145°F), or medium (150°F to 155°F), so that pink still shows in the meat. You can, if you prefer, cook it to well done (165°F), but it will be gray and quite dry. The following are approximate roasting times per pound: medium rare, 12 to 14 minutes; medium, 14 to 16 minutes; well done, 16 to 18 minutes. For easier slicing, cover the roast with foil and let it rest for 10 to 15 minutes.

Herbed Meat Rolls

If you prefer, substitute oregano for the sage and add 1 tablespoon grated Parmesan cheese.

2 pounds beef round, thinly sliced
1 cup plain (unseasoned) dry bread crumbs
¼ cup minced fresh parsley
 or 2 tablespoons dried
2 tablespoons minced fresh sage
 or 2 teaspoons dried
1 clove garlic, crushed
¾ teaspoon salt
¼ teaspoon pepper
½ cup olive oil

Preheat a broiler or prepare a charcoal grill. Pound the meat as thin as you can without breaking it. Cut it into portions 2½ to 3½ inches wide by 6 to 8 inches long.

Using a fork, mix the bread crumbs with the herbs, seasonings, and oil. Spread one side of each piece of meat thinly with the mixture; roll the meat and place it on skewers, setting the rolls close together until each skewer is filled.

Spread a little of the remaining crumb mixture over the top of the meat rolls and drizzle a little oil over all. Broil or grill the meat about 5 minutes on each side (it should be browned on the outside but slightly pink where the rolls touch each other). Makes 20 to 24 rolls, enough for 5 or 6 persons.

Beef Stew With Watercress

Plan to serve this stew as a one-dish meal.

2 tablespoons olive or vegetable oil
2 pounds stewing beef, cut in
 2-inch pieces
1 tablespoon flour
1 teaspoon salt
¼ teaspoon pepper
1 clove garlic, chopped
1 large onion, peeled and sliced
1 cup beef stock (see recipe page 409)
1 cup canned tomato sauce
3 whole cloves
1 tablespoon minced fresh marjoram or
 1 teaspoon dried
½ cup chopped watercress
1 bay leaf
½ cup red wine
6 potatoes, peeled and cut in quarters
6 carrots, peeled and cut in quarters
1 stalk celery, chopped

Heat the oil in a large enamel or stainless steel pan and brown the meat in it. Sprinkle the meat with the flour, salt, and pepper, and stir to coat. Stir in the garlic, onion, beef stock, tomato sauce, cloves, marjoram, watercress, and bay leaf. Cover; simmer for 3 hours.

Cook the carrots and potatoes in lightly salted water until crisp-tender (about 10 minutes); drain. Add them to the stew along with the wine and the celery. Simmer for another 30 minutes. Serve in large soup plates. Serves 6.

Chicken With Tarragon

This classic dish is easy to prepare.

1 3- to 4-pound frying chicken,
 cut into serving pieces
2 tablespoons chopped fresh tarragon
 or 2 teaspoons dried
2 tablespoons butter or margarine
1 tablespoon vegetable or olive oil
3 tablespoons minced shallots
Salt and pepper
½ cup dry white wine

With a knife, separate the skin of the chicken from the flesh on one or two edges. Using 1½ tablespoons of the tarragon, spread a little under the skin of each chicken piece. Melt the butter with the oil in an enamel or stainless steel sauté or frying pan. Over medium heat, brown the chicken on both sides. Remove the chicken and sauté the shallots in the pan for 30 seconds. Return the chicken to the pan; lightly salt and pepper it. Cook, covered, over low heat for 15 minutes. Add the wine; cook for another 15 minutes. Remove the chicken to a warm serving dish. Reduce the sauce slightly by boiling it; pour it over the chicken. Garnish with the remaining tarragon.

Marinated London Broil

The combination of wine and herbs makes the meat tender and flavorful.

1 cup red wine
½ cup vegetable oil
1 medium-size onion, chopped
¼ cup chopped parsley
1 tablespoon each chopped fresh marjoram and thyme or 1 teaspoon each dried
1 teaspoon salt
½ teaspoon pepper
1 clove garlic, crushed
3 pounds London broil

Mix all marinade ingredients in a bowl. Pour ¼ cup of the marinade into a deep dish. Place the meat in the dish and pour the remaining marinade over it. Cover and refrigerate for 24 hours or let stand at room temperature for 4 hours. Broil or barbecue the meat to the desired doneness, basting it with the marinade. Serves 8.

Tuna Casserole With Fennel

Fennel turns this quick and easy casserole into something special.

3 tablespoons butter
1 medium-size onion or 3 scallions, minced
¼ cup flour
2 cups milk
1 6½-ounce can tuna, packed in water
3 teaspoons minced fresh fennel leaves or 1 teaspoon fennel seeds, slightly crushed
Salt and pepper to taste
½ cup fresh bread crumbs
½ cup grated Swiss or Cheddar cheese

Over low heat, sauté the onion in the butter until translucent. Remove from the heat; stir in the flour. Return to the heat and cook for 1 minute more. Remove from the heat; add the milk slowly, stirring all the time. Break up the tuna and add it to the sauce along with the can liquid. Stir in the fennel; add salt and pepper.

Pour the mixture into a flameproof casserole. Mix the bread crumbs with the grated cheese and sprinkle over the top. Broil until golden (3 to 5 minutes). Serves 4.

Tortellini With Sage Sauce

This simple pasta dish can be served as a first course (in small portions) or as a main course. Tortellini are available fresh, frozen, or dried.

1 pound tortellini filled with meat
⅔ cup finely chopped fresh sage
½ cup (1 stick) sweet butter, melted

Bring a large potful of water to a boil and add the tortellini. Cook until soft but still firm (about 7 to 8 minutes). Meanwhile, chop the sage and add it to the melted butter. Drain the tortellini and toss with the sauce. Serves 4 as a first course or 3 as a main course.

Broiled Fish With Garlic, Parsley, and Oregano

Although not usually associated with fish, oregano combines well with it. This recipe is particularly suited to swordfish, but cod, halibut, tuna, or other fish steaks will do.

½ cup (1 stick) butter or margarine
2 cloves garlic, crushed
¼ cup minced fresh parsley or 2 tablespoons dried
2 tablespoons chopped fresh oregano or 2 teaspoons dried
4 fish steaks, about 1 inch thick
2 lemons

Melt the butter and add the garlic and herbs. Place the steaks on a foil-covered broiler pan and brush with the butter mixture. Broil for 5 minutes, turn, baste with more butter, and broil for another 5 minutes. Transfer the fish to a serving dish and keep it warm. Squeeze 1 lemon into the remaining butter and add the fish juice from the pan; simmer until slightly reduced. Pour the sauce over the fish. Garnish with the other lemon, cut into quarters.

Potato-Zucchini Frittata

A satisfying dish, this can be eaten hot or cold as a main dish or as an appetizer.

¼ cup olive oil
1 medium-size potato, peeled and thinly sliced
1 small zucchini, sliced
1 medium-size onion, thinly sliced
4 eggs
¼ cup fines herbes (see recipe page 408) or the same quantity of minced parsley, thyme, and basil combined
¼ teaspoon salt
1 tablespoon butter

Heat the olive oil in a heavy skillet. Over medium-high heat, fry the potatoes until brown on both sides; drain on paper towels. In the same skillet, sauté the zucchini until crisp-tender; remove with a slotted spoon and set aside. Turn the heat to medium-low and cook the onion until soft; remove with a slotted spoon and set aside.

Lightly beat the eggs with a whisk; add the minced herbs and salt. With the burner at medium-high, heat the butter in the skillet with the remaining olive oil. Add the potatoes, then the zucchini and the onions. Pour in the eggs. As the eggs cook, gently lift the sides with a spatula and tilt the pan so that uncooked egg runs underneath. When the eggs are no longer runny on top, hold a plate firmly over the pan and flip the pan over, so that the frittata is on the plate. Slide the frittata back into the pan and cook for another minute. (If you prefer not to flip the frittata, run it under the broiler for a few minutes to brown the top.) Serves 2 as a main dish or 4 as an appetizer.

Vegetables

Potato Casserole With Rosemary

Rosemary gives a delightful appeal to this simple casserole, which makes an ideal accompaniment for roasted meat or poultry, because it can be baked in the oven at the same time.

1 teaspoon salt
½ teaspoon black pepper
3 teaspoons fresh rosemary
  or 2 teaspoons dried
3 medium-size onions, peeled
  and thinly sliced
7 medium-size potatoes, peeled
  and thinly sliced
3 tablespoons melted butter or margarine
1 cup warm milk

Combine the seasonings. Put one-third of the onions on the bottom of a buttered ovenproof casserole. Sprinkle with a pinch of seasonings and drizzle on a little butter. Add one-third of the potatoes followed by more seasonings and butter. Layer the rest of the onions, potatoes, seasonings, and butter in the same way. Pour the milk over all. Bake at 375°F for 1¼ hours. (If you are roasting meat simultaneously at a different temperature, adjust the cooking time of the casserole accordingly.) Serves 6.

Cold Marinated Vegetables With Thyme, Parsley, and Basil

This recipe works well with almost any combination of fresh vegetables.

Marinade
3 cups beef or chicken stock
  (see recipe page 409)
1 cup dry white wine
1 cup vegetable or olive oil
¼ cup fresh lemon juice
¼ cup white vinegar
1 tablespoon chopped fresh thyme
  or 1 teaspoon dried
1 tablespoon chopped fresh basil
  or 2 teaspoons dried
2 tablespoons chopped fresh parsley
  or 1 tablespoon dried
1 teaspoon salt
½ teaspoon freshly ground pepper
Vegetables
2 cups green or yellow (wax) beans
2 sweet green or red peppers
  or 1 of each
1 medium-size yellow squash
1 medium-size zucchini
1 cucumber, sliced
1 cup cherry tomatoes

Combine all marinade ingredients in a heavy saucepan and bring to a boil. Cover and simmer for 30 minutes. Strain the marinade into a large bowl or pitcher. Return it to the pan and bring it again to a simmer.

Meanwhile cut the beans into 2-inch pieces and the peppers into ½-inch-wide strips. Cut the zucchini and yellow squash crosswise into 1-inch slices. Put the beans and peppers into the simmering marinade; cook for 3 minutes, then add the squash. Cook the vegetables until crisp-tender (another 5 to 7 minutes). Transfer them to a shallow bowl; add the cucumber and tomatoes. When the marinade is cool, pour it over the vegetables. Cover and refrigerate overnight. Drain the marinade, reserving a little. Arrange the vegetables on a platter and drizzle a little marinade over them. Serves 8.

Cabbage and Savory

Savory, winter or summer, imparts a peppery flavor that complements many vegetables.

1 medium-size head of cabbage
¼ teaspoon salt
3 tablespoons butter or margarine
3 tablespoons olive oil
2 tablespoons chopped fresh winter or
  summer savory or 2 teaspoons dried
1 clove garlic, crushed
Savory or parsley sprigs for garnish

Quarter and core the cabbage. Discard any discolored or tough outer leaves. Sprinkle the salt over the cabbage and bring it to a boil in about 1 inch of water. Cover and cook until crisp-tender (8 to 10 minutes). While the cabbage is cooking, melt the butter with the olive oil in a heavy saucepan. Add the savory and garlic and simmer for 3 minutes, stirring often. Transfer the cabbage to a warm serving platter. Spoon the sauce over it. Serve garnished with savory or parsley sprigs. Serves 4.

Stuffed Tomatoes With Basil

4 large ripe tomatoes
½ cup soft bread crumbs
¼ cup cubed mozzarella cheese
¼ cup chopped fresh basil
1 clove garlic, crushed
1 tablespoon minced onion
½ teaspoon salt
⅛ teaspoon pepper
5 tablespoons olive oil
2 tablespoons Parmesan cheese

Preheat the oven to 375°F. Halve the tomatoes and spoon their pulp into a bowl. Place the halves, cut side down, on paper towels to dry. Mix the bread crumbs, mozzarella cheese, basil, garlic, onion, salt, pepper, and 4 tablespoons of the oil with the pulp. Arrange the tomatoes, open side up, in a baking dish; fill with the pulp mixture. Sprinkle with Parmesan cheese and drizzle with the remaining oil. Bake for 20 minutes. Serves 4 or 8.

Salads and Salad Dressings

Summer Herb Salad

Here is a flavorful, aromatic salad.

**1½ quarts lettuce leaves—a bland type,
    such as Boston or romaine
¾ cup of the chopped fresh leaves of any
    of the following combinations:
    parsley, chives, basil
    parsley, tarragon, savory
    garden burnet, dill, chervil
8 nasturtium blossoms**

Wash, drain, and pat or spin dry the lettuce. Mix with the herbs. Toss with a favorite dressing. Garnish with nasturtium blossoms. Serves 4.

Sweet-Sour Dandelion Greens

Dandelion leaves are full of vitamins. Search out young plants (flowers should not yet have formed), preferably growing in rich garden soil, as these will be sweeter and more tender than the rugged survivors in your lawn. Make sure they have not been contaminated by chemicals or pets. (Note that seeds are commercially available these days for growing dandelions as a food crop.)

**4 cups young dandelion leaves
4 slices bacon
2 tablespoons sugar
¼ teaspoon powdered mustard
3 tablespoons cider vinegar
Salt and pepper to taste
3 hard-cooked eggs, sliced**

Wash the dandelion leaves thoroughly; pat or spin dry. Fry the bacon until crisp; remove it from the pan. Add the sugar, mustard, and vinegar to the bacon fat. Stir until the sugar is dissolved. Add salt and pepper.

Remove from the heat. Add the dandelion leaves; stir to coat them evenly. Put the leaves in a bowl. Sprinkle with crumbled bacon and decorate with hard-cooked eggs. Serves 4.

Weed and Flower Salad

Many of the plants that we now consider garden weeds were eaten by the first European settlers in America. In fact, many of these weeds were introduced here as a valuable source of food.

**2 cups young dandelion leaves
2 cups combined young leaves from any
    2 or 3 of the following: chickweed,
    chicory, plantain, violet, yarrow
½ cup walnut pieces
1 cup diced cooked chicken
¼ cup canned crushed pineapple
¼ cup plus 2 tablespoons mayonnaise
½ teaspoon pepper
A few violets, nasturtiums, or roses
    for garnish**

Wash the greens; pat or spin dry. Tear them into bite-size pieces and mix them in a large salad bowl. Add the walnuts, chicken, and pineapple; toss. Mix in the mayonnaise and pepper. Decorate each serving with flowers. Serves 4.

This recipe is also good with diced ham and grated cheese substituted for the chicken and pineapple; use an unseasoned oil and vinegar dressing instead of mayonnaise.

Cucumber-Mint Salad

This refreshing salad is of Middle Eastern origin.

**2 cups plain yogurt
2 tablespoons minced fresh mint or
    2 teaspoons dried
2 cloves garlic, crushed
2 large cucumbers, sliced
1 bunch watercress
6 radishes, sliced**

Combine the yogurt with the mint and garlic. Stir in the cucumber slices. Wash the watercress; pat or spin dry. Arrange each serving of cucumbers on a bed of watercress and garnish with the radish slices. Serves 6.

Lovage and Honey Dressing

Lovage has a sweet, celerylike taste that is good with either green or fruit salads.

**¼ cup honey
Juice of 1 lemon
1 cup salad oil
2 tablespoons herb vinegar (see recipe
    page 407), preferably spearmint
¼ cup minced fresh lovage leaves**

Put all ingredients except the lovage in a small mixing bowl or a 1-pint measuring cup. Whisk until blended. Stir in the lovage; spoon over salad greens or fruit. Makes about 1⅓ cups.

Green Goddess Salad Dressing

Parsley and chives give the "green" to this dressing, which can be used on vegetable or seafood salads.

**6 anchovy fillets, drained and minced
3 tablespoons minced fresh chives
    or 3 teaspoons freeze-dried
½ cup minced fresh parsley
    or ¼ cup dried
1 clove garlic, crushed
1 tablespoon lemon juice
3 tablespoons tarragon vinegar
1 cup sour cream
1 cup mayonnaise
⅛ teaspoon pepper**

Whisk together all ingredients until smooth, or mix them in a blender or food processor. Chill before using. Makes approximately 2¼ cups. Will keep in the refrigerator for about 1 week.

413

Sauces

Green Sauce

Serve green sauce with cold fish or meats.

1 tablespoon each chopped parsley,
  chervil, and tarragon
2 tablespoons each minced chives
  and celery
½ teaspoon grated horseradish
½ teaspoon anchovy paste
1 teaspoon dry mustard
1 tablespoon capers
3 tablespoons vinegar
½ cup olive oil

Whisk all ingredients together. Store them in a jar with a nonmetal lid. Makes about ¾ cup. Will keep up to 1 month in the refrigerator.

Aioli

This garlic sauce from the south of France is good with cold seafood, meat, or vegetables.

3 large cloves garlic, crushed
2 egg yolks
½ teaspoon salt
¼ teaspoon pepper
1 tablespoon lemon juice
1 cup olive oil

In a bowl, beat together the garlic, egg yolks, salt, and pepper with a whisk or electric mixer. Continuing to beat, add half the oil a drop or two at a time. The mixture will become thick and glossy. Beat in the remaining oil a tablespoon at a time; then add the lemon juice. Makes approximately 1¼ cups. Will keep about 1 week in the refrigerator.

Pizzaiola Sauce

A pungent combination of herbs transforms tomato sauce into zesty pizzaiola.

1 medium-size onion, chopped
2 tablespoons olive oil
1 bay leaf
1 28-ounce can plum tomatoes,
  chopped, with their juice
1½ tablespoons each chopped fresh
  thyme and oregano or 1½ teaspoons
  each dried
1 teaspoon salt
¼ teaspoon pepper
2 cloves garlic, minced

In a heavy saucepan over medium heat, cook the onion in the oil until translucent. Add the tomatoes, herbs, and seasonings. Bring the sauce to a boil. Reduce the heat, cover, and simmer for 45 minutes, stirring now and then. Shortly before serving, add the garlic and remove the bay leaf. If you want a smooth sauce, puree it in a food mill, blender, or food processor. Pour the sauce over 1 pound cooked pasta or use it for homemade pizza.

Herbed Steak Sauce

2½ cups beef stock (see recipe page 409)
1 small onion, peeled and sliced
1 teaspoon each chopped fresh thyme,
  marjoram, savory, sage, and basil
  or ¼ teaspoon each dried
⅛ teaspoon pepper
4 tablespoons butter or margarine
¼ cup all-purpose flour
1 tablespoon lemon juice
1 tablespoon minced fresh parsley
  or 2 teaspoons dried
Salt to taste

In a covered saucepan, simmer the stock, onion, herbs, and pepper for 15 minutes; strain through cheesecloth. Melt the butter in a saucepan; blend in the flour; cook, stirring, until thickened. Slowly mix in the stock and lemon juice, stirring until thickened. Simmer for 5 minutes. Add the parsley and salt. Makes about 2¼ cups. Serve with steaks or chops.

Pesto

Toss pesto with hot pasta for a first course, mix a small amount of it with a vinegar and oil dressing for salad, or stuff hollowed-out cherry tomatoes with it for a delicious appetizer.

2 cups fresh basil leaves
⅔ cup olive oil
3 cloves garlic, coarsely chopped
½ teaspoon salt
¼ cup pine nuts or chopped walnuts
⅓ cup grated Parmesan cheese
⅓ cup grated Romano cheese

Pack basil leaves loosely in the container of a blender or food processor. Add the oil, garlic, and salt; blend a few seconds at a time at low speed until the leaves are chopped and coated with the oil. Continue to blend at high speed until smooth. Add remaining ingredients; blend for another few seconds. If the paste seems too thick for pasta, add a little more oil. Makes enough sauce for 1 pound of cooked spaghetti.

If you want to freeze pesto, omit the cheese; add it to the thawed mixture before serving.

Sour Cream Sauces

Herbs and sour cream complement each other well. The following are suggestions to get you started. For fewer calories you can substitute plain yogurt for the sour cream.

Dill sauce. Mix 2 tablespoons minced fresh dill and 1 tablespoon mayonnaise with 1 cup sour cream. Add salt and pepper to taste. Use the sauce with cold poached fish, as a dip for raw vegetables, or to top baked potatoes.

Garden burnet sauce. Mix ¼ cup chopped fresh garden burnet with 1 cup sour cream. Serve with cold meat, seafood, or vegetables.

Breads and Stuffing

Herbed Cheese Bread

This is one recipe for which dried herbs are preferable to fresh.

1 cup milk
4 tablespoons (½ stick) butter or margarine
1½ teaspoons salt
1½ tablespoons sugar
1 egg
1½ packages dried yeast
½ cup warm water (105°F to 115°F)
½ cup grated sharp Cheddar cheese
1 teaspoon dried rosemary
1 teaspoon dried thyme
1 teaspoon dried sage
4½ cups all-purpose flour

Heat the milk to the boiling point. Add the butter, salt, and sugar and pour into a large mixing bowl. When lukewarm, beat in the egg. Dissolve the yeast in the warm water; stir it into the milk mixture. Add the grated cheese and herbs, then the flour, 1 cup at a time. As soon as the mixture becomes too heavy to stir, use your hands to mix in the remaining flour.

Transfer the dough to a floured board and knead it until smooth and elastic, about 10 to 15 minutes. Put it into an oiled bowl and turn to coat it with oil; cover the bowl with a damp cloth. Set the dough to rise in a warm, draft-free place (an oven that has been heated for about 1 minute is good) until doubled in bulk, 40 to 60 minutes. Punch it down.

Shape the dough into a loaf and put it in a greased and floured 9- by 5-inch loaf pan. Cover the pan loosely with a cloth and set in a warm place until doubled in bulk, about 40 minutes.

Before the dough finishes rising, preheat the oven to 400°F. Bake the bread for 40 to 50 minutes, or until it sounds hollow when tapped.

Sage-Dill Cornmeal Muffins

The dry ingredients can be mixed and kept in a jar or a can for quick last-minute preparation.

1 cup all-purpose flour
1 cup cornmeal
1 tablespoon baking powder
1 teaspoon baking soda
½ teaspoon salt
4 tablespoons butter or margarine
   (½ stick), melted
1 cup buttermilk
1 tablespoon sugar
2 eggs
2 tablespoons minced fresh sage
   or 2 teaspoons dried
2 tablespoons minced fresh dill
   or 2 teaspoons dried

Preheat oven to 425°F. Butter 12 2½-inch muffin cups. Sift together the flour, cornmeal, baking powder, baking soda, and salt.

In another bowl use a whisk to beat together the butter, buttermilk, sugar, and eggs until smooth. Stir in the sage and dill. Add the liquid ingredients to the dry ones, mixing just until the flour is moistened. Do not overmix.

Fill each muffin cup two-thirds full. Bake for 10 to 12 minutes.

Savory Herbed Biscuits

These are wholesome and flavorful and can be prepared in a matter of minutes.

2 cups all-purpose flour
¾ teaspoon salt
3 teaspoons baking powder
2 tablespoons wheat germ
3 tablespoons minced fresh winter or
   summer savory or 1 tablespoon dried
⅓ cup vegetable oil
⅔ cup milk

Preheat oven to 450°F. Sift the dry ingredients together into a bowl; stir in the savory. Make a well in the center of the dry ingredients. Pour the oil into a measuring cup and add the milk; do not stir. Pour the liquid all at once into the well. Mix with a fork until well blended, then knead the dough with your hands briefly until smooth. Put the dough on an *unfloured* board. Roll it out to ½ inch thick. Cut with a 2-inch round cutter. Place the rounds about 1 inch apart on an ungreased baking sheet. Bake 12 to 15 minutes, until golden brown. Makes 16 biscuits.

Chive-parsley biscuits. Substitute for the savory 1½ tablespoons each minced fresh chives and parsley or 2 teaspoons each dried.
Basil-marjoram biscuits. Substitute for the savory 1 tablespoon each minced fresh basil and marjoram or 2 teaspoons each dried.
Thyme biscuits. Substitute for the savory 3 tablespoons minced fresh thyme or 1 tablespoon dried.

Herbed Bread Stuffing for Poultry

This recipe makes enough stuffing to fill a 4-pound chicken; use multiples for larger birds.

4 tablespoons (½ stick) butter or margarine
1 small onion, minced
2 cups soft bread crumbs
   or dry bread cubes
2 teaspoons each minced fresh
   thyme, sage, and savory
   or ½ teaspoon each dried
2 tablespoons minced fresh parsley
¼ cup chopped walnuts

Melt the butter in a large pan. Cook the onion until translucent. Add the bread, herbs, and nuts; stir until blended. Just before roasting a chicken or turkey, stuff the mixture lightly into the cavities. Or bake the stuffing in a casserole for 45 minutes at 350°F.

Herbs in Drinks and Punches

Minted Lemonade

The cooling zest of mint is the classic antidote to a hot summer day.

Juice of 1 large lemon
Juice of 2 large juice oranges
1 cup apple juice
⅔ cup mint syrup (see recipe page 418)
Mint sprigs for garnish

Combine the juices and mint syrup; shake or stir well. Chill. Pour over ice cubes in glasses and garnish with the mint sprigs. Serves 2.

Herb and Strawberry Punch

This festive punch is ideal for serving at parties with both children and adult guests.

2 cups honey
3 tablespoons fresh rosemary
2 cups lemon juice
1 gallon water
1 pint (1 pound) fresh strawberries
2 cups lime juice
1 1-liter bottle carbonated
    mineral water or seltzer

Heat the honey, rosemary, and ½ cup of the lemon juice in 2 pints of the water. Bring to the boiling point and remove from heat. When lukewarm, strain into a punch bowl. Puree the strawberries. Stir them into the punch bowl. Add a block of ice. Pour in the remaining water, the lemon and lime juices, and the mineral water or seltzer.

Tomato-Cucumber Herb Juice

Use fresh herbs in summer, dried in winter.

1 large cucumber, peeled and sliced
3 sprigs fresh parsley leaves
    or 1 teaspoon dried
12 fresh basil leaves
    or 1 teaspoon dried
1 quart tomato juice
1 10½-ounce can beef consommé
    (undiluted)
2 tablespoons lemon juice
Hot pepper sauce to taste (optional)

Puree the cucumber and herbs with 1 cup of the tomato juice in a blender or food processor. Stir in the remaining tomato juice, the consommé, the lemon juice, and the hot sauce. Serve chilled over ice. Makes 6 7-ounce servings.

Violet Cooler

Make up a batch of violet syrup in the spring and keep it on hand for cool summer drinks. It's also good over ice cream.

Pick enough blossoms of deep purple wild violets to fill a glass jar. Rinse the blossoms in cold water; remove the green stalks and the calyxes. Put the violets in the jar and fill it almost to the brim with boiling water. Cover and leave it to stand overnight.

The next morning strain out the violets. For each cup of liquid add 2 cups granulated sugar and the juice of ½ a lemon. Bring this mixture to a boil. Pour it into a sterile bottle and refrigerate or freeze it. It should keep in the refrigerator for 6 months, but if it starts to ferment, throw it out.

Pour a little syrup over ice in a glass. Add water or carbonated water to taste.

Rose Geranium Wine Cup

This incorporates a variety of fragrant herbs.

12 rose geranium leaves
2 sprigs each sage and lemon verbena
1 short sprig rosemary
2 750-milliliter bottles sweet white wine,
    such as sauternes
1 quart (2 pounds) strawberries, fresh or
    frozen
2 tablespoons honey
1 bottle champagne or
    1 1-liter bottle seltzer

Bruise 4 of the rose geranium leaves and the other herbs in the bottom of a large bowl. Pour the wine over the herbs, cover and leave to steep at room temperature for at least 3 hours. Mash the strawberries and sweeten with honey. (If using sweetened frozen berries, omit the honey.) Chill for ½ hour, then add to the wine mixture. Chill the wine by adding a block of ice or a jug of crushed ice to the center of the bowl. Pour in the champagne or seltzer just before serving. Garnish with remaining rose geranium leaves. Makes about 20 4-ounce servings.

May Wine

This wine punch is traditional for celebrating May Day at European country festivals.

10 to 15 sprigs green-dried* sweet woodruff
    or ⅓ cup dried, packaged sweet woodruff
2 tablespoons superfine sugar
2 750-milliliter bottles sweet white wine,
    preferably a German one,
    such as a Moselle,
    or ½ gallon apple juice
Juice of 1 or 2 lemons
½ pint (½ pound) strawberries
1 bottle champagne or
    1 1-liter bottle seltzer

Steep the sweet woodruff overnight with the sugar in 2 cups of the white wine or apple juice. Strain. Add the rest of the wine or apple juice and lemon juice to taste. Pour over a block of ice in a punch bowl; add the strawberries and the champagne or seltzer.

*To green-dry sweet woodruff, put it in an earthenware or glass jar, covered with a cloth; leave it for 2 days.

Herbal Teas

Many herbs make delicious or beneficial teas. While some taste good brewed alone, others benefit from being blended with another herb or two for a more complex, balanced flavor; see the recipes below for complementary blends. If you do not have a wide variety available from your garden, you will find a good selection at health food stores and supermarkets. And by reading the labels of blends, you can obtain more ideas for creating your own mixtures.

Balm and catnip leaves make bracing afternoon teas; chamomile is a soothing drink late in the evening. Yarrow and peppermint make refreshing, invigorating teas. Horehound tea is ideal in cold weather, especially when a cold is threatening; see pages 434–435 for other good teas to drink for minor ailments. Not to be overlooked, also, are the possibilities of flavoring regular tea with herbs. Several mint, balm, or raspberry leaves added to a cup of black tea can provide a pleasant change of pace.

To obtain the most aromatic and flavorful tea, use pure spring water, if possible, and loose herbs; some of the subtler aromas are lost with tea bags. Most herbs brew well in the dried state; a few are definitely better when freshly picked. Quantities may vary for obtaining full flavor. Let your tastebuds be your guide. Don't try to brew a dark tea: herbal teas tend to be pale in color anyway and are generally better-tasting when on the mild, rather than the strong, side. Strength can also vary according to the amount of oils in the leaves when they were picked. When brewing an unfamiliar herb, start with 2 teaspoons dried or the fresh leaves from 2 or 3 sprigs for each measuring cup of water; allow the tea to steep for a minimum of 5 minutes. If necessary, add more herb. A longer steeping time might also be tried, but with some herbs long steeping releases bitter flavors.

The best way to brew tea is in a teapot made of glass, ceramic, or stainless steel (never aluminum or iron); the same is true for the kettle or pan in which you boil the water. Fill your teapot with hot water to warm it. Meanwhile, bring a kettle of fresh water to the boil (reboiled water has a flat taste). Empty the teapot and put in a measured amount of the herb. Pour in the boiling water, cover the pot, and leave it to steep for the specified time. Stir the brew and taste it. If necessary, allow to steep for another minute or two.

If you like, serve herbal tea with honey or sugar. Strong-flavored teas are even better when sweetened with brown sugar, maple syrup, or molasses. Milk clouds the flavor.

Herbal teas are best drunk in moderation; some can be harmful if consumed in large quantities over a long period. (See the appropriate article in the "Gallery of Medicinal Plants," pages 74–354, for comments on an herb's possible dangers.) When you first try an herbal tea, take just a small quantity to see whether you are sensitive to it.

Below are guidelines for brewing some of the more popular herbal teas. The quantities specified are for 1¼ cups of water, which will yield 2 teacups or one large mug of tea.

Balm. Refreshing in the afternoon. Try blending it with a few lavender flowers or rosemary or spearmint leaves. Pour boiling water over 2 tablespoons fresh or 3 teaspoons dried leaves.

Basil. Spicy and bracing. Pour boiling water over 2 teaspoons dried leaves or about 20 fresh leaves. Steep for 5 minutes.

Catnip. A pleasant afternoon tea. Pour boiling water over 2 teaspoons dried leaves. Steep for 5 minutes. Serve with lemon slices and honey.

Elderberry flower. Sweet and soothing. Pour boiling water over 2 tablespoons chopped fresh flowers. Steep for 5 minutes.

Fennel. Reminiscent of anise and peppermint flavors combined. Pour boiling water over 2 teaspoons dried leaves or 1 tablespoon fresh. Steep for 5 to 10 minutes.

Fenugreek. Slightly bitter but pleasant-tasting; blends well with mint. Pour boiling water over 1 teaspoon dried leaves or 1 tablespoon chopped fresh leaves. Steep for 5 minutes.

Hibiscus. Slightly tart; blends well with and imparts a warm, pinkish color to other teas. Pour boiling water over 1 teaspoon crumbled dried blossoms or 1 tablespoon chopped fresh blossoms. Steep for 10 minutes.

Mint. Invigorating and tangy; blends well with many herbs, including chamomile and balm. Pour boiling water over 2 teaspoons dried or the fresh leaves (at least 2 dozen) from 2 to 3 sprigs. Steep for 5 minutes.

Oswego tea. Sweet and fragrant. Pour boiling water over 2 teaspoons dried leaves. Steep for 5 minutes. Serve with a lemon slice and honey.

Roman chamomile. Delicate and soothing. Delicious blended with regular tea for an iced drink. Pour boiling water over 1 teaspoon dried flowers or 1 tablespoon fresh flowers. Steep for 5 to 10 minutes.

Rose hip (dog rose). Tangy and healthful because of its high vitamin C content; blends well with many herbs. The rose hip is the fruit of the dog rose. It should be picked in the fall, cut into pieces, and dried (see pages 406–407 for drying methods). Bring 1 tablespoon dried hips and 1¼ cups water to a boil. Remove from heat. Steep for 15 minutes.

Spicebush. Satisfying and spicy. Simmer 1 cup leaves, twigs, and bark in 2 cups water for 15 minutes. Sweeten with brown sugar.

Yarrow. An aromatic, tangy tea. Pour boiling water over ½ cup fresh flowers and leaves. Steep for 3 minutes. Serve with honey or sugar.

Desserts

Mint Syrup

Spoon this over fresh fruit or ice cream or use it as the basis for a refreshing summer drink.

½ cup mint leaves
½ cup water
1 cup sugar

Combine ingredients in a saucepan and bring to a boil. Reduce heat to low and cook until thickened (about 5 minutes). Strain, if desired. Makes about ⅔ cup.

Rich Chocolate Mint Cake

Mint adds a refreshing overtone to this rich cake. Serve it plain or iced and decorated with sugared mint leaves (recipe next column).

½ cup (1 stick) butter or margarine
2 cups granulated sugar
4 eggs
4 ounces (4 squares) baking chocolate
1 cup all-purpose flour
½ teaspoon salt
⅔ cup milk
2 teaspoons vanilla extract
1 teaspoon finely crumbled dried mint
1 cup chopped walnuts

Preheat the oven to 375°F. Cream the butter and sugar. Beat in the eggs one at a time. Melt the chocolate over a pan of boiling water; stir it into the butter-egg mixture. Sift the flour with the salt. Add the flour to the chocolate mixture alternately with the milk in small quantities. When the batter is smooth, stir in the vanilla, mint, and walnuts. Pour into an 8-inch-square cake pan. Bake for 50 minutes or until a toothpick inserted into the center comes out clean.

Orange Caramel Custard With Pineapple Sage

This is an easy yet special dessert. To dissolve caramel that remains in the pot after you empty it, fill the pot with water and bring to a boil.

¾ cup plus 2 tablespoons sugar
2 tablespoons water
2 large eggs
2 egg yolks
1½ cups milk
2 tablespoons grated orange rind
2 tablespoons minced pineapple sage
½ teaspoon vanilla

In a small saucepan, cook the water and ½ cup of the sugar over medium heat, stirring until the sugar is dissolved. Use a pastry brush dipped in water to wash down any sugar crystals from the side of the pan. Bring to a boil and cook, swirling the pan rather than stirring, until the sugar becomes a caramel color. Pour the hot caramel into 4 glass custard cups. Tilt the cups to cover the bottom evenly; cool.

Preheat the oven to 325° F. Whisk together the eggs, egg yolks, and remaining sugar. Heat the milk and add it in a stream while whisking the eggs and sugar. Beat in the orange rind, pineapple sage, and vanilla. Fill each cup. Set the cups in a baking pan and fill the pan with enough water to come halfway up the sides of the cups. Bake for 30 minutes or until a knife inserted near the center comes out clean. Cool the cups, then chill for at least 1 hour.

To serve, run a knife around the edge of the cups. Invert a dessert plate over each cup; turn the cup over. The custard and caramel will slide out. Garnish with pineapple sage leaves.

Fritters of Elderberry Flowers

Deep-fried in batter, elderberry blossoms make a light, delicately flavored dessert.

8 to 12 clusters of elderberry flowers
¼ cup flour
1 egg
1½ cups water
Oil for deep frying

Cut off all but a small stub of stalk from each flower cluster. Combine the flour, egg, and water in a blender or food processor or whisk the egg and water gradually into the flour.

In a heavy saucepan, heat oil, sufficient to cover the blossoms, to 375°F. (When the oil is the right temperature, a 1-inch cube of bread will brown in 1 minute.) Dip each cluster into the batter, then slip it carefully into the hot oil. Cook the flowers until golden brown, turning them with a slotted spoon. Remove and drain on paper towels. Serves 4.

Sugared Leaves and Flowers

Coat mint leaves, rose petals, whole borage or violet blossoms, or other edible flowers, and use them to decorate desserts.

1 cup leaves, petals, or blossoms
1 egg white
Superfine granulated sugar

Pick leaves and blossoms early in the day; rinse and dry them thoroughly. Separate rose petals and remove mint leaves from the stems.

Beat the egg white to soft peaks. Dip each leaf, petal, or blossom in the egg, coating it on all sides. Or paint on the egg white with a watercolor brush. Sprinkle the sugar over each piece, coating the surface as completely as possible. Lay the leaves and flowers on wax paper and leave them to dry for a day or two. For faster drying, lay them on a rack atop a cookie sheet. Put them in an oven preheated to 200°F, turn off the heat, and leave the oven door ajar. They should be dry in a couple of hours. Store the sugared items in an airtight container, separated by sheets of wax paper.

Herb Crafts

If you enjoy handicrafts, herbs present many possibilities for attractive and useful products. By following the directions on these pages, you can make dried flower arrangements, wreaths, tussie-mussies, pressed flowers, dyes, pomanders, potpourris, and sachets.

Creations With Dried Herbs

The decorative uses of dried herbs are numerous. To have on hand a variety suitable for drying, try to include in your garden planning some of the more showy herbs. Oswego tea (bergamot), chives, and yarrow, for example, have flowers that are very attractive for dried arrangements. For their leaves, plant bay, rue, lamb's-ears, lavender cotton, sage, and tansy.

To supplement these herbs, you may want to plant in your summer garden some of the everlastings—flowers that retain their true colors when dried. A few examples are cockscomb, larkspur (delphinium), cornflower (bachelor's-button), hydrangea, blue salvia, and strawflower. An excellent filler flower is baby's-breath.

Many wild plants are also excellent for drying. Some of the best are Chinese lantern, foxglove, milkweed, thistle, and teasel for their seedpods, and sea lavender (statice) and goldenrod for their flowers. It is best to wait a while before using seed heads in arrangements, because some release their seeds within a few weeks of becoming ripe.

Do not take endangered or threatened species. If you are not sure about the identification of a plant, select only from extensive stands; always cut stalks rather than uproot the plant.

Gathering and Air-Drying Plants

Gather plants on a dry day, preferably before noon, but after all moisture has dried. Choose flowers that are mature but not fully open (most will open as they dry, but full blooms will tend to fall apart later). Pick grasses and decorative leaves while still green. Take seed heads when brown but not yet weathered.

Strip the foliage from flowers and seed heads. With string or elastic bands, tie them in bunches near the base of their stalks and hang them upside down to dry in a warm, dark, airy place. If using string, fasten it with a slipknot; tighten it every few days as the plants shrink.

If you do not have room to hang flowers, a few, such as yarrow, goldenrod, lavender, and lavender cotton, can be be satisfactorily dried standing upright in containers. To dry grasses, delicate flowers, and leaves, lay them on screens and leave them in a warm, dark place where air can circulate around them.

Wire flowers with short or very thick stalks before drying. Snip off a short stalk close to the head; push thin florist's wire of the desired length through the stalk and flower, bend it to form a hook, then pull it back into the flower until it no longer shows. To wire flowers with thick stalks, snip them off ¾ inch from the head, loop green florist's wire through the stalk, and twist the wire around itself.

Drying Plants With Dessicants and Glycerin

A more complicated method than air-drying, but one particularly suited to thick blossoms, is the use of dessicants. Ground silica-gel crystals, available at florists, hobby shops, and garden centers, can be used, as can borax, perlite, or sand that has been washed and dried.

Put a 2-inch layer of dessicant in an airtight container. Cut off all but 1 or 2 inches of the flower stalks. Lay the flowers in the dessicant—cupped flowers faceup, radial flowers facedown, and sprays flat. Cover them completely with more dessicant. Close the container tightly. Most flowers will be dry within two or three days. When flowers are papery to the touch, attach wires for stalks (see page 421).

Another drying method, especially suited to leaves and grasses, is glycerin absorption. Mix one part glycerin, available at drugstores, with two parts hot water. Crush the ends of the plant stems and stand them in at least six inches of solution. Add water periodically to maintain the original level. When the leaves change color and are pliable and somewhat leathery, remove them from the solution and dry off the ends. The process takes from two to six weeks.

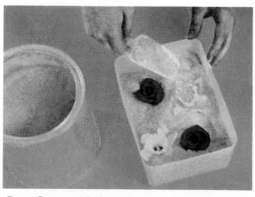

Cover flowers with dessicant and seal the container.

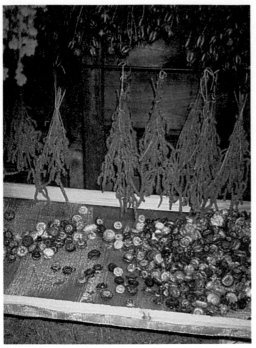

Dry flowers in bunches or on screens individually.

Dried Flower Arrangements

The beauty of a dried flower arrangement is that it can brighten an area too dark for living plants and will last for months or even years.

First decide where the arrangement will stand and select a suitable container. It should have a mouth wide enough to let you insert stems in a variety of positions. Baskets are particularly suitable. To hold the flowers in position buy a dry green foam available at florists. You will also need sharp scissors and a knife, florist's wire in suitable thicknesses, and florist's tape.

From your dried plants, choose two or three complementary colors or a range of tones of one hue. The colors should not only work well together but look good in the room where the

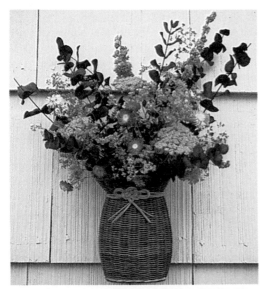

Dried flowers are a year-round treat for the eyes.

arrangement will stand. If in doubt about any particular color or material, leave it out.

Decide which large or clustered flowers or seed heads will form the main part of the design and which other flowers and leaves will fill it out. Try to include a variety of textures from fluffy to flat, globular to spiky. You will need more material than you would normally use for a fresh arrangement.

Before starting, weight your container with pebbles or sand so that it cannot be knocked over easily. Cut the foam to fit the top of the container snugly and push it into place. If necessary, use modeling clay to anchor the foam, or stabilize it with strips of florist's tape. Cover it with moss, if desired.

For a traditional balanced arrangement, start by placing three large stems to mark the height and width of the final shape, then fill it out with a variety of textures and colors within the range you have chosen. For the sides and front choose sprays or flowers that will curve or trail over to give a soft, natural appearance.

Wreaths of Leaves and Flowers

Wreaths of dried leaves and flowers make attractive decorations not only for holidays but the year round. Before starting a wreath, plan where you will hang it and what colors and materials will look best in that location.

For a foundation, buy a straw wreath from a

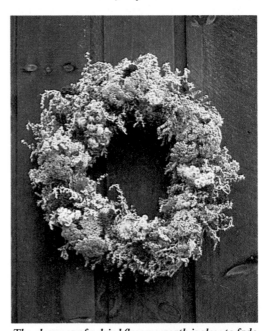

The elegance of a dried flower wreath is slow to fade.

florist or nursery. You will also need four to six dozen fern pins, three to four dozen floral picks, 18- and 20-gauge florist's wire, florist's tape, wire cutters, and scissors.

Select background material to cover the base. Goldenrod, southernwood, sea lavender, or knotweed would be a good choice. You will need a substantial amount of it. Make clusters of three to five stems; cut off all but about 2

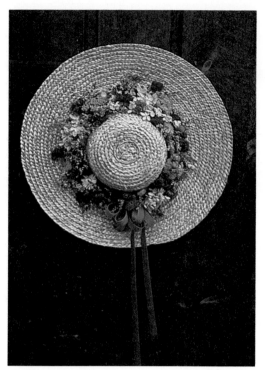

Flower clusters, glued to the crown, adorn a straw hat.

inches of the stems and wrap each cluster with wire. Before you start to cover the straw, wrap a double length of wire around it and make a loop by which to hang it later.

Starting on the inside edge of the frame, attach a background cluster with a fern pin. Attach the next cluster so that the stems of the first one are covered. Work around the wreath in this fashion, laying all clusters in the same direction. At the starting point, tuck the stems of the last bunch under the first one. Next, cover the face of the wreath, and finally the outside. Then you are ready to add such accent materials as flowers and seed heads, preparing them first with wires or florist's picks.

To attach wire to the stems, cut off all but 2 inches; lay a 6-inch length of wire next to the stem and wrap both with florist's tape.

To attach a florist's pick, use the same method as for wire, but cut the stem to 1 inch.

Arrange your accent materials around the wreath in a balanced design. To provide a focal point, group some in one spot at the bottom, top, or one side. When you are satisfied with the arrangement, insert the picks or wires of the accent plants carefully into the background material so that they are hidden. Finally, spray the wreath lightly with a clear floral fixative.

A wreath will stay fresh-looking for a longer time if you hang it where it will not be touched by direct sunlight, wind, or moisture.

Pressed Herbs

Pressed herbs make delightful decorations for greeting cards and stationery, or they can be arranged to make an attractive framed picture.

And nothing could be simpler to do. The leaves and flowers of many herbs are suitable: broom, fennel, lavender, maidenhair fern, thyme, and yarrow, to name a few. Many of these are fragrant as well as picturesque. In fact, the only plants that are not convenient for pressing are those with very fleshy leaves or very thick flowers. Even these can be pressed, however, if the petals are arranged separately.

The materials needed are wax paper, blotting paper, and heavy books. If you do much pressing, you may want to buy a press, or construct one like that described on pages 29–30.

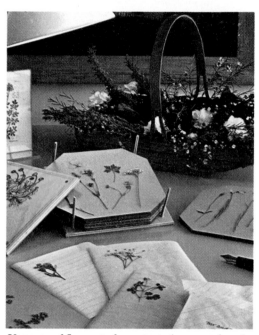

Use pressed flowers to decorate stationery and cards.

The basic technique is to gather the plants and press them as soon as possible. Put delicate sprays and flowers between two layers of wax paper, heavier ones between layers of blotting paper. Arrange sprays so that they are attractively, yet naturally, curved. Make sure that none of the plants are touching. Weight each layer with books or between cardboard sections of a press. Thin plants can be pressed satisfactorily between the pages of a heavy book. It takes two to four weeks for plants to dry thoroughly. The longer you leave them, the less they will fade when exposed to light. Drying too long, however, can result in brittleness.

If any of the plants are very moist, check them after a few days. You may have to replace the blotting paper with fresh sheets.

When the plants are sufficiently dry, you can store them for future use by putting them in transparent envelopes, available where photographic supplies are sold.

To attach your pressed plants to stationery or greeting cards, or to make a picture for framing, first mix white glue with a little water. Arrange your designs, then gently apply a little glue to the back of each plant with a watercolor brush and press the plant in place.

Tussie-mussies

A tussie-mussie is a small bouquet made with fresh or dried flowers. It makes a lovely gift or, placed upright in a small vase, a charming decoration. Making one is easy. Start with one perfect flower for the center, surround it with small-leaved sprays or tiny flowers or both, and then slip the stems through a doily or gather some starched lace around them at the base of the bouquet. If the flowers are fresh, wrap the stems with damp paper towels or wet absorbent cotton and a layer of foil. Wrap dried flower stems with floral tape.

Long ago tussie-mussies were carried to ward off bad smells and disease. In particular, rosemary, southernwood, thyme, and lavender were thought to be effective for this purpose. During Victorian times, tussie-mussies became part of the practice of sending flowers to convey certain sentiments. The list at the bottom of the page includes some of the old flower meanings. If you would like a tussie-mussie gift to communicate special sentiments, make it with one or more herbs selected from these lists. Be sure to attach a card explaining the significance of each herb.

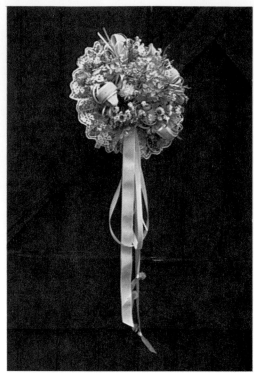

A tussie-mussie is just right for a special occasion.

The Language of Flowers

In 18th-century Turkey, as an English visitor observed, "you may quarrel, reproach, or send letters of passion, friendship, or civility, or even of news, without ever inking your fingers." The Turks' code was to use flowers and other objects as expressions of one's feelings. Every item—whether flower, fruit, feather, or piece of thread—had a meaning, and a properly constructed "letter" could express almost any combination of sentiments.

Such an intriguing custom soon traveled to France, where a Charlotte de La Tour—a pseudonym—devised a language composed entirely of floral symbols that was published in 1819 as *Le Langage des Fleurs*. This little handbook became a favorite reference on the subject. The new floral language appealed to the Romantic poets in England. "Sweet flowers alone can say what passion fears revealing," noted the poet Thomas Hood (1799–1845) in his poem "The Language of Flowers."

In Victorian times, the language of flowers became more complicated. Not only did flowers signify different feelings or conditions, but also the manner in which the flowers were offered and accepted could mean something. A single red rose in full bloom was a token of admiration for feminine beauty. But a rosebud offered with its thorns and leaves conveyed: "I fear, but I hope." If the recipient replied by coyly turning the bud upside down, the gesture implied, "You must neither fear nor hope." If the young lady receiving the flower placed it in her hair, her response signified caution, but if she put the blossom on her heart, the act implied love returned.

Flower	Meaning
Aloe	grief
Angelica	inspiration
Belladonna	silence
Broom	humility
Celandine	joys to come
Chickweed	rendezvous
Fennel	strength
Forget-me-not	true love
Foxglove	insincerity
Garden heliotrope	devotion
Hawthorn	hope
Hibiscus	delicate beauty

Flower	Meaning
Lady's-slipper	fickleness
Lavender	distrust
Lily of the valley	return of happiness
Maidenhair fern	discretion
Motherwort	secret love
Mugwort	happiness
Pansy	thoughts
Passionflower	belief
Raspberry	remorse
Red poppy	consolation
Sweet violet	modesty
Wood sorrel	joy

Mail-Order Suppliers of Herb Products

Many of the sources listed below carry a wide range of products. Others are more specialized. To find out what a supplier offers, write for a catalog; there may be a charge for it.

Preserved Herbs and Herb Derivatives

Aphrodisia Products, Inc.
282 Bleeker Street
New York, NY 10014

Caswell-Massey Co. Ltd.
Catalogue Division
111 Eighth Avenue
New York, NY 10011

Haussmann's Pharmacy
534 West Girard Avenue
Philadelphia, PA 19123

Indiana Botanic Gardens, Inc.
P.O. Box 5
Hammond, IN 46325

Nature's Herb Co.
281 Ellis Street
San Francisco, CA 94102

Penn Herb Co.
603 North Second Street
Philadelphia, PA 19123

To find herb suppliers near you, look in the yellow pages under "Herbs" and "Health Food." You can also send for *Herb Buyers' Guide* and other herbal publications, available for a small charge from:
Herb Society of America
2 Independence Court
Concord, MA 01742

Seeds and Plants

Carroll Gardens
P.O. Box 310
Westminster, MD 21157

Comstock, Ferre & Co.
263 Main Street
Wethersfield, CT 06109

Epicure Seed Ltd.
P.O. Box 450
Brewster, NY 10509

Meadowbrook Herb Garden
Route 138
Wyoming, RI 02898

Merry Gardens
P.O. Box 595
Camden, ME 04843

George W. Park Seed Co. Inc.
Greenwood, SC 29646

Wayside Garden Co.
Hodges, SC 29695

Nichols Garden Nursery
1190 North Pacific Highway
Albany, OR 97321

Rutland of Kentucky
P.O. Box 182
Washington, KY 41096

Sunnybrook Farms Nursery
9448 Mayfield Road
Chesterland, OH 44026

Taylor's Herb Garden, Inc.
1535 Lone Oak Road
Vista, CA 92083

Well-Sweep Herb Farm
317 Mount Bethel Road
Port Murray, NJ 07865

Any store with a good selection of vegetable and flower seeds is likely to carry seeds for the more popular herbs as well. The major seed companies also offer a variety of common herbs in their catalogs.

Chemical Supplies

Handweavers Guild of America, Inc.
65 LaSalle Road
West Hartford, CT 06107
(They do not sell supplies, but publish *Shuttle, Spindle & Dyepot*, which has information on equipment for dyers, spinners, and weavers.) Also consult the *OPD Chemical Buyers Directory*, available at many local libraries. It may lead you to a chemical supply house in your area that sells small, retail quantities.

Scented Goods

Whether intended to ward off illness and bad odors, to keep away pesty insects, or simply to make a person or place smell nice, scented goods have long been associated with the herbalist's craft. The best known of these scented items are toilet waters. They are easy to make if you use essential flower oils and mix them with an inexpensive, domestic vodka, the closest thing to plain, unadulterated grain alcohol that is widely available. Indeed, you can make a simple toilet water with any essential flower oil by blending about a tablespoon of the oil with a cup of vodka. Allow the mixture to mature for a month or two before using it.

Although they require a moderate investment of time, potpourris, sachets, and pomanders are also easy to make.

A *potpourri* is a mixture of preserved flower petals and other aromatic plant parts that you can use to give a room a delightful floral fragrance.

A *sachet* is a similar mixture, crushed and put into a small sack.

A *pomander* was originally a pierced silver or gold ball or a perforated box filled with herbs and spices. Nowadays it is usually a citrus fruit stuck with cloves and coated with ground spices.

Potpourris and Sachets

The chief ingredient of a potpourri is rose petals. Roses are one of the few flowers that retain most of their fragrance after they are dried. Ideally, the petals should come from the older red or pink species, such as damask and cabbage roses; they have a richly perfumed odor that tends to be missing in modern hybrids. *Rosa gallica* varieties retain both their color and scent well.

Lavender, tuberose, and rose geraniums also have a lasting fragrance. Any of them can add an interesting overtone to a rose-based potpourri or to a sachet or can be a mixture's main ingredient. Petals from other pleasantly scented flowers can contribute to a potpourri's or sachet's fragrant bouquet. You can also include less fragrant flowers simply to add bulk and color. The fixative, normally added to help retain fragrance, also adds it own distinctive odor. The fixative in these recipes is orrisroot, the violet-scented root of white iris; you can buy it from perfumers and specialty pharmacies.

Besides flowers, potpourris and sachets often include some other strongly aromatic plant ingredients, such as dried citrus peel, cloves, cinnamon bark, bay leaves, vanilla bean, rosemary, and allspice. Both spicy items and fixative should be added with restraint, since they can easily overwhelm the fragrance from the flowers.

What Kind of Potpourri?

You can make two kinds of potpourris: moist or dry. To produce a moist potpourri, you layer the flower petals and other plant materials with salt and let the mixture sit until it ferments. This is the way that potpourris were first made. Indeed, the original French name *pot-pourri* translates literally as "rotten pot." A moist potpourri produces a strong, enduring fragrance, which can last for years if the potpourri is used sparingly and kept tightly covered at other times. Because of its generally uninviting appearance, a moist potpourri is kept in an opaque container. It usually has two covers: a perforated one to release the scent and a second, solid cover to conserve the scent. However, you can use any china or crockery container that can be closed tightly.

Today, dry potpourris are more common. They are easier to prepare and emit a subtler scent.

Picking and Drying Flowers

Pick flowers in the morning after the dew has dried. Work on a sunny day, preferably at least three days since the last rain. Avoid flowers that are past their prime.

Petals for a dry potpourri or for sachets should be dried until they are crisp. Select a spot that is warm, dry, and out of direct sunlight. Spread the petals in a single layer on newspapers or on a window screen made of fiberglass or some other nonmetallic mesh. If the petals tend to blow away, cover them with a fine cheesecloth weighted along the edges. Shift the petals every couple of days to hasten drying. It can take up to two weeks for the flowers to dry completely. If you dry a small amount of petals at a time, store them in a tightly sealed jar until you have enough to make the potpourri or sachets. For a moist potpourri, dry the petals just until leathery.

A Basic Dry Potpourri

Use a container that you can seal tightly. The potpourri should fill it only about halfway.

1 quart dried rose petals
2–4 cups dried petals from other
** fragrant flowers**
2–3 tablespoons ground orrisroot
2–3 tablespoons well-crushed spices
** (cloves, cinnamon, for example)**
2–3 tablespoons crushed aromatic leaves
** (rosemary, bay leaf, for example)**
1–2 tablespoons grated citrus peel
** (optional)**
6–10 drops aromatic oil (good choices
** include rose, lilac, patchouli, jasmine,**
** tuberose, rosemary, and neroli)**

Put the dried flower petals in a large jar and

carefully mix them together. Then gently mix in the orrisroot, spices, aromatic leaves, and citrus peel. Finally, sprinkle the aromatic oil on top and seal the jar tightly. Let the mixture stand in a dark place for 6 weeks or so to allow the odors to blend and mellow. Agitate the mixture every 3 or 4 days by gently shaking it and turning it from side to side. Divide the mixture into smaller glass containers that you can set around the house. Keep them covered when they are not in use.

To make sachets, crush the mixture. Place a small amount in a frilly handkerchief tied with a ribbon. Or sew up some bags using tightly woven fabric, preferably a natural type, such as cotton, silk, or linen. If you like, add embroidery, appliqué, or lace edging. Slip sachets into pockets, attach them to hangers, or put them between layers in a drawer.

A Basic Moist Potpourri

You can add flower petals a batch at a time.

**Same ingredients as a dry potpourri
(see previous recipe)
2 cups or so noniodized salt**

Spread a layer of mixed flower petals on the bottom of a large, wide-mouthed crock. Sprinkle a couple of tablespoons of salt over them. Continue to alternate layers of petals and salt until you use up the batch. Then put a weighted plate on top to compress the petals. Whenever you add a new batch, stir the petals with a wooden spoon, breaking up any crust that has formed. Then layer the new petals with salt and cover again with the plate. If a dark liquid forms as the petals ferment, just stir it back in. After adding the last batch, let the mixture stand for at least 2 weeks to harden into a cake. Then break up the cake into small pieces and add the orrisroot, spices, aromatic leaves, citrus peel, and oils. Stir everything together thoroughly. Cover this mixture with the plate and let it mature for another 2 weeks or longer. The longer the potpourri stands, the stronger and more mellow the scent it provides.

Moth-Repellent Sachets

In this recipe, you can use either a single herb or a mix of them, depending on availability. A sachet of rue is reputed to keep fleas out of a dog's bed. Dry plants for sachets in the same way as flowers for dry potpourri, described on the preceding page.

**6 ounces dried insect-repelling herbs
(lavender, southernwood, tansy,
wormwood, rue, lavender cotton,
costmary, rosemary, most mints)
½ ounce ground orrisroot
½ ounce ground spice (cloves,
cinnamon, coriander)**

Grind the dried herbs almost to a powder in a blender or food processor or with a mortar and

pestle. Then mix in the orrisroot and spice. Before putting the mixture into bags, store it in a sealed jar for a day or two to let any liquid be reabsorbed and to let the scents blend.

A Spicy Pomander

The key to making a successful pomander is letting the fruit dry slowly in a dry, warm place. If it dries too quickly, the outer part will harden, leaving the inside to decay. If it is exposed to excess heat or humidity, it may mildew. During drying, the fruit will shrink to almost half its original size. Although the recipe calls for an orange, a lemon can be made into a pomander in the same way; just use narrower tape and ribbon.

**1 unblemished orange, preferably
thin-skinned
Plastic tape, ½ inch wide
2 ounces whole cloves
2 ounces mixed ground cinnamon,
nutmeg, and allspice
2 ounces orrisroot
1 yard ribbon, ½ inch wide**

Roll the fruit in your hands for a couple of minutes to soften the skin. Wrap tape around it, dividing it in half; then wrap a second piece around it, dividing it in quarters. Working in rows, insert whole cloves in the fruit except for the taped areas. If the skin is tough, make holes first with a toothpick or a large needle. To allow for shrinkage as the fruit dries, leave a space equal to one head between cloves.

Mix the ground spices with the orrisroot; then put them in a small box lined with tissue paper and roll the fruit in them. Cover the box and let the fruit dry for 4 to 6 weeks in a warm (not hot), dry place. When you remove the pomander, shake off the excess spice mixture. Then remove the tape and replace it with the ribbon. For hanging, attach a loop or a hook.

Florida Water

Variations of this citrus-scented toilet water have been popular for over a hundred years.

**½ teaspoon oil of lavender
½ teaspoon oil of lemon
1 teaspoon oil of jasmine
1½ teaspoons oil of bergamot
2 drops each oils of cloves, cinnamon,
and neroli
1 teaspoon tincture of musk
1⅓ cups vodka
2 tablespoons plus 2 teaspoons rose water**

Blend the oils and tincture of musk thoroughly into ¼ cup of the vodka. Slowly add the rest of the vodka and the rose water, stirring all the while. Pour the mixture into a bottle and cap tightly. Let it stand for a month or two to mature. Shake well every 3 or 4 days. If it becomes cloudy, strain it through a coffee filter in a funnel until it is clear.

Making Natural Dyes

Extracting and using the dye colors available in plants is a bit of work, but rewarding if you are partial to lovely, subtle, and varied colors.

In natural dyeing, many conditions affect the results: the maturity of the plants, the time of year when they are harvested, the kind of mordant (color fixative) used, and the type of material being dyed; it can be impossible to duplicate a color exactly for a second batch.

The water that is used can also affect dye color. Best results are obtained with soft water. If your tap water is hard (you can check with your utility or have it tested), add commercial softener before using it to mordant or dye.

Basic equipment for dyeing should include at least one enamel or stainless steel pot (other metals will affect the dye color) with a minimum capacity of 5 gallons; a glass, stainless steel, or wooden stirrer; a strainer; some cheesecloth; and rubber gloves. A kitchen scale is also useful for weighing dye materials and mordants when recipes are given in ounces.

Only natural fibers—wool, silk, linen, and cotton—will take natural dyes. Wool, especially yarn, is the easiest to work with; all instructions on these pages are for dyeing wool. (One pound of knitting worsted makes a large-size child's or a small-size woman's sweater.) It is better to have some experience before attempting to dye cotton, linen, or silk.

Preparing the Material To Be Dyed

For a dye to penetrate evenly, all finishes and oils must first be removed from the fiber by scouring. Undyed wool yarn may already have been scoured (inquire at the time of purchase); other yarns and fabrics you will have to scour yourself. Before treating yarn, wind it into circular skeins of 2 to 4 ounces each. You can do this by winding it around a chair back or your hand and elbow. Tie each circle in three or four places to keep it from tangling.

To scour 1 pound of wool, put 3 to 4 gallons of soft water in your large pot and add enough mild soap or detergent to form suds. Put in the wool, bring the water slowly to a simmer, and leave the wool in the simmering water for at least 45 minutes. Allow the soapy water to cool, then rinse the wool thoroughly. If you are not going to mordant or dye the scoured material right away, spin it dry in a washing machine, then hang it to dry.

To make natural dye permanent, a mordant is needed. The ones most commonly used are called by dyers alum (potassium aluminum sulfate), chrome (potassium dichromate), tin (stannous chloride), copperas (iron sulfate), and blue vitriol (copper sulfate). Sometimes cream of tartar is combined with a mordant.

Alum has little effect on colors; chrome, used mostly with yellows, mellows them. Tin brightens colors; copperas dulls them (it is often applied after dyeing material treated previously with another mordant). Blue vitriol, used with greens, will intensify them.

Alum is the most popular mordant; it is less expensive and easier to use than the others. Mordants are available at some drugstores, craft stores, and chemical supply houses. Their purity and prices vary. Technical grades, in powdered or granular form, are adequate.

Mordant chemicals are poisonous: never apply them in a utensil used for cooking; use them in a well-ventilated area and cover the pot; store them well out of the reach of children.

Mordant is applied before, during, or after the dye bath, but most often before. To mordant 1 pound of scoured wool with alum, dissolve 4 ounces in a little hot water, then stir it into 4 gallons of soft water. Put in the yarn or fabric, which has already been soaked for at least 30 minutes in warm water, and gradually bring the water to a simmer. Leave the wool completely submerged in the water for 1 hour. Let it cool, then rinse and dye it. Follow the same procedure to mordant with other chemicals but use these quantities in 4 gallons of water: **chrome,** ½ ounce; **tin,** 4 ounces; **copperas,** ½ ounce; **blue vitriol,** 1 ounce.

Preparing the Dye

In general, fresh materials yield the strongest dyes. However, because large quantities are needed for most projects, you may want to dry or freeze some materials for future use. A dye source such as onion skins can be saved in the refrigerator over a period of several months; leaves and twigs can be dried on screens in a warm, dark, airy place; berries can be frozen.

For best results, pick stalks, twigs, and leaves when they are mature, flowers at their prime, and berries fully ripe. Plan on about 1 pint of leaves and stalks or flowers, or ½ to 1 ounce of roots, for each ounce of fabric or yarn to be dyed. Chop up flowers and leaves. Cut twigs, stalks, and roots into pieces and soak any tough or woody parts overnight. Break bark into pieces; soak it for several days.

To extract the color, cook the plants in soft water—fresh leaves, stems, and flowers for about 30 minutes, dried or tougher materials for an hour or more. For easy removal, tie the plants in cheesecloth; otherwise strain the cooked material. After removing the plants, add enough water to the dye bath to cover the wool, generally 4 gallons for 1 pound.

Dyeing the Wool

If you dried the yarn or fabric after mordanting, soak it in warm water until it is thoroughly wetted, then immerse it in the dye. Gently push the material around to facilitate even penetration of the dye, and slowly bring the liquid to a simmer. When most of the color has been absorbed from the water, usually in 30 minutes to 1 hour, lift the yarn or fabric from the dye and submerge it in rinse water that is only a few degrees cooler than the dye bath. Continue to rinse it in gradually cooler water, until no more color washes out. Or let it cool in the dye bath, then rinse it in cool water.

Plants Suitable for Making Dyes

Almost any plant material, when boiled, will yield some type of dye, but the plants listed below are rich sources. Each is accompanied by an approximation of the color it can be expected to yield if used with the designated mordant. These plants can be found in the "Gallery of Medicinal Plants," pages 74–354, in "Growing Herbs," pages 396–398, or both.

Dye Sources and Mordants

Plant	Part Used	Mordant	Color
Agrimony	leaves and stalks	alum	
Alkanet	roots	none	
Bloodroot	roots	alum	
Broom	flowers	alum	
Celandine	flowers	alum	
Comfrey	leaves	tin	
Comfrey	leaves	chrome	
Dandelion	flowers	tin	
Dandelion	roots	alum	
Elderberry	berries	alum	
Elderberry	berries	tin	
Fenugreek	seeds	alum	
Goldenrod	flowers	alum	
Heather	tips	alum	
Hyssop	leaves	alum	
Lily of the valley	leaves and stalks	alum	
Lily of the valley	leaves and stalks	chrome	
Mullein	leaves and stalks	alum	
Onion (yellow)	skins	alum	
Onion (red)	skins	tin	
Parsley	leaves	alum	
Privet	leaves and twigs	chrome	
Queen Anne's lace	flowers and stalks	alum	
Smartweed	entire plant except roots	alum	
Stinging nettle	entire plant except roots	alum	
Tansy	flowers	alum	
Yarrow	flowers	alum	

Herbs for Beauty

Herbs have been used as beauty aids throughout recorded history. Ancient Egyptians employed plant extracts to outline their eyes, to redden their lips and cheeks, and to anoint and perfume their bodies. Romans applied herbal face packs and soaked in flower-scented baths. The basic recipe for cold cream dates to the Greek physician Galen in the second century A.D. Indeed, until mass-produced cosmetics became widespread in this century, most beauty products were concocted at home from herbs and other natural ingredients. The art of making beauty preparations in the kitchen is far from dead. Many people still prefer to make their own, both to save money and to have the assurance that the ingredients they are using are natural and pure. The chief advantage of making beauty preparations yourself, however, is that you can experiment with ingredients to find the combinations that work best on your skin and hair or to find the fragrances that are most agreeable to you.

The recipes given here and on the following pages cover facials, skin lotions, shampoos, conditioners, rinses, scented baths, and herbal soaps. All of the ingredients are widely available. Many are sold at drugstores or supermarkets. The rest can be obtained from a specialty druggist or a well-stocked herbal store. (See page 423 for mail-order sources.) Nearly all of the recipes can be prepared in a short time. A few do need to be prepared ahead and allowed to stand so that the herbs can surrender their essences. In making any of these recipes, keep in mind that they are only starting points. Feel free to change the ratio of the ingredients and to substitute other herbs in much the same way as you would modify a dish you are cooking to suit your taste. There are many other possible variations besides the ones suggested.

When making any beauty preparation, use utensils and containers that are thoroughly clean. Most preparations that you make yourself will not keep as long as cosmetics off the shelf. Lotions and creams made from essential oils and other distilled herbal essences will generally last several weeks, especially if they are kept in the refrigerator. Vinegars and soaps will keep much longer. Any facial, shampoo, rinse, or other preparation made with an herbal tea or decoction should be thrown out if not used up after three or four days.

If you suffer from hay fever or other plant allergies, it is a good idea to test a preparation before using it. Put a small amount on the inside of your forearm; wait 24 hours to see if you get a reaction.

Herbal Face and Skin Care

Herbal ingredients can do much to help your skin to look and feel better. As the recipes on this and the facing page show, you can use ingredients derived from plants to produce bracing astringents, soothing emollient lotions and creams, and deep-cleaning masks and steam facials. But remember that the health of your skin depends on a number of factors—age, diet, heredity, stress, exercise, and sleeping habits as well as environmental influences such as humidity and sun exposure.

Sage Astringent

This can be especially refreshing if kept in the refrigerator and applied while cold. Tincture of benzoin, a preservative, is sold by specialty druggists. This preparation is for external use only and should not be taken internally.

½ **cup dried sage**
½ **cup vodka**
4–5 **drops tincture of benzoin**

Put half the sage in a jar and pour the vodka over it. Cap the jar tightly and let it stand for a week. Strain, reserving the liquid and discarding the sage. Put the rest of the sage in the jar, add the liquid, and let it stand for another week. The liquid should have a strong herbal odor. If you would like it to be stronger, repeat the process, using another ¼ cup sage. Strain the astringent into a clean bottle, using a fine filter, such as a coffee filter. Add the tincture of benzoin, cap the bottle tightly, and shake well.

This astringent is even better made with fresh sage. Use about ½ cup, loosely packed, each time you fill the jar.

A milder astringent. Dilute with distilled water or substitute a less astringent herb, such as chamomile.

A more bracing astringent. Add from 2 to 4 tablespoons of witch hazel extract or substitute a more astringent herb, such as yarrow.

Rose Water–Glycerin Lotion

Quite likely a favorite of your grandmother, this traditional mix makes an effective basic moisturizer and hand lotion. A version is sold at any drugstore, but if you make your own, you can vary the proportions to suit your skin and its seasonally changing condition.

½ **cup rose water**
¼ **cup glycerin**

Use prepared rose water or make it by adding 1 teaspoon soluble rose oil to ½ cup distilled water. Blend the rose water with the glycerin until you have a smooth, creamy mixture. Pour it into a clean bottle and cap.

A thinner lotion, for oily skin. Mix ⅔ cup rose water with 2 tablespoons glycerin.

A thicker lotion, for dry skin. Mix ⅓ cup rose water with ⅓ cup or more glycerin.

Rose water–glycerin gel. Dissolve 1 teaspoon plain gelatin in ½ cup hot water; blend in 1 teaspoon oil of rose and 3 tablespoons glycerin.

Aloe Vera Cold Cream

Aloe adds an interesting texture to this traditional cleansing and moisturizing cream. An 18-century-old formula calls for expensive oil of roses, but olive oil and rose water make a good, moderate-priced substitute. Anhydrous (waterless) lanolin is available from specialty druggists. Beeswax can be found where sewing notions are sold. Pick a favorite essential oil for scent: oil of rose or lavender will heighten the cream's floral fragrance; oil of eucalyptus or peppermint will give it a refreshing, healthful smell.

  1 tablespoon aloe vera gel
  ⅓ cup olive oil
  1 tablespoon white beeswax
  2 tablespoons anhydrous lanolin
  2 tablespoons rose water
  2–3 drops essential oil (rose,
      lavender, eucalyptus, peppermint)

Use a wire whip or a blender to mix the aloe gel thoroughly into the oil. Set the mixture aside. Melt the beeswax with the lanolin in the top of a double boiler. Slowly stir in the oil mixture. Then remove the pan from the heat and stir in the rose water and the essential oil. Keep stirring as the mixture cools and thickens. Just before it begins to solidify, pour it into a jar with a screw-on lid.

An Herbal Steam Facial

Steaming moisturizes the skin, cleans out the pores, and increases the surface blood flow. Herbs can make it both more stimulating and soothing. For the ingredients below you can substitute other aromatic or astringent plants, such as dried sage and yarrow leaves, lavender flowers, and fresh or dried parsley. Make herbal steam baths in a large bowl instead of the sink; the herbs can clog the sink's drain.

  1 tablespoon fennel seeds
  1 tablespoon dried peppermint
      or dried spearmint
  2 tablespoons dried chamomile flowers
  1 tablespoon dried elderberry flowers
  2 teaspoons powdered licorice root
  1 quart boiling water

Crush the fennel seeds with a spoon. Then put them together with the other herbs in a large heat-proof bowl, and pour the water over them. Put your face over the bowl and cover your head with a towel, forming a tent. Keep your face about 12 inches from the water.

Steam for 5 to 10 minutes. Then pat your face dry and apply a moisturizing cream to keep the absorbed moisture from evaporating.

An Oatmeal Face Mask

This recipe combines two ingredients—oatmeal and almonds—traditionally regarded as deep-cleansing agents that are highly beneficial to the complexion. You can use prepared almond meal or you can make it by grinding almonds to a fine powder in a blender or food processor. For a smoother-textured mask, substitute the special colloidal oatmeal sold at the drugstore. Refrigerate the leftover infusion and use it as a face wash.

  ½ cup boiling water
  1 teaspoon dried rosemary leaves
  1½ tablespoons regular oatmeal
  1 tablespoon almond meal

Pour the boiling water over the rosemary, steep for 15 minutes, and strain. In a separate bowl, crumble the dried oatmeal with your fingers; then mix in the almond meal. Add just enough of the rosemary infusion to make a thick paste. To use the mask, first wash your face and steam it or apply a warm, wet washcloth for a few minutes. Gently spread the paste on your face, avoiding the eyes and lips. Leave the mask on for 15 to 30 minutes, letting it dry completely. Wash it off with a soft cloth soaked in lukewarm water.

An astringent mask. For oily skin, substitute an astringent, tannin-rich herb such as agrimony, lady's-mantle, raspberry leaf, or yarrow for the rosemary.

A stimulating mask. Instead of rosemary, use peppermint, elderberry flower, eucalyptus leaf, or some other herb that has an invigorating effect on the skin.

A smoothing mask. To help soften rough, dry skin, heat 1 or 2 teaspoons flaxseed, kelp, or another mucilage-rich herb in water until it thickens. Then add it to the oatmeal-almond mixture instead of the rosemary infusion. Dampen the dry mixture with a little water first. Aloe vera gel can also be substituted.

A richer mask. For dry skin, substitute an egg yolk mixed with ¼ cup honey for the rosemary infusion. If the mask is too thick to apply easily, add a little milk or yogurt.

Papaya Skin Treatment

The enzyme in papaya (a fruit that resembles a melon) helps remove dried flaky skin. Do not leave the papaya on your face too long, since it also tends to dry the skin.

  1 wedge of papaya fruit

Cut a wedge from a ripe fruit and save the rest to eat. Scrape off the seeds. Scoop out the fruit pulp and mash it. Smooth the pulp over your face. After a couple of minutes, wipe it off with a washcloth. Splash your face with cool water.

Herbal Hair Care

Herbs have long been associated with hair care and are often ingredients in conditioners, shampoos, and rinses. The most highly regarded herb for the hair is rosemary, reputed to be a good general conditioner that leaves the hair silky, shiny, fragrant, and very slightly darker. Two other hair herbs that have had many devoted fans over the centuries are sage, prized as a darkener and conditioner, and chamomile, believed to brighten fair hair and soften all hair. Mullein's golden flowers are also supposed to intensify blond highlights. Tradition also asserts that parsley thickens hair and enriches its color, southernwood increases growth, burdock root controls dandruff, and stinging nettle conditions hair as well as helps cure dandruff. Any number of plants, ranging from kelp to yarrow, will supposedly curb hair loss and stimulate growth—but none, unfortunately, has been scientifically proved effective. Other herbs, such as lavender, simply leave the hair with a delightful scent.

As with the beauty preparations on the preceding pages, the recipes here are starting suggestions meant to show how you can use herbal preparations. Experiment to find the best combination of ingredients for your hair. The ingredients are all common plant or household items.

Before using a recipe, put a small amount of it on the inside of your elbow. If you get an itching or burning reaction within the next 24 hours, do not use the preparation; you are probably allergic to one of the ingredients.

Herbal Conditioning Oil

To give this conditioning oil time to absorb the herbal essences, prepare it a week before you intend to use it. You can substitute any of the traditional hair herbs mentioned above—or other plant oils such as sunflower, soy, corn, peanut, and jojoba. Olive oil can be substituted if it is not too robust in odor, but avoid strong-smelling sesame oil. Once you find a combination you like, double or triple the quantities and store the extra in a capped bottle.

½ cup dried chamomile flowers
¼ cup dried rosemary leaves
1 cup safflower oil

Put the herbs in the top of a double boiler and add the oil. Heat the mixture for 30 minutes; then pour it into a wide-mouthed jar. Cover the jar with a couple of layers of muslin, held by a string or rubber band. Let the jar stand in a warm place for a week or so. Stir every day. When the oil has a pronounced herbal aroma, strain it into a clean container.

Warm ⅓ to ½ cup of the oil (depending on the thickness and length of your hair) over very low heat for a few minutes. Wet your hair with hot water and squeeze it out. Then, spread the warm oil through your hair with your fingers until it is fully coated. Cover your hair with a plastic bag or a shower cap; pin it up first, if necessary. To keep the oil warm, soak a heavy towel in hot water; then wring it out and wrap it securely over the plastic covering. When the towel cools, wet it again. Treat your hair for 20 to 30 minutes. Shampoo it twice.

Herbal Egg Conditioner

Use this conditioner following the procedure described in the previous recipe. Or simply warm it and apply it to the hair for 15 minutes before shampooing.

2 teaspoons lemon juice
1 heaping teaspoon honey
1 egg
2–3 drops oil of rosemary
¼ cup safflower or other vegetable oil

Add the lemon juice and honey to the egg and beat them together. Pour the mixture into the top of a double boiler and heat, stirring, until it is warm and creamy. Let it cool. Then mix the rosemary oil in the vegetable oil and slowly add it to the egg mixture while whipping with a whisk to blend. You can substitute ¼ cup of Herbal Conditioning Oil (see previous recipe) for the vegetable oil and the rosemary oil.

Bouncing Bet Natural Shampoo

The lathering herb bouncing Bet is often called soapwort. You can substitute 2 tablespoons of the more sudsy dried bouncing Bet root, if it is available. For variety, replace chamomile with rosemary, southernwood, or lavender—or sage for dark hair. Expect to use more of this natural shampoo and to see less suds than you would with a commercial preparation. Pure-grade borax is sold in drugstores.

3 tablespoons dried bouncing Bet herb
1½ tablespoons dried chamomile
   flowers
1 teaspoon pure-grade borax
2 cups boiling water

Put the bouncing Bet herb, chamomile flowers, and borax in a heat-proof jar or other container that you can cover tightly. Pour in the boiling water and stir well. Let the mix steep, loosely covered, until cool. Then cap the container and shake well. Let it stand for a day or so, shaking every few hours. Strain.

Herbal Castile Shampoo

Made from olive oil–based castile soap, this shampoo lathers as profusely as commercial shampoos, cleans well, rinses off easily, and is much gentler. Use pure castile soap—either powdered or flaked or grated from a solid bar.

Liquid castile soaps usually have peppermint or other ingredients already added to them. Use chamomile if your hair is light; sage if it is dark. Feel free to add a tablespoon of southernwood, stinging nettle, or another traditional hair herb. Or add an aromatic ingredient such as lemon or orange peel.

¼ cup dried chamomile flowers
    or 1 tablespoon dried sage leaves
2 tablespoons dried rosemary leaves
1 tablespoon dried peppermint
2¼ cups distilled water
2 ounces castile soap
3 drops oil of peppermint or eucalyptus
2 tablespoons vodka

Put the dried herbs in a heavy saucepan. Add the distilled water and bring it to a boil. Reduce the heat and simmer for 10 minutes. Then cover and steep for about 30 minutes. Strain the liquid into a mixing bowl; squeeze the herbs to remove all the liquid before discarding them. Put the castile soap in the saucepan and pour in the herbal brew. Simmer over low heat until the soap dissolves completely; stir regularly with a wooden spoon. Let the mixture cool; it should be thin and creamy. Then mix the drops of peppermint or eucalyptus oil into the vodka and stir into the shampoo mixture. Pour the mixture into a jar and cap it. Let stand in a warm place for 3 or 4 days before using.

Quick Herbal Shampoo

The fastest and easiest way to make an herbal shampoo is to mix a strong infusion of an hair herb with a mild shampoo.

1 heaping teaspoon dried sage,
    rosemary, or stinging nettle or
    1 tablespoon dried chamomile flowers
¼ cup boiling water
¼ cup baby or other mild shampoo

Add herbs to the water. Turn off heat, steep for 30 minutes, strain, and mix into shampoo.

Blond Highlighting Rinse

For best results, use this rinse regularly and dry your hair in bright sunlight. Shampoo and rinse well with plain water first.

2 cups water
½ cup dried chamomile flowers
2 tablespoons dried mullein flowers
1 tablespoon orange blossom water
Juice of ½ lemon

Bring the water to a boil; then lower the heat and stir in the chamomile and mullein flowers. Simmer for 30 minutes; then cover and steep for several hours or overnight. Strain, squeezing the liquid from the herbs. Then stir in the orange blossom water and lemon juice. Pour the rinse through your hair several times, catching the liquid in a large bowl.

Deepening Rinse for Dark Hair

Use as a final rinse after shampooing and rinsing well with plain water.

2 cups boiling water
2 tea bags of regular beverage tea
¼ cup dried sage leaves
2 tablespoons dried rosemary leaves
1 tablespoon dried stinging nettles

Pour the water over the tea bags and steep covered for 15 minutes. Remove the tea bags, squeezing out the liquid. Reheat the tea to the boiling point. Then pour it over the dried herbs. Cover and steep for 30 minutes to an hour. Strain. Pour the rinse through your hair several times, catching the liquid in a bowl.

Herbal Vinegar Rinse

This rinse helps to restore the hair's natural acid balance and to remove dulling traces of soap. If bergamot is not available, you can substitute another fragrant herb from the mint family, such as basil or peppermint.

¼ cup dried rosemary leaves
¼ cup dried bergamot
2 cups clear cider vinegar

Put the dried herbs in wide-mouthed jar. Heat the vinegar until it is just about to boil and pour it over the herbs. After the vinegar cools, cap the jar. If the lid is metal, screw it on with a couple of layers of plastic wrap under it, so that the acidic vinegar will not react with the metal. Let it stand in a warm place for a week. Shake vigorously every day. Using fine cheesecloth in a funnel, strain the vinegar into a bottle and cap it. To use, dilute ⅓ cup of the vinegar with 2 or 3 cups of warm water and pour it over the hair one or two times as a final rinse.

Quick Herbal Rinse

Any infusion made with an hair herb can be used as a quick rinse. Let the infusion cool to lukewarm before using it.

1 to 2 tablespoons dried sage, rosemary,
    or stinging nettle
2 cups boiling water

Put the herbs in the boiling water, turn off the heat, and allow them to steep for 15 minutes. Strain and apply as a rinse.

Flaxseed Setting Lotion

Try combing in this mixture to give body to thin, limp hair.

⅓ cup flaxseeds
1 cup water

Crush the flaxseeds with a spoon. Bring the water to a boil in a saucepan. Then reduce the heat and stir the flaxseeds into the simmering water, a teaspoon at a time, until the mixture thickens. Strain out the seeds and thin the mixture to the desired consistency.

Herbal Baths and Soaps

You can enjoy the luxury of bathing with herbs by simply steeping dried herbs in the bathwater. Not only will they make your bath more fragrant but they can also make it more invigorating or soothing. Virtually any combination of dried leafy fragrant herbs—or any single herb—can be used for an herbal bath. The secret, as the recipe on this page shows, is to tie the herbs in cloth. This keeps them from clinging to your skin and the sides of the tub and from clogging the drain.

Another way to use herbs when bathing is to incorporate them in soap. Ordinarily, soap-making is a time-consuming process, requiring the cautious handling of a caustic ingredient. But an array of delightfully scented herbal soaps can be made by simply melting bars of plain soap, adding the herbal ingredient, and remolding them. Essential oils are the easiest addition, but you can also mix in such traditional ingredients as oatmeal, almond meal, lanolin, cold cream, or honey to change the texture and feel of the soap.

An Herbal Bath

Some ingredients commonly used for herbal baths are listed below. Select about a cupful of any of these in dried form, mixing and matching from different categories as you please. You may want a combination that emphasizes floral and other sweet-smelling ingredients, or you may want one that has a cleaner or more bracing scent. Even when stressing one category, however, it is often best to add an ingredient or two from another category just to obtain a more interesting aroma. Once you have found a mixture that you like, prepare a large quantity and keep it ready for use in a large, attractive jar.

Sweet and fragrant. Chamomile (Roman or German), elderberry, linden, lavender, and rose flowers and angelica, rose geranium, and rosemary leaves.

Stimulating and clean-smelling. Basil, eucalyptus, peppermint, and thyme leaves.

Spicy and citrus-smelling. Balm, lemon verbena, and southernwood leaves. Strips of fresh lemon and orange peel can also be added.

Mix the ingredients together, crushing them slightly to help release their fragrance. Put the mixture in the center of a piece of clean muslin about 9 inches square. Bring the edges of the muslin together to form a sack around the mixture and secure it with a string or a rubber band. Hang the bag from the bathtub tap. Using hotter water than usual, let the water run over the bag as you fill the tub. Then drop the bag in the filled tub and let it steep for 5 minutes or until the water is cool enough for you to get into it. You can leave the bag in the tub while you soak and bathe.

Herbal Bath Oil

4 parts safflower, olive, corn, or almond oil*
1 part oil of bergamot, thyme, cloves, lavender, or eucalyptus
1 part vodka

Put all the ingredients in a bottle that can be capped tightly. Shake well before using. Add 1 teaspoon to the bathwater.

The oil will make the tub slippery. Make sure that you use a rubber bath mat, and get in and out of the tub carefully.

*Almond oil is the most pleasing ingredient, but it is much more expensive than the others.

French Bouquet Soap

Traditional *savon au bouquet*, or perfumed soap, can be varied by changing the scenting ingredients. Besides the oils and waters suggested below, oils of bergamot and cinnamon are favorite additions. If you have no soap molds, use custard cups, food molds, or similar containers.

If you want to color the soap, blend a few drops or shavings of candlemaking dye (sold at craft stores) into the melted mixture.

14–16 ounces unscented hard white soap (castile soap is excellent)
¼–½ cup water
½ teaspoon each oils of clove and thyme

Grease soap molds with petroleum jelly. Grate the soap and put it in a heavy enameled saucepan. Melt it over low heat, adding just enough water to keep a sticky film from forming on the pan. When the soap is smooth and about the consistency of whipped cream, remove it from the heat. Let it cool slightly, stirring to keep it smooth; add the aromatic oils.

Pour the soap into the molds and cover them with a heavy cloth or cardboard. Remove the soap from the molds after 24 hours. Put the cakes on a rack in a dry, well-ventilated spot. Leave them for 3 or 4 weeks to dry and harden. The harder the soap gets, the longer it will last.

Orange blossom or rose soap. Omit the water and essential oils. Stir ⅓ cup orange blossom or rose water into the soap as it melts.

Oatmeal soap. Thoroughly blend ⅔ cup of regular uncooked oatmeal into the melted soap along with the scenting ingredients. Oatmeal is beneficial to the skin and makes the soap mildly abrasive. Almond meal and bran are two other abrasives you can add to beauty soaps.

Other variations. For a smoother texture, add a couple of teaspoons of cold cream, beeswax, lanolin, glycerin, or aloe vera gel. Melt beeswax or lanolin first in a double boiler. A couple of teaspoons of honey will make the soap less alkaline and less harsh. A teaspoon of lemon juice will make it more astringent.

Herbs for Health

A great many traditional herbal remedies are completely fanciful. Their reputations are based on hearsay, dubious theories, the coincidental recovery of a few patients, and the never-ending hope of the sick that a cure exists for their illness. Still, there are many herbal preparations that really do seem to work. A few are potent and dangerous—or just unwise—to use. But many others are safe and may help ease minor ailments. Indeed, many of the symptom-easing preparations lining the aisles of drugstores are little more than modified or synthetic versions of herbal remedies.

A number of the safer and more soundly based herbal preparations are given on the following pages. None of them will cure a disease. But they may be able to relieve symptoms and ease the discomfort of ordinary, nonserious conditions such as mild digestive problems, colds, and irritated or itchy skin. The preparations include stomach-calming teas, soothing cough drops, mild washes, and bracing liniments. All achieve their effect as a result of a particular physical property—such as astringency or a high mucilage content. In most cases the effective ingredient works externally on the skin or the mucous membranes or else it passes through the digestive system without being absorbed. Overall, the herbal preparations outlined here are probably less potent than many over-the-counter products.

Since they are less potent, however, they may not be as effective as a product from the drugstore. An herb's strength, too—unlike that of a manufactured product—may vary, depending on how much sunlight it received, how it was dried, how it was stored, and how long ago it was harvested. A freshly picked herb can also vary in strength from a dried one. As a result, a particular herbal preparation may help at one time and not another. Or it may work for one person and not for another.

Taking Reasonable Precautions

Never try to substitute an herbal remedy for proper medical attention. A serious condition should be treated by a doctor. Even a minor disorder that is persistent should receive a doctor's attention. Also consult with a doctor before using an herbal remedy if you have a chronic condition, are pregnant, or are on medication.

Even though the herbal preparations described on the following pages are generally safe, remember that some individuals may be allergic to certain herbs. Before using an herbal preparation for the first time, always try a small amount and wait a couple of days to see if you have a reaction. It is also best as a rule to start with weaker concentrations and work up to stronger ones. If you develop any unusual symptoms while you are using an herbal preparation, stop using it at once. Anyone who suffers from hay fever or any other plant allergies should be especially careful about using herbal preparations.

Herbal Remedies to Avoid

Some herbs that are widely available should not be taken internally because the safety of their prolonged use has been questioned. *The common herbs you should avoid consuming are alfalfa, coltsfoot, comfrey, pennyroyal, goldenseal, sassafras, sweet flag, and tansy.* Alfalfa contains a hormonelike substance that is potentially dangerous. Coltsfoot, comfrey, sassafras, and sweet flag are suspected or known to contain cancer-causing agents. In large quantities, pennyroyal may cause convulsions and tansy may be fatal, while goldenseal may be dangereous to pregnant women and people with high blood pressure. Both European pennyroyal (*Mentha pulegium*) and American pennyroyal (*Hedeoma pulegioides*) are considered unsafe in large doses.

Some other herbal remedies should be avoided because there is no sound reason to use them. Look with suspicion on any remedy based on outmoded, unfounded theories. The traditional uses of many herbs were determined by the idea that an herb's appearance, rather than its chemical or physical properties, was the clue to its effectiveness. Thus the eyebright flower's bloodshot appearance was a sure sign of its ability to clear up eye irritations.

Also be wary of sweeping claims. Even for herbs that are not considered panaceas, you can usually find lengthy, often contradictory, lists of disorders that they are supposed to cure. In times past, any herb that became part of an herbalist's repertory stood a good chance of being prescribed for almost any disease—to be applied externally sometimes, to be taken internally at other times.

Avoid remedies that call for mixing herbs together. Again, once an herb was on an herbalist's shelf, it was likely to be combined with other herbs in recipes with only the most whimsical logic to support them. There is no real proof that combining one herb with another will increase either's effectiveness or lessen the adverse effects of one. Of course, it is all right to make a tart or bland preparation more palatable by adding honey or a fragrant herb.

Obtaining Herbs

Some of the herbs called for on the next few pages are culinary herbs available at the supermarket or at a food specialty shop. A few are found in preparations sold in your local drugstore. You can obtain most of the others from a well-stocked herbal or health food store or a specialty druggist. Since the common names of herbs can vary, look for packages that also carry the plant's two-word Latin scientific name. The label should also specify the plant part—roots, flowers, leaves. On these labels, "herb" usually means just the parts of the plant above the ground, while "plant" means the entire plant, roots and all. Many herbs come as powders as well as in regular dried form; essential oils are also available.

You can also use fresh or dried herbs from your garden or the wild. If you pick wild herbs, be absolutely sure that they have not been sprayed and that you have identified them accurately. If you substitute fresh herbs for dried ones, the general rule is to use two to three times the specified amount.

Digestive Aids

Taken as liquid brews, many herbs can aid digestion and help calm mild digestive disorders. Depending on the herb, they may be able to perk up a flagging appetite, ease intestinal gas and cramps, control mild diarrhea, or relieve constipation. Leaves, flowers, or seeds — fresh or dried—are prepared by the regular tea-making process known as **infusion**: they are simply steeped in freshly boiled water. Tougher roots, bark, and stems need to be boiled or simmered to release their active ingredients, a process known as **decoction**. Whether infused or decocted, an herbal brew used as a tonic or symptom-easing preparation is usually made stronger than one used as a beverage. But the wisest course is to start with a weak, beverage-strength infusion or decoction and then make increasingly stronger ones until you find the most effective. As when making a beverage, you will get best results if you use loose ingredients rather than tea bags, and fresh spring or distilled bottled water rather than chlorinated tap water. As always, herbal brews should be made in a ceramic teapot or in glass, enameled, or stainless steel cookware. Never use a container made from aluminum, which might react with an herb.

Appetite-Stimulating Tonics
People once swore by tart-tasting spring tonics, believing the herbal preparations cleansed the blood, which had grown sluggish over the winter. We now know that the healthy afterglow many attributed to such tonics was more likely the result of their restorative effect on a listless digestive system. Bitter substances, research suggests, stimulate gastric secretions, increasing the desire to eat and facilitating digestion. Depending on its strength, a half or full cup of bitter tonic taken about half an hour before mealtime seems to be effective.

You can produce a bitter tonic from dried dandelion leaves by simple infusion. It has a mildly laxative effect in quantity and is sometimes taken to promote regularity.

Dandelion Leaf Tonic
1–2 teaspoons dried dandelion leaves
1 cup boiling water

Put the dandelion leaves in a teapot and pour the water over them. Let them steep for 5 minutes; then strain the tea into a cup. Let it cool until it is lukewarm.

If you use fresh dandelion leaves, double or triple the amount (chop the leaves before measuring) and follow the recipe for fresh mint tea on the next page. Do not pick leaves in an area that has been sprayed or where pets have roamed.

You can also make bitter tonics by the method above using the dried whole plant of flowering European centaury or the leaves and stems of horehound. Centaury is especially tart. Mix it with a sweet herb, such as peppermint. Or add a spoonful of brown sugar or honey. Although it is more fragrant than bitter, an infusion of Roman chamomile also seems good for the appetite and digestion.

Gentian Root Tonic
When a bitter tonic is made from roots, it is usually prepared by decoction, as in this recipe for a gentian root tonic.

The gentian root sold in herbal shops is more likely to come from the European *Gentiana lutea* or other gentian species than from Sampson's snakeroot, shown on page 291. Feel free to substitute Sampson's snakeroot if it is available. The peppermint in this recipe is optional; it helps lessen the bitter brew's bite.

1–2 teaspoons chopped dried gentian root
1 teaspoon dried peppermint leaves
1 cup water

Put the gentian root in a saucepan with the water. Bring the water to a boil; then reduce the heat and simmer for 15 minutes. Turn off the heat and add the peppermint. Cover and let it steep for 5 minutes. Strain it into a cup. Let it cool until it is lukewarm.

If you prefer to use powdered gentian root, blend ½–1 teaspoon into a paste, then mix it into one cup of water and steep.

Dandelion root and chicory root are also believed to stimulate the appetite. Both of these longtime coffee substitutes are sold roasted and ground. Like gentian root, they can be prepared by decoction, although chicory is often brewed in a drip coffee pot, using half the amount you would of coffee.

Stomach-Settling Brews

A surprising number of herbs seem to relieve or ease digestive problems, especially excess gas. The ones with this capacity for reducing flatulence are primarily aromatic herbs rich in essential oils, and researchers believe that the oils' active ingredients are responsible for the effect. Most are common culinary herbs sold in supermarkets and gourmet shops or easily grown in the garden; it should be easy for you to experiment and find the most effective ones.

Among these gas-relieving herbs are angelica and lovage roots, which can be made into a decoction by following the preceding recipe for gentian root. The mint family supplies many useful aromatic leaves, including basil, marjoram, rosemary, sage, and savory as well as both peppermint and spearmint. Dill and flowering European centaury plant also seem to be effective in easing gas. Any of these can be made into an infusion, following the recipe for dandelion tonic on the previous page. Fresh leaves can be prepared as in this recipe for mint tea.

Fresh Mint Digestive Tea

This refreshing drink seems to aid digestion as well as ease gas. It is stronger than a mint tea taken as a beverage.

4–5 stems of peppermint or spearmint
1 cup of boiling water

Rinse the mint leaves, pick them off the stems, and pat them dry with a paper towel. You should have about four dozen leaves. Put them in a teapot, pour the water over them, and let them steep for 5 minutes. Strain into a cup.

With herbs such as dill, rosemary, and savory, which do not have large leaves that can easily be picked off, you can substitute an equal quantity of stems with the leaves on them.

Fennel Seed Digestive Tea

Seeds are especially rich in essential oils that help ease gas. Many come from popular members of the carrot family: anise, caraway, celery, dill, and fennel. Fenugreek seeds, a popular Middle Eastern spice sold in herbal stores, are also a good source of a gas-controlling essential oil. You can make any of these seeds into a tea by infusion, as in this recipe for fennel tea. The licorice-tasting fennel has been used since antiquity for digestive relief.

1–1½ teaspoons fennel seeds
1 cup boiling water

Crush the seeds lightly with a spoon. Put them into a teapot and pour the water over them. Allow them to steep for 5 to 7 minutes; then strain the tea into a cup.

Besides relieving gas, fennel seed tea also seems to ease a sometimes related disorder —intestinal cramping. Other widely available herbs that appear to have this antispasmodic quality are German chamomile flowers and thyme leaves—and probably elecampane root and rosemary leaves.

When you do not have the time or facilities to brew an herb, you can in some cases use the concentrated essential oil of the herb to make a kind of instant substitute tea. Thyme, rosemary, and peppermint are commonly available as essential oils. To use them, simply stir three or four drops of oil into a cupful of lukewarm water. *Never take these potent essential oils undiluted and never use more than a few drops.*

Bowel-Controlling Preparations

Because purging the system was long a major concern of herbal medicine, the laxative powers of many herbs are well documented. Today, however, we know that the powerful purgatives used in the past were not only of questionable value but downright dangerous. You should even avoid using milder laxatives regularly, since your system can become overly dependent on them. For chronic constipation, you can obtain safer, long-term results by changing to a diet with a higher fiber and liquid content and by strengthening your abdominal muscles through exercise.

If a doctor does recommend a laxative, however, there are some classic herbal preparations you might consider. One of the safest is powdered psyllium seed husks. Sold in drugstores as "natural fiber laxative," the powdered psyllium stimulates the bowel by increasing the bulk in it. Typically a teaspoon of powder is simply mixed with a glass of water.

On a doctor's recommendation, two other herbs that you might consider are senna and cascara sagrada. Both are common ingredients in commercial laxatives. Taken as teas or decoctions, they cause an increase in intestinal contractions by irritating the bowel wall. Leaves and pods from wild senna and related species can be made into a tea by infusion. Do not be frightened if your urine turns red after taking senna tea—it is a common, harmless side effect. Cascara sagrada bark can be made into a decoction. Be sure to use only the dried bark; the fresh bark can make you nauseated. The barks from two species closely related to cascara sagrada—buckthorn and alder buckthorn—are often suggested as laxatives by herbalists, but they are stronger and are best avoided. Be sure to allow several hours for a laxative brew to take effect, and do not take it more often than your doctor recommends.

Mild cases of diarrhea can often be controlled by teas made from herbs with a high tannin content, since the astringent property of the tannin has a binding effect on the bowel. Safe tannin-rich herbs include agrimony herb, purple loosestrife herb, meadowsweet plant, powdered bistort rootstock, and raspberry leaves. Common barberry bark and cranesbill root are also rich in tannin; the powdered form of either can be made into a decoction.

Easing Cold Symptoms

No herbal preparation and no medicine can cure the common cold. Whether you take something or not, the worst part of a cold will pass in a few days. Many herbal preparations, however, can help to relieve symptoms such as coughing, sore throat, and congestion of the nose and upper chest—whether they are caused by a cold or some other mild respiratory problem. Indeed, traditional herbal ingredients form the basis of many popular over-the-counter cough syrups, lozenges, gargles, and inhalants, and you can prepare safe, effective substitutes directly from the herbs themselves. Most have physical properties that work on the tissue surface to relieve a condition—to soothe irritation, for example, or to loosen phlegm.

Throat-Soothing Cough Syrups

A sore throat that accompanies a cold will often feel much better after you take a syrup with a high mucilage content. Bland, with a thick gluelike consistency, the mucilage coats the raw, irritated throat membranes, soothing and protecting them. The same preparations will also often relieve a bout of coughing—when it is the result of throat irritation, as is frequently the case during a cold. But remember that some coughing is good for you. Coughing is a natural reflex that helps clear phlegm and foreign matter from the respiratory tract.

Herbal preparations for soothing a sore throat are usually taken as a syrup, rather than a tea, for the simple reason that the syrup's thick consistency enhances the soothing effect of the mucilage. No doubt the sweet taste has also helped to make syrups popular—and palatable to ill, cranky youngsters who would recoil from a bitter-tasting brew. Most herbalists recommend taking homemade cough syrup a teaspoonful at a time as needed. Throw out any that is left over after three or four days.

Hyssop Cough Syrup

Tart, minty-tasting hyssop has been used to ease respiratory problems since ancient times. The anise in this recipe adds a pleasant licorice flavor that offsets the pungent taste of the hyssop without diminishing its effect.

Do not give this syrup or any preparation containing honey to a child less than a year old. Honey is sometimes contaminated with bacteria that can cause food poisoning in a young child.

1 cup honey
¼ cup water
2 tablespoons dried flowering hyssop tops
1 teaspoon aniseeds

Pour the honey into a heavy saucepan and stir in the water, a tablespoon at a time, until the consistency is like that of pancake syrup. Bring the honey slowly to a boil over medium heat and skim off any scum that forms. Dampen the dried hyssop with a tablespoon or so of water and crush the aniseeds with a spoon; then stir both into the honey. Cover and simmer over very low heat for 30 minutes. Uncover the syrup and let it cool slightly; then while it is still warm enough to flow easily, strain it into a jar or bottle with a screw-on lid. Put the lid on only after it cools completely.

If you have fresh hyssop, substitute about ⅓ cup of chopped flowering tops.

Marshmallow Root Cough Syrup

The orange juice in this recipe adds a bit of acidity that helps keep the syrup from crystallizing. It also adds flavor; marshmallow syrup by itself has a bland, undistinctive taste. If you want a syrup that is more tangy, substitute the juice of one lemon.

1½–2½ teaspoons chopped dried marshmallow root
2 cups water
2 cups refined sugar
¼ cup orange juice

Stir the marshmallow root into the water and bring it to a boil. Lower the heat and simmer for 20 minutes. Strain the decoction into another saucepan; you should have about a cup. Over low heat, gradually stir in the sugar, so that a thick syrup forms. Simmer the mixture for another 5 minutes. Make sure the grains are fully dissolved. Stir in a small amount of water if the mixture gets too thick. Let the mixture cool slightly; then gradually mix in the orange juice. Pour the syrup into a sealable container and cover it when it is cool.

Wild cherry cough syrup. Decoct 1 teaspoon of wild cherry bark along with the marshmallow and add ⅓ teaspoon cream of tartar to the sugar. Leave out the orange juice.

Other variations. You can make syrups in the same way from decoctions of flaxseed, high mallow root, and slippery elm bark—all rich sources of mucilage. Crush the flaxseeds before decocting them. With a powdered herb, use about half the amount; blend it into a paste with water and simmer for only 10 minutes.

Leaves with a high mucilage content—from horehound, hyssop, and marshmallow—can be made into syrups too. Steep 1 tablespoon of the dried leaves in 1½ cups of water for 10 to 15 minutes; then strain and slowly add about 2 cups of sugar, stirring over low heat. Mullein herb can also be infused to produce mucilage; use about 2 teaspoons and strain the tea through fine cheesecloth or muslin to remove the velvety plant's tiny hairs. Another source rich in mucilage for syrups is seaweeds, such as bladderwrack and kelp. Use 1 tablespoon of the chopped dried seaweed or 1 teaspoon of the powdered to make an infusion.

You can make a syrup even more easily by blending an infusion or decoction of any of the above herbs into honey. Simply stir about ½ cup of the hot, strong brew into 1 cup honey.

Lozenges

An herb with a high mucilage content can also be made into hard candy lozenges, or cough drops, and used to ease a sore throat and the coughing related to it. The advantage of a lozenge is that it releases its throat-soothing mucilage and sugar more slowly. Equally important, it stimulates the flow of saliva, which also coats the throat membranes. The traditional herb for making lozenges is horehound. It has been used for relieving throat soreness for centuries, but its musty, mouth-puckering flavor is an acquired taste.

Horehound Cough Drops

1 cup boiling water
¾ cup dried horehound herb
2 cups refined sugar
⅓ teaspoon cream of tartar

Pour the boiling water over the horehound; cover and let steep for 30 minutes. Strain the infusion into a heavy saucepan, pressing to extract all the liquid. Add the sugar and cream of tartar and stir over low heat until the sugar is fully dissolved. Cover the pan and let it cook for 3 or 4 minutes until the steam has melted any sugar crystals clinging to the pan's side. Then remove the lid and cook the mixture, without stirring, over high heat; skim off any scum. When it reaches the hard-crack stage— when a candy thermometer reads 300°F or when drops form brittle threads in ice water— immediately remove it from the heat. Brush a marble slab or a baking sheet with butter or oil and pour out the mixture. As it begins to set, score it into small squares with a sharp knife. Cut it along the lines when it is cold and brittle. Store the pieces in an airtight container.

Gargles

Gargles can also help to ease throat soreness; they are good alternatives if you are concerned about the extra calories or the potentially damaging effect of sugar on your teeth. A strong tea prepared from any mucilaginous herb makes a good gargle. Try infusions of herbs and leaves such as horehound, hyssop, mullein, and kelp or decoctions of harder plant parts such as marshmallow and high mallow root, slippery elm bark, and flaxseeds. If you like the taste, also try them as teas; warm liquids tend to soothe sore membranes.

You can make gargles from herbs that are astringent as well. They have a tightening effect on the membranes, which can sometimes temporarily alleviate a tickle in the throat or a feeling of rawness. The astringent ingredient is usually tannin, and a number of herbs can produce tannin-rich brews. Among them are meadowsweet plant, powdered bistort rootstock, and purple loosestrife leaves. All can be prepared by simple infusion, as in this recipe for an astringent gargle made from a commonly available high-tannin herb, raspberry leaf, also called red raspberry leaf.

Raspberry Leaf Gargle

1 tablespoon dried raspberry leaves
2 cups boiling water
1–3 teaspoons honey

Put the raspberry leaves in a teapot and pour the water over them. Let them steep for 10 minutes. Strain into a container and add the honey, if desired, to temper the tartness. Let it cool to room temperature before using. Store in an airtight container in the refrigerator. Throw out if not used up in 3 days.

Powdered cañaigre root and cankerroot also have a high tannin content and can be used to produce astringent gargles. Just prepare them by decoction.

Congestion-Easing Inhalants

Other cold symptoms—a clogged nose and tight chest—can often be eased by the traditional practice of inhaling steam. The steam usually comes from a basin filled with freshly boiled water, and frequently an aromatic ingredient is added—usually a few drops of a volatile plant oil. Inhaling the steam helps increase the amount of fluid in the respiratory tract. This dilutes the mucus, making it thinner and much easier to discharge. At the same time, the oil in the steam acts as an expectorant —an agent that helps loosen the mucus. As a side benefit, the warmth and moisture have a soothing effect on irritated tissues. Although menthol and camphor are more traditional ingredients, the essential oils of eucalyptus, pine, rosemary, and thyme are more likely to be effective. Eucalyptus has an especially pleasant, refreshing odor.

Eucalyptus Steam Inhalant

4 cups boiling water
3–4 drops oil of eucalyptus

Pour the water into a heat-proof bowl and stir in the eucalyptus drops. Put a towel over your head to form a tent to contain the steam. Breathe in the vapors for about 10 minutes. Repeat two or three times a day.

Teas Rich in Vitamin C

Whether or not vitamin C helps a cold is hotly disputed. At best, it seems, the vitamin may lessen the severity and duration of a cold a bit. If you want to try it, rose hips and cleavers are rich sources that can be infused into a tea.

Externally Applied Preparations

Herbal medicine has a long tradition of oils and ointments, liniments and lotions, and poultices and plasters that are applied directly to the skin to cure ailments ranging from burns to rheumatism. Many of these concoctions merely felt good as they went on the skin, reinforcing the user's belief that they were effective. But some herbal preparations seem to be genuinely capable of easing conditions such as mild itching, irritation, and soreness. Many are the basis for common over-the-counter symptom relievers. In applying preparations to the skin remember it is generally best to avoid ointments and lotions that leave a water-repelling coating, especially if the skin is raw or broken. Such coatings can seal in infectious agents, and thus can make the condition worse.

Relieving Lotions and Pastes

The bothersome itching caused by insect bites, prickly heat, and similar mild skin problems can often be relieved by wiping the area with an astringent solution, which tightens and contracts the skin. You can use an infusion or decoction of any herb with a high tannin content, such as raspberry leaves, purple loosestrife herb, and the powdered roots of bistort and cañaigre. The most popular herbal preparation by far, however, is a solution made from witch hazel, which is especially effective in creating a tingly sensation as it puckers and shrinks the skin's surface. It is easiest to use the commonly available witch hazel extract, which is made by boiling the plant for hours, steam distilling the essence, and then adding alcohol to enhance its astringency. If you live in an area where witch hazel trees and shrubs grow, you may want to try making your own version of this zesty-feeling compound. The leaves are especially rich in tannin.

Witch Hazel Lotion

A handful of fresh witch hazel leaves
2 cups water
½ cup rubbing alcohol

Rinse the leaves well to remove all dirt and other foreign matter, and chop them coarsely. You should have about ¼ cup loosely packed. Bring the water to a boil in a porcelain or enameled saucepan and add the leaves. Lower the heat and simmer for 15 minutes. Let it steep until cool; then strain. Add the alcohol. Apply with cotton or clean sheeting material. Keep any leftover solution in a capped container in the refrigerator; throw it out if it is not used up in 3 or 4 days.

You can prepare a decoction of witch hazel twigs and bark in the same manner. Use about 2 tablespoons of the roughly chopped material and simmer for at least half an hour.

While witch hazel acts as an astringent, other herbal preparations work to lessen your awareness of itching and minor irritation by creating a competing sensation. Any preparation that has this distracting effect is known as a **counterirritant,** and many preparations used on the skin fall into this category. One herbal product that acts as a counterirritant by producing a refreshing, stimulating effect is the essential oil of peppermint. As it is absorbed by the skin, it stimulates the nerve endings so that you feel a sensation of coolness replacing the itching or irritation. A mild peppermint lotion is easy to prepare.

Peppermint Lotion

Oil of peppermint contains menthol, which is toxic if consumed internally in quantity. But it is safe to use in externally applied preparations like this.

½ cup water
½ cup rubbing alcohol
3–4 drops peppermint oil

Put the water and alcohol in a bottle that you can cap tightly. Add the oil and shake well. Apply with cotton or clean sheeting.

The same procedure will yield refreshing, itch-relieving lotions from oil of eucalyptus and from oil of cade, a tarry-smelling essence derived from the bark of a juniper tree. Before applying any counterirritant for the first time, check your skin's sensitivity by dabbing a bit of the lotion on the inside of your wrist. Wait a few hours to see if it causes a reaction.

Oatmeal Paste

For a small, localized area of itching, such as an insect bite, you might want to apply a soothing paste of oatmeal.

2 teaspoons regular oatmeal
1–2 tablespoons warm tap water

Crumble the oatmeal with your fingers into fine particles. Stir in a teaspoon of water and let the mixture stand for a few minutes until it thickens. Then add more water, a few drops at a time, until the mixture is thick and gelatinous. Just before applying the paste, desensitize the area by applying a compress of hot water. Using tap water hot enough to be uncomfortable but not so hot as to scald you, wet a cloth and press it against the area for a few seconds. Then smooth on the paste.

Some researchers believe that another herbal product can be highly effective in easing itching from an insect bite. Any of the widely available meat tenderizers produced from papaya fruit contains an enzyme, papain, that not only makes tough cuts of meat more palatable but also apparently helps break down the toxins insects inject into the skin.

Papaya Tenderizer Paste for Insect Bites

⅓ teaspoon papaya meat tenderizer
½–1 teaspoon warm tap water

Put the tenderizer into a small container and mix in a drop or two of water at a time until the paste has a smooth consistency. Rub the paste on the bite and let it dry.

Discomfort-Easing Baths

When discomfort and itching from rashes, hives, allergic reactions, or other mild skin conditions cover a larger area of the body, a bath is often the easiest way to obtain some temporary relief. Again, the best agent for soothing the skin is oatmeal.

Oatmeal Bath

You can use regular uncooked oatmeal straight from the kitchen, if you crumble it into fine particles first. But it is better to buy special colloidal oatmeal at the drugstore. Meant to be used for baths, the powdery colloidal oatmeal becomes uniformly suspended in the water.

A tubful of lukewarm water
1 cup colloidal oatmeal

As you fill the tub, mix the oatmeal with the running water. Stir the water with your hand to make sure the oatmeal is well mixed before you get in. *An oatmeal bath is extremely slippery.* Line the bottom of the tub with a towel to help keep you from slipping. Be extra careful getting in and out of the tub, and make sure there is a mat you can step out onto. Soak for 15 to 20 minutes. Gently pat yourself dry, leaving a thin coat of the mixture on your skin.

Another plant product, cornstarch, can produce a bath that soothes irritation, especially from sunburn. Mix 1 cup of cornstarch with a quart of water until it is thoroughly dissolved; then stir the mixture into a tub of lukewarm to cool water. Cool water feels best on a sunburn.

Soothing Emollients for Dry Skin

If you have widespread itching that results from dry or chapped skin, a better way to relieve the discomfort may be to take a bath with an oil and then apply an emollient to the skin. Together they help soften the skin and make it more pliant. At the same time, they give it a protective coating that helps retain moisture. For the bath, add 2 or 3 ounces of mineral oil to the running water as the tub fills or use any theraputic bath oil as directed. Herbal Bath Oil (page 432) can also have a soothing effect on dry skin.

Although you can make an emollient by preparing a very strong decoction of a plant with a high mucilage content, the easiest herbal emollient to apply after the bath is the jelly-like sap of aloe vera. You can get bottles of it at most herbal shops. But if you have an aloe plant, you can just break off a leaf and rub the juice directly on the skin.

Aloe may also be of help on mild burns. Some researchers believe that it contains an ingredient that helps them heal faster. When you get a mild burn, first soak the affected part in cold water for 20 to 30 minutes—or apply cold compresses—until the initial pain subsides. Then gently pat the area dry and lightly rub it with the aloe juice. *Do not use aloe or any other preparation on a burn that is blistered or raw.* See a doctor immediately with a burn that covers more than about a square inch or that seriously damages the skin.

Liniments for Aches and Pains

Rubbing a stimulating liniment into the skin is a popular way to treat sore muscles, stiff joints, and other minor aches and pains. Most liniments are made from herbal products or synthetics based on them. And like the itch-relieving lotions described above, they work as counterirritants, producing a competing sensation that makes you less aware of pain. Indeed, the ingredients in many liniments, such as menthol and camphor, are the same ones used in lotions. The chief difference is that the concentrations are much stronger. As a result, they have a much more stimulating effect on the area. They create a warm, tingling sensation and draw blood to the area—an effect that, many researchers believe, may help speed healing. Since a liniment is stronger, it is even more important to check first that your skin is not sensitive to the active ingredient.

Wintergreen oil seems to make an especially good liniment. Besides acting as an counterirritant, it contains an aspirinlike ingredient, methyl salicylate, that may help ease pain when it is absorbed by the skin. Ordinary cider vinegar makes a good vehicle, since it is mildly astringent. Never apply a liniment to broken skin. Do not use more than four times a day.

Wintergreen Liniment

Natural wintergreen oil is rare today. The wintergreen oil commonly sold is a synthetic, sometimes labeled methyl salicylate. *Never take wintergreen oil internally except under a doctor's direction.*

1 cup white cider vinegar
½ teaspoon wintergreen oil

Put the vinegar and the wintergreen oil in a bottle you can seal tightly. Shake well.

Peppermint oil and pine oil can be made into liniments in the same manner. Essences derived from mustard or cayenne pepper can be especially strong and should be avoided or used very sparingly.

Glossary

The words and terms that follow serve as both reminders and extensions of the material covered in MAGIC AND MEDICINE OF PLANTS. The botanical terms round out the information given in the section called "The Anatomy of Plants," pages 32–41, and will give the reader confidence to approach even more advanced botanical texts. Similarly, enough medicinal and therapeutic terms have been included to provide the reader with a ready reference vocabulary for further investigations into the fascinating world of herbalism. A word that is printed in SMALL CAPITAL letters is defined under that heading in another part of the glossary.

NOTE: The spellings of many words (e.g., *abortifacient*) are the same for both adjectives and nouns, and thus definitions for such terms are a guide to both types of usage.

A

abortifacient bringing on an abortion.

acaulescent lacking or appearing to lack a stem.

acetylsalicylic acid chemical name of aspirin.

achene a dry INDEHISCENT fruit having one seed.

acicular needlelike, as the leaf of pine.

active principle chemical or chemical compound in a plant that has a medicinal effect.

acuminate tapering abruptly to a sharp point, as the leaf of the slippery elm.

adjuvant aiding the action of a medicinal agent or medical treatment.

adventitious arising at other than the usual place; e.g., adventitious buds or roots.

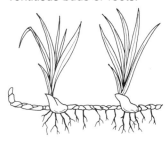

algin any of a group of substances obtained from marine algae, some of which are used as emulsifiers and stabilizers.

alkaloid any of a large class of nitrogen-containing organic compounds found especially in seed plants. Alkaloids, which include codeine and morphine, have many medicinal applications.

allantoin a nitrogen-containing organic compound found in many plants (and in the urine of many mammals) and used to treat wounds and ulcerated tissue.

allopathy medical practice using any treatment that seems to fight against a disease—including such harsh treatments as the use of silver nitrate against gonorrhea, which would not always be approved by practitioners of HOMEOPATHY, another system of medicine. Allopathy is sometimes defined as conventional medical practice exclusive of homeopathy.

alterative medicine that favorably alters the course of an ailment.

alternate describing leaves that arise singly along the stem, in contrast to OPPOSITE.

analeptic having a restorative or stimulating effect, as on the central nervous system.

analgesic relieving pain.

anaphrodisiac reducing capacity for sexual arousal.

anesthetic inducing loss of feeling or consciousness.

angiosperm any of a class of seed-bearing plants whose ovules are enclosed in an ovary; e.g., orchids, roses.

annual completing the life cycle from seed to seed production in one year.

anodyne an agent that relieves pain or promotes general comfort, usually externally.

anorectic (anoretic, anorexic) lacking appetite.

anthelmintic killing or expelling intestinal parasitic worms.

anther pollen-bearing part of a stamen, or male reproductive organ.

anthesis the action of a flower's opening or the period when it opens.

anti- (ant-, anth-) prefix meaning opposed to, against.

antiasthmatic relieving asthma.

antibilious easing stomach distress; reducing excessive secretion of bile, a condition that often results from a disorder in liver function.

antibiotic literally, life-killing; in modern medicine, a substance that will kill disease-causing microorganisms.

anticoagulant inhibiting the clotting of blood.

antidiarrheal preventing or controlling diarrhea.

antidote substance that counteracts the effects of a poison.

antidyspeptic relieving dyspepsia, or indigestion.

antiemetic stopping emesis, or vomiting.

antihemorrhagic controlling hemorrhaging, or copious bleeding.

antihypertensive reducing high blood pressure.

anti-inflammatory controlling inflammation, a reaction of the body to injury or infection, which is typically marked by swelling, redness, pain, heat, and other symptoms.

antipyretic reducing fever.

antirachitic preventing or curing rickets, a childhood bone disease associated with lack of exposure to sunlight and inadequate intake of vitamin D.

antirheumatic easing the discomfort of or preventing rheumatism, a condition that causes inflammation and pain in the joints and muscles.

antiscorbutic preventing the disease scurvy, caused by a deficiency of vitamin C.

antiscrofulous treating scrofula, or tubercular swellings of the lymph glands, usually those of the neck.

antiseptic preventing sepsis, or putrefaction that results from bacterial infection; germ-killing.

antispasmodic calming nervous and muscular spasms.

antitussive controlling or preventing cough.

antiuric counteracting excessive acidity in the urine.

aperient mildly laxative.

aperitive stimulating the appetite for food.

apoplexy "stroke"; sudden lessening or loss of consciousness, muscular control, or feeling because of a clot or rupture in a brain artery.

arbutin a plant chemical of the GLYCOSIDE group extracted from the leaves of bearberry and other plants and sometimes used to treat urinary-tract disorders.

aril an outgrowth around the seed in some plants.

aromatic having a pleasant or spicy odor, a quality often valued in medicinal preparations.

astringent causing soft tissues to draw together, or pucker; an agent that diminishes either external or internal secretions. Astringents are used externally in herbal medicine to check minor bleeding and internally to control diarrhea.

atropine a drug derived from belladonna and other plants of the nightshade family and used to stop spasms and to dilate the pupil of the eye.

axil the upper angle formed by a leaf or branch as it arises from a main axis, or stem.

axillary located or growing in the AXIL.

axis a plant stem; more generally the line of growth of a stem or any of its branching parts that carry flowers, other branches, or leaves.

B

bacteriostatic stopping the multiplication of bacteria.

balsamic having the odor of an aromatic substance called balsam, which is derived from various plants and used in medicinal preparations.

basal growing at the base of a stem.

beak a long, pointed tip on a fruit or seed that may be an aid in its dispersal.

bechic relieving or curing a cough.

berberine a plant chemical of the ALKALOID group found in the roots of barberry and other plants and used in certain tonics and eye preparations.

berry in everyday usage, a small, edible fruit such as a strawberry or raspberry; botanically, a fruit that arises from a single ovary, contains one or more seeds but no stone (in contrast to a DRUPE), and is fleshy or pulpy throughout, such as the banana, grape, tomato.

bi- prefix meaning two or twice.

biennial completing the life cycle in two years.

bipinnate twice PINNATE; i.e., a pinnately divided leaf whose leaflets are themselves pinnately divided.

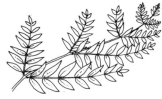

bitter a substance that stimulates the secretion of saliva and gastric juices. In herbal medicine bitter tonics are taken to increase appetite.

blade the part of a leaf other than the stalk; a leaflet of a COMPOUND leaf.

blood purifier an old term for any substance that was supposed to cleanse the blood of impurities and toxic substances and thus restore or maintain good health.

brachycardiac (or bradycardiac) making the heart beat slower.

bract a modified leaf often found outside the CALYX or at the base of a flower stalk.

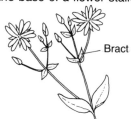
Bract

bud a small growth on the end or sides of a stem that may develop into a flower, leaf, or branch. The terminal bud is the one at the growing end of the main axis, or stem.

bulb a modified underground stem having one or more buds enclosed in fleshy modified leaves or scales, which supply nourishment when the bud or buds begin a new period of growth; e.g., hyacinth, lily, onion, tulip.

bulbil a secondary or small bulb.

bulk laxative bowel-moving agent (laxative) combined with a bulk-forming agent that absorbs water and swells, thus softening the stool, giving it bulk, and promoting gentle evacuation. Bulk laxa-

tives derived from plants include cellulose, agar, Irish moss, and psyllium seeds.

C

caducous dropping off before its usual time, as a leaf or flower. Compare PERSISTENT.

calyx collective term for SEPALS; the calyx encloses the flower bud.

campanulate bell-shaped, as the flowers of many nightshades.

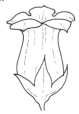

canaliculate having grooves or channels, as a canaliculate petiole (leafstalk).

capsule in plants, a dry, DEHISCENT fruit.

carcinogenic cancer-causing.

cardi- prefix denoting heart.

cardiac of or relating to the heart.

cardiac depressant slowing the action of the heart.

cardiokinetic regulating or strengthening the heartbeat.

cardiotonic keeping the heart functioning normally.

carminative causing the release of stomach or intestinal gas.

carpel the simplest flower structure that can perform the function of a PISTIL (the female reproductive organ). The two terms, carpel and pistil, are sometimes used interchangeably, but a flower may have many carpels forming one pistil.

catarrh a condition in which the mucous membranes of the nose and breathing passages are inflamed, often chronically.

cathartic acting to move the bowels. The word is often used to imply action harsher than that of a laxative.

catkin an often drooping inflorescence (flower cluster) with stalkless unisexual flowers along its main axis; e.g., that of willows and walnuts.

caulescent having an aboveground stem.

cauline on the stem.

caustic having the power to

eat away by chemical action.

chenopodium oil an essential oil obtained from wormseed (*Chenopodium ambrosioides*) and related species, which has been used to expel intestinal worms.

cholagogue an agent that increases the flow of bile from the gallbladder.

choleretic stimulating the liver to produce more bile.

cicatrizing promoting the growth of a cicatrix (scar tissue) over a wound.

-cide suffix meaning killing.

cirrhosis loss of function of tissue of an organ, often applied to liver tissue.

colchicine a plant chemical of the ALKALOID group that is obtained from the corms and seeds of autumn crocus (*Colchicum autumnale*) and is used in treating gout.

colic acute abdominal pain; of or relating to the colon.

complete flower one having both STAMENS and PISTILS, that is, male and female reproductive parts, as well as PETALS and SEPALS.

composite of or associated with the Compositae, a large family of plants that includes asters, daisies, dandelions, goldenrods, and sunflowers. The daisy has a structure, called a flowerhead, typical of many composites: its "eye," or central "button," is composed of many individual DISC FLOWERS, and each of the petallike structures around the "eye" is an individual flower known as a RAY FLOWER.

compound leaf a leaf divided into two or more leaflets; e.g., the leaf of the horse chestnut, ash, walnut, hop.

condiment something that adds flavor to food.

cone a seed-bearing elongated mass of overlapping scales. Pine, spruce, and fir are typical cone-bearing trees.

coniferous "cone-bearing"; coniferous plants (called conifers for short) are the large group of GYMNOSPERMS that includes the yew family, which has somewhat imperfect cones, and the pine family, which has more perfect cones. Most conifers, but not all, are evergreen. Some authorities put the cypress family, Cupressaceae, together with the yews and pines as conifers.

conserve as a noun, a mixture of fruits prepared in some way to preserve them for later use; much the same as a fruit preserve.

contusion an injury to tissue that does not break the skin; a bruise.

cordial a medicine or drink that stimulates good health or the feeling of good health.

corm a bulblike stem, differing usually from a true BULB in that it is solid and sends down a root when a new growing season begins.

corolla collective term for the PETALS of a flower.

corrective herbalist's term meaning an additive that improves the taste or smell of a medication or food.

corymb a flat-topped or somewhat rounded inflorescence (flower cluster) in which the outer flowers open first.

cotyledon a seed leaf; the leaf of an embryonic plant within the seed, which often emerges atop the sprout.

coumarin a plant chemical, smelling like new-mown hay, used in soap and perfume.

counterirritant an agent that causes local inflammation of an area (e.g., the skin) for the purpose of lessening the effects of inflammation in an underlying or adjacent area. Sometimes a counterirritant simply diverts attention from the pain of an inflammation elsewhere.

crenate describing a leaf with scalloped edges, such as that of many members of the *Coleus* genus, of the mint family.

cryptogam plant that does not have seeds or flowers and reproduces by spores; e.g., ferns and mosses.

cutaneous of the skin.

cutting a plant part that, if placed in a favorable environment, will generate new individual plants. Stem cuttings are known as slips.

cyanide a highly poisonous chemical. In nature it may be present in the seeds of certain plants, such as the pits of wild cherries.

cyme a branching, usually flat-topped flower cluster at the end of a stem, in which the central flower opens first.

D

deciduous shedding leaves at the growing season's end.

decoction an extract made by putting a plant or its parts in water, bringing the mixture to a boil, and allowing it to boil or simmer for a time. The liquid is then cooled and strained for use.

decongestant relieving congestion, as of the mucous membranes.

decurrent describing a leaf whose base extends downward along the stem and is wholly or partly fused with it.

dehiscent opening at maturity to discharge seeds or spores.

demulcent soothing an inflammation, especially an inflammation of the mucous membranes. The soothing action may be helpful in relieving coughs.

dentate shaped like a tooth or teeth; referring to a leaf or other structure with toothed edges.

depurative BLOOD PURIFIER.

dermatitis irritation or inflammation of the skin.

detergent cleansing.

di- prefix meaning twice or double.

diaphoretic increasing the amount of perspiration.

dichotomous dividing or forking in two parts, as a branch or terminal shoot.

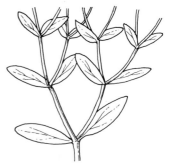

dicotyledon a member of one of the two great subclasses of ANGIOSPERMS; its typical members (called dicots for short) have two COTYLEDONS attached to the embryo. Magnolias, mustards, cacti, legumes, composites, and most deciduous trees are dicots.

MONOCOTYLEDONS are the other great group of angiosperms.

dicoumarol a plant chemical that is formed in rotted sweet clover and that hinders blood clotting.

digestive improving digestion or relating to it.

digitalis a medicine obtained from leaves of the foxglove, *Digitalis purpurea*, and prescribed for certain heart ailments, especially heart failure.

digitate looking like a finger; arranged like the fingers on a hand; e.g., a digitate leaf.

dioecious having male parts (stamens) and female parts (pistils) on separate plants of the same species. English holly is a dioecious plant.

diosgenin a plant chemical obtained from Mexican yams and used in the synthesis of steroid hormones such as cortisone.

disc flower one of the individual tubular flowers that usually make up the dense central head, or "button," characteristic of most members of the composite family, such as daisies, dandelions, and asters.

discutient removing tumorous, diseased, or dead tissue.

distillation in herbalism, a liquid made by condensing the vapor from a heated mixture of herbs and water.

diuretic increasing urine flow.

dropsy an old-fashioned term for EDEMA.

drug any medicine or medication; a substance that causes addiction or mental or emotional distortions.

drupe a fleshy fruit containing one seed enclosed in a hard-walled stone that is embedded in a juicy pulp covered by an outer skin; e.g., cherries, olives, peaches.

dysmenorrhea painful menstruation.

E

ecbolic tending to increase contractions of the uterus and thus facilitate childbirth. The ergot fungus is a source of chemicals with ecbolic action.

edema fluid retention by the body causing swelling and discomfort. Edema is not a disease but a symptom of other disorders or diseases.

elixir a liquid containing alcohol and a medicinal substance and sweetened, usually with sugar.

elliptical shaped like an ellipse, as a leaf.

emetic producing vomiting.

emmenagogue an agent that regulates and induces normal menstruation.

emollient softening and soothing to the skin or other exposed tissue.

ephedrine a plant chemical of the ALKALOID group obtained from various ephedras, especially mahuang, or Chinese ephedra, and used for the relief of asthma, hay fever, and nasal congestion.

epicalyx on some flowers, an additional whorl of BRACTS outside the CALYX, which it resembles.

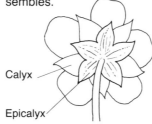

Calyx

Epicalyx

epiphyte one of many kinds of "air plants" without attachment to the soil, which grow on other plants but are not parasitic.

erose unevenly notched.

errhine bringing on sneezing and increasing the flow of mucus in the nasal passages.

escharotic a caustic substance that creates a mass of dead cells, or scab.

essence a preparation of an herbal medicine in concentrated form. A typical essence would be an ounce of herbal product dissolved in a pint of alcohol.

essential oil any of the large class of volatile (readily vaporizing), usually scented plant oils that are constituents of many herbal medications.

estrogenic affecting female functions.

eupeptic aiding digestion.

euphoriant producing a sense of bodily comfort and well-being and the absence of pain or distress. The effect of any euphoriant substance is always temporary and almost always potentially addictive and dangerous.

excipient a substance mixed with a drug to give it a stable form.

expectorant facilitating the expulsion of phlegm from the respiratory tract by making the mucus less dry or sticky. Expectorants are sometimes given to help alleviate coughs or to ease bronchitis.

extract in herbalism, the desired constituents withdrawn from a plant by physical or chemical means or both.

F

family a classification category that is below an order and above a genus. Typically, a botanical family includes more than one genus. Members of the same plant family share characteristics but not as many as do members of the same genus.

fascicle a close cluster of flowers, stems, leaves, or other similar parts.

febrifuge an agent that relieves fever.

felon a deep infection around the nails of toes or fingers.

fertilization union of female and male reproductive cells.

fibrous of a root system, having roots all about the same size, with no single dominant root; also describing one of these roots.

filament the stalk in a stamen (a flower's male reproductive part) that bears the anther (pollen-bearing part).

filiform threadlike.

fistula an abnormal, or sometimes surgically constructed, opening from an internal organ to the body's surface, or between two internal organs.

floret a "little flower"; specifically, the flowers in the inflorescences (flower clusters) of daisies and other members of the composite family.

flower an organ for sexual reproduction in ANGIOSPERMS. Most flowers have a self-contained bisexual reproductive system including both stamens (male parts) and pistils (female parts).

flowerhead a dense inflorescence (flower cluster), such as that found in the composite family.

flowering plant one bearing flowers, fruits, and seeds; in general the same as ANGIOSPERM.

follicle a dry DEHISCENT fruit

that splits open along one side; e.g., a milkweed pod.

fomentation a hot compress made by dipping a cloth in a medicinal DECOCTION or INFUSION, wringing out the cloth, and then applying it where indicated.

frond leaf of a fern; also describing various large, compound leaves, such as those of palms.

fruit mature product of a fertilized ovary or ovaries.

-fuge suffix meaning driving out.

fungicide an agent that kills fungal growths.

G

galactogenic (or **galactagogic)** promoting the flow of milk.

galenic (or **galenical)** a medicine, such as a TINCTURE, made from plants according to the principles and procedures set forth by the second-century A.D. Greek physician Galen.

gam- (or **gamo-)** prefix meaning joined.

gamete a reproductive cell, or sex cell (i.e., an egg or a sperm), that can fuse with another gamete to form a new individual.

genus a classification category that is below a family but above a species. Members of the same genus generally share more characteristics than do those of the same family. A genus may include many species. The genus name—always capitalized— is the first word of a plant's scientific name.

glucoside a GLYCOSIDE that when chemically broken down yields the type of sugar called glucose.

glycoside any of the large group of plant compounds that are described chemically as sugar derivatives and that are the source of many substances that have medicinal uses. When glycosides are broken down chemically, they yield various types of sugars.

-gogue (-agogue, -ogogue) a suffix indicating secretion or expulsion of the substance identified by the prefix; e.g., a sialagogue promotes the flow of saliva, an emmenagogue promotes normal menstrual flow.

gravel small, hard deposits in the urinary bladder or in the kidneys.

gum any of various plant-derived substances useful for their adhesive properties. Gum arabic, from trees and shrubs of the genus *Acacia,* is a common example.

gymnosperms the class of plants that, in contrast to the ANGIOSPERMS, do not have their ovules enclosed in an ovary. Coniferous, or cone-bearing, plants such as pines are gymnosperms.

H

hallucinogenic producing hallucinations.

head sometimes used to mean FLOWERHEAD.

heart palpitations abnormally rapid and irregular beating of the heart.

hem- (or **haem-)** prefix meaning blood.

hemagogue an agent that promotes the flow of blood; an EMMENAGOGUE.

hematinic stimulating the formation of blood cells and hemoglobin.

hemolytic destructive to red blood cells.

hemostatic controlling or stopping blood flow.

hepatic having to do with the liver.

herb a plant that does not have permanent woody tissue and dies down at the end of its growing season, although the plant may have a biennial or perennial life span; a plant or plant part used medicinally or for its flavor or aroma in other applications such as food preparation.

herbaceous having to do with herbs; specifically, having a nonwoody stem that dies back after the growing season.

herbal a guidebook to plants, especially one concerned with their medicinal and healing properties.

herbalism the practice of identifying and using plants that have aromatic, flavoring, and, particularly, medicinal properties. The claims for the plants' therapeutic value may be based on scientific fact, folklore, myth, or conjecture.

herbalist (or **herb doctor** or **herbist)** broadly, a collector and grower of herbs; in the sense of "herb doctor," one who uses herbs to treat diseases and discomforts.

herbarium a collection of plants or plant parts that are picked, pressed, and dried and then mounted for permanent reference.

hermaphroditic said of a flower having both male (stamens) and female (pistil) reproductive parts.

herpetic treating skin eruptions, such as those associated with herpes simplex and ringworm.

hip in botany, the receptacle of a rose, enclosing many ACHENES. Rose hips are a source of vitamin C.

homeopathic dose the smallest amount of medicine required to achieve a desired effect. Administration of such doses is an important principle of the system of medicine called HOMEOPATHY.

homeopathy a system of medicine that stresses the administration of very small doses of medicines that, when given to a healthy person, would produce symptoms of the disease. The system is based on the principle of "like cures like"; e.g., a fever-producing medication or treatment will combat a fever.

husk a usually dry outer covering, often composed of BRACTS, of a fruit or seed.

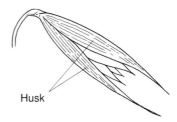

Husk

hybrid in botany, the issue of crossbreeding two different species; loosely, the offspring of crossbreeding varieties of the same species.

hydrogogue an agent that produces watery stools; a strong laxative.

hyoscyamine a poisonous plant chemical of the ALKALOID group, found in plants of the nightshade family and used to make both ANTISPASMODICS and drugs that dilate the pupils.

hyper- prefix meaning excessive, excessively, higher than normal.

hypericin a plant chemical

found in St. John's wort that can cause hypericism (a skin disorder characterized by increased sensitivity to light).

hypertensive tending to raise blood pressure; of or relating to high blood pressure or a person with it.

hypnotic inducing sleep or a state resembling sleep.

hypo- prefix meaning less or lower than normal.

hypoglycemant lowering the level of blood sugar in the body.

hypotensive tending to lower blood pressure; of or relating to low blood pressure or a person with it.

I

indehiscent a seed-bearing plant part that does not open at maturity; e.g., a walnut. Compare DEHISCENT.

indusium on fern fronds, a small flap of tissue protecting the spore clusters, or sori.

inflorescence a cluster of flowers growing together, rather than singly, on a stalk or stem. Depending on their shape or other characteristics such as the arrangement of flowers, inflorescences are called by many different names, including FLOWER-HEAD, PANICLE, RACEME, SPIKE, UMBEL.

infusion medicinal fluid made by pouring boiling water on an herb (or herb parts) or adding a plant extract to boiled water; similar to a tea.

insecticide killing insects.

intermittent fever a regularly recurring fever; e.g., malaria.

intestinal worm any of various worms, such as tapeworms, that can live as parasites in the human intestines; such an infestation is often called worms.

involucel a small, secondary INVOLUCRE, most commonly found on flower clusters of members of the carrot family.

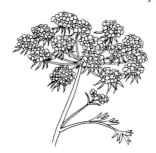

involucre a ring of BRACTS or small leaves around the base of a flower or flower cluster, as in asters, chrysanthemums, daisies, marigolds, and other members of the composite family.

irritant an agent that causes inflammation.

itch mites collective name for chiggers, harvest mites, red bugs, and other small pests that cause skin irritations for which a number of herbal treatments exist.

J

jaundice yellowing of the skin and other tissues caused by the presence of bile pigments. Once found, the underlying causes are treatable.

K

kidney stone small, hard stone that may form in the kidneys and cause intense pain. Various methods are used to dissolve them or break them into smaller parts so that they may be passed.

L

laciniate fringed with deep, irregularly cut lobes.

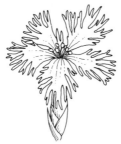

lactation the secretion of milk by mammals; many herbal remedies are meant to control or increase lactation.

lactifuge increasing the secretion of milk.

lanceolate describing a leaf that tapers at one or both ends to the shape of a lance head.

latex milky fluid produced by several kinds of plants, including milkweeds, rubber plants, and poppies.

leaf a primary appendage of most higher plants, usually the chief site of photosynthesis. Bracts, bulb scales, petals, and sepals are often considered specialized leaves.

leaflet division of a COMPOUND LEAF; a small leaf.

lenticel an opening in the stem bark of a woody plant through which gases can be exchanged.

lesion a wound; any detectable evidence of injury, inflammation, or underlying disorder.

ligule tongue-shaped appendage of the sheath of a blade of a grass leaf; a structure like a ray flower in the composite family.

liniment a liquid or thin paste applied to the skin to work as a pain reliever or COUNTERIRRITANT.

lobe any distinct rounded shape on the margin of a leaf or other organ.

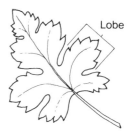
Lobe

local in medicine, confined to one area, rather than involving the whole body or a large part of it.

M

macerated soaked so as to be softened and dissolved.

margin the outside edge, as of a leaf.

masticatory a substance that is chewed to increase the flow of saliva.

materia medica literally in Latin, "medical matter": drugs and medicines of all kinds, collectively; a branch of medical science devoted to the study of these substances.

menarche the first menstrual period in the life of a woman.

mericarp a part of a fruit that seems to be a separate fruit, as the two CARPELS in fennel and other plants in the Umbelliferae, or carrot family.

methyl salicylate a plant chemical of the ESSENTIAL OIL

type that has a strong winter-green odor and is used as a flavoring, in perfumes, and as a COUNTERIRRITANT medicinally; known also as winter-green oil and sweet birch oil.

mon- (or **mono-**) prefix meaning one or single.

monocotyledons one of the two great subclasses of ANGIOSPERMS; its members (called monocots for short) have only one COTYLEDON, or leaf, attached to the embryo. Grasses, palms, lilies, orchids, and many aquatic herbs are monocots. DICOTYLEDONS are the other great group of angiosperms.

monoecious having separate pistillate (female) flowers and staminate (male) flowers on the same individual plant. Compare DIOECIOUS.

mucilage a gooey, sticky substance derived from seaweeds and other plants and often used for both its soothing action on skin and its adhesive properties.

mucilaginous sticky, containing MUCILAGE; in herbalism, mucilaginous substances are used to soothe inflamed areas of the body.

mucous membrane a lining of many of the body's passages, either internal or leading from the outside in, which is moistened and protected by secretions of mucus.

mucronate having a short, needlelike tip.

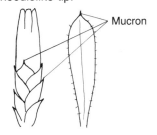

Mucron

mydriatic causing dilation of the pupil of the eye.

N

narcotic inducing drowsiness, sleep, or stupor and lessening pain.

naturalized describing a plant that has arrived from somewhere else and that now grows in the wild along with the rest of the local flora.

necrotic dead or dying, especially in reference to tissue of a certain area.

nectary specialized part of a flower that secretes nectar.

needle a rigid, elongated, pointed leaf, such as those of pines or firs.

nerve tonic a medicinal preparation that is meant to stimulate and "tone up" the nervous system and thus give a feeling of healthy well-being.

nervine NERVE TONIC.

nit the egg or young adult of a louse or other parasitic insect, which can cause various kinds of inflammation.

node a point on a stem from which one or more leaves grow or have grown. The part of the stem between nodes is called the internode.

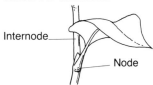

Internode

Node

nut hard, usually single-seeded, dry INDEHISCENT fruit.

O

oblong describing a leaf that is more long than wide, with nearly parallel sides and rounded ends.

obovate describing a leaf that is oval, with the end farthest from the stalk wider than the attached end.

obtuse describing a leaf tip that does not taper to a point.

official in medicine or pharmacy, sanctioned for medicinal use by virtue of being listed in a PHARMACOPEIA.

ointment a solid medication applied to the skin for soothing or healing.

oleoresin a natural plant product combining an ESSENTIAL OIL (oleo) with a resin (e.g., turpentine). Oleoresins are usually aromatic and have both medicinal and industrial applications.

opposite describing leaves arranged in pairs on opposite sides of the stem.

oval describing a leaf or fruit that is egg-shaped, with the narrower end away from the base.

ovary in ANGIOSPERMS, the portion of the pistil (female reproductive part) that contains an OVULE or ovules.

ovary, inferior an ovary joined to the basal parts of the flower or to the tip of the peduncle (flower stalk).

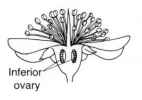

Inferior ovary

ovary, superior an ovary standing free of the basal parts of the flower.

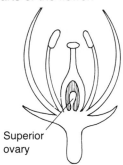

Superior ovary

ovoid oval; usually referring to a three-dimensional structure, such as a fruit.

ovule the part of the ovary containing a female sex cell or cells, which can develop into a seed after fertilization.

oxalic acid a poisonous plant chemical derived from various plants and used in bleaching, cleaning, and making dyes.

oxymel a mixture of honey and acetic acid (one of the chief constituents of vinegar), used as an EXPECTORANT.

P

palmate (or **palmatifid**) describing a leaf that has the shape of a hand, with fingers radiating from the palm. Palmately compound leaves have leaflets that issue from a single point on the leafstalk. Compare PINNATE.

panicle a branched, compound flower cluster, with the individual clusters forming RACEMES, especially common in grasses.

parasorbic acid a form of SORBIC ACID.

parenchyma the ground tissue of higher plants, made up of photosynthetic, storage, and other kinds of nonspecialized cells.

parturient (or **parturifacient**) inducing the contractions of labor at childbirth.

pectoral affecting the chest, lungs, or bronchial passages.

pedicel stalk of a solitary flower or of a flower in a cluster.

pediculocide an agent that kills body lice.

peduncle the stalk supporting an inflorescence (flower cluster); stalk of a single flower.

peltate describing a leaf whose stalk or support is attached to the leaf's dorsal (back) side instead of its base.

perennial in botany, having a life cycle of more than two years.

perianth the outside envelope of a flower, i.e., PETALS and SEPALS collectively.

pericarp a structure developed from the ovary wall and enclosing the seed in ANGIOSPERMS; more specifically, the collective term for the outer layers around the seed in the kind of fleshy fruit called a DRUPE. The cherry's pericarp, for example, consists of three layers, which from outside in are called the epicarp, mesocarp, and endocarp.

persistent retained beyond the usual period, as opposed to CADUCOUS.

petal one of the modified leaves that together form the corolla of a flower. Petals are often the most colorful part of the flower.

petiole the stalk of a leaf.

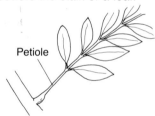

Petiole

petiolule the stalk of a leaflet of a COMPOUND leaf, as on walnuts and horse chestnuts.

pharmacognosy a branch of pharmacy that deals with drugs and medicines obtainable from natural sources such as plants.

pharmacology the study of drugs and MATERIA MEDICA, including their administration and healing properties.

pharmacopeia (pharmacopoeia) a publication listing and describing medicines and drugs and their uses; e.g., the *U.S. Pharmacopeia* and the *National Formulary*.

photosensitive reacting to light; commonly describing a heightened sensitivity of the skin and eyes to sunlight, caused by some food, drug, or environmental factor.

phytotherapy treating sickness by the use of plants and of plant-derived substances.

pinnate having the structure of a feather in that similar parts occur on opposite sides of an axis. A pinnate leaf is divided into numerous leaflets that grow along either side of the leafstalk and have their own stalks (petiolules), as in ferns.

pistil the part of a flower comprising the female reproductive organs, including usually a STIGMA, a STYLE, and an OVARY containing OVULES.

pistillate having PISTILS; sometimes, having pistils but lacking stamens (male reproductive parts).

plaster a medication applied externally by placing it over a body part and covering with a cloth or towel.

plume a featherlike plant part, as a single tuft of the dandelion seed head.

plumose plumelike; feathery.

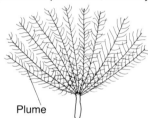

Plume

pollen grains produced in the ANTHER of a flower, and containing male sex cells.

pollinate to cause the transfer of pollen from the ANTHER to the STIGMA of a flower or from one flower's anther to another's stigma.

potion a liquid dose.

poultice a PLASTER that is applied hot and wet.

powder in herbal medicine, crushed, dried plants or plant parts.

principle *See* ACTIVE PRINCIPLE.

purgative strong laxative; cathartic.

pyxidium a DEHISCENT fruit CAPSULE whose splitting creates a cap-shaped part.

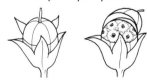

R

raceme an INFLORESCENCE (flower cluster) consisting of stalked flowers arranged along the sides of a central stalk, or RACHIS.

rachis (or rhachis) the main axis, or stalk, of an inflorescence (flower cluster) or compound leaf.

radical of or relating to roots; the area where the stem meets the root; basal.

ray flower one of the flat, usually petallike florets that are part of the flowerheads of most members of the composite family, or Compositae. Typically, as in asters, daisies, and sunflowers, the ray flowers edge the central disc, which is made up of DISC FLOWERS.

receptacle the part of the flower to which the PERIANTH is attached; the enlarged end of a stalk bearing an inflorescence (flower cluster), as in the flowerheads of the composite family.

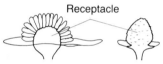

Receptacle

recurring fever INTERMITTENT FEVER.

refrigerant making cooler.

renal relating to the kidneys.

resin any of various solid or nearly solid, usually aromatic, yellowish, and translucent, gummy and sticky substances secreted by plants such as conifers. Resins are widely used in making paints, varnishes, printing inks, and other commercial products. In medicine, resins have been used for their astringent, antispasmodic, diuretic, and stimulant properties.

resolvent dissolving tumors; or reducing inflammation.

resorptive aiding reabsorption of blood from bruises.

reticulate having a network of fibers or veins, as a reticulate leaf.

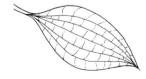

rheadine (or rhoeadine) a plant chemical of the ALKALOID group found in red poppies and other plants. It is a mild sedative and has been used in syrups to ease coughs and treat bronchitis.

rhizome a horizontal underground stem, often with thickened portions holding stored food for the plant's growth, that can send out both aerial shoots and roots into the ground.

root the part of a plant, usually below ground, that anchors it and absorbs water and dissolved nutrients for the plant's maintenance and growth.

rosette a circle, or whorl, of leaves around the stem of a plant; a basal rosette occurs at the base of the stem.

rubefacient literally, "making redder"; having the action of a COUNTERIRRITANT.

runner a long, slender STOLON; a twining vine, as in the name scarlet runner, a climbing bean plant.

S

safrole a poisonous plant chemical obtained from sassafras and used, after modifying treatment, in flavoring and perfume.

salicin a plant chemical of the GLYCOSIDE group obtained from certain poplars and willows. It is related to synthetic substances, such as aspirin, that alleviate pain and reduce fever.

salivation the making of saliva; the term is usually used to mean an abnormally copious flow of saliva.

salve same as OINTMENT.

samara the dry, INDEHISCENT, "winged" fruit of ashes, elms, maples, and other plants. A samara is also called a key.

sap the fluid that circulates through a plant, carrying water and nutrients to all tissues.

saponin plant chemical of the GLYCOSIDE group that produces froth and foam when mixed in water. Bouncing Bet contains saponins.

scabies a skin condition marked by severe itching and crusty sores.

scale a modified leaf, such as one of those that make up a plant bulb; a name for various kinds of BRACTS.

scopolamine a poisonous plant chemical of the ALKALOID group obtained from plants of the nightshade family and used as a sedative in medicine, usually in combination with other drugs. Scopolamine has also been used as

a "truth serum" because it makes people under its influence talk openly about subjects they would not normally discuss.

scrofula swellings of the lymph glands in the neck, caused by tuberculosis.

scutellarin a plant chemical obtained from various skullcaps, of the mint family, and used by herbalists to make a nerve tonic.

sedative acting on the central nervous system to produce sleep.

seed a fertilized and mature OVULE; characteristically a resting phase in the reproductive cycle of plants, ready to sprout given favorable environmental conditions.

seed plant SPERMATOPHYTE.

sepal one of the set of floral leaves that occur outside the petals; sepals are often green or greenish, but in many plants, such as buttercups and monkshoods, they are the most colorful part of the flower.

sessile having no stalk, as a leaf or a flower.

sheath in certain plants, the lower part of a leaf enveloping the stem or stalk.

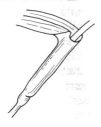

shoot new plant growth; especially an aerial stem or trunk growing upward with its leaves and other parts emerging.

shrub usually, a woody plant that does not attain a height of more than a few feet and has no dominant stem or trunk. No widely accepted distinction exists between a shrub and a tree other than size and the fact that a tree has one dominant stem.

sialagogue an agent that increases saliva flow.

simple a medicinal herb without strong effects.

simpling the practice of identifying, collecting, and using medicinal herbs.

soporific inducing sleep.

sorbic acid an oily, volatile, liquid plant chemical found in unripe berries of the mountain

ash and used as a fungicide and food preservative.

sorus a cluster of spores on the underside of a fern frond (leaf).

spadix the thick, fleshy flower spike borne by members of the arum family, usually surrounded by a SPATHE.

spasm an abnormal muscle contraction that is often accompanied by pain and may signal an underlying disorder.

spasmolytic helping to relieve cramps and other muscle contractions.

spathe a BRACT or bracts that sheathe the base of a flower cluster such as a SPADIX.

spatulate spatula-shaped.

species a classification category that is below GENUS and contains all the individuals capable of interbreeding. Within a species there may be many varieties that look very different, as in rose species.

specific of or relating to species; a drug that is useful against a particular disease.

spermatophyte any of the group of plants that produce seeds; namely, ANGIOSPERMS and GYMNOSPERMS.

spice a food flavoring. Many herbs are used as spices.

spike a flower cluster with SESSILE (stalkless) flowers arranged along an axis.

spore the one-celled, asexual reproductive body of algae, ferns, mosses, and other CRYPTOGAMS.

spur a tubelike projection from the petal, as in the larkspur.

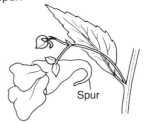

Spur

stamen the male (pollen-producing) organ of a flower, consisting of the anther, which bears the pollen, and the filament, which supports the anther.

staminate having STAMENS (male reproductive parts) but lacking pistils (female parts).

stem the main axis of a plant, on which buds, leaves, and branches develop.

sternutatory ERRHINE.

steroid any of a large group

of chemicals, many of which occur in plants and have medicinal uses. For example, the cardiac stimulant and diuretic digitoxin, obtained from the common foxglove, is a steroid, as are the D vitamins.

stigma the part of a flower's pistil (female reproductive part) that receives pollen.

stimulant making a body organ or system work faster.

stipule leaflike outgrowth found at the base of the petiole (leafstalk) in many plants; its function is protective in the bud stage.

stolon a branch or stem that creeps out horizontally above ground from the base of a plant and tends to root and produce a clone plant.

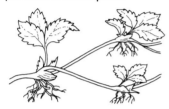

stomachic aiding the stomach and digestion.

stone hard inner part of a DRUPE, such as the peach.

stupefacient inducing stupor; narcotic.

style necklike part of a flower's pistil (female reproductive part) joining the ovary to the stigma (the pistil's pollen-receiving part).

styptic tending to stop bleeding; ASTRINGENT.

sucker shoot a shoot from the lower part of the stem.

sudorific acting to increase perspiration.

synergistic producing more than the predictable effect of two or more agents working together.

syrup a water and sugar solution to which are added flavoring, medicinal, or some other desired ingredients.

T

taeniacide (or **teniacide**) an agent that kills tapeworms.

taeniafuge (or **teniafuge**) an agent that expels tapeworms from the body.

tannic acid TANNIN.

tannin any of a group of chemicals from a wide variety of plants that are used in tanning, dyeing, and making ink and medicines. In herbal medi-

cine, tannins are used for their ASTRINGENT properties.

tea a dried substance, usually a plant or plant part, steeped in hot water for drinking. Many medicinal plants are administered as teas, or INFUSIONS.

tendril coiling, stemlike organ, as of passionflowers, grapes, and peas, that attaches itself to objects, supporting the plant and allowing it to climb.

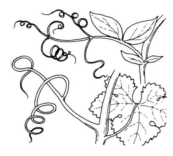

tetrahydrocannabinol (or **THC**) a plant chemical found in hemp plant resin; it is the main intoxicating substance in marijuana.

thorn a sharp, rigid projection on a plant; a woody plant bearing thornlike briers or spines, as the *Crataegus* genus of the rose family.

thrombosis a blood clot that may partially or wholly block the flow of blood through a blood vessel.

tincture a medication that has its medicinal agent dissolved in alcohol.

tisane a weak tea or infusion.

tonic as defined by one herbalist, "an agent that is used to give strength to the system," that is, restore or maintain health in the whole body or its individual organs.

toxic poisonous.

tranquilizer drug employed to calm or sedate people or animals.

tree a large woody perennial plant, usually having a dominant axis, or trunk. A tree's dominant stem and its larger size at maturity are the only clear-cut distinctions between it and a shrub.

trifoliate having a compound leaf with three leaflets.

trilobar having three lobes.

triturated crushed, pulverized.

tuber thickened portion of an underground stem, as the common white potato.

U

umbel a type of flower cluster with a flattish top, in which the individual stalks radiate from a central point like the ribs of an umbrella; if the stalks end in separate umbels, the cluster is a compound umbel; e.g., Queen Anne's lace.

unguent OINTMENT.

urticaria itching, inflamed skin caused by an allergic reaction to a drug, food, or substance in the environment; also called hives.

uterine sedative an agent that relaxes the muscles of the uterus.

V

valve one of the pieces into which a DEHISCENT fruit splits at maturity.

variety a member or group of members of a species that has characteristics that distinguish it from other members of the species but do not qualify it as a separate species.

vascular in plants, relating to the circulatory system of channels that carry water, nutrients, and other materials around the plant. A VEIN, for example, is a vascular body.

vasoconstrictor an agent that narrows blood-vessel openings, restricting the flow of blood through them.

vasodilator an agent that expands blood vessels, allowing more blood to flow through them.

vein in plants, the passageway for water and nutrients to and from a leaf; also the mechanical support system.

venate veined, having veins.

vermifuge an agent that rids the body of worms; also called an ANTHELMINTIC.

vesicant a COUNTERIRRITANT strong enough, in some cases, to cause blistering.

volatile oil as generally used in regard to plant substances, an ESSENTIAL OIL.

vulnerary soothing or healing wounds and sores.

WXYZ

wash liquid medicinal preparation for external use; lotion.

whorl ring of leaves, BRACTS, or flowers radiating out horizontally from a common point on a stem.

Index

A

Abies balsamea, 91
Aborigines, Australian, 372
Absinthe, 348
Acacia, false, 107
Acacia greggii, 374
Acacias, African, 44
Acacia senegal, 374
Acetylsalicylic acid, 109, 333
Achenes, 41
Achillea millefolium, 350
Achilles, 232, 350
Aconite, 52, 63
Aconitum uncinatum, 357
Acorns, 331
Acorus calamus, 314
Actaea pachypoda, 358
Actaea rubra, 358
Adair, James, 126
Adderwort, 101
Adiantum capillus-veneris, 240
Adventitious root stysems, 32, 33, 34
Aeneid (Virgil), 17
Aerial stems, 33, 34
Aesculapius, 53, 205
Aesculus hippocastanum, 219, 356
Agar, 360
Aggregate fruits, 41
Agrimonia eupatoria, 79
Agrimony, 79
Agropyron repens, 153
Ague grass, 144
Ague tree, 292
Agueweed, 116
Aioli, 414
Air-drying plants, 419
Aiton, William Townsend, 46
Ajuga reptans, 124
Alabama Indians, 152
Alchemilla vulgaris, 19, 230
Alchemy, 57–58, 230
Alder, 46, 172
Alder buckthorn, 80, 133
Alehoof, 204
Aletris, 144
Aletris farinosa, 144
Alexanders, 86
Alexander the Great, 362
Alfalfa, 72, 81
Alfred the Great, 60
Algae, 34, 43. *See also* Seaweeds.
Algonquin Indians, 94, 105
Aliens, 27
Alkali grass, 356
Alkaloids, 42, 43, 44
Alkanet, 82
Alkanna tinctoria, 82
Alleluia, 19
Allgood, 200
Allheal (garden heliotrope), 192
Allheal (heal-all), 207
Allium cepa, 261
Allium sativum, 194
Allium schoenoprasum, 396
Allopathy, 55
Allspice, wild, 305
Alnus glutinosa, 172
Aloe, 51, 83
Aloeroot, 144
Aloe vera, 71, 83
Aloe vera cold cream, 429
Alpine plants, 26
Alpinia berries, 72

Alternate leaves, 37
Althaea, 244
Althaea officinalis, 244
Alum, 426
Alumroot, 155
Amanita muscaria, 52
Amber, 16
Amber touch-and-heal, 290
American ash, 329
American aspen, 322
American chestnut, 174
American cowslip, 245
American Family Physician (King), 106
American ginseng (five-fingers), 44, 68, 72, 84, 399
American ginseng (misnomer for cañaigre), 129
American hemp, 210
American licorice, 337
American Medical Botany (Bigelow), 270
American Medical Record, 279
American mistletoe, 85, 356
American saffron, 288
American sanicle, 110
American sarsaparilla, 306
American senna, 338
American sloe, 106
American spikenard, 306
American upland cotton, 152
American valerian, 231
American wormroot, 224
American wormseed, 347
American yew, 356
Amino acids, 34, 43
Ammi visnaga, 378–379
Amor seco, 73
Amwebe, 72
Amyroot, 210
Ananas comosus, 384–385
Anatomy, plant, 32–41
Andromachus, 54
Anemone patens, 265
Angelica, 21, 45, 72, 86
Angelica archangelica, 86
Angelica tree, 270
Anise, 44, 87, 394, 396
Aniseed, 53, 87
Annual mercury, 212
Annuals, 33
Antennaria neglecta, 277
Anthemis nobilis, 284
Anther, 37
Anthriscus cerefolium, 396
Antibiotics, 44, 52
Antimony, 58, 63, 67, 68
Apium graveolens, 136
Apocynum cannabinum, 210, 356
Appetite-stimulating tonics, 434
Appetizers, 408
Apple-of-Peru, 226
Apples, 40
Apricot vine, 266
Aqua hirundinum, 19
Arabia tea, 365
Aralia nudicaulis, 306
Aralia racemosa, 306
Archangel, 160
Arctium lappa, 201
Arctostaphylos uva-ursi, 94
Areca catechu, 362
Argemone mexicana, 272
Argentine, 297

Aristolochia serpentaria, 324
Aristotle, 53–54, 55, 57
Armstrong, 229
Arnica, 88, 356
Arnica fulgens, 88
Arnica montana, 88, 356
Arrangements, dried flower, 420
Arrowwood, 80
Artemisia absinthium, 348, 356
Artemisia dracunculus, 319
Artemisia tridentata, 97
Artemisia vulgaris, 258
Art of Simpling, The (Coles), 62
Ascharius, Erik, 46
Asclepias syriaca, 249
Asclepias tuberosa, 125
Ash, poison, 189
Ash, white, 329
Asiatic ginseng, 44
Aspen, trembling, 322
Asperula odorata, 317
Aspirin, 42, 109, 247, 333
Ass-ear, 147
Asthma weed, 225
Astringent, sage, 428
Astrology, 61–62
Atropa belladonna, 20, 96, 356
Atropine, 96, 211, 372, 382
Attila the Hun, 362
Autumn crocus, 89, 356
Avena sativa, 260
Avicenna, 56–57, 58, 90
Axillary buds, 35
Axils, 35
Ayurveda, 52
Azafran, 288
Aztecs, 22, 315, 368, 384

B

Babylonians, 51
Bachelor's-button (cornflower), 40, 151
Bachelor's-button (feverfew), 182
Baillon, Henri Ernest, 46
Baker, John Gilbert, 46
Baldness, 119, 240
Bald's Leechbook, 60
Balfour, John Hutton, 46
Balm, 46, 90, 394, 396, 406
tea, 417
Balm, field, 204
Balm, horse, 310
Balm, Indian, 100
Balm, lemon, 90
Balm, sweet, 90
Balm of Gilead, 109
Balm of Gilead fir, 91
Balm tea, 417
Balsam, 315, 361
Balsam fir, 17, 44, 57, 91
Balsam of Peru, 360–361
Balsam poplar, 109
Baneberry, red, 358
Baneberry, white, 358
Baptisia, 336
Baptisia tinctoria, 336
Barbados aloe, 83
Barbara, Saint, 342
Barbarea vulgaris, 342, 356
Barberry, 148
Barefoot doctors, 72
Barley, 16
Barton, Benjamin Smith, 46

Credits and Acknowledgments

The editors wish to thank Mrs. Lothian Lynas and Mrs. Jane Brennan of the New York Botanical Garden Library and Ms. Pearl Spears, Administrative Assistant for the Program for Collaborative Research in the Pharmaceutical Sciences, the University of Illinois at Chicago, for their invaluable assistance in the research for this book.

Grateful acknowledgment is made for permission to use and adapt recipes from the following sources:
TEA ROOM RECIPES by Sandy Greig. Copyright © 1984 by Sandy Greig. Reprinted by permission. *HERBS WITH EVERYTHING* by Sheila Howarth. Copyright © 1976 by Sheila Howarth. Reprinted by permission of Holt, Rinehart and Winston, Publishers. *COOKING WITH THE HEALTHFUL HERBS* by Jean Rogers. Copyright © 1983 by Rodale Press. *RODALE'S BASIC NATURAL FOODS COOKBOOK* edited by Harles Gerras. Copyright © 1984 Rodale Press. Adapted by permission. *THE FORGOTTEN ART OF GROWING, GARDENING, AND COOKING WITH HERBS* by Richard M. Bacon. Copyright © 1981 by Yankee, Inc. Reprinted by permission of Yankee Publishing, Incorporated.

Contributing illustrators to the Gallery of Medicinal Plants, pages **79** through **354**: David Baxter: page **86**. Françoise Bonvoust: pages **101**, **146**, **151**, **178**, **193**, **205**, **219**, **259**. Luc Bosserdet: pages **112**, **148**, **167**, **171**, **172**, **177**, **180**, **184**, **196**, **202**, **206**, **237**, **248**, **307**, **351**. Pierre Brochard: page **79**. Jean Coladon: pages **90**, **93**, **94**, **143**, **185**, **200**, **203**, **216**, **312**. François Collet: page **349**. Philippe Couté: pages **109**, **149**, **313**. Françoise de Dalmas: pages **241**, **290**, **314**. Maurice Espérance: pages **103**, **111**, **131**, **134**, **138**, **160**, **187**, **220**, **228**, **236**, **240**, **278**, **288**, **350**. Ian Garrard: pages **141**, **168**, **217**, **229**, **247**, **273**, **322**, **326**. Odette Halmos: pages **215**, **268**. Madeleine Huau: pages **120**, **123**, **170**, **190**, **227**, **257**, **277**, **328**. Mette Ivers: pages **80**, **117**, **159**, **232**, **235**, **255**, **293**, **294**, **296**, **300**, **311**, **320**, **327**. Mary Kellner: pages **81**, **83**, **84**, **85**, **91**, **92**, **95**, **97**, **100**, **104**, **105**, **106**, **113**, **114**, **115**, **116**, **121**, **125**, **126**, **127**, **128**, **129**, **130**, **132**, **133**, **137**, **144**, **145**, **150**, **152**, **154**, **155**, **156**, **157**, **165**, **179**, **189**, **192**, **197**, **198**, **199**, **210**, **214**, **222**, **224**, **225**, **231**, **246**, **249**, **253**, **260**, **261**, **262**, **264**, **266**, **267**, **270**, **271**, **272**, **275**, **279**, **281**, **291**, **292**, **295**, **298**, **299**, **301**, **303**, **305**, **306**, **310**, **315**, **324**, **325**, **329**, **330**, **331**, **332**, **334**, **335**, **336**, **337**, **338**, **341**, **343**, **345**, **353**, **354**. Josiane Lardy: pages **82**, **102**, **135**, **142**, **153**, **161**, **174**, **175**, **182**, **263**, **283**, **284**, **316**, **323**, **333**, **347**, **352**. Annie Le Faou: pages **99**, **110**, **118**, **163**, **173**, **201**, **209**, **221**, **234**, **239**, **289**, **308**, **340**, **342**, **346**. Yvon Le Gall: page **119**. Nadine Liard: pages **98**, **108**, **186**. Guy Michel: pages **147**, **181**, **207**, **208**, **213**, **244**, **250**, **282**, **304**. Daniel Moncla: pages **164**, **254**. Marie-Claire Nivoix: pages **122**, **139**, **183**, **212**, **280**, **297**, **339**. Britt-Mari Norberg: pages **87**, **89**, **96**, **188**, **194**, **211**, **226**, **242**, **251**, **286**, **319**. Alain d'Orange: page **124**. Robert Rousso: pages **136**, **169**, **204**. Jean-Paul Turmel: pages **191**, **195**, **218**, **223**, **233**, **245**, **252**, **269**, **287**. Denise Weber: pages **88**, **107**, **140**, **158**, **162**, **166**, **176**, **230**, **238**, **243**, **256**, **258**, **265**, **274**, **276**, **285**, **302**, **309**, **321**, **344**, **348**.

6 *top & middle* Ibn Botlân, Tacuinum Sanitatis, Faksimilupplaga, Kungliga Biblioteket; *bottom* The New York Public Library, Rare Book Division. **7** *top* Ibn Botlân, Tacuinum Sanitatis, Faksimilupplaga, Kungliga Biblioteket; *bottom* Ira Block. **8–9** Ibn Botlân, Tacuinum Sanitatis, Faksimilupplaga, Kungliga Biblioteket. **10** Städelsches Kunstinstitut, Frankfurt am Main. **11** Mary Evans Picture Library. **12** The Bettmann Archive. **13** The New York Public Library, Picture Collection. **14** The Metropolitan Museum of Art. **15** Scala. **16** Kungliga Biblioteket. **17** Apotekarsocieteten-Farmacevtiska Föreningen/Stina Brockman. **18** John Bauer, Bland Tomtar och Troll, 1912. **20** Per Adolphson. **21** Apotekarsocieteten-Farmacevtiska Föreningen/Stina Brockman. **22** Painting by Gérard Valcin from the Kurt Bachmann Collection. **24–25** Ibn Botlân, Tacuinum Sanitatis, Faksimilupplaga, Kungliga Biblioteket. **26** Gerald Ferguson. **27** Gerald Ferguson. **28** *top* Gerald Ferguson; *bottom* Naturhistoriska Riksmuseet. **29** Gerald Ferguson. **30** Edward Lipinski. **31** Ingmar Fröhling. **32–41** & **43** Maurice Espérance. **48–49** The New York Public Library, Rare Book Division. **50** Larousse, Paris. **51** Cliche Musées Nationaux. **52** *top* National Archaeological Museum, Athens; *bottom* Mary Evans Picture Library. **53** *top left & right* Dioscorides, De Materia Medica, Faksimilupplaga, Kungliga Biblioteket; *lower* Medicina Antiqua, Faksimilupplaga, Kungliga Biblioteket. **56** *top* Musée d'Unterlinden, Colmar; *bottom* Bayerische Staatbibliothek. **57** *upper* Topkapi Saray Museum, Istanbul/Haluk Doganbey; *bottom* Österreichische Nationalbibliothek, Vienna. **59** *top* Bildarchiv Preussischer Kulturbesitz; *bottom* Giambattista Porta, Phytognomonica, Naples 1589, Kungliga Biblioteket. **60** *top* Fotostudio Jahn, Bingen; *bottom* E. Rosslin, Kreuterbuch, Apotekarsocieteten-Farmacevtiska Föreningen/Stina Brockman. **61** From the Gunnar Göthbergs Collection/Ingmar Fröhling. **62** Blauel Kunst-Dias. **63** From the Gunnar Göthbergs Collection. **64** *top* F. Hoffman La Roche & Co.; *bottom* Ullstein Bilderdienst. **65** Andrea Friederici Happe, Botanica Pharmacevtica, 1788, Biomedicum/Stina Brockman. **66** Institut vor Tax zool, Amsterdam. **67** *top* Alexander Roslin, Carl von Linné; Statens Porträttsamlingpå Gripsholms slott; *bottom* The New York Public Library, Rare Book Division. **68** *top right* David K. Stone; *top left & bottom* The New York Public Library, Rare Book Division. **69** *top* Minnesota Historical Society; *bottom* Nebraska State Historical Society. **70** National Museum of History & Technology, Smithsonian Institution. **73** The New York Public Library, Picture Collection. **74–75** Ibn Botlân, Tacuinum Sanitatis, Faksimilupplaga, Kungliga Biblioteket. **79** M. Keraudren-Aymonin. **80** Heather Angel. **81** Donald Specker/Earth Scenes. **82** C. de Klemm/Jacana. **83** Library, New York Botanical Garden, Bronx, New York. **84** Wendy Neefus/Earth Scenes. **85** Library, New York Botanical Garden, Bronx, New York. **86** R. Longo **87** Sven Samelius **88** Binois/Pitch. **89** J.-C. Hayon. **90** G. Lacz-E. Lemoine. **91** Richard B. Fischer. **92** Anita Sabarese. **93** P. Briolle. **94** Heather Angel. **95** Kent and Donna Dannen. **96** P. Delaveau. **97** Willard Luce/Earth Scenes. **98** J. Six. **99** Ruffier-Lanche/Jacana. **100** Wendy Neefus/Earth Scenes. **101** J.-C. Hayon/Pitch. **102** O. Polunin. **103** M. Buzzini. **104** Anita Sabarese. **105** Pamela Harper. **106** Pamela Harper. **107** Binois/Pitch. **108** P. Delaveau. **109** R. P Bille. **110** Heather Angel. **111** J. Burton/Bruce Coleman Ltd. **112** O. Polunin. **113** Library, New York Botanical Garden, Bronx, New York. **114** Richard B. Fischer. **115** Library, New York Botanical Garden, Bronx, New York. **116** Anita Sabarese. **117** M. Brosselin. **118** P. Lieutaghi. **119** Frédéric/Jacana. **120** J. Vincent/Photothèque. **121** Robert and Linda Mitchell. **122** Ruffier-Lanche/Jacana. **123** M. Brosselin. **124** J.-C. Hayon. **125** Anita Sabarese. **126** Doel Soejarto. **127** Theodore Niehaus. **128** Brian Milne/Earth Scenes. **129** Library, New York Botanical Garden, Bronx, New York. **130** Richard B. Fischer. **131** R. Longo. **132** Library, New York Botanical Garden, Bronx, New York. **133** Doel Soejarto. **134** P. Lieutaghi. **135** J.-C. Hayon. **136** R. Longo. **137** Robert and Linda Mitchell. **138** J.-C. Hayon. **139** M. Brosselin. **140** M. Buzzini. **141** P. Lieutaghi. **142** J-.C.Hayon/Pitch. **143** M. Brosselin. **144** Pamela Harper. **145** George H. H. Huey/Earth Scenes. **146** J.-C. Hayon. **147** J.-C. Hayon/Pitch. **148** Heather Angel. **149** J.-F. Gonnet/Jacana. **150** Richard F. Trump/Photo Researchers. **151** C. Rives/Cedri. **152** Anita Sabarese. **153** J.-P. Germain/SRD. **154** Richard Kolar/Earth Scenes. **155** Anita Sabarese. **156** Pamela Harper. **157** Doel Soejarto. **158** Binois/Pitch. **159** J.-C. Hayon. **160** M. Brosselin. **161** Heather Angel. **162** C. Nardin/Jacana. **163** Heather Angel. **164** S. C. Porter/Bruce Coleman Ltd. **165** Gerald Ferguson. **166** J. Prissette/Pitch. **167** M. Buzzini. **168** M. Brosselin. **169** M. Bibin/Jacana. **170** M. Brosselin. **171** J. Vincent/Photothèque. **172** M. Buzzini. **173** R. Volot/Jacana. **174** D. Lecourt/Jacana. **175** J. Vincent/Photothèque. **176** M. Buzzini. **177** Binois/Pitch. **178** I. and L. Beames/Ardea. **179** Irvin L. Oakes/Photo Researchers. **180** J. Vincent/Photothèque. **181** O. Polunin. **182** P. Briolle. **183** B. Mallet/Jacana. **184** J. Markham/Bruce Coleman Ltd. **185** M. Buzzini. **186** M. Brosselin. **187** Heather Angel. **188** P. Delaveau. **189** Anita Sabarese. **190** IBL AB. **191** M. Brosselin. **192** Mary M. Walker/New England Wild Flower Society. **193** M. Brosselin. **194** Sven Samelius. **195** Archivio Foto. **196** M. Brosselin. **197** Doel Soejarto. **198** Robert P. Carr/Bruce Coleman Inc. **199** Anita Sabarese. **200** Ruffier-Lanche/Jacana. **201** J.-P. Champroux/Jacana. **202** C. Nardin/Jacana. **203** P. Lieutaghi. **204** J.-C. Hayon. **205** C. de Klemm/Jacana. **206** H. Veiller/Jacana. **207** M. Buzzini. **208** M. Buzzini. **209** J.-P. Germain/SRD. **210** Jean Baxter/New England Wild Flower Society. **211** Sven Samelius. **212** J.-C. Hayon. **213** M. Buzzini. **214** Derek Fell. **215** M. Buzzini. **216** M. Brosselin. **217** Heather Angel. **218** P. Lieutaghi. **219** D. Lecourt/Jacana. **220** P. Lieutaghi. **221** J.-C. Hayon. **222** Derek Fell. **223** R. P. Bille. **224** Pamela Harper. **225** Library, New York Botanical Garden, Bronx, New York. **226** Finn Sandberg. **227** Frédéric/Jacana. **228** F. Bricout/Pitch. **229** Heather Angel. **230** J. Vincent/Photothèque. **231** Pamela Harper. **232** A. Malvina/Pitch. **233** M.-C. Noailles/Jacana. **234** Ruffier-Lanche/Jacana. **235** J.-C. Hayon. **236** M. Brosselin. **237** I. and L. Beames/Ardea. **238** R. Volot/Jacana. **239** P. Delaveau. **240** C. de Klemm/Jacana. **241** A. Margiocco. **242** Sven Samelius. **243** J.-P. Champroux/Jacana. **244** M. Keraudren-Aymonin. **245** M. Buzzini. **246** Library, New York Botanical Garden, Bronx, New York. **247** Lieutier/Jacana. **248** B. Mallet/Jacana. **249** Anita Sabarese. **250** C. Nuridsany. **251** Sven Samelius. **252** M. Buzzini. **253** Pamela Harper. **254** A. Malvina/Pitch. **255** R. Longo. **256** R. Engel/Pitch. **257** M. Brosselin. **258** Sven Samelius. **259** P. Pilloud/Jacana. **260** E. R. Degginger/Earth Scenes. **261** Anita Sabarese. **262** Library, New York Botanical Garden, Bronx, New York. **263** J.-P. Ferrero/Pitch. **264** Anita Sabarese. **265** J.-P. Champroux/Jacana. **266** Pamela Harper. **267** J. Shaw/Bruce Coleman Inc. **268** J.-C. Hayon. **269** A. Malvina/Pitch. **270** Pamela Harper. **271** G. Lacz-E. Lemoine. **272** Pamela Harper. **273** M. Brosselin. **274** J.-P. Germain/SRD. **275** Doel Soejarto. **276** J. Vincent/Photothèque. **277** Heather Angel. **278** A. Malvina/Pitch. **279** Library, New York Botanical Garden, Bronx, New York. **280** F. Peuriot/Pitch. **281** Pamela Harper. **282** J. Vincent/Photothèque. **283** J.-C. Hayon. **284** Bevilacqua/Cedri. **285** M. Buzzini. **286** Ruffier-Lanche/Jacana. **287** Heather Angel. **288** M. Buzzini. **289** G. Lacz-E. Lemoine. **290** C. de Klemm/Jacana. **291** Paul Martin Brown/Photo/Nats. **292** U. S. National Arboretum. **293** Frédéric/Jacana. **294** J. Bosser. **295** Pamela Harper. **296** M. Brosselin. **297** J. Markham/Bruce Coleman Ltd. **298** Mary M. Thacher/Photo Researchers. **299** Richard Parker/Photo Researchers. **300** P. Lieutaghi. **301** Doel Soejarto. **302** C. Nardin/Jacana. **303** Mary M. Walker/New England Wild Flower Society. **304** P. Pilloud/Jacana. **305** Library, New York Botanical Garden, Bronx, New York. **306** Frank Bramley/New England Wild Flower Society. **307** Orjan Nilsson. **308** C. de Klemm/Jacana. **309** N. Fox-Davies/Bruce Coleman Ltd. **310** Doel Soejarto. **311** Heather Angel. **312** C. Nardin/Jacana. **313** C. Nardin/Jacana. **314** C. Nardin/Jacana. **315** Library, New York Botanical Garden, Bronx, New York. **316** A. Malvina/Pitch. **317** M. Buzzini. **318** P. Pilloud/Jacana. **319** Sven Samelius. **320** J.-P. Champroux/Jacana. **321** A. Malvina/Pitch. **322** D. and J. Bartlett/Bruce Coleman Ltd. **323** M.-C. Noailles/Jacana. **324** Library, New York Botanical Garden, Bronx, New York. **325** M.-C. Noailles/Jacana. **326** M.-C. Noailles/Jacana. **327** M. Buzzini. **328** C. Nuridsany. **329** J. Six. **330** Library, New York Botanical Garden, Bronx, New York. **331** E. R. Degginger/Earth Scenes. **332** Library, New York Botanical Garden, Bronx, New York. **333** Heather Angel. **334** Pamela Harper. **335** Richard B. Fischer. **336** Jean Baxter/New England Wild Flower Society. **337** Library, New York Botanical Garden, Bronx, New York. **338** Anita Sabarese. **339** R. Volot/Jacana. **340** M.-C. Noailles/Jacana. **341** Paul Martin Brown/Photo/Nats. **342** J. Vincent/Photothèque. **343** Pamela Harper. **344** J. Six. **345** U. S. National Arboretum. **346** R. Longo. **347** Grands-Augustins/SRD. **348** M. Buzzini. **349** O. Polunin. **350** M. Buzzini. **351** C. Nardin/Jacana. **352** F. Peuriot/Pitch. **353** Pamela Harper. **354** Pamela Harper. **355** Hortus Sanitatis, Lübeck, 1520. **356** *left* Gwen Leighton; *upper right* Wayne Trimm; *lower right* Elizabeth McClelland. **357** *bottom left* Wayne Trimm; *upper left* Allianora Rosse; *remainder* Gwen Leighton. **358** *middle left* Wayne Trimm; *bottom right* Elizabeth McClelland; *remainder* Gwen Leighton. **359** From *Dragon Tree,* John Gerards Herball, London, 1957. **360** *left* Elizabeth McClelland; *lower right* Library, New York Botanical Garden, Bronx, New York/Photo by James A. McInnis. **361** Kohler, Medizinal-Pflanzen, Apotekarsocieteten-Farmacevtiska Föreningern/Stina Brockman. **362** *left* Library, New York Botanical Garden, Bronx, New York/Photo by James A. McInnis; *right* S. C. Porter/Bruce Coleman Ltd. **363** Finn Sandberg. **364** *left* Heather Angel; *right* J. Six. **366** Library, New York Botanical Garden, Bronx, New York/Photo by James A. McInnis. **367** *left* J.-P. Champroux/Jacana; *right* J. Six. **368** Starfoto/Zefa. **369** *left* K. Scholz/Zefa; *right* E. G. Carle/Zefa. **370** W. Schacht/Roebild. **371** J.-M. Pelt. **372** *left* Finn Sandberg; *right* Britt-Mari Norberg. **373** Library, New York Botanical Garden, Bronx, New York/Photo by James A. McInnis. **374** Y. Delange. **375** *left* Köhler, Medizinal-Pflanzen, Apotekarsocieteten-Farmacevtiska Föreningern/Stina Brockman; *right* Elizabeth McClelland. **376** Library, New York Botanical Garden, Bronx, New York/Photo by James A. McInnis. **377** Köhler, Medizinal-Pflanzen, Apotekarsocieteten-Farmacevtiska Föreningern/Stina Brockman. **379** *left* J.-M. Pelt; *right* Y. Delange. **380** *left* C. Errath/Jacana; *bottom* Daniel Moncla. **381** *left* Shostal; *right* Library, New York Botanical Garden, Bronx, New York/Photo by James A. McInnis. **382** Library, New York Botanical Garden, Bronx, New York/Photo by James A. McInnis. **383** Brooklyn Botanic Garden/Photo by James A. McInnis. **384** *left* Library, New York Botanical Garden, Bronx, New York/Photo by James A. McInnis; *right* L. Carle/Shostal. **385** Köhler, Medizinal-Pflanzen, Apotekarsocieteten-Farmacevtiska Föreningern/Stina Brockman. **386** W. Rauh. **387** Library, New York Botanical Garden, Bronx, New York/Photo by James A. McInnis. **388** *left* Roebild; *right* Brooklyn Botanic Garden/Photo by James A. McInnis. **389** R. König/Jacana. **390** *right* W. Schacht/Roebild. **391** Library, New York Botanical Garden, Bronx, New York/Photo by James A. McInnis. **392–393** ® Ira Block **399** Suzanne O'Connell. **400–401** Mary Kellner. **402** *top* Gerald Ferguson; *bottom* M.C. Dobelis. **403** *top* M.C. Dobelis; *bottom* Santi Visalli. **404** *upper* Mary Kellner; *bottom left* The New York Public Library, Rare Book Division; *bottom right* photo and garden by Debbie Peterson. **419** *bottom* Joseph Barnell. **420** M.C. Dobelis. **421** *left* M.C. Dobelis; *right* Courtesy of *Cuisine* Magazine/Photo by Don Levy. **422** M.C. Dobelis. **440–449** Maurice Espérance.

Picture Editor: Robert J. Woodward
Associate Picture Editor: Richard Pasqual
Text Rights and Permissions: Dorothy M. Harris

Library of Congress Cataloging in Publication Data
Main entry under title:
Magic and medicine of plants.
At head of title: Reader's digest.
Includes index.
1. Botany, Medical. 2. Plants, Useful. 3. Plants, Useful—Identification. 4. Plants—Identification.
I. Reader's Digest Association. II. Reader's Digest.
QK99.A1M325 1986 615'.321 85-30101
ISBN 0-89577-221-3